# Recreational Therapy

# and

# The International Classification of Functioning, Disability, and Health

Heather R. Porter, Ph.D., CTRS

*Idyll Arbor's Recreational Therapy Practice Series*

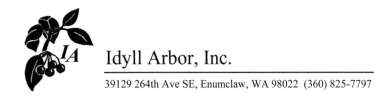

Idyll Arbor, Inc.

39129 264th Ave SE, Enumclaw, WA 98022 (360) 825-7797

Idyll Arbor's Recreational Therapy Practice Series Editor: Heather R. Porter, Ph.D., CTRS
Idyll Arbor, Inc. Editor: Thomas M. Blaschko
Cover design: Curt Pliler

To the best of our knowledge, the information and recommendations of this book reflect currently accepted practice. Nevertheless, they cannot be considered absolute and universal. Guidelines suggested by federal law are subject to change as the laws and interpretations do. Recommendations for a particular client must be considered in light of the client's needs and condition. The authors and publisher disclaim responsibility for any adverse effects resulting directly or indirectly from the suggested therapy or management practice, from any undetected errors, or from the reader's misunderstanding of the text.

**ISBNs paper 9781882883950, e-book 9781611580563**

*This book is dedicated to*
*Mary Cary & Mary Elizabeth*

# Contents

# ICF Contents

## Chapter 2 The Eye, Ear, and Related Structures ........................................... 160

## Chapter 3 Structures Involved in Voice and Speech.............................................. 161

## Chapter 4 Structures of the Cardiovascular, Immunological, and Respiratory Systems.....................................162

# Editor and Author

**Heather R. Porter, Ph.D., CTRS**
Associate Professor
Department of Rehabilitation Sciences
Temple University
Philadelphia, PA

# Contributor

**Yoshitaka Iwasaki, Ph.D.**
Professor, Director, and Associate Dean (Research)
Community-University Partnership for the Study of Children, Youth, and Families (CUP)
University of Alberta
Edmonton, Alberta, Canada

# Reviewers

A special thank you to these individuals who graciously gave of their time to review the 2006 edition and provide feedback for re-shaping this edition.

**Jo Ann Coco-Ripp, Ph.D., LRT/CTRS**
Associate Professor
Therapeutic Recreation Program Coordinator
School of Education and Human Performance
Winston-Salem State University
Winston-Salem, NC

**Jennifer A. Piatt, Ph.D., CTRS**
Assistant Professor
Department of Recreation, Park, and Tourism Studies
School of Public Health
Indiana University
Bloomington, IN

**Thomas K. Skalko, Ph.D., LRT/CTRS**
Professor
Recreational Therapy
College of Health and Human Performance
East Carolina University
Greenville, NC
and
Honorary Professor
College of Health Sciences
University of KwaZulu-Natal
Durban, South Africa

# Research and Editing Assistants

The following individuals volunteered their time to be research and editing assistants. Their dedication to assist with recreational therapy research is highly commendable.

Rebecca Baro
Recreational Therapy Student
Temple University

Genee Bower
Recreational Therapy Student
Temple University

Joshua Cino
Recreational Therapy Student
Temple University

Morgan Ferrante
Recreational Therapy Student
Temple University

Tonya D. Fromm
Recreational Therapy Student
Temple University

Kristen Hartman
Recreational Therapy Student
Temple University

Tracy Ann Jastrzab
Recreational Therapy Student
Temple University

Lea Peterson
Recreational Therapy Student
Temple University

Erin Kate MacElroy
Recreational Therapy Student
Temple University

Yekaterina Mishin
Recreational Therapy Student
Temple University

Marianella Sanchez
Recreational Therapy Student
Temple University

Alexa Szal
Psychology Student
Temple University

Mandi Shearer
Recreational Therapy Student
Temple University

Rachel L. Thomas
Recreational Therapy Student
Temple University

# Foreword

In 2002, Heather R. Porter and joan burlingame embarked upon a major project — to consolidate recreational therapy practice into a handbook for students and clinicians, and explain it using the International Classification of Functioning, Disability, and Health (ICF). The project took four years and the first edition of the *Recreational Therapy Handbook of Practice: ICF-Based Diagnosis and Treatment* was published in 2006. The 770-page text was well received in the field, and earned special recognition by the Centers for Disease Control as being the first book, other than the ICF itself, to describe the ICF as a basis for healthcare practice.

Author joan burlingame moved onto other endeavors, so in 2010 I took on the task of developing an updated version of the book. The first edition needed significant revision, as it was primarily based upon clinical experiences. For the new edition I reached out to many content experts in the field of recreational therapy and asked them to contribute to the new evidence-based practice edition with the aim of making the text reflective of the entire profession.

As the project went forward, the publisher and I realized that there was too much information to fit into one book. We decided to create three books, one covering diagnoses (*Recreational Therapy for Specific Diagnoses and Conditions*), another looking at treatment modalities (*Recreational Therapy Basics, Techniques, and Interventions*), and this book describing the ICF. This book offers an in-depth review of the over 1,400 ICF codes, as well as coding procedures related to recreational therapy practice. When we tie our practice to the set of international standards provided by the ICF, it is clear that what we do is at the cutting edge of healthcare practice. We are doing so much more than treating medical conditions. We are finding ways to restore the minds, bodies, and spirits of our clients to the best possible levels of personal, interpersonal, societal, and environmental well-being.

This book is an essential resource for the education of recreational therapists, as well as a reference manual for practicing clinicians and researchers, in guiding the provision of quality evidence-based care aimed at maximizing health, function, and participation. It is with great appreciation that I thank the authors who have contributed to this set of books, especially Yoshitaka Iwasaki, Ph.D., who wrote the section on Personal Factors for this book. Their hard work, passion, and dedication to the profession serve as an inspiration to all in the field and those to follow.

— *Heather Porter*

# I. Introduction

The *International Classification of Functioning, Disability, and Health* (ICF) from the World Health Organization represents a major shift in healthcare. It looks at health, not from the perspective of disease, disorder, or injury, but from the perspective of how a person's health fits in with the rest of his or her life, the kinds of things the person does, and the environment the person lives in.

This is what recreational therapists have been saying all along.

*Recreational Therapy and the International Classification of Functioning, Disability, and Health* was written to bring together the ideas that are already well understood in recreational therapy practice and the model of healthcare represented by the ICF. Some of the terminology is different and there are a few differences in perspective, but if recreational therapists take the time to understand and use the ICF, they will find it to be an excellent tool both for improving practice and for demonstrating the importance of the work we do.

This book includes all of the codes in the 2016 version of the ICF.

# Introduction to the ICF

The *International Classification of Functioning, Disability, and Health* (called the ICF for short) was released by the World Health Organization (WHO) in May 2001. It provides a consensual, meaningful, and useful framework that governments, providers, and consumers can use to describe a person's health and health-related domains including body functions, body structures, activities and participation, and the person's interactions with the environment. It is both a model that guides how we view disability and health, and a classification system to describe what needs to be done to improve the health of our clients.

The ICF is a biopsychosocial model based on systematic theory. (See Figure 1.) The model depicts six components all connected with each other. The arrows show the systematic nature of the model where all of the components interact and are influenced by the others. The biopsychosocial model encompasses all the ways in which health and disability are viewed and fuses them together to provide a more holistic and systematic viewpoint. If everyone throughout the world adopts this view of functioning, disability, and health, we will have a common understanding to guide research and practice.

In addition to a model, the ICF is a classification system with codes for recording the current condition of clients. The terms in the model and the classification system provide a common language for describing functioning and health. Having a common language across disciplines and countries allows comparison of data, which can strengthen research, policy, and practice.

WHO identified five major applications for the ICF: (1) as a statistical tool to collect and record data; (2) as a research tool to measure outcomes, quality of life, or environmental factors; (3) as a clinical tool in needs assessment to match treatments with specific conditions, vocational assessment, rehabilitation, and outcome evaluation; (4) as a social policy tool in social security planning, compensation systems, and policy design and implementation; and (5) as an educational tool in curriculum design and to raise awareness and undertake social action (WHO, 2007).

The discipline of recreational therapy, although continuing to grow, is relatively small compared with other healthcare professions. Consequently, use of the ICF model and classification system will afford us

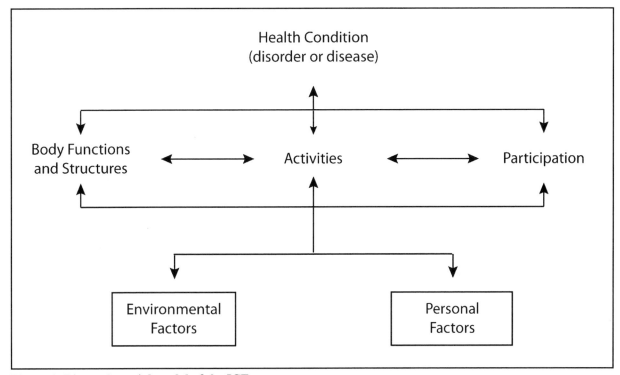

**Figure 1: Biopsychosocial model of the ICF**

3

opportunities to share and better compare practice outcomes and research; thus strengthening evidence-based practice and research.

## The ICF and the ICD-10

Much of our healthcare system uses or will soon be transitioning to the World Health Organization's *International Classification of Diseases, 10<sup>th</sup> edition* (ICD-10) to classify health problems. When a person is diagnosed with a disease, disorder, or injury, it is recorded in the healthcare system as a code (e.g., S62.7 Multiple Fractures of Fingers). This type of classification reflects a medical model based on disease.

Recreational therapists need to understand the ICD-10, but they are not the ones who code the diagnosis. When a person sees a doctor, the doctor assigns a diagnosis and related ICD-10 code to the client. This code is entered into a national computerized healthcare database. The ICD-10 codes are primarily used for the purpose of reimbursement and gathering statistics about a population's health status and needs, such as the number of people who were diagnosed with breast cancer in 2015.

The ICF is an additional classification system to complement, not replace, the ICD-10. Instead of just coding the disease, disorder, or injury, the ICF provides codes that health professionals score on a Likert scale to reflect a client's level of impairment with a body structure (e.g., moderate impairment of the left elbow), level of difficulty with a body function (e.g., severe difficulty with short-term memory), level of difficulty with a specific life activity (e.g., mild difficulty with walking long distances), and barriers and facilitators that affect impairment and difficulty (e.g., attitude of family is a moderate facilitator, financial assets are a severe barrier). The addition of these codes to a healthcare database will give us a much greater understanding of the relationship between a client's health problems (ICD-10 codes) and a client's level of functioning (ICF codes).

In the near future, it is anticipated that recreational therapists, as well as other healthcare professionals, will use the ICF to describe their client's functioning. Professional organizations such as the American Therapeutic Recreation Association, American Psychological Association, American Physical Therapy Association, and American Occupational Therapy Association are currently working on how to incorporate the ICF into current clinical practice and introducing their professions to the new terminology and guidelines in preparation for the implementation of this new classification system. As professional organizations review the classification, recommendations for revisions will be made and some of those recommendations may be implemented prior to using the ICF in our healthcare system.

## Overview of the ICF

The World Health Organization (WHO) published two books of ICF codes (2001, 2007). The first book, simply titled "The International Classification of Functioning Disability and Health" (ICF), contained codes to be used with an adult population. Later, in 2007, the WHO published its second ICF code book titled, "The International Classification of Functioning, Disability, and Health: Children and Youth Version" (ICF-CY) in response to requests for additional codes to reflect the functioning of children (birth to 18 years old). The ICF-CY book contained all of the codes from the original ICF book and added further descriptions for the codes to reflect how they relate to the younger population. Several new codes were also added to reflect the functioning of children, such as d8802 Parallel Play. The 2012 WHO resolution (WHO, 2014) made the decision to merge the ICF-CY back into the ICF. As this book is going to press, the ICF-CY codes are not available in the ICF reference material, but the ICF is an evolving document. Changes and possible additions to the system should be expected.

The ICF is divided into two parts as shown in Table 1.

**Table 1: Overview of the ICF**

**Part I: Functioning and Disability**

*Component 1:* Body Functions and Structures

*Domains:* Body functions and body structures

*Constructs:* Change in body functions (physiological) and change in body structures (anatomical)

*Positive aspect:* Functional and structural integrity (functioning)

*Negative aspect:* Impairment

*Component 2:* Activities and Participation

*Domains:* Life areas (tasks, actions)

*Constructs:* Capacity (executing tasks in a standard environment) and performance (executing tasks in the current environment)

*Positive aspect:* Activities and participation (functioning)

*Negative aspect:* Activity limitation and participation restriction (disability)

**Part II: Contextual Factors**

*Component 1:* Environmental Factors

*Domains:* External influences on functioning and disability

*Constructs:* Facilitating or hindering impact of features of the physical, social, and attitudinal world

*Positive aspect:* Facilitators

*Negative aspect:* Barrier or hindrance

*Component 2:* Personal Factors

*Domains:* Internal influences on functioning and disability

*Constructs:* Impact of attributes of the person

*Positive aspect:* not applicable

*Negative aspect:* not applicable

(WHO, 2001, p.11)

## *ICF Part One*

Part One is called Functioning and Disability and it has two components called "Body Functions and Structures" and "Activities and Participation."

*Body Functions (BF):* Body Functions are the physiological and psychological functions of the body. It is a component of the ICF that recreational therapists will need to become familiar with since many of the codes in this component fall into the scope of recreational therapy practice. EXAMPLE: A client had a heart attack and became anoxic (lack of oxygen to the brain). As a result he has short-term memory and attention problems. The recreational therapist finds the code for each of the problems (b1440 Short-Term Memory, b1400 Sustaining Attention), and scores the client's level of difficulty with the function. Body Functions codes all begin with a lower case b. If a person has difficulty with a body function, it is called an impairment.

*Body Structures (BS):* Body Structures provides a list of anatomical parts of the body such as organs, limbs, and their components. Typically, a physician or nurse practitioner codes a client's level of impair-

ment in Body Structures. EXAMPLE: If a client had a heart attack, the physician would refer to Body Structures, find code s4100 Heart, and score the level of impairment in the structure. It is not anticipated at this time that recreational therapists will be scoring Body Structures. A list of Body Structures codes is provided in this book without elaboration. This list is provided for completeness so therapists who are reading a clinical note that lists Body Structures codes and scores will know what they mean without having to find another source of information. Body Structures codes all begin with a lower case s. If a person has difficulty with a body structure, it is called an impairment.

*Activities and Participation (A&P):* "Activity" is the execution of a task or action by an individual. "Participation" is involvement in a life situation. The codes for activities and participation are the same. Activities and Participation lists the activities that people commonly perform in real life, such as taking care of plants, maintaining health, handling stress, preparing meals, swimming, shopping, using transportation, recreation and leisure, and spirituality. The scores assigned by the therapist reflect a client's ability to engage or participate in those activities in a standardized environment (capacity) and in his/her current real-life environment (performance). Activities and Participation is different from Body Functions. Body Functions reflects the function in isolation, while Activities and Participation reflects the client's ability to do an activity. For example, a client may have moderate difficulty with short-term memory but no difficulty managing a daily routine. The Activities and Participation component allows us to look at the level of difficulty that a client has with a specific activity, not just the level of body function impairment. As therapists, we know that impairments do not always mean that there will be difficulty with activities or that the level of difficulty with an activity will be the same as the level of the impairment. This type of coding guides our current health system into a new way of looking at the health and functioning of people. Recreational therapists predominantly assess and address skills within the context of an activity, so most of the codes that the recreational therapist will use will be in this section. Activities and Participation codes all begin with a lower case d. If a person has difficulty in executing an activity, it is referred to as an "activity limitation."

If a person has difficulty with involvement in a life situation, it is referred to as a "participation restriction."

### ICF Part Two

Part Two of the ICF is Contextual Factors. Contextual Factors is divided into two components called Environmental Factors and Personal Factors.

*Environmental Factors (EF)*: Environmental Factors are things in the person's environment that affect his/her health and functioning, such as adaptive equipment, attitudes of other people, or physical structures of buildings. Recreational therapy practice has a long history of identifying and addressing environmental factors that pose problems for clients. These problems are called barriers. In the ICF, however, not only will therapists score the extent that environmental factors are barriers to specific activities, but will also score the extent that environmental factors are facilitators for activities. The Environmental Factors codes bring attention to specific factors that are causing a problem or increasing the level of difficulty in an activity scored with Activities and Participation codes. It also brings attention to the specific Environmental Factors that are strengths (facilitators) in the person's life, which are supporting the person's ability to participate in activities that are scored with the Activities and Participation codes. Using these codes provides justification for including environmental factors in the treatment plan. Recreational therapists will most likely attach Environmental Factors codes to Activities and Participation codes to show these connections. For example financial assets may be a moderate barrier and immediate family may be a substantial facilitator to engagement in arts and culture. Environmental Factors codes all begin with a lower case e.

*Personal Factors (PF)*: Personal Factors are things that have to do with a person's life and living. They are not part of a health problem, but rather attributes of a person and his/her way of life that could affect health and functioning. Examples of Personal Factors identified by the ICF include gender, race, age, other health conditions, fitness, lifestyle, habits, upbringing, coping styles, social background, education, profession, past and current experience, overall behavior pattern and character style, and individual psychological assets. Personal

Factors, although recognized by the ICF as being influential on a person's health and functioning, are not coded in the ICF. According to the ICF, they are not classified because of the large social and cultural variances associated with them. It is also possible, although not discussed in the ICF book, that personal factors are often made into facilitators or barriers by other environmental factors, body structures, body functions, and activities and participation. Consequently, therapists should take this cue and look at environmental factors that might be changed to yield a positive result. For example, it may be the attitudes of others that impact a woman's participation in activity, not that she is a woman. Changing the attitudes of others, an Environmental Factor, will allow the client to participate with fewer barriers. Although Personal Factors are not currently coded in the ICF, and many cannot be changed, therapists are attentive to personal factors that hinder or facilitate functioning and revise therapy plans and interactions accordingly.

### Terminology in the ICF

When you look through the ICF codes, you will notice that the terminology is quite simple. For example, health professionals use the term "ambulation" to describe the action of moving from one place to another using the legs assisted or not by other people and/or devices. They might write, "The client is able to ambulate 50' with minimal assistance and a rolling walker." The ICF does not recognize the term "ambulation." It uses the basic term "walking" instead. Therapists need to be aware of the terminology changes so that they can find the correct codes. The language chosen by the WHO was chosen for good reason. The terms are simple so that they can be translated and understood by all cultures, all over the world. To help you make this transition, we have included common therapy terms that will guide you to the ICF term. See Table 2.

### Table 2: Translation of Common Therapy Terms

ambulation: d450 Walking
balance (dynamic): b755 Involuntary Movement Reaction Functions, d410 Changing Basic Body Position
balance (static): d415 Maintaining a Body Position

community mobility: d460 Moving Around in
   Different Locations, d465 Moving Around
   Using Equipment
direction following: d210 Undertaking a Single Task,
   d220 Undertaking Multiple Tasks
endurance: b740 Muscle Endurance Functions, b455
   Exercise Tolerance Functions
fine motor skills: d440 Fine Hand Use
gross motor skills: d445 Hand and Arm Use, d435
   Moving Objects with Lower Extremities, b760
   Control of Voluntary Movement Functions
initiation: d210 Undertaking a Single Task, d220
   Undertaking Multiple Tasks
leisure skill development: d155 Acquiring Skills for
   learning how to acquire skills and d810 Informal
   Education for learning the actual skills
range of motion: b710 Mobility of Joint Functions
sequencing: b176 Mental Functions of Sequencing
   Complex Movements
standing tolerance: d4154 Maintaining a Standing
   Position
strength: b730 Muscle Power Functions
transfers: d420 Transferring Oneself

## ICF in RT Practice, Education, and Research

The American Therapeutic Recreation Association (ATRA) adopted the ICF in 2005:

> The concepts and terminology of the ICF are compatible with recreational therapy practice. ATRA supports the use of ICF language and terminology in recreational therapy practice guidelines, standards of practice, curriculum development, public policy, international relations, and research. ATRA also acknowledges the significance of the use of the ICF classification and coding system as a vehicle to clarify and enhance practice and research in recreational therapy (ATRA, 2005, p. NA).

As a result of this statement, many recreational therapists, educators, and researchers have adopted the ICF model and classification system in practice, education, and research.

It is uncertain when the ICF will be fully adopted into the U.S. healthcare system, even though other countries are moving forward. For example, Australia, Canada, Italy, India, Japan, and Mexico are

piloting the ICF in rehabilitation, home-care, age-care, and disability evaluation (WHO, 2012, p. NA). Even though the ICF codes are not yet part of the U.S. electronic healthcare coding system, the ICF model and terms are often used in healthcare and disability literature. A Google Scholar search using the term "International Classification of Functioning Disability and Health" yielded over 17,000 results. Recreational therapy has contributed about 200 of those papers. Increased use of the ICF in practice will contribute to increased ICF research and larger numbers of publications. In addition, if more recreational therapists use the ICF in practice, we can combine our data, thus strengthening evidence-based practice and research.

Below are a few suggestions on how to incorporate the ICF into recreational therapy practice, education, and research:

- *Adopt the ICF model*: Adopt the ICF model into your practice, curriculum, and research. As a practitioner, use the ICF model to guide your assessment and treatment plan. As an educator, teach the ICF model to students as a basis for understanding health and functioning. As a researcher, use the ICF model as a framework for research studies.

- *Incorporate ICF terminology*: As a practitioner, incorporate the ICF terminology into your clinical documentation. As an educator, use the terminology when teaching basic therapy concepts. As a research, use the terminology in scholarly publications.

   o Use the term "impairment" when talking about a problem a client has with a body structure or function.

   o Use the term "capacity" when talking about a client's ability to do an action or task in a standardized testing environment, such as a clinic setting. If the client has difficulty with this, refer to it as an "activity limitation."

   o Use the term "performance" when talking about a client's ability to engage in a real-life situation. If the client has difficulty with this, refer to it as a "participation restriction."

   o Use the term "environmental factor" when talking about things in the environment that hinder or facilitate a person's functioning or health.

o   Use the term "personal factor" when talking about things that have to do with the person, such as culture or beliefs, that hinder or facilitate a person's functioning or health.

o   Use the term "barrier" when talking about things that hinder a person's capacity or performance.

o   Use the term "facilitator" when talking about things that help a person's capacity or performance.

•   *Use ICF scaling*: Incorporate ICF scaling whenever possible to describe impairments, activity limitations, participation restrictions, and barriers or facilitators. Scales for each component of the ICF are described in the text.

•   *Educate*: Teach your colleagues about the ICF, seek out and attend ICF training workshops or conferences, and keep up to date on ICF changes.

•   *Collaborate*: Encourage colleagues to use the ICF model, terms, scaling, and codes. Share, combine, and publish data.

## Introduction to ICF Codes and Scoring

First it is important to note that the ICF is a classification system, not an assessment tool. Therapists and other health professionals will continue to use observation, clinical judgment, and various informal and formal assessment tools to identify the specific problems and strengths of a client. Once the problems or strengths are identified, the therapist will then need to find the appropriate ICF code and score it.

### How do I find the correct code?

When looking at the ICF for the first time, the number of codes can be overwhelming. However, the more you look through it and the more you use it, the more you will understand it and be able to quickly identify the correct code. There are several ways you can find a specific code.

•   *Thumbing*: Thumb through the ICF component that best fits the problem you would like to code. Remember that the codes you are most likely to use will be found in Body Functions or Activities and Participation. If you are looking for a code to

describe a specific impairment, such as a personality impairment, look in the Body Functions component. If you are looking for a code to describe a problem that a client is having with a specific activity, such as shopping or play, look in the Activities and Participation component. And finally, if you are looking for a code to describe an external variable that is affecting a client's level of impairment or difficulty, look in the Environmental Factors component.

•   *Index*: Look for the name of the specific impairment or activity in the index of this book. It will refer you to the location of a code.

•   *Online*: A copy of the ICF codes that can be searched by keyword is available on line at http://apps.who.int/classifications/icfbrowser/

### How do I score the identified code?

How you score the code will depend on the ICF component. Each component of the ICF (Body Functions, Body Structures, Activities and Participation, and Environmental Factors) is scored differently, although there are some similarities in how they are expressed. The introductions in this book for each of the components give specific scoring instructions.

### When will I score the codes?

It is currently unclear how often the recreational therapist will score the ICF codes. It is possible that the therapist will score the ICF codes after each encounter, such as assessment and treatment, at admission and again at discharge, or in relation to predefined documentation. One important emphasis in healthcare is connecting treatment to diagnosis. For each treatment session, the therapist should refer to the ICF codes in the diagnosis that are being treated.

### Are there specific ICF forms?

The World Health Organization (WHO) developed a clinical ICF form that is publicly available, but it does not reflect all of the ICF categories that are pertinent to the scope of recreational therapy practice. It is important to note that the clinical ICF form is not a finalized document, but rather a working form that will most likely be adapted to meet the needs of a discipline or a facility. The form can be downloaded by selecting the ICF Checklist option on the ICF website: http://www.who.int/classifications/icf/icfapptraining/en/index.html

### What are ICF Core Sets?

ICF "core sets" have been developed for specific diagnoses and conditions. A core set is a list of ICF codes that are commonly used for a particular diagnosis. The brief and the comprehensive lists can be helpful to clinicians because they identify the most relevant codes for the diagnosis. However, the use of core sets is controversial. Those in favor of core sets find they are helpful in guiding the clinician to commonly used codes. This can save time and serve as a guide for what should be covered in the assessment and treatment plan. Others, while recognizing these benefits, believe that core sets can be limiting. The utilization of a core set has the potential for clinicians to fall into the trap of using it as a sole reference and not considering other codes that might be relevant.

Core sets are a good starting point for identifying codes related to specific diagnoses, but recreational therapists should not limit themselves to core sets only. Recreational therapists look holistically at a client's lifestyle and functioning, which will often require a broader array of codes. Recreational therapists also recognize that people are more than their diagnosis. Consequently, there may be other relevant codes impacting the person's health and functioning that lie outside of the primary diagnosis. And finally, people often have more than one diagnosis, resulting in the need to reference several core sets. The combination of several diagnoses may also result in additional issues not listed on either core set.

The current set of ICF core sets is provided in the companion book, *Recreational Therapy for Specific Diagnoses and Conditions*. Core sets continue to be revised and developed. To find a core set for a particular diagnosis go to Google and search "ICF core set for [insert name of diagnosis or condition]."

### Cross References

ICF codes are featured in both of the companion books discussing recreational therapy practice, *Recreational Therapy for Specific Diagnoses and Conditions* and *Recreational Therapy Basics, Techniques, and Interventions*. At the end of each ICF code discussion there is a list of where the code is mentioned in the other books. In addition to the discussions at the end of each three-digit code, the initial discussion for each chapter lists places where the whole chapter is referenced in the companion books.

# References

American Therapeutic Recreation Association. (2005). Position statement on the ICF. Accessed via website http://www.atra-online.com/displaycommon.cfm?an=1&subarticlenbr=86

World Health Organization. (2001). International classification of functioning, disability, and health. Geneva, Switzerland: World Health Organization.

World Health Organization. (2006). International classification of functioning, disability, and health: Children and youth version. Geneva, Switzerland: World Health Organization.

World Health Organization. (2012). ICF application areas. Accessed via website http://www.who.int/classifications/icf/appareas/en/index.html

World Health Organization. (2014). WHOFIC resolution 2012: Merger of ICF-CY into ICF. Accessed via website http://www.who.int/classifications/icf/whoficresolution2012icfcy.pdf?ua=1

# II. ICF Codes and Recreational Therapy Practice

The ICF classification is comprised of over 1,400 codes. Each code is listed and described as it appears in the official ICF online reference. A further description of each code is provided as it relates to recreational therapy practice. A complete list of all ICF codes without descriptions is available at the beginning of the book after the table of contents.

# Body Functions

*Heather R. Porter*

Body functions include physiological and psychological functions that are used to indicate the extent of a client's impairments in these areas. The codes are divided into eight chapters.

## Scoring

Recreational therapists will routinely score Body Functions codes in most practice settings.

*Body functions* are the physiological functions of body systems, including psychological functions.

*Impairments* are problems in body functions or structures representing a significant deviation or loss.

To score a Body Functions impairment the therapist first identifies the appropriate code to score using the General Coding Guidelines shown below.

## General Coding Guidelines (WHO, 2001)

- Choose the appropriate codes that best reflect the client's functioning as it relates to the purpose of the encounter.
- Only choose codes that are relevant to the context of the health condition. For example, if a person has impairments with involuntary movement functions (e.g., b7651 Tremor) but is being evaluated for cognitive functioning, only cognitive functioning should be coded.
- Do not make inferences or assumptions about a client's functioning in other areas based on a Body Functions impairment. Each function should be evaluated and then scored separately. For example, just because a person has a moderate impairment with b1641 Organization and Planning, it does not mean that the client will have difficulty with d230 Carrying Out Daily Routine.
- Only choose codes that reflect the specific predefined timeframe. Functions that relate to a timeframe outside of the predefined timeframe should not be coded.
- Use the most specific code possible. For example, if a client has an impairment with sustaining attention, score the specific code of b1400 Sustaining Attention rather than the broader code of b140 Attention Functions.

The code is written down in its entirety. This includes the letter and number. All Body Functions codes begin with the letter b. A decimal point is placed after the code. After the decimal point, the extent of the client's impairment is recorded. This is the only qualifier for Body Functions. The scoring for the qualifier is shown in Table 3.

### Table 3: Body Functions Qualifier (WHO, 2001)

| Qualifier 1. Extent of Impairment |
| --- |
| 0: NO impairment, 0-4% (none, absent, negligible…) |
| 1: MILD impairment, 5-24% (slight, low…) |
| 2: MODERATE impairment, 25-49% (medium, fair…) |
| 3: SEVERE impairment, 50-95% (high, extreme…) |
| 4: COMPLETE impairment, 96-100% (total) |
| 8: not specified |
| 9: not applicable |

*Example*: A client has moderate short-term memory problems. The code for short-term memory is b1440 Short-Term Memory. The qualifier is a 2 for moderate impairment. The appropriately written code would look like this: b1440.2. It is possible to have a different score for different situations (e.g., in quiet vs. noisy environment). The situation may be noted after the score.

# Chapter 1 Mental Functions

This chapter is about the functions of the brain: both global mental functions, such as consciousness, energy, and drive, and specific mental functions such as memory, language, and calculation mental functions.

*Sample Scoring of Mental Functions*

- A client is unable to identify approximately 75% (severe impairment = 3) of his family members and friends (b11421 Orientation to Others). The correct scoring of b11421 Orientation to Others would look like this: b11421.3.
- A client is unable to immediately recall (b1440 Short-Term Memory) two out of six items (moderate impairment = 2) after the therapist says the names of the items. The correct scoring of b1440 Short-Term Memory would look like this: b1440.2.

Mental functions have a direct relationship with health, other abilities, and quality of life. This chapter covers all of the function of the brain divided into global and specific mental functions. Global functions include overall functioning, such as consciousness and orientation, temperament, personality, energy, and sleep. Specific mental functions are the ability to perform specific tasks, such as attention, memory, emotions, perceptions, thought, language and calculation skills, sequencing movement, and experience of self.

Some of the research demonstrating the relationship between mental functions and the client's quality of life are shown below. These studies explain why treatment in this area is so important.

A study of 2,349 older adults found that global and executive cognitive functions predict declines in gait speed (Atkinson et al., 2007). The authors theorize that this may have occurred because "maintenance of an efficient gait may require specific cognitive capacities [such as] memory, visuospatial skills, cognitive processing speed, and executive cognitive skills [which] may be differentially important to the planning, initiating, and maintaining of walking" (p. 848). They additionally note that this could be due to vascular or degenerative lesions affecting both cognition and physical performance.

These findings were supported by Inzitari et al. (2006) who conducted a study of 1,052 older adults and found that attention and executive dysfunction predicts motor performance decline.

Mental functions also play a role in life satisfaction and quality of life. A study by Edwards et al. (2006) found that adults who had a mild stroke reported disability and diminished life satisfaction despite full independence in basic self-care and mobility as measured by the *Functional Independence Measure*. The authors noted that depression, impaired executive function, and attention seem to play a greater role in life satisfaction. In another study of adults with stroke, cognitive impairment predicted less satisfaction. Unilateral neglect was the most predictive for long-term depressive symptoms. Reduced quality of life was associated with problems in visual perception and construction (Nys et al., 2006).

Halligan (2006) reviewed four aspects of consciousness and awareness, also known as insight, to help healthcare professionals understand, measure, and improve deficits in this area including: neurogenic factors (malfunctions in monitoring systems), psychosocial factors (response to illness influenced by the psychosocial environment in which behaviors are elicited and understood), psychogenic factors (defense mechanism, coping strategy), and nonmedical factors (symptom exaggeration or malingering to avoid potential consequences of illness and the sick role, such as medication, childcare custody, etc.). The authors note that lack of insight and awareness is associated with poor recovery and recommend a holistic approach to its evaluation and treatment.

Mental functions also play a role in community integration. For example, a study by McCabe et al. (2007) found that cognitive rehabilitation and interventions using cognitive strategies improved the percentage of individuals with acquired brain injury returning to full time vocational activity, satisfaction with community reintegration, and cognitive functioning outcomes.

*Assessment of Mental Functions*

Recreational therapists utilize various methods to assess mental functions including but not limited to interview, observation, functional testing, and standardized assessments. The skills in this section are significantly different from one another. Consequently the assessment methods chosen will vary greatly. For example, assessment methods chosen to evaluate orientation will be quite different from those chosen to evaluate temperament and personality functions. See the individual codes for more specific information.

*Treatment of Mental Functions*

Treatment for mental functions will vary depending upon the client's diagnosis, severity of symptoms, therapy time allotted, and resources available, both in the therapy setting and after discharge. Depending upon the above, the therapist will utilize a restorative/development approach or a compensation approach. In some instances, the therapist may choose to utilize both approaches by utilizing a restorative approach for one aspect of the activity and a compensation approach for another aspect of the activity. Cognitive Retraining and Rehabilitation in the companion book, *Recreational Therapy Basics, Techniques, and Interventions*, provides specific information on how to choose a mental functions intervention. It also provides detailed protocols and processes for a variety of interventions, including internal and external strategies, errorless learning, spaced retrieval, chaining, predict-perform procedure, time-pressure management training, and caregiver education and training.

*Evidence Review*

Reviews of several studies are provided below to highlight evidence-based practice related to mental functions. This is only a sample of the evidence. Further review of the literature may be needed to identify evidence-based practice interventions that address a particular deficit.

Physical exercise has been found to improve mental functions. For example, a study of older adults who participated in a six-month physical activity program showed improvement in cognition (Lautenschlager et al., 2008).

Horgan and MacLachlan (2004) conducted a review of the literature related to psychosocial adjustment of adults with lower-limb amputation.

Better psychosocial adjustment is associated with greater time since amputation, more social support, greater satisfaction with prosthesis, active coping techniques, optimistic personality disposition, lower level of amputation, and lower levels of phantom limb pain and stump pain. Social discomfort and body image anxiety have been found to be associated with increased activity restriction, depression, and anxiety.

Potter and Keeling (2005) conducted a study of 31 adult male shift workers. Baselines were recorded for memory at various times of the day. The subjects were instructed to take a brisk self-paced walk for 10 minutes at different times during their workday. After doing brisk walking, participants' memory showed significant improvements. The authors note that "regular bouts of exercise have been shown to increase growth hormone concentrations, increase neurogenesis in the hippocampus, improve memory performance … and also bring about improvements in executive function in humans" (p. 123).

Vance and Crowe (2006) propose a model to improve cognitive reserve in older adults through taking advantage of neuroplasticity and modifying factors that influence this process. The model illustrates six paths to increase cognitive reserve including modifiable health factors, education, social support, positive affect, stimulating activities with novel experiences, and cognitive training. "Encouraging a healthy lifestyle that includes a combination of regular exercise, taking steps to reduce stress and negative affect, engaging in novel and stimulating activities, having educational pursuits, and participating in cognitive training may be beneficial for maintenance of cognitive reserve in older adulthood" (p. 75).

Fisher et al. (2010) conducted a study on 32 clinically stable individuals with schizophrenia. They found that "a total of 50 hours of neuroplasticity-based computerized cognitive training is sufficient to drive improvements in verbal learning, memory, and cognitive control that endured six months beyond the intervention" (p. 869).

Davis et al. (2007) conducted a study of 94 sedentary, overweight children who were randomized into low dose (20 minutes per day exercise, five days per week, 15 weeks), high dose (40 minutes per day exercise, five days per week, 15 weeks), or control group. The exercise interventions were aerobic with a heart rate greater than 150 beats per minute. The *Cognitive Assessment System* (CAS) was administered to each participant before and after the intervention. Following the intervention, planning scores for the high-dose group were significantly greater than those of the control group. "Exercise may prove to be a simple, yet important, method of enhancing aspects of children's mental functioning that are central to cognitive and social development" (p. 510).

### Cross References

In *Recreational Therapy for Specific Diagnoses and Conditions, First Edition,* ICF code b1 Mental Functions and its subcategories are listed in 39 chapters: Amputation and Prosthesis, Attention-Deficit/Hyperactivity Disorder, Autism Spectrum Disorder, Back Disorders and Back Pain, Borderline Personality Disorder, Burns, Cancer, Cerebral Palsy, Cerebrovascular Accident, Chronic Obstructive Pulmonary Disease, Diabetes Mellitus, Epilepsy, Feeding and Eating Disorders, Fibromyalgia and Juvenile Fibromyalgia, Gambling Disorder, Generalized Anxiety Disorder, Guillain-Barré Syndrome, Hearing Loss, Heart Disease, Intellectual Disability, Major Depressive Disorder, Multiple Sclerosis, Neurocognitive Disorders, Obesity, Oppositional Defiant Disorder and Conduct Disorder, Osteoarthritis, Osteoporosis, Parkinson's Disease, Post-Traumatic Stress Disorder, Pressure Ulcers, Rheumatoid Arthritis, Schizophrenia Spectrum and Other Psychotic Disorders, Sickle Cell Disease, Spina Bifida, Spinal Cord Injury, Substance-Related Disorders, Total Joint Replacement, Traumatic Brain Injury, and Visual Impairments and Blindness.

See the Cognitive Retraining and Rehabilitation chapter in the *Recreational Therapy Basics, Techniques, and Interventions* book for more mental function techniques and interventions (e.g., strategies to improve insight; problem solving strategies such as Stop, Think, Plan; metacognitive strategies; internal/external memory strategies; errorless learning; spaced retrieval; chaining; emotional perception training; predict-perform procedure; time pressure management training).

In *Recreational Therapy Basics, Techniques, and Interventions, First Edition,* treatment for ICF code b1 Mental Functions and its subcategories are discussed in 37 chapters: Activity and Task Analysis, Adjustment and Response to Disability, Consequences of Inactivity, Education and Counseling,

Parameters and Precautions, Participation, Psychoneuroimmunology, Stress, Activity Pattern Development, Adaptive Sports, Adventure Therapy, Anger Management, Animal Assisted Therapy, Aquatic Therapy, Assertiveness Training, Balance Training, Behavior Strategies and Interventions, Bibliotherapy, Cognitive Behavioral Counseling, Cognitive Retraining and Rehabilitation, Errorless Learning, Group Psychotherapy Techniques, Leisure-Based Stress Coping, Leisure Education and Counseling, Life Review, Medical Play and Preparation, Mind-Body Interventions, Montessori Method, Neuro-Developmental Treatment, Physical Activity, Reality Orientation, Reminiscence, Sensory Interventions, Social Skills Training, Therapeutic Thematic Arts Programming, Values Clarification, and Walking and Gait Training.

## Global Mental Functions (b110 - b139)

### b110 Consciousness Functions

General mental functions of the state of awareness and alertness, including the clarity and continuity of the wakeful state.

Inclusions: functions of the state, continuity and quality of consciousness, loss of consciousness, coma, vegetative states, fugues, trance states, possession states, drug-induced altered consciousness, delirium, stupor

Exclusions: orientation functions (b114); energy and drive functions (b130); sleep functions (b134)

- *b1100 State of Consciousness*
  Mental functions that when altered produce states such as clouding of consciousness, stupor, or coma.

- *b1101 Continuity of Consciousness*
  Mental functions that produce sustained wakefulness, alertness, and awareness and, when disrupted, may produce fugue, trance, or other similar states.

- *b1102 Quality of Consciousness*
  Mental functions that when altered effect changes in the character of wakeful, alert, and aware sentience, such as drug-induced altered states or delirium.

- *b1108 Consciousness Functions, Other Specified*
- *b1109 Consciousness Functions, Unspecified*

To evaluate consciousness functions, the recreational therapist observes the client's reaction to single and multimodal stimuli in order to determine a baseline. Multimodal stimuli means stimulation using more than one sense at a time, such as sense of touch combined with sense of hearing. Once a baseline level of functioning is determined, the therapist focuses on an approach that increases the client's ability in this area. If a client's consciousness skills are not fully recovered, the therapist will then change his/her approach to work on adaptations and modifications that will maximize the client's independence, function, and safety.

For the clinical observation the therapist presents the client with single or multimodal stimuli and observes the client's response. These may include withdrawal from stimuli; approach toward the stimuli; or reactions such as eyebrow raise, hand squeeze, smile, or moan. Appropriate stimuli include:

- *Tactile stimuli*: Stimulation of the skin through touching the client with the hand (light touch, deep touch, massage), objects (washcloth, feather, lotion, blankets on or off), water (different temperatures), and air (breeze, burst of cold air, fan).
- *Vestibular stimuli*: Stimulation of the sensation of movement through rocking, bending, rolling, movement of rolling bed, etc.
- *Auditory stimuli*: Stimulation of the sense of hearing through sounds such as voice (saying hello, client's name, telling a story), music (pleasant and noxious), familiar sounds from client's life (voices of family, lawnmower, daughter playing guitar, telephone ringing), varied sound volumes (soft, loud), and varied sound speeds (slow music, fast upbeat music).
- *Visual stimuli*: Stimulation of vision through objects of varied color, size, and familiarity (home, family, hobbies), and people (family, staff).
- *Olfactory stimuli*: Stimulation of the sense of smell through oil extracts, food, lotions, perfumes, soaps, body sprays, and room freshener.
- *Gustatory stimuli*: Do this only if client can swallow safely. Stimulation of the sense of taste through small tastes such as placing a swab in the mouth that was rubbed in something sweet (melted chocolate), sour (lemon juice), salty (salt), or bitter (coffee). Place swab on area of tongue associated with each taste. Sweet is the tip of tongue; sour is the lateral edges, midway between the tip and back; salty is the lateral edges, proximal and distal to the sour sensors; and bitter is the back portion.

The therapist documents the specific stimuli presented, along with the:

- *Specific response observed*: e.g., opens eyes on command (b1100.0), no reaction to loud noise or light touch (b1100.4).
- *Length of time the behavior was observed*: e.g., client's continuity of consciousness was five consecutive minutes within a 30-minute session (b1101.3).
- *Level of cueing client required to invoke a response to the stimuli in relation to a specific task*: e.g., client requires maximal verbal and tactile cues to open eyes and turn head in direction of therapist (b1100.3).

If a client is in a coma, sensory stimulation techniques as described above are helpful in monitoring changes in the state of consciousness. For example, if a client is in a coma (Rancho Los Amigos Level I), an eye-opening response to stimuli may signal a positive change in the client's status to a Rancho Los Amigos Level II.

The evaluation of other consciousness functions is assessed through behavior observation, as described below.

Fugue state: A state in which the person denies memory of activities for a period of hours to weeks (Segen's Medical Dictionary, 2012a).

Trance state: An altered mental state in which the body is still or movements are jerky, the limbs feel "heavy," the eyelids flicker due to rapid eye movements, the eyeballs roll upwards (as occurs when one is asleep), the eye tears, the pupils dilate, and speech pattern changes (Segen's Medical Dictionary, 2012b).

Possession state: The individual's behavior is reflective of being possessed; spirit possession (Littlewood, 2004).

Pharmacologically (drug) induced altered consciousness: A change in the person's alertness, awareness, orientation, and responsiveness to the environment as a consequence of medication or drugs.

Delirium: A syndrome, or group of symptoms, caused by a disturbance in the normal functioning of the brain. There is a reduced awareness of and responsiveness to the environment, which may be manifested as disorientation, incoherence, and memory disturbance. It is often marked by hallucinations, delusions, and a dream-like state (Gale Encyclopedia of Medicine, 2008).

Stupor: A state of impaired consciousness in which the person shows a marked diminution in reactivity to environmental stimuli and can be aroused only by continual stimulation (Farlex Partner Medical Dictionary, 2012).

There are many factors that can influence the client's level of consciousness, such as time of day, fatigue, and depression. Consequently, the therapist must be consistent when measuring consciousness to be able to accurately reflect changes. For example, if a therapist assesses the client's baseline for continuity of consciousness in the late morning, then his/her follow-up assessments should also be conducted in the late morning.

The recreational therapist has one standardized testing tool that fits well with this type of therapy intervention and documentation. The *FOX — Activity Therapy Skills Baseline* measures six areas in what it terms the "social" domain. The six areas are (1) the client's reaction to others, (2) the client's interactions with objects, (3) the client's seeking attention from others to manipulate the environment, (4) the client's interactions with objects, (5) the client's concept of self, and (6) the client's interactions with others.

Recreational therapists also utilize a variety of scales to indicate consciousness functions including the *Glasgow Coma Scale* (GCS), the *Glasgow-Liege Scale* (GLS), the *Grady Coma Scale*, the *Wessex Head Injury Matrix* (WHIM), the *JFK Coma Recovery Scale*, the *Coma Recovery Scale—Revised*, and the *Sensory Modality Assessment and Rehabilitation Technique* (SMART) (Majerus et al., 2005).

Some clients, especially those with severe brain injury, may be unarousable initially. They are not in a coma, just very low functioning. The client may not open his/her eyes, respond physically to a stimuli (e.g., turn his head toward the stimuli), or even acknowledge the presence of a stimuli in any manner (e.g., shooing away the therapist with an arm, looking away, leaning toward stimuli). Since the client at this level is unable to engage in a task, the therapist is to provide stimulation to invoke a response with the goal of having the client show simple signs of arousal. Some techniques that have been helpful with this type of client include:

- Rubbing a cold washcloth on the back of the client's neck (the back of the neck is sensitive to temperature).
- Turning the lights off and then on again.
- Clapping loudly.
- Changing voice tone when giving a command (e.g., say "open your eyes" sweetly, commandingly, or matter-of-factly).
- Using touch alone or in conjunction with another stimulus (e.g., squeeze the client's hand or touch the client's upper back when saying the client's name).
- Calling the client by his/her name. Some clients may respond better to a nickname if it was commonly used by friends and family (e.g., client may respond to "Nick" but not to "Nicholas"). Some clients, however, respond to formal names better despite having been commonly addressed by a nickname.
- Using fresh air (especially cold or cool air). Cool or cold fresh air commonly invokes an eye opening response (e.g., turn on a fan so that client feels the breeze, open an outside door or window so that the client gets a burst of cold air, use an air-conditioned room that is kept cooler than the rest of the facility).

Other ideas can also be useful for treatment of consciousness functions. O'Sullivan and Schmitz (1988) recommended the following to promote arousal or consciousness.

- Implement short periods of stimulation (5-10 minutes) and intersperse them throughout the day to balance rest with activity.
- Use different types of stimulation (auditory, visual, tactile, olfactory, gustatory) by themselves or in combination, e.g., provide an auditory stimuli of saying "hello" and stating the client's name or provide auditory and tactile stimuli together by saying "hello," stating the client's name, and touching the client's shoulder.
- Use activities that are important to the client. Activities that are important and attractive to the client increase motivation and initiation skills.

- Avoid over-stimulating the client. If the client is over-stimulated by an overwhelming amount of stimuli in the environment, s/he may react in one of two ways: shut down by withdrawing inwardly or express over-stimulation through agitation and outbursts. Agitated clients who demonstrate excessive levels of arousal also benefit from a controlled application of sensory techniques. Frequently, sources of stimulation from the environment precipitate bouts of agitation and disorganization. The client is generally unable to process stimuli effectively and is similarly unable to control responses, which are often bizarre and combative.
- Careful assessment can reveal offending stimuli and those that have a calming influence. Therapists should (1) eliminate or reduce irritating stimuli; (2) use a quiet, non-distracting environment and gradually build up the client's tolerance to a more stimulating environment; (3) minimize unexpected surprises since they can precipitate outbursts; (4) establish a predictable routine and structure to the day (e.g., therapies are held on the same day, at the same locations within the facility, and as much as possible involve the same task or activity); (5) if a new activity is used, the therapist carefully explains the activity to the client before it is attempted and provides verbal reassurance and manual guidance during the execution of the new activity; and (6) if an agitated outburst occurs, the therapist calmly redirects the client's attention away from the cause of irritation.
- Verbal explanations should be kept brief and to the point to keep the client focused on the specific stimuli.
- Keep a 24-hour record of the types of sensory stimuli used, the individuals who applied them, and the client's responses.

Often selection of a task over which the client has some control will help the client regain composure. The therapist should provide a model for calm, controlled behavior by speaking slowly and calmly at a moderate volume that conveys understanding and control and reward each of the client's successful efforts with positive reinforcement.

Treatment for other consciousness functions such as fugue states, trance states, possession states, pharmacologically (drug) induced altered consciousness, delirium, and stupor will vary depending upon the underlying cause. Underlying causes could include mental illness, substance use or abuse, medication, and neurological impairments (including brain tumors). Depending on the cause, the therapist may implement interventions to reduce or minimize any causative behaviors, such as substance abuse. As part of the medical team, however, therapists routinely monitor and record such behaviors.

### Cross References

In *Recreational Therapy for Specific Diagnoses and Conditions, First Edition*, ICF code b110 Consciousness Functions is listed in 11 chapters: Attention-Deficit/Hyperactivity Disorder, Cerebrovascular Accident, Chronic Obstructive Pulmonary Disease, Diabetes Mellitus, Epilepsy, Heart Disease, Multiple Sclerosis, Parkinson's Disease, Spinal Cord Injury, Substance-Related Disorders, and Traumatic Brain Injury.

In *Recreational Therapy Basics, Techniques, and Interventions, First Edition*, treatment for ICF code b110 Consciousness Functions is discussed in three chapters: Consequences of Inactivity, Parameters and Precautions, and Aquatic Therapy.

### b114 Orientation Functions

General mental functions of knowing and ascertaining one's relation to self, to others, to time, and to one's surroundings.

Inclusions: functions of orientation to time, place, and person; orientation to self and others; disorientation to time, place, and person

Exclusions: consciousness functions (b110); attention functions (b140); memory functions (b144)

- *b1140 Orientation to Time*
  Mental functions that produce awareness of day, date, month, and year.
- *b1141 Orientation to Place*
  Mental functions that produce awareness of one's location, such as one's immediate surroundings, one's town or country.
- *b1142 Orientation to Person*
  Mental functions that produce awareness of one's own identity and of individuals in the immediate environment.

o   *b11420 Orientation to Self*
Mental functions that produce awareness of one's own identity.

o   *b11421 Orientation to Others*
Mental functions that produce awareness of the identity of other individuals in one's immediate environment.

o   *b11428 Orientation to Person, Other Specified*

o   *b11429 Orientation to Person, Unspecified*

- *b1148 Orientation Functions, Other Specified*
- *b1149 Orientation Functions, Unspecified*

With clients who are able to answer questions, the therapist assesses the client's functioning by challenging the client with one or more orientation questions in each sphere (time, place, and person). The therapist must already know the answers to the questions to be able to determine the accuracy of the client's answers.

*Time*: What time of day is it? Which meal did you just eat? What activity are you going to next? What day of the week is it? What month is it? What season is it? What is the year?

*Place*: What city and state are we in? What is the name of this facility? What floor are you on? What is your room number? Which way is your room? Where is the dining area? Topographical orientation (also known as spatial orientation) is a form of orientation to place. Topographical orientation is the mental function that produces awareness of where one is in relation to the environment using both visual and non-visual input to understand the layout of one's world. For example, if a client is standing in front of the hospital cafeteria, she should be able to form a "mental map" of where she is in relation to her room.

*Person*: What is your name? How old are you? Are you a grandfather? Do you have any brothers, sisters, or children? What are their names? How old are they? Show the client pictures of his/her family and ask the client to tell you who they are.

The therapist also observes the client's behavioral responses to assess orientation, especially for clients who are unable to speak or whose expression of speech is impaired. Some observations the therapist may make provide answers to questions like: Does the client seem to be aware of being a separate individual? Does the client get lost easily when walking around the hospital floor and/or is the client unable to find his/her room? Does the client attempt to put on a heavy coat when it is 80°F outside? Does the client's facial expression look puzzled or fearful when someone in his/her immediate family is standing in front of him/her?

The most common method of documenting orientation is the scale called *Orientation x3*. As burlingame and Blaschko (2010) point out, the protocols for determining orientation x3 are not well developed, so the scores should always be taken as a general measurement of orientation and not as specific orientation. Similarly to consciousness, variability in orientation is seen as the day progresses. In addition to noting the time of day that the therapist is measuring orientation, the therapist should measure the client's response in the following ways:

- *Terms of sphere*: e.g., client is oriented to person without cueing, but is not oriented to time (b1142.0), client is alert and oriented in all five spheres (b114.0). If a client is not alert, it is very hard for him/her to be oriented.
- *Percentage of orientation*: e.g., client is oriented to place at 50% — this means that the client was able to answer only 50% of the orientation questions about place or that the client was observed being disoriented to place about half the time through behavioral observation (b1141.3).
- *Type and extent of cueing needed*: e.g., client requires moderate verbal cues to orient to place (b1141.2).
- *Relation to task dysfunction*: e.g., client requires moderate verbal cues to locate the cafeteria secondary to poor place orientation (b1141.2).

Once a baseline level of functioning is determined, the therapist focuses strategies to enhance the client's functioning. If a client's orientation is not fully recovered, the therapist also includes an approach that identifies specific adaptations and modifications that will maximize the client's independence, functioning, and safety.

Improving functioning should be done in a clinically correct sequence. Orientation to self is the most basic function. Orientation to person seems to come back before orientation to place. And orientation to place seems to come back before orientation to time. Orientation to person is a retrograde memory function having to do with a client's ability to remember information that occurred before the injury, while orientation to place and time require the client to learn, retain, and recall new information. Problems with retrograde memory may resolve due to the normal healing process of the brain, whereas the ability to learn, retain, and recall new information are more complex skills that take longer to recover.

Therapists enhance the skills of orientation by challenging the client with orientation tasks. This is done in accordance with cognitive retraining strategies. Some of the techniques commonly used include:

- *Asking the client one specific orientation question* (e.g., "What is the name of this facility?"). If the client says, "I don't know" or gives a wrong answer, provide the client with cues to identify the right answer (e.g., It's a rehab hospital in Malvern. It begins with the letter B.). The therapist should refrain from giving the client the specific answer whenever possible to promote cognitive restructuring.
- *Developing and adhering to a daily routine for the client.* A structured and consistent routine will help to orient the client because it will be predictable and repetitive. For example, the client always goes to speech therapy at nine in the morning, followed by recreational therapy at ten in the morning. As a result of this schedule, the client may begin to associate therapy with a specific time, thus increasing the client's orientation to time. In addition, the client will travel the same route, the client's room to the speech clinic, the speech clinic to the recreational therapy clinic, the recreational therapy clinic back to the client's room. A consistent travel pattern will assist the client in remembering the environmental layout. (The environment can be confusing if you are always coming and going from different places and from different directions.) This will help to orient him/her to place.
- *Organizing the client's personal environment* so that it consistently enhances orientation. Examples include shoes that are always inside the closet on the floor or orientation materials are always kept in a binder on the side of the wheelchair.
- *Making and posting clear signage* for specific locations, perhaps a big arrow and a picture of a toilet that points to where the bathroom is lo-

cated and then a big picture of a toilet on the outside of the bathroom door.

- *Teaching the client to look for landmarks.* These could be paintings on the wall or finding familiar locations such as the lobby area and then learning directions from there.
- *Using orientation materials* such as a calendar on the wall in the client's room, using maps, using pictures with labels for family members, making sure the client has and uses a watch and a clock, and/or using a memory book or logbook.
- *Using a daily orientation group* that focuses on cognitive remediation techniques for orientation. Many facilities run a reality orientation group first thing in the morning, either before or after breakfast, to orient clients to the day and to help them prepare their orientation materials for the day. This could include reviewing each client's therapy schedule and making sure it is put in the memory book and checking the correctness of the calendar inside the memory book.
- *Using cognitive remediation techniques* to orient the client at the beginning of each treatment session. For example, ask the client what his/her name is, what therapy s/he is now attending, what is typically done at this therapy, what the name of the hospital is, what time of day it is.

If a client does not fully recover orientation functions, the therapist will have to adapt or modify the client's environment and tasks to maximize functioning. The therapist shifts from a restorative approach to an adaptation approach. In addition, the therapist will need to educate the client's caregivers on how to promote further recovery of orientation after discharge. Adaptation and modification of the client's environment are very important for the client's safety, functioning, and emotional health. If the client is not properly oriented, injury could result. For example, the client could become lost without place orientation. Another consideration is that of functioning. If a client is not properly oriented to time of day, then the client's sleep cycle could become disturbed and activities might be initiated at inappropriate times. Finally, disorientation can affect the emotional health of clients. Being told, "No, you're wrong. That's not right." can take a toll on the client's self-esteem and self-confidence, possibly leading to depression.

Compensatory strategies for disorientation are not very different from what a therapist uses to enhance the skills of orientation. Compensatory strategies used during treatment are kept and carried over into the client's daily routine outside of the hospital setting. The therapist is responsible to assess assimilation of the compensatory strategies into the client's "real life" and make changes as necessary to promote best functioning. Changes should be as minimal as possible. For example, a client may have used a large binder to hold reference papers for orientation in the hospital setting, but now finds it difficult to constantly carry around the large binder for community tasks such as grocery shopping, hiking with the kids, and bike riding. The therapist may suggest using a backpack to carry the binder so that the client's hands are free for activity. The client may be able to alter the shape and content of the memory book without additional disorientation into a smaller date book organizer. Then it would fit in a waist pack, back pants pocket, or pocket book. It is not unusual for a client to have a large binder in the home environment and a small date book organizer in the community environment. If the client is able to use an electronic device, such as a PDA or smart phone, the problems related to the size are easily eliminated.

### Cross References

In *Recreational Therapy for Specific Diagnoses and Conditions, First Edition*, ICF code b114 Orientation Functions is listed in nine chapters: Attention-Deficit/Hyperactivity Disorder, Autism Spectrum Disorder, Borderline Personality Disorder, Cerebrovascular Accident, Chronic Obstructive Pulmonary Disease, Intellectual Disability, Multiple Sclerosis, Neurocognitive Disorders, and Traumatic Brain Injury.

In *Recreational Therapy Basics, Techniques, and Interventions, First Edition*, treatment for ICF code b114 Orientation Functions is discussed in eight chapters: Activity and Task Analysis, Education and Counseling, Animal Assisted Therapy, Life Review, Medical Play and Preparation, Reality Orientation, Social Skills Training, and Therapeutic Thematic Arts Programming.

### b117 Intellectual Functions

General mental functions, required to understand and constructively integrate the various mental functions, including all cognitive functions and their development over the life span.

Inclusions: functions of intellectual growth; intellectual retardation, mental retardation, dementia

Exclusions: memory functions (b144); thought functions (b160); higher-level cognitive functions (b164)

Intellectual functions refer to the normal healthy growth and maintenance of integrative cognitive processes. This ICF code will most likely be scored for individuals that have a developmental disability, intellectual disability, learning disability, dementia, or other disability that affects intellectual functioning.

Therapists assess intellectual functions through clinical interview, observation, functional assessment, and standardized assessment tools (e.g., *Developmental Assessment of Young Children, Version 2, Montreal Cognitive Assessment, Mini-Mental State Exam*). Impairments in intellectual functions are documented in terms of:

- *Stage of functioning*: e.g., client is performing at Piaget's sensorimotor stage.
- *Type of deficit*: e.g., client's intellectual abilities are moderately compromised by dementia (b117.2). Specific deficits should be scored in the relevant categories of b114 Orientation Functions.
- *Level of assistance*: e.g., client needs total assistance to find any location outside the home (b117.4).
- *Prognosis*: e.g., client is expected to progress to some concrete reasoning ability through training with Montessori materials.

The work therapists do with intellectual functions falls into two broad categories: helping in the development and mitigating loss.

Helping in the development of intellectual functioning occurs primarily in school settings and with individuals that have a developmental or intellectual disability. It may also apply in some psychiatric situations. In these cases the therapist's goal is to follow the normal course of intellectual development and provide challenges that allow the client to progress to higher levels of functioning. This can be done in group or individual settings by using activities that teach more mature thought processes. The therapist can present situations, such as appropriate touching, and use social stories to help individuals learn how a person decides what is appropriate. At one level there are rules to be followed. At a higher level there are reasons for the rules. A therapist in this case would explain the concept of looking for the reasons behind the rules, give the clients practice in finding reasons for the things they do, and teach ways to use the reasons to come up with appropriate rules in novel situations. Similarly the therapist can teach concepts from the next developmental stage in any of the areas covered by intellectual functioning.

Therapists mitigate the loss of intellectual function when there is damage to the brain. This includes TBI, stroke, and dementia. Losses may also occur from psychological trauma. If it is possible to improve the intellectual function, the process is similar to helping the development as described above.

The additional complication in the case of loss is dealing with the client realizing that some ability has been lost. When restoration of intellectual function is not expected, as in the case of dementia, the therapist's responsibility is to find adaptations that the client or the client's caregivers can use to reduce the harmful effects of the loss. This includes appropriate restrictions on the client's activities (e.g., they may no longer be allowed to make investment decisions) and dealing with the feelings of loss that accompany these restrictions. It is important to support the client as much as possible in making decisions and not take away choices when it is not necessary. Finding the appropriate balance of autonomy and support for the client's current (and changing) mental abilities is the goal of this treatment.

### Cross References

In *Recreational Therapy for Specific Diagnoses and Conditions, First Edition*, ICF code b117 Intellectual Functions is listed in seven chapters: Attention-Deficit/Hyperactivity Disorder, Hearing Loss, Intellectual Disability, Major Depressive Disorder, Multiple Sclerosis, Neurocognitive Disorders, and Substance-Related Disorders.

In *Recreational Therapy Basics, Techniques, and Interventions, First Edition*, treatment for ICF code b117 Intellectual Functions is discussed in two chapters: Animal Assisted Therapy and Therapeutic Thematic Arts Programming.

### b122 Global Psychosocial Functions

General mental functions, as they develop over the life span, required to understand and constructively integrate the mental functions that lead to the formation of the interpersonal skills needed to establish reciprocal social interactions, in terms of both meaning and purpose.

Inclusions: such as in autism

For evaluation and treatment refer to Activities and Participation d7 Interpersonal Interactions and Relationships. Document using this code and other codes, as required.

### Cross References

In *Recreational Therapy for Specific Diagnoses and Conditions, First Edition*, ICF code b122 Global Psychosocial Functions is listed in eight chapters: Attention-Deficit/Hyperactivity Disorder, Autism Spectrum Disorder, Intellectual Disability, Multiple Sclerosis, Neurocognitive Disorders, Spina Bifida, Substance-Related Disorders, and Traumatic Brain Injury.

In *Recreational Therapy Basics, Techniques, and Interventions, First Edition*, treatment for ICF code b122 Global Psychosocial Functions is discussed in one chapter: Therapeutic Thematic Arts Programming.

### b126 Temperament and Personality Functions

General mental functions of constitutional disposition of the individual to react in a particular way to situations, including the set of mental characteristics that makes the individual distinct from others.

Inclusions: functions of extraversion, introversion, agreeableness, conscientiousness, psychic and emotional stability, and openness to experience; optimism; novelty seeking; confidence; trustworthiness

Exclusions: intellectual functions (b117); energy and drive functions (b130); psychomotor functions (b147); emotional functions (b152)

- *b1260 Extraversion*
  Mental functions that produce a personal disposition that is outgoing, sociable, and demonstrative, as contrasted to being shy, restricted, and inhibited.

- *b1261 Agreeableness*
  Mental functions that produce a personal disposition that is cooperative, amicable, and accommo-

dating, as contrasted to being unfriendly, opposi-tional, and defiant.

- *b1262 Conscientiousness*
  Mental functions that produce personal disposi-tions such as in being hard-working, methodical, and scrupulous, as contrasted to mental func-tions producing dispositions such as in being lazy, unreliable, and irresponsible.

- *b1263 Psychic Stability*
  Mental functions that produce a personal disposi-tion that is even-tempered, calm, and composed, as contrasted to being irritable, worried, erratic, and moody.

- *b1264 Openness to Experience*
  Mental functions that produce a personal disposi-tion that is curious, imaginative, inquisitive, and experience-seeking, as contrasted to being stag-nant, inattentive, and emotionally inexpressive.

- *b1265 Optimism*
  Mental functions that produce a personal disposi-tion that is cheerful, buoyant, and hopeful, as contrasted to being downhearted, gloomy, and despairing.

- *b1266 Confidence*
  Mental functions that produce a personal disposi-tion that is self-assured, bold, and assertive, as contrasted to being timid, insecure, and self-effacing.

- *b1267 Trustworthiness*
  Mental functions that produce a personal disposi-tion that is dependable and principled, as con-trasted to being deceitful and antisocial.

- *b1268 Temperament and Personality Functions, Other Specified*
- *b1269 Temperament and Personality Functions, Unspecified*

Temperament and personality are common de-scriptors used by recreational therapists in documen-tation, as well as common areas for treatment goals. Impairments in temperament and personality are typically seen in mood disorders such as bipolar disorder, personality disorders such as borderline personality disorder, organic disorders such as dementia, childhood disorders such as autism, drug abuse, alcohol abuse, childhood abuse of any kind, and learned behaviors.

Therapists who note a change or oddity in a cli-ent's temperament or personality functions should request an evaluation by a psychologist, psychiatrist, or neuropsychologist as appropriate.

In addition to studying the extent of tempera-ment and personality impairment observed by other members of the treatment team, the recreational therapist documents additional information including:

- The specific function and extent of impairment: e.g., client has severe distrust in others (b1264.3), the client's psychic stability is moder-ately compromised secondary to dementia (b1263.2).
- The impact of the impairment on activity: e.g., client's extreme shyness (b1260.3) prevents her from forming friendships thus limiting her circle of support, client's lack of optimism (b1265.3) is seriously limiting his ability to participate in therapy sessions.
- Functionality of the subcategory on performance: e.g., client exhibits confidence (b1266.0) in his approach to outdoor community walking.
- Effect of treatment on impairment: e.g., client has shown a 50% increase in optimistic verbali-zations since initiation of expressive writing therapy, progressing from severe impairment (b1265.3) to mild impairment (b1265.1); child has become more conscientious of caring for play toys as evidenced by putting them away correctly at the end of the day, progressing from moderate impairment (b1262.2) to mild impair-ment (b1262.1).
- The context of the behavior: e.g., in group therapy sessions, when confronted by another person, client becomes completely defiant (b1261.4).
- The percentage of the time the behavior is observed: e.g., client exhibited self-confidence in 80% of situations (b1266.1).
- The type and extent of cueing needed to move the behavior in a more positive direction: Client required maximum verbal prompting to try a new activity (b1264.3)

Once a root cause of the problem has been iden-tified, treatment is prescribed. Treatment may include:

- *Medication*: such as medication for psychic stability.

- *Specially designed experiences*: such as use of "new games" or adventure therapy to facilitate development of trust; activities that will facilitate feelings of success to promote confidence.
- *Journaling*: such as writing three positive things that happened each day in a journal to promote optimism.
- *Behavior modification*: such as positive rewards for conscientious behavior.
- *Group work*: such as using a jigsaw approach in a group project that requires the individual to cooperate with others to complete a task by dividing required resources among group members.
- *Social skills*: Working on the development of a particular social skill and providing opportunities to apply learned skills. Making friends is a social skill that affects several of the personality functions.
- *Opportunities for leadership*: Be sure success is highly likely.
- *Challenges*: to promote openness to experience such as participation in new activities or socializing with a different peer group.
- *Role-playing*: such as practice reacting to situations in a more positive and healthy manner including responding in an appropriate way to constructive criticism.

A positive and reinforcing approach is best in most situations. Situations where there is a risk of failure are typically avoided until the client has built up a basic faith in his/her abilities. Risk is slowly increased so that the client can continue to have an overall sense of being able to recover from failure and try the activity again.

Despite interventions, temperament and personality functions may not change or fully resolve. Healthcare professionals who are working with clients who have organic changes, such as dementia, that impair temperament and personality functions may need to alter the client's environment, educate caregivers about the cause of the impairment, teach how to best respond to temperament and personality that is not typical of their loved one, and put safety measures in place when appropriate.

### Cross References

In *Recreational Therapy for Specific Diagnoses and Conditions, First Edition*, ICF code b126

Temperament and Personality Functions is listed in 35 chapters: Attention-Deficit/Hyperactivity Disorder, Autism Spectrum Disorder, Back Disorders and Back Pain, Borderline Personality Disorder, Burns, Cancer, Cerebral Palsy, Cerebrovascular Accident, Chronic Obstructive Pulmonary Disease, Epilepsy, Feeding and Eating Disorders, Fibromyalgia and Juvenile Fibromyalgia, Gambling Disorder, Generalized Anxiety Disorder, Guillain-Barré Syndrome, Hearing Loss, Heart Disease, Intellectual Disability, Major Depressive Disorder, Multiple Sclerosis, Neurocognitive Disorders, Obesity, Oppositional Defiant Disorder and Conduct Disorder, Osteoarthritis, Osteoporosis, Parkinson's Disease, Post-Traumatic Stress Disorder, Rheumatoid Arthritis, Schizophrenia Spectrum and Other Psychotic Disorders, Sickle Cell Disease, Spina Bifida, Spinal Cord Injury, Substance-Related Disorders, Traumatic Brain Injury, and Visual Impairments and Blindness.

In *Recreational Therapy Basics, Techniques, and Interventions, First Edition*, treatment for ICF code b126 Temperament and Personality Functions is discussed in 30 chapters: Adjustment and Response to Disability, Education and Counseling, Parameters and Precautions, Participation, Psychoneuroimmunology, Stress, Activity Pattern Development, Adaptive Sports, Adventure Therapy, Anger Management, Animal Assisted Therapy, Aquatic Therapy, Assertiveness Training, Bibliotherapy, Cognitive Behavioral Counseling, Disability Rights: Education and Advocacy, Group Psychotherapy Techniques, Leisure-Based Stress Coping, Leisure Education and Counseling, Life Review, Medical Play and Preparation, Mind-Body Interventions, Montessori Method, Physical Activity, Reality Orientation, Reminiscence, Sensory Interventions, Social Skills Training, Therapeutic Thematic Arts Programming, and Values Clarification.

### b130 Energy and Drive Functions

General mental functions of physiological and psychological mechanisms that cause the individual to move towards satisfying specific needs and general goals in a persistent manner.

Inclusions: functions of energy level, motivation, appetite, craving (including craving for substances that can be abused), and impulse control

Exclusions: consciousness functions (b110); temperament and personality functions (b126); sleep functions (b134); psychomotor functions (b147); emotional functions (b152)

- *b1300 Energy Level*
  Mental functions that produce vigor and stamina.

- *b1301 Motivation*
  Mental functions that produce the incentive to act; the conscious or unconscious driving force for action.

- *b1302 Appetite*
  Mental functions that produce a natural longing or desire, especially the natural and recurring desire for food and drink.

- *b1303 Craving*
  Mental functions that produce the urge to consume substances, including substances that can be abused.

- *b1304 Impulse Control*
  Mental functions that regulate and resist sudden intense urges to do something.

- *b1308 Energy and Drive Functions, Other Specified*
- *b1309 Energy and Drive Functions, Unspecified*

These descriptors have to do with a client's mental functions that impact energy level, motivation, appetite, craving, and impulse control. Mental functions that control these issues can be affected by injury (e.g., traumatic brain injury), disease processes (e.g., chronic fatigue syndrome, cancer), and physiological changes in the body that alter chemical and hormonal balance (e.g., depression, prescription medications, illegal substance abuse). A client's behavior can also affect mental functions, such as lack of exercise, sleep, or proper nutrition.

### Energy Level

Low energy should be expected and allowed for when a client has a major illness or disability. Changes in sleep, eating, and exercise patterns are commonly affected by low energy, as well as psychological and physiological changes related to illness. When the immune system is compromised by illness, energy is directed to healing rather than to outside activity.

Therapists carefully evaluate the client's history and behavioral patterns to identify modifiable variables, such as exercise, nutrition, sleep, and coping skills; underlying disorders, such as depression, chronic fatigue syndrome, multiple sclerosis, and reduced energy level from chemotherapy for cancer; and current medications and substances, such as substance abuse or drowsiness as a side effect of a medication, that could be affecting energy levels. Baselines of functioning are determined and goals are established.

Low energy levels are commonly a result of the interaction of many factors. For example, the client experiences fatigue from multiple sclerosis but also does not exercise regularly, adapt adequately for energy-demanding tasks, and get good quality sleep. Therapists should refer to specific diagnoses for more information about the problems contributing to low energy levels.

Energy level can be measured by amount of time (e.g., participated in social activity for 15 minutes prior to fatigue), descriptors of poor, fair, good, and excellent (e.g., exhibited poor motivation for therapy), and type and extent of cueing (e.g., requires moderate verbal encouragement to perform task).

Treatment for energy level issues is usually done in conjunction with the rest of the treatment team. There are times when a client's energy will be low as a result of the illness or treatment. The therapist needs to make sure that other issues discussed in this set of functions, especially a lack of motivation, are not being mistaken for a lack of energy.

The therapist can work on making sure that the client has adequate nutrition, sleep, and time to rest during activities. Activities themselves can be energy enhancing as discussed in the *Vitality Through Leisure* assessment.

### Motivation

"Motivation is a state of being that produces a tendency toward action. The state may be one of deprivation (e.g., hunger), a value system, or a strongly held belief (e.g., religion). In the mediation of learning and perception, biological mechanisms play an important role in motivating behavior. An organism tries to maintain homeostasis or internal balance against any disturbance of equilibrium (e.g., a thirsty animal is motivated to find water and drink). Social motives, such as the need for recognition and achievement, also account for behavioral patterns (e.g., studying to get good grades). But the intensity of motivation to master any task in a particular situation is determined by at least two different factors: the achievement motive (desire to achieve) and the likelihood of success" (Sadock & Sadock, 2003, p 148).

People's motivation for goals and objects vary according to the value that they place on different things. For example, one person may strongly value academics, another may strongly value social status within a peer group, and yet another may value restoring his/her level of independence. Understanding what motivates a client is important when identifying activities and life events to address in therapy. Therapists are aware that clients may have motivations that stay constant for long periods of time, such as a client who desires to finish school and get a job at a major law firm. Therapists are also aware that motivators fluctuate as a person's views, situations, and life experiences change. For example, a person currently attending college full time may highly value graduating with a high grade point average in the hope of landing a good job. However, if she just had a skiing accident and damaged her spinal cord, a high grade point average, although still important to her, may take second place to achieving independence in self-care activities.

One of the most challenging issues for recreational therapists is motivating a client to address issues that the client is not fully ready to embrace. For example, often when a recreational therapist walks into a client's room and proceeds to talk with the client about his/her lifestyle, the response is, "I'm not really interested in that right now. I just want to be able to walk, use the bathroom, and get back home."

Abraham Maslow has created a hierarchy of needs that helps in understanding this situation. The basic idea is that people will be motivated by basic physiological needs such as hunger and thirst until those needs are satisfied. After that they care about safety, love and belonging, self-esteem, and self-actualization. Getting back to normal life takes top priority. The recreational therapist should acknowledge that and work on issues that will help the client reach his/her immediate goals.

Once people have met the needs in the first two levels of Maslow's hierarchy, their motivations become more complex. There are several ways for the therapist to evaluate the client's motivation.

Motivation can be assessed through a client interview with questions such as: What do you value in your life? What is important to you right now? What would you like to accomplish while you're here? If you could do anything you wanted to do, what would it be? Therapists also use observation of the client's verbalizations and behavior, such as the client's concern about being able to care for his children or the client asking when she can play golf again. One of the most common methods is to identify the leisure interests of the client through brainstorming.

The therapist should also consider formal assessments including the *Leisure Interest Measure, Leisure Satisfaction Measure, Leisure Motivation Scale, Leisurescope Plus*, and the *Free Time Boredom* measure. Each of these assessments measures some aspect of what motivates a client to pursue leisure and recreational activities.

Once the therapist determines the motivational level of the client, the therapist verbally reflects to the client an understanding of his/her situation and validates the client's concerns and feelings. This in turn shows the client that the therapist truly understands how s/he is feeling and facilitates the development of the client-therapist relationship.

Therapists may go on to talk about the importance of these activities or the need to further develop or alter activities to positively affect the client's health condition (e.g., "You are really lucky that your stroke was so mild. To decrease your risks of having another stroke, which could be a lot worse, we really need to get some exercise into your schedule.").

When therapists establish goals with their clients, the focus needs to be on what motivates the client. Establishing small incremental goals that are success driven will help keep up the motivation. For example, if a client requires moderate assistance to perform floor to chair transfers and does not believe that he will ever be independent, his motivation for the task is low and his perceived level of success is low. Knowing that the client is motivated by spending time with his children and that one of the activities that the client enjoys doing with his children is fishing on a lake in a small boat, the therapist incorporates the activity into the task of a chair to floor transfer. The therapist validates the client's value of spending time with his children and fishing and sets a one-foot tall block in front of the chair. The client is to transfer onto the block (a smaller task than directly onto the floor) and then from the block onto the floor, all the while visualizing that the goal of the transfer is not just to get down onto the floor but onto a boat dock so that the client can then transfer into the boat. The goal of achieving this skill is turned into a goal that has personal value to the client.

If the client does not feel that his/her values are being addressed, the client may become non-compliant with therapy. A re-evaluation of the client's values is conducted if this is suspected and goals are re-established as appropriate. For example, a client in a rehabilitation hospital may value being able to walk and therefore refuse all therapy except physical therapy. The recreational therapist discusses the RT treatment plan with the client and puts added focus on walking during functional activities both in the home and in the community.

Other factors that can also contribute to or influence non-compliance included behavior issues, disorientation, delusions, depression, fear, and anxiety. A holistic view of the client's motivation will help the therapist during treatment.

### Appetite

A person's appetite can fluctuate depending on various factors:

- Discomfort or pain with eating or digesting food.
- Prescription medications, including those used for chemotherapy.
- Illegal drugs.
- Psychological issues, such as depression, mania, and stress, that suppress or stimulate appetite.
- Personal perception of certain foods, such as "food looks unappetizing."
- Level of physical activity.
- Likes and dislikes of certain foods.
- Availability of foods.
- Influences of perceived consequences of consuming foods, such as those associated with anorexia and bulimia.
- Injury to the area of the brain that controls appetite.
- Learned eating behaviors and patterns.
- Psychiatric diagnosis of anorexia, bulimia, or binge eating.
- Psychiatric diagnoses with an eating disorder that are commonly comorbid, such as intermit-

tent explosive disorder and obsessive-compulsive disorder.

A healthy appetite can be defined by calories consumed and balance of food groups chosen. The number of calories and the balance of different foods will vary depending on the needs and health of the client (e.g., calorie restricted for weight loss, avoidance of certain foods secondary to irritated bowel).

Therapists document the health of a client's appetite by noting the amount of food eaten at a given time (e.g., client ate 50% of breakfast), the type of foods eaten (e.g., client reports having eaten only a piece of celery for the entire day), the number of meals eaten (e.g., client ate two complete meals today), reaction to foods eaten (e.g., client vomited after eating half a turkey sandwich), client's behavior related to food (e.g., client angry at being watched during meals), and general reports of the client about his/her appetite (e.g., client reports having a poor appetite/ravenous appetite).

Treatment involves addressing the underlying conditions that affect appetite, such as detoxification from drugs, medication to control mental illness, nutrition education, increased physical activity level, or counseling to address body image. Referrals to other healthcare practitioners, such as a nutritionist, psychologist, or gastroenterologist, are initiated as needed. Where health is severely compromised, as in anorexia, the treatment team will need to work together on a plan and each member of the team will need to observe the client carefully when in charge of the client's treatment to make sure the plan is being carried out.

### Craving

Craving is defined as the mental functions that produce an urge to consume substances such as tobacco products, illegal drugs, and legal drugs. A craving is more than a mere thought. The craving for a substance can be strong enough that it takes priority over other life activities. Cravings can be mild, as when a client reports a slight craving for a cigarette when wearing a nicotine patch, to severe, as when meeting basic hygiene, nutrition, and sleep needs take a backseat to finding and using heroin.

Craving is assessed through (1) single-item assessment questions (e.g., on a scale of 0 to 10 with 0 being no craving for alcohol and 10 being extreme craving for alcohol, how would you rate your current craving?), (2) observation of craving behaviors (e.g., asking for the item, seeking behaviors), and (3) standardized assessment tools, such as the *Alcohol Craving Questionnaire, Marijuana Craving Questionnaire, Tobacco Craving Questionnaire*, and the *Obsessive-Compulsive Drinking Scale*. See the Alcohol and Drug Abuse Institute Library for more screening and assessment instruments: http://lib.adai.washington.edu/dbtw-wpd/exec/dbtwpub.dll

Cravings can be controlled or minimized with medication. Therapists also help clients to recognize craving triggers, how to reduce their exposure to triggers, and how to cope with triggers when experienced. For example, a client may feel triggered to use a substance when with certain friends or when particular emotions are experienced. For more information about specific interventions, refer to Substance-Related Disorders in the companion book, *Recreational Therapy for Specific Diagnoses and Conditions*.

### Impulse Control

Mental dysfunction related to impulse control is most commonly seen in clients with traumatic brain injury, dependencies and addictions, schizophrenia, kleptomania, mania, delusional disorders, depression, bingeing, and/or anger management problems such as intermittent explosive disorder.

Impulse control problems are believed to be related to neurobiological mechanisms, psychodynamic factors, and psychosocial factors. Biologically, parts of the brain that control a person's ability to not act on an impulse may be impaired, such as in traumatic brain injury. Psychodynamically, a person may act on impulses to avoid emotional pain, as when impulsive action becomes a coping mechanism in kleptomania or bingeing. Impulse control problems may also be related to psychosocial issues, such as in learned behavior from improper role modeling or violence in the home. Whether or not psychodynamic and psychosocial issues truly affect the mental functions of the brain to control impulses is difficult to say, however it cannot be excluded.

Impulse control is commonly measured by the amount of times that an inappropriate impulse is experienced, the amount of times the client is able to resist the impulse, and the intervention used by the therapist and/or client to reduce or extinguish each

impulse. For example, "Client decreased from six to three episodes of impulsive walking away from the treatment session resulting in a 50% reduction. Therapist stated the remaining time of the treatment session to the client when signs of impulsiveness appeared. On two occasions the client self-initiated looking at the clock and self-controlled the impulse to walk away from the treatment session."

Fatigue, over-stimulation, and psychological trauma can lower a person's ability to control impulses (Sadock & Sadock, 2003). Therefore, therapists should seek to minimize these issues whenever possible. Treatment to minimize or extinguish unhealthy impulses may include the use of pharmacology, social support, and behavior modification interventions. If a specific disability or illness is identified, the therapist should refer to that diagnosis for more specific interventions.

### Cross References

In *Recreational Therapy for Specific Diagnoses and Conditions, First Edition*, ICF code b130 Energy and Drive Functions is listed in 32 chapters: Attention-Deficit/Hyperactivity Disorder, Autism Spectrum Disorder, Back Disorders and Back Pain, Borderline Personality Disorder, Burns, Cancer, Cerebrovascular Accident, Chronic Obstructive Pulmonary Disease, Diabetes Mellitus, Epilepsy, Feeding and Eating Disorders, Fibromyalgia and Juvenile Fibromyalgia, Gambling Disorder, Hearing Loss, Heart Disease, Intellectual Disability, Major Depressive Disorder, Multiple Sclerosis, Neurocognitive Disorders, Obesity, Osteoarthritis, Parkinson's Disease, Post-Traumatic Stress Disorder, Pressure Ulcers, Rheumatoid Arthritis, Schizophrenia Spectrum and Other Psychotic Disorders, Sickle Cell Disease, Spina Bifida, Spinal Cord Injury, Substance-Related Disorders, Total Joint Replacement, and Traumatic Brain Injury.

In *Recreational Therapy Basics, Techniques, and Interventions, First Edition*, treatment for ICF code b130 Energy and Drive Functions is discussed in 26 chapters: Adjustment and Response to Disability, Consequences of Inactivity, Education and Counseling, Parameters and Precautions, Participation, Psychoneuroimmunology, Stress, Activity Pattern Development, Adaptive Sports, Adventure Therapy, Anger Management, Animal Assisted Therapy, Aquatic Therapy, Assertiveness Training, Bibliotherapy, Cognitive Behavioral Counseling, Group

Psychotherapy Techniques, Leisure Education and Counseling, Life Review, Mind-Body Interventions, Montessori Method, Reality Orientation, Reminiscence, Social Skills Training, Therapeutic Thematic Arts Programming, and Values Clarification.

### b134 Sleep Functions

General mental functions of periodic, reversible, and selective physical and mental disengagement from one's immediate environment accompanied by characteristic physiological changes.

Inclusions: functions of amount of sleeping, and onset, maintenance, and quality of sleep; functions involving the sleep cycle, such as in insomnia, hypersomnia, and narcolepsy

Exclusions: consciousness functions (b110); energy and drive functions (b130); attention functions (b140); psychomotor functions (b147)

- *b1340 Amount of Sleep*
  Mental functions involved in the time spent in the state of sleep in the diurnal cycle of circadian rhythm.

- *b1341 Onset of Sleep*
  Mental functions that produce the transition between wakefulness and sleep.

- *b1342 Maintenance of Sleep*
  Mental functions that sustain the state of being asleep.

- *b1343 Quality of Sleep*
  Mental functions that produce the natural sleep leading to optimal physical and mental rest and relaxation.

- *b1344 Functions Involving the Sleep Cycle*
  Mental functions that produce rapid eye movement (REM) sleep (associated with dreaming) and non-rapid eye movement sleep (NREM) (characterized by the traditional concept of sleep as a time of decreased physiological and psychological activity).

- *b1348 Sleep Functions, Other Specified*
- *b1349 Sleep Functions, Unspecified*
  The ability to initiate sleep, maintain a healthy amount and quality of sleep, and keep to a healthy sleep-wake rhythm is influenced by many factors including chemical changes in the brain. Behavior can influence chemical changes in the brain. Inade-

quate amounts and quality of sleep can affect energy levels, attention, concentration, and mood. Sleep is also needed to promote healing. When sleeping, the body is able to direct more energy to healing.

Sleep functions are affected by

- Schedules.
  - o Jet lag.
  - o Changes in work schedule, as from a day shift to a night shift.

- Psychological issues and disorders.
  - o Stress and anxiety: can cause difficulty in relaxing enough to sleep.
  - o Night terrors: can be caused by psychological stress, medications, withdrawal from substance use, or posttraumatic stress disorder.
  - o Avoidance behavior: excessive sleeping may be an avoidance behavior.
  - o Depression: insomnia, multiple awakenings, and hypersomnia (excessive sleeping) are common symptoms of depression.
  - o Mania: a decreased amount of time sleeping is a common symptom of mania.
  - o Neurological disorders: including dementia and Parkinson's.

- Environment.
  - o Environmental changes: such as sleeping in a new room, needed nursing care during the night, common noises at bedtime being absent such as the sound of a fan, and room temperature. Although many of these issues are related to things that are outside of the brain, it is important to note that these things can influence the chemicals in the brain that help to regulate sleep.
  - o Noise, as from nurses in the hallway or construction.

- Pregnancy: can cause sleep function problems due to hormonal changes and discomfort.
- Substances.
  - o Stimulants: such as caffeine and cocaine that keep the person awake outside of normal sleep patterns thus impacting a person's circadian rhythm.

o Depressants and muscle relaxants: cause drowsiness and may induce sleep outside of typical sleep patterns.

o Alcohol withdrawal: Insomnia is a common problem associated with alcohol withdrawal. It can last for several weeks or longer. Medication to aid with sleep is to be avoided due to addictive tendencies.

o Withdrawal from psychoactive drugs: resulting in extremely vivid and frightening dreams.

o Smoking: High doses of nicotine can interfere with sleep onset. Nicotine withdrawal can cause either drowsiness or arousal.

• Urinary incontinence or urgency during the night.

Therapists may document:

• *Ability to fall asleep*: e.g., client fell asleep in 10 minutes after relaxation exercises (b1341.1).

• *Number of sleep hours*: e.g., client had six hours out of the recommended eight hours of continuous sleep (75% of hours obtained, 25% of hours not obtained — b1342.2).

• *Clock time slept*: e.g., 10:00 PM to 6:00 AM.

• *Number of times woken during the night*: e.g., client reports waking up at 1:00 AM and 3:00 AM during the night with night terrors, which resulted in only obtaining half of recommended sleep hours (b1342.3).

• *Techniques used to assist with healthy sleep*: e.g., as per client report, client independently initiated relaxation-training exercise of progressive muscle relaxation at 10:00 PM and was able to fall asleep by 10:30 PM (b1341.1).

Recreational therapists identify variables that affect a client's sleep and aim to reduce or eliminate the problems. This may include helping the client develop a consistent routine. This is a very common problem for people who are adjusting to life changes. For example, prior to injury the client woke up at 7:00 AM and went to bed at 10:00 PM to be able to work during the day. After a disability or life changing event where the normal events of the day are disrupted, sleep is often affected. For example, the client doesn't have to wake up at 7:00 AM to go to work so she sleeps in to 10:00 AM and stays up to 2:00 AM. Maintaining sleep cycles in a healthcare setting is very important for infants and toddlers to promote healthy development. Therefore therapists should coordinate therapy sessions to allow appropriate breaks for rest and sleep periods.

Therapists can alter the environment to help the client fall asleep and maintain sleep. Possibilities include turning on a fan if that is what the client is used to listening to at bedtime, playing soft music, darkening the room, shutting the door to minimize noise, and having an appropriate number of covers and pillows available. Therapists can recommend that clients who have difficulty falling asleep avoid caffeinated drinks and foods, alcohol, and tobacco for at least six hours before bedtime. Stress management and relaxation training may be helpful.

Other recommendations that can help sleep functions include management of underlying causes of sleep impairments, such as antidepressant medication for major depressive disorder, keeping a consistent sleep-wake schedule every day, only lying in bed when it is time to sleep, avoiding daytime naps, exercising regularly in the morning, avoiding stimulation or strenuous exercise close to bedtime, engaging in relaxing activities prior to bedtime, a long hot shower or bath before bedtime, no nighttime snacking, and making the bedroom a quiet and comfortable space to help induce relaxation.

***Cross References***

In *Recreational Therapy for Specific Diagnoses and Conditions, First Edition*, ICF code b134 Sleep Functions is listed in 20 chapters: Attention-Deficit/Hyperactivity Disorder, Back Disorders and Back Pain, Burns, Cancer, Cerebrovascular Accident, Chronic Obstructive Pulmonary Disease, Epilepsy, Fibromyalgia and Juvenile Fibromyalgia, Generalized Anxiety Disorder, Intellectual Disability, Major Depressive Disorder, Multiple Sclerosis, Neurocognitive Disorders, Obesity, Osteoarthritis, Parkinson's Disease, Post-Traumatic Stress Disorder, Rheumatoid Arthritis, Sickle Cell Disease, and Substance-Related Disorders.

In *Recreational Therapy Basics, Techniques, and Interventions, First Edition*, treatment for ICF code b134 Sleep Functions is discussed in eight chapters: Parameters and Precautions, Psychoneuroimmunology, Stress, Adaptive Sports, Aquatic Therapy, Bibliotherapy, Mind-Body Interventions, and Physical Activity.

### b139 Global Mental Functions, Other Specified and Unspecified

Any other Global Mental Function, whether specified or unspecified, not mentioned in the previous categories are scored under this code. Therapists make a notation of the impairment to the right of the scored code.

## Specific Mental Functions (b140 - b189)

### b140 Attention Functions

Specific mental functions of focusing on an external stimulus or internal experience for the required period of time.

Inclusions: functions of sustaining attention, shifting attention, dividing attention, sharing attention; concentration; distractibility

Exclusions: consciousness functions (b110); energy and drive functions (b130); sleep functions (b134); memory functions (b144); psychomotor functions (b147); perceptual functions (b156)

- *b1400 Sustaining Attention*
  Mental functions that produce concentration for the period of time required.

- *b1401 Shifting Attention*
  Mental functions that permit refocusing concentration from one stimulus to another.

- *b1402 Dividing Attention*
  Mental functions that permit focusing on two or more stimuli at the same time.

- *b1403 Sharing Attention*
  Mental functions that permit focusing on the same stimulus by two or more people, such as a child and a caregiver both focusing on a toy.

- *b1408 Attention Functions, Other Specified*
- *b1409 Attention Functions, Unspecified*

The therapist observes all of the attention functions of the client in both a non-distracting and distracting environment. The therapist will need to have a clear view of a clock or be wearing a watch to note the time when attention to the task begins and when it ends to determine a total length of time that the client was able to attend to the task.

For example, give the client a wood project that needs to be sanded. Provide the client with only the piece of wood and one piece of sandpaper. Observe the client's ability to remain focused on the task at hand (sustained attention). Next, give the client the written directions that go with the woodworking project. Observe the client's ability to shift his attention between the directions and the project (shifting attention). Next, have the client perform a physical skill that is part of the client's treatment plan while working on the wood project. For example, have the client stand while working on the wood project and direct him to pay attention to his posture (standing tall, maintaining desired weight bearing on a lower extremity, etc.). Observe the client's ability to pay attention to two things at the same time (dividing attention). Lastly, assist the client with a portion of the wood project, such as assembling the pieces, and observe the client's ability to attend to the project appropriately with the therapist (sharing attention). Some things to watch for in this example include: does the client notice that the therapist has a piece of the project that he is looking for, does the client exhibit behavioral changes when sharing a task, etc.?

The therapist measures the client's response in terms of:

- *Length of time*: e.g., client is able to sustain attention to a task for 30 minutes in a highly distracting environment (b1400.0).
- *Percentage of task*: e.g., client is able to sustain attention to a simple task at 50% — meaning that the client is able to sustain attention to 50% of the task or sustain attention to the task 50% of the time (b1400.3).
- *Type and extent of cueing*: e.g., client requires moderate verbal cues to shift attention from one task to another in a minimally distracting environment (b1401.2).
- *Dysfunction related to task*: e.g., client requires moderate tactile cues for grooming at the bathroom mirror secondary to poor divided attention skills (b1402.2).

There are a variety to issues that affect a client's attention functions including stimulus intensity, novelty, past experience, memory, motivation, expectancy, complexity of task demands, distractions, and fatigue. The therapist should be aware of these issues and try to account for these issues within sessions:

- Choose a treatment time when the client is not fatigued.

- Vary the complexity of the task to observe attention changes. Does the client's ability to focus on a task vary depending on the complexity of the task? For example, a client is asked to sand a piece of wood and he is able to attend to the task for 30 minutes. However, when he is asked to do a task that involves reading, such as reading instructions for the wood project, he is highly distracted and requires moderate verbal cues to attend to the task. The therapist needs to explain the variability in the amount of assistance needed. In this example, reading is a more complex task than sanding a piece of wood. Reading requires the individual to be able to read words, remember the previous sentences to be able to see the whole scope of the material, have good vision, and have adequate attention functions for reading. Therefore, therapists must be aware of the inherent characteristics of each task and discover the specific problem or problems for the client.
- Choose tasks that are attractive to the client.
- Consider the inherent stimulus of the activity. A stimulus that has an action component is inherently easier to attend to. For example, a toy that sings and dances will draw more attention than a piece of wood that sits on the table and does nothing.

The therapist works on increasing a client's attention functions by designing treatment sessions that slightly challenge the client beyond his/her current level. Some recommendations are to:

- Use graduated tasks. The therapist chooses activities that require slightly more skill than the client's current baseline. For example, if the client's baseline for sustained attention is five minutes, then the therapist should choose modalities that inherently require 10 minutes. More than 10 minutes is not advised in this case because the therapist risks frustrating the client by asking for something far beyond the client's ability. It could also cause the client to feel inadequate or angry and possibly affect the client-therapist relationship and the client's motivation to attend and participate in therapy. Tasks should not be simple. They should be possible to accomplish, but progressively more challenging. However, in cases, such as dementia, where functions are being lost, the therapist must progressively reduce the complexity of tasks to the level appropriate for the client.
- Manipulate the environment. The session could start out in a quiet and non-distracting environment and have gradually increasing distractions from the environment.
- Choose activities initially that are familiar and enjoyable to the client and gradually transition to advanced activities of daily living that are not as attractive or familiar to the client yet are realistic parts of the client's activity pattern after discharge.
- Choose simple repetitive activities and increase the complexity by adding activities that require more diverse skills and increased attention functions. For example, sanding a wood project is a simple repetitive physical motion that requires less sustained attention than the task of reading directions about which parts to sand.
- Use treatment sessions of an appropriate length. Treatment sessions may need to be short and multiple rather than one long session, especially if the client's attention span is shorter than five minutes.
- Use a variety of interventions to help the client maintain attention, such as verbal cues, demonstrations, pictorial illustrations, videos, gestural cues, and computer software programs.
- Provide the client with immediate positive feedback. For example, "You are doing a wonderful job. Do you know that you paid attention to the game for 20 minutes without me saying a word! Yesterday you were only able to pay attention for 15 minutes."
- Encourage the client to maintain eye contact during social tasks, such as conversations, to help with paying attention to the task and being able to divide attention.
- Structure or limit information presented to the client. Good verbal commands using adequate volume and inflection can provide an effective means of directing attention. Clearly identify the key task elements and the order the client should do them in.
- Break the task into simple components if the task is complex. As learning progresses, the whole task and its component parts should be practiced.

Providing increased distractions will promote the development of advanced skills.

Some clients with severe attention function deficits perseverate on one action, verbalization, or thought. This means that the client gets stuck on a particular action (e.g., snapping fingers, tapping hand on table), verbalization (e.g., a name, curse word), or a thought (e.g., Client asks, "Where is my mom? She said she would be here." Therapist replies, "She is coming at 3:00 PM." Two minutes after this conversation the client asks the therapist the same question again.). The problem of perseveration is caused by deficits in attention functions and memory functions. Use of activities that are interesting to the client and have a well-defined sequence can help reduce perseveration incidents because they help to keep the client's attention focused. Should a client begin to perseverate, the recreational therapist gently guides the client back to the task.

If the client's attention functions are not fully recovered or do not reflect the appropriate developmental level of the client, the therapist will need to adapt activities to maximize the client's functioning, independence, and safety. Some recommendations include:

- Teach the client's caregivers how to manipulate the client's environment to reduce distractions, provide appropriate cueing to redirect the client back to a task, and use adaptive aids such as a recorder that plays a general verbal cue to encourage attention to a simple repetitive task. For example, a tape recorder that plays, "Nancy, keep eating, you're doing a good job" every three minutes might allow the caregiver time to get dressed in the morning without having to continually cue the client to eat her breakfast.
- Encourage the client to use self-talk in preparation for the task (e.g., "I have to really concentrate on this and read this sentence.") and during the task ("First, I am going to open up the checkbook. Now I am going to find the right page," etc.).
- Encourage caregivers and friends to speak slowly and in short phrases and sentences with pauses to allow time for processing and then have the client paraphrase what s/he just heard. Caregivers need to repeat the information, as needed, until the client understands it.

- Reduce environmental stimuli competing for attention.
- Reduce internal stimuli competing for attention.
- Emphasize information to draw increased attention, such as highlighting words in a document.

Because of the kind of tasks s/he is concerned with, the recreational therapist is in a very good position to help the client with real-world attention functions. The therapist's ability to increase attention skills in the client will help all of the members of the treatment team in their work with the client.

### Cross References

In *Recreational Therapy for Specific Diagnoses and Conditions, First Edition*, ICF code b140 Attention Functions is listed in 16 chapters: Attention-Deficit/Hyperactivity Disorder, Autism Spectrum Disorder, Borderline Personality Disorder, Cerebral Palsy, Chronic Obstructive Pulmonary Disease, Epilepsy, Fibromyalgia and Juvenile Fibromyalgia, Hearing Loss, Intellectual Disability, Major Depressive Disorder, Multiple Sclerosis, Neurocognitive Disorders, Oppositional Defiant Disorder and Conduct Disorder, Spina Bifida, Substance-Related Disorders, and Traumatic Brain Injury.

In *Recreational Therapy Basics, Techniques, and Interventions, First Edition*, treatment for ICF code b140 Attention Functions is discussed in 11 chapters: Activity and Task Analysis, Stress, Adaptive Sports, Adventure Therapy, Aquatic Therapy, Behavior Strategies and Interventions, Bibliotherapy, Montessori Method, Social Skills Training, Therapeutic Thematic Arts Programming, and Walking and Gait Training.

### b144 Memory Functions

Specific mental functions of registering and storing information and retrieving it as needed.

Inclusions: functions of short-term and long-term memory, immediate, recent, and remote memory; memory span; retrieval of memory; remembering; functions used in recalling and learning, such as in nominal, selective, and dissociative amnesia

Exclusions: consciousness functions (b110); orientation functions (b114); intellectual functions (b117); attention functions (b140); perceptual functions (b156); thought functions (b160); higher-level cognitive functions (b164); mental functions of language (b167); calculation functions (b172)

- *b1440 Short-Term Memory*
  Mental functions that produce a temporary, disruptable memory store of around 30 seconds duration from which information is lost if not consolidated into long-term memory.

- *b1441 Long-Term Memory*
  Mental functions that produce a memory system permitting the long-term storage of information from short-term memory and both autobiographical memory for past events and semantic memory for language and facts.

- *b1442 Retrieval of Memory*
  Specific mental functions of recalling information stored in long-term memory and bringing it into awareness.

- *b1448 Memory Functions, Other Specified*
- *b1449 Memory Functions, Unspecified*

In order to commit something to memory, information needs to be encoded so the brain can effectively store the information. Incoming information is encoded in several ways:

- *Acoustic encoding*: remembering something by its sound, such as words or noises.
- *Visual encoding*: remembering something by the way it looks, such as shape, color, and size.
- *Semantic encoding*: remembering something based on a mental representation of an experience, such as translating written information into their meaning (Bernstein et al., 2007).

Once information has been encoded, it goes into short-term memory. The short-term memory is able to hold about seven items for 20-30 seconds (Hockenbury & Hockenbury, 2008). Information is only transferred into the long-term memory when it is rehearsed and utilized. Information that is pulled from the long-term memory is called memory retrieval.

In addition to the categories of short-term and long-term memory, there are different types of memory including:

- *Episodic memory*: memory of a specific event.
- *Semantic memory*: generalized knowledge that doesn't revolve around a particular event.

- *Procedural memory*: how to do things.
- *Sensory memory*: information about the environment (Bernstein et al., 2007; Hockenbury & Hockenbury, 2008).

The therapist challenges the client's memory functions and assesses the client's response. There are many ways to test memory functions. Some examples include:

- *To test short-term memory functions*: Ask the client to immediately recall a list (utilizes acoustic encoding) or a group of objects (utilizes visual encoding). Teach the client a new auditory or visual task (e.g., a short song on the piano, how to put together a mosaic puzzle) and have the client repeat back, verbally or via performance, how to do the task (utilizes procedural encoding). The therapist might find that the client has stronger short-term memory skills based on the type of encoding. For example, some clients might have a better memory for auditory information than for visual information.
- *To test long-term memory*: Ask the client to recall personal history, such as vacations, birth of children, activities one did at school last year. Therapists will need to verify the accuracy of the information provided.
- *To test retrieval of memory*: Teach the client a new task and ask the client to perform the new task at a later date. Note that the tests of long-term memory (above) also test the retrieval functions. It is nearly impossible to test long-term memory without using the retrieval process.

Memory can be measured by:

- *Scales:* e.g., poor, fair, good, excellent.
- *Percentage of memory function:* e.g., client's immediate recall is 60% of material presented (b1440.2).
- *Ratio:* e.g., client is able to recall 4:6 (four out of six) items after five minutes (b1442.2).
- *Type and extent of cueing:* e.g., client requires moderate verbal cues to recall family members (b1441.2).
- *Dysfunction related to task:* e.g., client requires minimal verbal cues to gather needed items at the grocery store secondary to memory function impairment (b1442.1).

The recreational therapist enhances memory functions predominantly through repetition, graduated tasks, and cueing. Attention skills are required in order to focus on information. Consequently therapists typically address attention and memory simultaneously (O'Sullivan & Schmitz, 2007). Therapists begin by working on encoding skills to help the client move the information to memory. Such techniques might include rehearsal, such as using the same steps to do a task every time the task is done, and repetition with the use of vanishing cues. Other techniques to facilitate memory skills and compensate for poor memory skills include:

- *Chunking or grouping*: Provide a way of organizing information to be recalled. It doesn't have to be written. For example, the client might remember that she needs to buy purple flowers at the store by repeating to herself that the top of the letter P in purple is round, just like a flower, and also like the container that she wants to plant them in. Therefore, she is using the shape of a circle to help her remember what she needs to buy at the store. Items and information can be grouped by color, size, shape, function, origins, etc.

- *Mental retracing*: This is mentally going through past actions to trigger a memory. For example, I can't find my keys. I thought they were on the table. Let me think. When I came home, I took the mail out of the mailbox and then opened the door. I walked inside and put the mail down on the hutch. Oh, I put the keys down with the mail on the hutch.

- *Visual imagery*: Client closes his/her eyes and pictures in the mind's eye the information, the task, or the action. For example, the client pictures herself in the locker room at the YWCA and walks through the process of re-dressing to help her to remember all of the items she needs to take with her — hairdryer, towel, change of clothes, lock for the locker, soap, etc.

- *Story method*: The client forms a story about the words or phrases s/he is to remember. For example, if a client has to remember to call his friend Dave, buy dog food, and call the water department, he might remember it by making up the story: Dave ate the dog food and then needed a drink of water.

- *Association*: Two new pieces of information can be associated or new information can be associated with old information. Associations can be gained from all sensory modalities. An emotional association can also assist in recall. For example, remembering a name can be easier if the client thinks about all of the other people she knows with the same name and associates the new person with the other people.

- *Pegging*: Develop a word from the first letters of things that need to be recalled (e.g., DEEP: D: deep breathing, E: eat right, E: exercise, P: play).

If the client's memory functions are not adequate, external aids may be developed and used to enhance functioning and safety, such as paper or electronic organizers, schedules, logs, lists, pictures, directions, watches, and alarms. Clients might also use a voice recorder, sticky notes, or labels.

### Cross References

In *Recreational Therapy for Specific Diagnoses and Conditions, First Edition*, ICF code b144 Memory Functions is listed in 13 chapters: Attention-Deficit/Hyperactivity Disorder, Cerebral Palsy, Epilepsy, Fibromyalgia and Juvenile Fibromyalgia, Intellectual Disability, Major Depressive Disorder, Multiple Sclerosis, Neurocognitive Disorders, Post-Traumatic Stress Disorder, Pressure Ulcers, Spina Bifida, Substance-Related Disorders, and Traumatic Brain Injury.

In *Recreational Therapy Basics, Techniques, and Interventions, First Edition*, treatment for ICF code b144 Memory Functions is discussed in six chapters: Stress, Animal Assisted Therapy, Errorless Learning, Montessori Method, Reality Orientation, and Therapeutic Thematic Arts Programming.

### b147 Psychomotor Functions

Specific mental functions of control over both motor and psychological events at the body level.

Inclusions: functions of psychomotor control, such as psychomotor retardation, excitement and agitation, posturing, catatonia, negativism, ambitendency, echopraxia and echolalia; quality of psychomotor function

Exclusions: consciousness functions (b110); orientation functions (b114); intellectual functions (b117);

energy and drive functions (b130); attention functions (b140); mental functions of language (b167); mental functions of sequencing complex movements (b176)

- *b1470 Psychomotor Control*
  Mental functions that regulate the speed of behavior or response time that involves both motor and psychological components, such as in disruption of control producing psychomotor retardation (moving and speaking slowly, decrease in gesturing and spontaneity) or psychomotor excitement (excessive behavioral and cognitive activity, usually nonproductive and often in response to inner tension as in toe-tapping, hand-wringing, agitation, or restlessness).

- *b1471 Quality of Psychomotor Functions*
  Mental functions that produce nonverbal behavior in the proper sequence and character of its subcomponents, such as hand and eye coordination, or gait.

- *b1478 Psychomotor Functions, Other Specified*
- *b1479 Psychomotor Functions, Unspecified*
  Recreational therapists should also score concerns in these areas with the related codes in Activities and Participation. Possibilities include d4 Mobility and d7 Interpersonal Interactions and Relationships. Recreational therapy treatment for b147 Psychomotor Functions codes will most often be done using the effects of those deficits as noted in Activities and Participation codes.

*Cross References*

In *Recreational Therapy for Specific Diagnoses and Conditions, First Edition*, ICF code b147 Psychomotor Functions is listed in nine chapters: Attention-Deficit/Hyperactivity Disorder, Cerebral Palsy, Epilepsy, Fibromyalgia and Juvenile Fibromyalgia, Major Depressive Disorder, Multiple Sclerosis, Neurocognitive Disorders, Spina Bifida, and Traumatic Brain Injury.

In *Recreational Therapy Basics, Techniques, and Interventions, First Edition*, treatment for ICF code b147 Psychomotor Functions is discussed in six chapters: Stress, Adventure Therapy, Neuro-Developmental Treatment, Physical Activity, Sensory Interventions, and Therapeutic Thematic Arts Programming.

## b152 Emotional Functions

Specific mental functions related to the feeling and affective components of the processes of the mind.

Inclusions: functions of appropriateness of emotion, regulation and range of emotion; affect; sadness, happiness, love, fear, anger, hate, tension, anxiety, joy, sorrow; lability of emotion; flattening of affect

Exclusions: temperament and personality functions (b126); energy and drive functions (b130)

- *b1520 Appropriateness of Emotion*
  Mental functions that produce congruence of feeling or affect with the situation, such as happiness at receiving good news.

- *b1521 Regulation of Emotion*
  Mental functions that control the experience and display of affect.

- *b1522 Range of Emotion*
  Mental functions that produce the spectrum of experience of arousal of affect or feelings such as love, hate, anxiousness, sorrow, joy, fear, and anger.

- *b1528 Emotional Functions, Other Specified*
- *b1529 Emotional Functions, Unspecified*
  The appropriateness, regulation, and range of emotion can be affected by changes in the brain (e.g., traumatic brain injury, stroke), life experiences (e.g., taught in childhood not to show emotion), culture (e.g., Italians often have a colorful and dramatic show of emotions), psychological trauma (e.g., abused child has a restricted range of emotions), psychological illness (e.g., major depressive disorder, bipolar disorder), and the current social situation (e.g., being in a social situation that requires the individual not to engage in conflicts).

  If emotional deficits are suspected, the recreational therapist can further assess the client by observing emotional functions in various contexts, such as therapy groups or when interacting with specific people. Depending on the underlying cause of the emotional dysfunction, behaviors may differ from context to context, and the level of insight the client has into the dysfunction might also vary.

  When evaluating b1520 Appropriateness of Emotion the therapist looks for congruence among the client's verbalizations, behavioral actions, and the current situation. When evaluating b1521 Regulation of Emotion the therapist looks for any difficulties the client might have in controlling emotions. For example, a client may scream loudly when communicating in a quiet room with the therapist, while another client may be unable to control constant variability in emotional expression. When evaluating b1522 Range of Emotion the therapist looks for the client's ability to show a complete spectrum of emotions. Depending on the context of the observation, evaluating a range of emotion might be difficult in a single observation.

Emotional functions are commonly measured by:

- *Description of incongruence*: e.g., client's emotional expression is not congruent with verbalizations (b1520.4). Client's words express sadness, yet affect is upbeat and cheerful.
- *Percentage*: e.g., client is able to regulate emotional responses within treatment sessions 75% of the time b1521.2)
- *Type and extent of cueing*: e.g., with minimal verbal distraction from the current situation, the client is able to halt emotional lability events (b1521.1).
- *Dysfunction related to task*: e.g., client requires moderate verbal cues to express emotion of anger within a conflict (b1522.2).

A therapist can utilize a variety of approaches to help a client enhance emotional functioning including:

- *Drama*: Client portrays a character that expresses the emotional goals of the client. For example, a client who lacks the ability to show sadness portrays a client who is sad about the loss of her sister. Psychodrama is a type of drama therapy that enables the client to act out a specific interaction that holds psychological meaning. It allows the client the opportunity to try out new behaviors in a safe therapeutic environment. For example, the therapist portrays the abusive parent and the client portrays himself in the context of a typical interaction that the client has with the parent. Roles are often reversed so the therapist plays the client and client portrays the parent. Giving a client a safe environment to explore and express emotions that had negative consequences can be helpful to increase the client's emotional range.

- *Social skills training*: Social skills training is covered in Recreational Therapy Basics, Techniques, and Interventions.
- *Other creative arts*: Like drama, creative arts such as music, dance, writing, clay, painting, and crafts provide an alternative form of emotional expression, thus providing the client with the psychological benefits of such expression. It may also help client to express the emotion since it can be, for example, easier to write about anger than to talk about it. Refer to the Bibliotherapy and Therapeutic Thematic Arts chapters in *Recreational Therapy Basics, Techniques, and Interventions* for more techniques and interventions. Also see Nathan and Mirviss (1998) *Therapy Techniques Using the Creative Arts*.
- *Direct feedback*: Providing the client with direct and immediate feedback about his/her emotional expression may increase the client's awareness of the behavior, thus allowing the client to incorporate techniques to change his/her emotional response. For example, if a client is screaming a conversation in a quiet room with the therapist, the therapist should say to the client, "Do you realize that you are screaming loudly?" Once the client becomes aware of the behavior in a therapy setting, the therapist can teach him how to become aware of the behavior in other settings and how to modify the behavior to express emotions more appropriately and effectively. Repetitive use of a technique in functional tasks can help in learning the strategies.

Therapists need to be aware, though, that the above approaches are not appropriate for all clients. There may be other issues that need to be resolved before the client is ready to allow himself/herself to have a full range of emotions. There may also be physical causes, such as brain injury, that need time to heal before the client can be expected to display a normal range of emotions. Clients who continue to have a flat affect, who are emotionally labile, who are unable to regulate their emotions, or who have a limited range of emotions despite interventions may benefit from the following adaptations.

- *Pharmacology*: Certain medications can be helpful in controlling mood, thus increasing the client's appropriateness, regulation, or range of emotions.

- *Distraction*: Distracting the client for a moment from the conversation or task at hand can be very helpful to halt an emotional lability event. For example, if the client is crying during a game of checkers and you know that the client is emotionally labile, asking the client "What time is it?" may disrupt the event and halt the behavior.

- *Direct feedback*: Teach caregivers how to provide feedback to the client to facilitate awareness of emotional expressions. Some clients may respond negatively to direct feedback and therefore it may be contraindicated. If this is the case, behavior modification techniques may be helpful. Refer to the Behavior Strategies and Interventions chapter in the *Recreational Therapy Basics, Techniques, and Interventions* book for more techniques and interventions.

### Cross References

In *Recreational Therapy for Specific Diagnoses and Conditions, First Edition*, ICF code b152 Emotional Functions is listed in 27 chapters: Attention-Deficit/Hyperactivity Disorder, Autism Spectrum Disorder, Back Disorders and Back Pain, Borderline Personality Disorder, Burns, Cancer, Cerebral Palsy, Cerebrovascular Accident, Feeding and Eating Disorders, Fibromyalgia and Juvenile Fibromyalgia, Generalized Anxiety Disorder, Guillain-Barré Syndrome, Hearing Loss, Heart Disease, Major Depressive Disorder, Multiple Sclerosis, Neurocognitive Disorders, Obesity, Oppositional Defiant Disorder and Conduct Disorder, Osteoarthritis, Osteoporosis, Post-Traumatic Stress Disorder, Schizophrenia Spectrum and Other Psychotic Disorders, Spina Bifida, Spinal Cord Injury, Total Joint Replacement, and Traumatic Brain Injury.

In *Recreational Therapy Basics, Techniques, and Interventions, First Edition*, treatment for ICF code b152 Emotional Functions is discussed in 22 chapters: Adjustment and Response to Disability, Parameters and Precautions, Participation, Psychoneuroimmunology, Stress, Adaptive Sports, Adventure Therapy, Anger Management, Aquatic Therapy, Assertiveness Training, Behavior Strategies and Interventions, Bibliotherapy, Cognitive Behavioral Counseling, Leisure Education and Counseling, Life Review, Medical Play and Preparation, Mind-Body Interventions, Montessori Method, Reality Orientation, Reminiscence, Social Skills Training, and Therapeutic Thematic Arts Programming.

### b156 Perceptual Functions

Specific mental functions of recognizing and interpreting sensory stimuli.

Inclusions: functions of auditory, visual, olfactory, gustatory, tactile, and visuospatial perception, such as hallucination or illusion

Exclusions: consciousness functions (b110); orientation functions (b114); attention functions (b140); memory functions (b144); mental functions of language (b167); seeing and related functions (b210 - b229); hearing and vestibular functions (b230 - b249); additional sensory functions (b250 - b279)

- *b1560 Auditory Perception*
  Mental functions involved in discriminating sounds, tones, pitches, and other acoustic stimuli.

- *b1561 Visual Perception*
  Mental functions involved in discriminating shape, size, color, and other ocular stimuli.

- *b1562 Olfactory Perception*
  Mental functions involved in distinguishing differences in smells.

- *b1563 Gustatory Perception*
  Mental functions involved in distinguishing differences in tastes, such as sweet, sour, salty, and bitter stimuli, detected by the tongue.

- *b1564 Tactile Perception*
  Mental functions involved in distinguishing differences in texture, such as rough or smooth stimuli, detected by touch.

- *b1565 Visuospatial Perception*
  Mental function involved in distinguishing by sight the relative position of objects in the environment or in relation to oneself.

- *b1568 Perceptual Functions, Other Specified*
- *b1569 Perceptual Functions, Unspecified*
  Perception is "the ability to select those stimuli that require attention and action, to integrate those stimuli with each other and with prior information, and finally to interpret them. The resulting awareness of objects and experiences within the environment enables the individual to make sense out of a complex and constantly changing internal and external sensory environment" (O'Sullivan & Schmitz, 2007, p. 1150).

The categories in this section do not address whether the client has the ability to receive sensory input. Those issues are dealt with in Body Functions b2 Sensory Functions and Pain. The functions described in this chapter deal with the ability to process sensory stimuli once they have reached the brain.

When assessing a client's function in a task, careful attention should be given to sensory and perceptual problems. If sensory or perceptual problems are suspected, further evaluation will be needed. It can be very difficult to separate perceptual problems from other problems. For example, if the therapist asks a client to pick up a pencil from the table and the client does not respond, the problem could lie in the area of language processing (maybe the client has receptive aphasia — words spoken sound like gibberish), visual object agnosia (unable to identify common objects), visual neglect (pencil is on the left side of the table and the client has left neglect), severe attention problems (unable to follow one-step directions), etc. To do the assessment well the therapist must have:

- A full knowledge of the deficits associated with specific disabilities. For example, a client with a right stroke is prone to having left neglect.
- The ability to rule out other possible deficits. For example, place the pencil on right side of the table, show the client a picture of a pencil and then put the palms of your hands in the air to express the question of "Where is it?", move the client into a quiet and then a highly distracting environment to find out if distractions play a role in being able to attend to the verbal command of picking up the pencil, etc.
- Good observational skills
- The ability to manipulate environmental factors
- Understanding of the findings of other health professionals.

Once the therapist knows that sensory function itself is intact and can make the instructions clear to the client, presenting examples of stimuli in any of the sensory modes in this chapter is relatively straightforward. It is mostly a matter of having an appropriate set of examples. See b110 Consciousness Functions for examples of how to stimulate each of the senses to determine if there are any difficulties with sensory perception. A variety of

specific testing tools for perceptual problems are clearly reviewed in Zoltan's book *Vision, Perception, and Cognition* (2007).

Recreational therapists document the deficits in the following ways:

- *Percentage of behavior*: e.g., client has visual object agnosia, however client is able to identify common objects through tactile perception at 25%. In other words, when the client is presented with visual objects, the client is able to identity 25% of the objects presented using tactile perception. To score this observation using the ICF requires determining the client's ability to recognize shape, size, color, and other ocular stimuli. This code does not score the ability to find the name of an object. For this code the therapist needs to look at the aspects of the object rather than its identity.
- *Dysfunction related to task*: e.g., client requires moderate assistance when going up and down stairs due to problems with depth perception (b1565.2). Client requires supervision when traveling to and from school due to inability to successfully compensate for color agnosia (1561.3).
- *Descriptors*: Poor, fair, good, excellent, e.g., client exhibits poor figure-ground perception (1565.3).
- *Type and extent of cueing*: e.g., client requires gestural cueing 20% of the time to recognize that a ringing telephone signals a phone call, possibly 1560.2, but the therapist needs to rule out other possible impairments in hearing the ring and understanding the purpose of the phone.

Treatment for deficits in perceptual functions consists of trying to increase the client's ability to recognize and correctly interpret sensory stimuli and finding adaptations for functionality that is not currently present.

Increasing abilities is most often done through repeated practice. Techniques for focusing attention are appropriate for all of these deficits because part of the problem is that the brain has lost the ability to focus a particular type of attention. Here are some ideas for the specific modalities discussed in the ICF:

- *Auditory perception*: Practice identifying sounds that are important to the client's lifestyle, such as a smoke detector, telephone, doorbell, or teakettle whistle. If the deficit includes problems with understanding speech, the recreational therapist should work on matching spoken words with objects or pictures to help rebuild an aural vocabulary.

- *Visual perception*: There are several common visual deficits. If the problem is recognizing objects by sight, hand the client objects repetitively in treatment sessions and say the name of the object. Ask the client to repeat the name of the object. Label each object with its name. Have the client try to pick out the object from a variety of objects on a table. See the discussion on form discrimination, below, for more ideas. If the problem is identifying faces, practice matching names with faces that are familiar to the client. If the problem is identifying colors, which is important in the community for actions like crossing streets, practice naming and identifying colors.
- *Olfactory perception*: Practice with odors that are important for the client. Oil-based olfactory stimuli are usually better than alcohol-based.
- *Gustatory perception*: Practice tastes. Start with simple tastes (salty, sweet) and move on to food tastes (apples, hamburgers).
- *Tactile perception*: Practice identifying shapes and textures without using vision. As always, start with simple forms and textures (wooden blocks, warm water) before moving to more subtle objects.
- *Visuospatial perception*: To improve perception of the relationship between objects in the whole visual field, practice combining parts of the task into a whole through multimodal cues.

If the deficits are interfering with advanced activities of daily living or creating a safety issue, the therapist should make adaptations that will help the client deal with the deficit. One of the most important adaptations to consider is the use of a companion animal. Companion animals are usually thought of as appropriate for sensory deficits, but they can help the client with perceptual function deficits as well. Examples of other adaptations include:

- *Auditory perception*: Change sounds to a visual cue, such as a flashing light on a telephone. For speech issues, teach the client how to cue others that they need to speak more slowly and allow more time for the client to process the conversation.
- *Visual perception*: If the problem is recognizing objects by sight, put labels on items that will be used for functional tasks so the client can recognize the object by its name. If the problem is identifying faces, provide names on pictures and teach acquaintances to say their name when greeting the client. If the problem is identifying colors, recommend that assistance be provided, especially if the client is unable to judge the color of the traffic light by evaluating traffic patterns or the location of the lights relative to one another.
- *Olfactory perception*: Make sure the client has support so that he does not come to harm by not being able to smell. Two examples are being sure not to eat spoiled foods by mistake and being aware of smoke alarms since the client can't smell smoke.
- *Gustatory perception*: As with olfactory perception, make sure that spoiled foods aren't eaten.
- *Tactile perception*: Use vision as a compensatory strategy. Teach the client to use vision to tell the shape and texture of items. If heat and cold are an issue, make sure the client is protected from dangerous situations, such as scalding water and hot stoves.
- *Visuospatial perception*: Simplify tasks that a client regularly performs into singular components. Reduce the number of objects the client needs to deal with at one time.

### *Visuospatial Perception*

Visuospatial perception deficits require special consideration from recreational therapists because they can cause significant problems when participating in community activities. For that reason recreational therapists need a better understanding of the whole scope of the deficit. There are several types of spatial relation disorders including figure-ground discrimination, form discrimination, spatial relations, position in space, topographic disorientation, depth and distance perception and vertical disorientation (O'Sullivan & Schmitz, 2007; Zoltan, 2007). The following information looks at each of these deficits.

### **Figure-Ground Discrimination**

Problems with figure-ground discrimination cause an inability to distinguish the foreground from the background. Items in the environment appear to blend together and it is difficult for the client to separate different objects. Practice with attention is one of the best ways to help the client reduce this deficit. Place several objects into a box so that the objects overlap each other. Ask the client to identify what s/he sees. Gradually increase the number of items in the box.

Adaptations include keeping the environment neat and organized so that items are clearly differentiated from one another. Use high contrast backgrounds whenever possible. For example, if a client wants to paint on a white piece of paper, place a dark colored tablecloth on the table so that the client is able to clearly see the edges of the paper. In addition, paint the handles of the paintbrushes white so that they too stand out on the dark tablecloth. Use a white mug to hold the water, etc.

### Form Discrimination

Form discrimination is an inability to attend to variations in form (e.g., mistaking a water pitcher for a urinal). Some additional ideas for addressing the deficit include: practice sorting objects, encourage the use of tactile perception to distinguish items. In addition to using labels on objects, you can also use these additional ideas for making form discrimination easier. Keep items in the same place as much as possible. The more organized things are, the more familiar the client will become with the items. Shapes are best recognized when they are in upright positions, so try to put commonly used items in this position, such as hanging toothbrushes on the wall and using "stand up" toothpaste containers.

### Spatial Relations

Spatial relations is the ability to relate objects to one another. When there is a deficit, objects are seen as separate entities without relation to other objects in the environment. For example, when looking at a standard wall clock, the client recognizes the hands on the clock and the numbers on the clock, but is unable to put the two together to tell the time. Therapists should encourage and practice relational tasks, such as putting together pieces to make a puzzle.

### Position in Space

Position in space impairment is when the client has difficulty with spatial concepts such as up, down, under, over, in, out, in front of, and behind. This impairment can greatly hinder activity participation where positional directions are required, such as hide under the blanket or get the bucket from under the table. To enhance this skill, the therapist can have the client practice placing items into positions and retrieving items from various positions. The therapist could also take several objects and have the client identify the objects by position. For example, when cleaning up from a craft activity, place all of the paintbrushes in the art box and leave one paintbrush behind the art box. Ask the client to identify which brush is in a different position compared to the others and to describe its position and the position of other brushes. Then have the client place the odd item in the art box. Encourage verbalization and description of locations.

### Topographic Disorientation

Topographic disorientation is when the client has difficulty understanding and remembering the relationship of one location to another. This leads to difficulty in getting from one place to another, even if a map is present. The client might not be able to find his/her room, specific places in the building, or places in his/her neighborhood despite being familiar with the area or being shown repeatedly. When asked, the client is unable to describe the environmental characteristics of the route or place, such as the cafeteria walls or a landmark at a corner. Practice going from one place to another. Begin with simple routes and progress to more complex routes. Have the client describe the environment and directions along the route, such as turn left at the nursing desk, look at the room numbers, find number 304A. If a client continues to have difficulty with this, compensatory strategies can be employed, such as indoor signage. Safety issues should also be addressed, including providing supervision to prevent the client from getting lost.

### Depth and Distance Perception

Depth and distance perception is the ability to perceive the third dimension of depth. This is necessary for actions such as climbing stairs, driving, and grasping objects. To provide therapy for the deficit, have the client use tactile perception to identify distances between or among items. For example, if a client is going to make a craft project, line up the supplies perpendicular to the client. Have the client feel each craft supply in its place in line. Play games that require depth perception, including any game that has objects that approach the client. Adaptations include encouraging the client to rely on tactile perception to identify distances. Environmental adaptations to promote safety may also be helpful.

**Vertical Disorientation**

Vertical disorientation is when the client is unable to determine the vertical orientation of an object. For example, the doorway may not look straight up and down to the client. It may look like it is slanted to the right so the client adjusts his/her posture to the perceived orientation of the doorway and leans to the right. The client might also have difficulty knowing if his/her body is in a vertical orientation. The therapists provides feedback to the client about his/her orientation, encourages the client to seek feedback from the environment to better understand the vertical orientation of the environment, and to adjust his/her posture accordingly. When working on seated or standing activities, the therapist might also use a long mirror to provide additional feedback about posture.

*Cross References*

In *Recreational Therapy for Specific Diagnoses and Conditions, First Edition*, ICF code b156 Perceptual Functions is listed in 13 chapters: Attention-Deficit/Hyperactivity Disorder, Autism Spectrum Disorder, Chronic Obstructive Pulmonary Disease, Fibromyalgia and Juvenile Fibromyalgia, Guillain-Barré Syndrome, Hearing Loss, Intellectual Disability, Multiple Sclerosis, Neurocognitive Disorders, Schizophrenia Spectrum and Other Psychotic Disorders, Spina Bifida, Substance-Related Disorders, and Traumatic Brain Injury.

In *Recreational Therapy Basics, Techniques, and Interventions, First Edition*, treatment for ICF code b156 Perceptual Functions is discussed in five chapters: Activity and Task Analysis, Stress, Balance Training, Sensory Interventions, and Social Skills Training.

### *b160 Thought Functions*

Specific mental functions related to the ideational component of the mind.

Inclusions: functions of pace, form, control, and content of thought; goal-directed thought functions; non-goal directed thought functions; logical thought functions, such as pressure of thought, flight of ideas, thought block, incoherence of thought, tangentiality, circumstantiality, delusions, obsessions, and compulsions

Exclusions: intellectual functions (b117); memory functions (b144); psychomotor functions (b147); perceptual functions (b156); higher-level cognitive functions (b164); mental functions of language (b167); calculation functions (b172)

- *b1600 Pace of Thought*
  Mental functions that govern speed of the thinking process.

- *b1601 Form of Thought*
  Mental functions that organize the thinking process as to its coherence and logic.

  Inclusions: impairments of ideational perseveration, tangentiality, and circumstantiality

- *b1602 Content of Thought*
  Mental functions consisting of the ideas that are present in the thinking process and what is being conceptualized.

  Inclusions: impairments of delusions, overvalued ideas, and somatization

- *b1603 Control of Thought*
  Mental functions that provide volitional control of thinking and are recognized as such by the person.

  Inclusions: impairments of rumination, obsession, thought broadcast, and thought insertion

- *b1608 Thought Functions, Other Specified*
- *b1609 Thought Functions, Unspecified*

Thought function impairments are generally seen in mental health disorders such as schizophrenia, bipolar disorder, delusional disorders, phobias, depression, dementia, and obsessive-compulsive disorder, as well as physical disabilities that impair the brain including dementia, traumatic brain injury, and cerebrovascular accident.

Thought is the process of putting together ideas and associations, while content includes the specific things the person is thinking about. Formal thought disorders identified by Sadock and Sadock (2003) include:

- *Circumstantiality* (trouble getting to the point): When trying to relay an idea, the client lacks the ability to relay the thought in a goal-directed manner. Irrelevant thoughts and ideas are unnecessarily explained. The client eventually comes back to his/her main thought.

- *Clang associations* (rhyming): Thoughts are associated by the sound of words rather than by their meaning, e.g., through rhyming or assonance.
- *Derailment* (synonymous with loose associations): A breakdown in both the logical connection between ideas and the overall sense of goal directedness. The words make sentences, but the sentences don't make sense.
- *Neologism*: The invention of new words or phrases or the use of conventional words in idiosyncratic ways.
- *Perseveration*: Repetition out of context of words, phrases, or ideas.
- *Tangentiality*: The client loses the thread of the conversation and pursues divergent thoughts that are influenced by internal and external stimuli. The client does not return to the original thought. For example, a client begins to talk about wanting a specific food. Before telling the therapist the specific food he wants, he thinks about the nurse who brought the food the last time. He begins to talk about the nurse and does not return to telling the therapist the specific food he wants.
- *Thought blocking*: A sudden disruption of thought or a break in the flow of ideas. The client may say that s/he is unable to remember what s/he wanted to say or is unable to recall what s/he was talking about.

Common measurement descriptors of thought functions include:

- *Pace of thought*: Typically described as being slow, fast, or hesitant. For example, client's hesitant pace of thought impairs his ability to effectively problem solve for simple tasks (b1600.3).
- *Form of thought*: Described by type of formal thought disorders such as those described by Sadock and Sadock. For example, client's form of thought is tangential when describing difficult family relations (b1601.2).
- *Content of thought*: Described by dominant patterns, such as delusions; preoccupations; obsessions; compulsions; phobias; plans, intentions, or recurrent ideas about suicide or homi-

cide; symptoms of hypochondria; and specific antisocial urges (Sadock & Sadock, 2003). For example, client obsessed about washing her hands throughout the 30-minute treatment session (b1602.4).
- *Control of thought*: Described by who or what the person believes is controlling his/her thoughts. For example, client reports that he fights with a demon for control of his thoughts (1603.2).

Scoring b160 Thought Functions using the ICF can be done by identifying the situation as descried above. This means there will be different scores for different situations. When anxiety is high, content of thought impairment might be high. When anxiety is low, content of though impairment might be low. Thought functions can also be affected by the environment. For example, a quiet environment without distractions might exacerbate control of thought impairment, whereas an environment that provides meaningful distractions might lower control of thought impairment. An alternative method of scoring is to combine observations to find an overall frequency of occurrence for the specific thought function. If the client experiences control of thought impairment approximately 60% of the time, the overall score would be b1603.3. Both methods of scoring can provide useful information for determining treatment direction.

In general, pharmacology can be helpful to minimize or extinguish invasive, unhealthy thoughts, such as delusions or obsessions. Cognitive behavioral interventions can help to change distorted thought patterns, such as phobias or negative thought patterns about the self. Other psychological interventions may be helpful depending on the level of dysfunction and orientation of the client. For example, existential counseling for exploration of life meaning may help alleviate feelings of depression thus reducing or eliminating recurrent ideas of suicide.

### Cross References

In *Recreational Therapy for Specific Diagnoses and Conditions, First Edition*, ICF code b160 Thought Functions is listed in 16 chapters: Attention-Deficit/Hyperactivity Disorder, Autism Spectrum Disorder, Back Disorders and Back Pain, Burns, Feeding and Eating Disorders, Fibromyalgia and Juvenile Fibromyalgia, Generalized Anxiety Disorder,

Guillain-Barré Syndrome, Major Depressive Disorder, Multiple Sclerosis, Neurocognitive Disorders, Post-Traumatic Stress Disorder, Schizophrenia Spectrum and Other Psychotic Disorders, Spina Bifida, Substance-Related Disorders, and Traumatic Brain Injury.

In *Recreational Therapy Basics, Techniques, and Interventions, First Edition*, treatment for ICF code b160 Thought Functions is discussed in eight chapters: Activity and Task Analysis, Parameters and Precautions, Stress, Balance Training, Bibliotherapy, Cognitive Behavioral Counseling, Social Skills Training, and Therapeutic Thematic Arts Programming.

### *b164 Higher-Level Cognitive Functions*

Specific mental functions especially dependent on the frontal lobes of the brain, including complex goal-directed behaviors such as decision-making, abstract thinking, planning and carrying out plans, mental flexibility, and deciding which behaviors are appropriate under what circumstance; often called executive functions.

Inclusions: functions of abstraction and organization of ideas; time management, insight, and judgment; concept formation, categorization, and cognitive flexibility

Exclusions: memory functions (b144); thought functions (b160); mental functions of language (b167); calculation functions (b172)

- *b1640 Abstraction*
  Mental functions of creating general ideas, qualities or characteristics out of, and distinct from, concrete realities, specific objects, or actual instances.

- *b1641 Organization and Planning*
  Mental functions of coordinating parts into a whole, of systematizing; the mental function involved in developing a method of proceeding or acting.

- *b1642 Time Management*
  Mental functions of ordering events in chronological sequence, allocating amounts of time to events and activities.

- *b1643 Cognitive Flexibility*
  Mental functions of changing strategies, or shifting mental sets, especially as involved in problem-solving.

- *b1644 Insight*
  Mental functions of awareness and understanding of oneself and one's behavior.

- *b1645 Judgment*
  Mental functions involved in discriminating between and evaluating different options, such as those involved in forming an opinion.

- *b1646 Problem-Solving*
  Mental functions of identifying, analyzing, and integrating incongruent or conflicting information into a solution.

- *b1648 Higher-Level Cognition Functions, Other Specified*
- *b1649 Higher-Level Cognition Functions, Unspecified*

Each of the ICF subheadings is discussed below. Note that these functions are intertwined. Reading through all of them will help the therapist understand their complexity and interrelatedness. In addition, ideas in one section will often be useful in evaluating a skill or teaching a technique in another section.

#### *Abstraction*

To think abstractly is to conceptualize. It is an integration of skills that requires the client to generate ideas, to compare and differentiate, to recognize relationships, and to categorize. It also has components of memory, attention, cognitive flexibility, and problem solving. A client that is able to think abstractly would be able to recognize that a paintbrush and a jar of paint are both painting supplies or that a sarcastic remark from another client was a consequence of the disagreement they had five minutes ago.

Contrasted with thinking abstractly is thinking concretely. The client who is thinking concretely is only able to recognize objects or verbalizations in isolation. He would have no connection to other things or be able to conceptualize a higher level of thinking. For example, a client would see a paintbrush as simply a paintbrush. It would hold no connection to the other art supplies that surrounded him. And, if a sarcastic remark was directed towards him from another client, he would react to the remark as if it held no connection to the disagreement that just occurred.

If a client may be having problems with abstraction, the therapist would assess this ability through:

- Observing the client's verbal responses. Does the client view events in isolation? Is he able to see the consequences of an action or that the event is related to another action? For example, if the client is told that she is not allowed to drive, does she see this limitation as only not being able to operate the car, or does she see the consequent lack of mobility in the community?
- Observing the client's behavioral responses. For example, ask the client to gather gardening supplies from the closet. If the client looks confused, becomes frustrated or agitated with the task, brings out a variety of items from the closet that are unrelated to gardening supplies, or replies to the request by asking for clarification, then the therapist may suspect that the client has problems with abstraction.
- Asking the client specific questions to test his/her ability to compare categories (how are a pear and an apple alike?), differentiate (what is the difference between a hammer and a screwdriver?), generalize specific items to abstract categories (a pear is a ___ [fruit], a spoon is a ____ [utensil]), and identify what does not belong within a category (what does not belong: parakeet, swan, crow, poodle?).

Once deficits in abstraction have been identified, the therapist must determine a baseline of functioning. Abstraction functions can be measured in terms of:

- *Descriptors*: poor, fair, good, excellent.
- *Percentage*: e.g., Client is able to categorize items correctly 50% of the time (b1640.3). Client is able to form logical relationships between two items 75% of the time (b1640.2).
- *Type and extent of cueing*: e.g., Client requires moderate verbal cues to separate items into two categories (b1640.2). Client requires moderate verbal cues to form logical relationships between two items (b1640.2).
- *Dysfunction related to task*: e.g., Client requires minimal verbal cues to place clothing into appropriate drawers secondary to difficulty with categorization of clothing items (b1640.1). Cli-

ent requires close supervision in woodworking area secondary to safety issues resulting from poor formation of logical relationships (b1640.2).

To enhance development or restoration of abstraction skills the therapist can:

- *Use cognitive remediation techniques*: Challenge the client to sort items into categories, compare and differentiate among items, and form logical relationships. Some possibilities include: Have the client organize supplies in the woodworking room. Have the client organize items that have been purposely put into a box for the client to organize. Ask the client to name what does not belong on the table for the task at hand, when the therapist has purposely placed something on the table that is not needed. Ask the client to name what is missing to complete the task at hand, such as having a paintbrush and paper, but no paint.
- *Provide challenges*: Challenge the client to apply abstraction skills in a functional environment. For example, identify a specific store on the mall directory with a directory that is divided into categories. Order a complete meal from a menu where the client has to refer to categories of food items and form relations of food items to one another. Prepare a simple meal in a kitchen where the client is challenged to know categories of supplies — I need a fork, a fork is a utensil, utensils are in the drawer — as well as form relationships of parts to make a whole — to make a scrambled egg I need milk, salt, pepper, etc.

If the client does not develop or recover adequate abstraction skill for functional tasks, the therapist can:

- Make up cheat sheets of all the parts that are needed for tasks. The therapist may also find it helpful to develop audiotapes that describe the task.
- Educate caregivers about the client's problem with the skill of abstraction and describe specifics of how it will affect the client's functional life skills. The list may include having trouble finding things at stores, missing parts necessary for a task because of difficulties forming associations, having trouble linking events together and forming consequences. The therapist should teach the

caregivers how to give the client supervision and cueing.

### Organization and Planning

Organizing and planning are not isolated skills. They require integration of many skills including conceptualizing change, relating objectively to the environment, conceiving alternatives, weighing alternatives and making choices, estimating the difficulty of the task, and creating a framework to carry out the plan. They also require the ability for abstract thought, cognitive flexibility, memory, strategizing, and the basic ability to understand and have awareness (Zoltan, 2007).

Zoltan (2007) gives the therapist a working outline for assessing this function through clinical observation and activity analysis. General guidelines for evaluation:

- Determine whether the client is aware that he has a planning deficit. Defective planning often is revealed by asking the client what he intends to do.
- Observe the client in a number of settings and activities during the day. Can the client plan for activities requiring two-step operations? Three-step? More complex operations?
- Give the client a complex task without instructions. If the client begins the task without a plan, ask him to create one and begin the task again. The client's plan can then be evaluated for organization and completeness.
- Establish functional baseline measures. Consider the duration and frequency of the problem. Select relevant functional tasks as the basis of evaluation and reassessment.

Specific areas and questions to evaluate:

- Is the client logical and consistent in his/her approach to the task?
- How reliable is his/her chosen method?
- Is there a common problem or consistently faulty planning strategy that is generalized to several activities?
- Can the client conceptualize change from the present, as evidenced through verbal or other means of communication?
- Can the client present alternatives and make a choice based on his/her judgments?
- Can s/he weigh alternatives and make a choice based on his/her judgments?

- Does s/he appear to have a framework for the plan or direction s/he is demonstrating for task completion?
- Can s/he accurately estimate task difficulty?

Note that questions and observations such as these can be applied to both functional and cognitive perceptual motor tasks. For example, inability to complete block designs and layout of graphic designs can indicate poor planning and task organization.

These and similar questions can be incorporated into a checklist or used in conjunction with a frequency rating scale. To improve validity, rule out decreased attention, poor memory, decreased mental flexibility and abstraction, impaired problem solving, and aphasia as causes of poor performance.

Once deficits in organization and planning have been identified, the therapist must determine a baseline. Organization and planning can be measured in terms of:

- *Frequency*: e.g., always, sometimes, rarely, never.
- *Percentage*: e.g., client is able to complete 50% of a three-step organization and planning task (b1641.3).
- *Level of assistance*: e.g., client requires minimal assistance for planning and organizing simple tasks (b1641.1).
- *Dysfunction related to task*: e.g., client requires moderate assistance to develop next semester's college course schedule secondary to difficulty with organizing information (b1641.2).

To enhance planning and organizing functions the therapist can:

- Start with simple planning tasks that require only two or three steps and gradually progress to more complex tasks using graduated tasks.
- Ask the client to verbalize the sequential steps of a task before it is performed.
- Pose questions to the client to help him/her develop organizational and planning skills. Possible questions include: What do we need next? How are we going to do that? What should we do if X happens? What are we trying to accomplish?
- Repeat organizational and planning skills to improve processes.
- Teach the client organizational and planning skills by helping the client to identify and break

down main categories. For example: To plan a two-day trip to the shore, we have to find out when the shore house is available, make reservations, pack, and then drive there. Let's look at each one separately. The first one is to find out when the shore house is available, so let's make a list of what we have to do to find this out. What do you think we should write down? Find the realtor's phone number, call the realtor, and ask for availability of two consecutive days in June.

If the client does not fully develop or recover adequate organization and planning functions for functional tasks, the therapist can:

- Educate the client's caregivers about the client's deficits in this area and the type and amount of assistance needed.
- Identify specific compensatory strategies to maximize the client's independence and functioning. This may include the use of lists, day planners, calendars, and specific task worksheets. For example, if the client has to travel often, the therapist may help the client develop a checklist of tasks before each trip including a packing list. Students should be encouraged to use day planners and to make notations to help with planning and organizing class requirements. For example, the student should not only mark down when a paper is due, but should also make notations of when to begin research for the paper, when to begin typing the paper, etc.

### Time Management

Many of the ideas described in organization and planning also apply to time management. The three basic requirements for time management are to understand how long a task is going to take, to create a schedule that has enough time for each of the tasks the client plans to do, and to allow appropriate amounts of time for transitioning between tasks.

Deficits in time management can be measured in terms of:

- *Descriptors*: poor, fair, good, excellent.
- *Percentage*: e.g., client allows enough time for transitioning between tasks 20% of the time. For a score looking just at transitioning this would be b1642.3. Since transitioning is a relatively small part of overall time management, the score for complete time management would show less impairment (b1642.1).

- *Level of assistance*: e.g., client requires moderate assistance for scheduling a day with four or more tasks (b1642.2).
- *Dysfunction related to task*: e.g., client expects to be able to do two tasks at the same time in different locations (b1642.4).

Teaching time management requires techniques similar to teaching organization and planning:

- Help the client analyze the requirements of a task, specifically looking at how long each step is going to take.
- Plan parts of a day, working up to a full day, to teach how to allow time for each task and how to estimate the time for transition between tasks. For example, getting dressed and seeing a friend for breakfast requires time for dressing and travel time between home and the restaurant, as well as the time spent eating and getting to the next activity.
- Teach the client how to use a day planner to schedule events. This is not usually considered an adaptation because it is typical for people to use day planners to keep track of their activities.
- Teach the client how to estimate transition times, including how long a drive will take at different times of the day.

Adaptations include detailed activity sheets as described in Organization and Planning that include the time to complete an activity, help from caregivers in filling in a day planner, and lists of tasks that need to be done on a regular basis, so they can be added to the client's schedule.

### Cognitive Flexibility

Cognitive flexibility refers to the ability of the client to change strategies and shift mental mindsets, especially as involved in problem solving. Zoltan (1996, p. 167) explains that "the [client] with poor mental flexibility will have difficulty releasing a particular stimulus from his attention. The [client's] behavior appears perseverative and an appropriate set of responses may be followed by a set of inappropriate responses. This occurs because the [client] continues to respond to prior cues that are no longer relevant. The [client] may show poor association ability and have difficulty in evaluating the relevance of the result obtained from a given problem. This stimulus-bound or perseverative behavior makes it difficult for the [client] to generalize knowledge for future problem solution." A client who has difficulty shifting mental mindsets and changing strategies in accordance with a changed mindset will have difficulty solving problems, theorizing concepts, and seeing things from a different point of view. Clients may also have problems forming and maintaining social relationships.

If problems with cognitive flexibility are suspected, the therapist should evaluate by:

- Choosing a task that can be manipulated to test the client's cognitive flexibility. For example, give the client a word search puzzle with horizontal and vertical letters evenly spaced over the page. The usual goal is to find predetermined words in the puzzle. For this evaluation, the puzzle is not used in this way. Instead, ask the client to cross out every 'A'. About a quarter of the way through the puzzle, ask the client to stop crossing out the letter 'A' and begin crossing out the letter 'D', and so on. Evaluate whether or not the client is able to shift from one task to another.
- During a conversation with the client, abruptly switch topics of conversation to evaluate the level of difficulty with cognitive flexibility. For example, when talking about the goals of the session, say, "Oh, I forgot, I wanted to ask you about your therapy schedule for tomorrow. What is your schedule like?"
- Ask the client to sort a pile of change by type of coin. After the client begins to do this task, change the request often to evaluate the client's ability to shift from one task to another. The therapist could ask the client to sort the change into piles of seven cents, then take one cent from each of the piles of seven cents.

The therapist can document cognitive flexibility with:

- *Dysfunction*: e.g., client was minimally frustrated when asked to change tasks for the third time (b1643.1). Client took 10 seconds to answer a question not related to the current task (a normative score would be used to determine the extent of impairment).
- *Level of assistance*: e.g., client required a question not related to task to be repeated twice before answering (b1643.1)

The above-mentioned tasks can be used to further enhance cognitive flexibility, although using real-life tasks and situations is better. Some ideas include changing tasks in a home environment, such as making a sandwich while giving directions to another person on setting the table, reading a map or written directions while keeping track of road signs, and appropriately engaging in social conversation while following directions for a craft project. It can be difficult to differentiate between divided attention, shifting attention, and cognitive flexibility. Attention to a task does not equal understanding of a task, whereas cognitive flexibility requires the client to understand and respond to the changing task or situation.

Clients who continue to have difficulty with cognitive flexibility will typically show better outcomes in less stimulating environments. Written responses that the client can reference might also be helpful for common, everyday activities. Family members should be educated to not bombard the client with multiple tasks but to provide the client with one request or topic of conversation at a time. Adequate time should be provided after the end of one task or situation to allow the client to "clear" for the next task or situation. It is recommended that the client and family seek to minimize common tasks or situations that compete for the client's attention, such as organizing the morning routine to make it as simple as possible so that multiple tasks do not have to be completed simultaneously.

### *Insight*

Insight is the client's awareness of himself or herself. A client who is insightful recognizes his/her strengths and weaknesses, whereas a client who lacks insight has a diminished or absent awareness of abilities and limitations. Consequently, the client who lacks insight may not recognize, and may adamantly deny, that deficits are present, thus putting himself/herself at an increased risk for injury and negative outcomes. Clients with impaired insight about their deficits can become hostile and agitated when confronted about an observed problem, have a very low tolerance for tasks that challenge deficit areas, exhibit impulsive behavior, have poor safety awareness, have an inability or diminished ability to compensate for deficits depending on the extent of impaired insight, exhibit poor social skills and defiant personality traits, blame an observed problem on an external source, such as saying, "I can't remember what you told me because it wasn't important. I only remember things that are important," and/or refuse to attend or participate in therapy because nothing is wrong with them.

The client who experiences difficulty achieving self-established goals may blame failure on others. One example is displaced failure, where the client might say, "They think I'm dumb, but I know better. My mom doesn't want me living in my own apartment because she wants to see me more." They may also internalize failure due to other variables, such as, "No one likes me. That's why they are sending me to live at the nursing home." This could lead to the development of other psycho-emotional issues including low self-esteem, poor internal locus of control, depression, and anger.

Barco et al (1991) suggests that there are three levels of awareness (insight) that form a basis for evaluation and treatment.

- *Intellectual awareness*: the cognitive capacity of the client to understand to some degree that a particular function is diminished from premorbid levels.
- *Emergent awareness*: the ability of clients to recognize a problem when it is actually occurring.
- *Anticipation awareness*: the ability to anticipate that a problem is going to happen because of some deficit.

If problems with insight are thought to be present, the therapist can assess the client's awareness by:

- *Intellectual awareness*: Ask the client a general question during the evaluation that gives the client an opportunity to convey his/her deficits. For example, "Tell me what you notice is different about yourself since you had the motorcycle accident."
- *Emergent awareness*: Observe how the client reacts while in the midst of a problem. Does she recognize that there is a problem? Does she attempt to fix or solve the problem? Is she able to identify the source of the problem? At what level is the client aware (if aware) of her deficits that are affecting the situation? Does the client become angry, agitated, or hostile? Does the client blame poor performance on an external source? Does the client deny having the problem?

- *Anticipatory awareness*: Ask the client questions about what types of problems s/he thinks may occur with specific tasks. The therapist could ask a client who lacks insight into his problems with math, "Do you think you will have any trouble balancing the checkbook?" A client who lacks insight into problems with walking up and down steps can be asked, "Do you think you will have any trouble getting into the house?" A client who is not allowed to return to driving and who used to drive back and forth to the grocery store might be asked, "How do you plan on doing the grocery shopping when you get home?"

Documenting insight can be done in the following ways:

- *Dysfunction*: e.g., client is not aware of problems with time management even when he has missed an appointment (b1644.4).
- *Type and extent of cueing*: e.g., client requires minimal prompting to anticipate problems with tasks, especially when supplies are running out (b1644.1).
- *Reaction to dysfunction*: e.g., client blames all difficulties with utilizing the bus during a community outing on therapist's incomplete instructions (b1644.4). Client becomes angry when left-side neglect is pointed out. The anger might be scored with b1521 Regulation of Emotion. The extent of the client's difficulty with insight depends on the reason for the anger. If the client is angry because he knows he can't do the task, there is not a deficit in insight.

The therapist can assist the client in developing greater insight by using the strategies reviewed below:

- Develop a list of the strengths and weaknesses of the client and review them at each session.
- Provide direct, clear, and concrete feedback about the client's performance. For example, "There is a mistake in the checkbook. Can you find it?" Give the client adequate time to review the work. Give the client a clue as to where the problem is located. "It is on the second line of the checkbook." Again, give the client adequate time to review the work. If the client is unable to identify the problem, point out the specific problem. "Right here the addition is wrong. Two plus six is eight. You wrote down a four." Observe the

client's reaction to the feedback. Give the client measurable feedback. "So far, we have found six errors on one page. Last session, you had 15 errors to a page. You are doing much better, but you are still having some trouble with math. Do you agree? Do you think that mistakes in balancing your checkbook will cause any problems?" If the client is not able to anticipate problems, the therapist must tell the client what problems could occur. "If your checkbook is misbalanced you may overdraw your account. An important check might bounce. You will have to pay additional fees not only to the bank for the bounced check but possibly to the company who you wrote the check to because it would be documented as being late. If these incidents continue to happen regularly, let's think worst-case scenario and say your rent check bounces continually, your landlord may terminate your lease."

- Teach the client how to deal with feelings of anger in a healthy way by teaching anger management strategies. Have the client practice applying these techniques in treatment sessions when feelings of frustration surface.
- Provide positive feedback to the client when insight is displayed.
- Consider the use of videotaping or role-playing to provide a different type of feedback to the client about his/her performance.

If the client has absolutely no insight into his or her deficits, the strategies described above are not appropriate. However, the therapist should continue to monitor the client for a positive change in insight. For clients who are unable to demonstrate adequate insight into deficits, the therapist shifts his/her focus from a developmental or restorative approach to an adaptive approach. Adaptations for insight include:

- Educating caregivers about the client's impaired insight into his/her deficits. This can be a hard concept for caregivers to understand. They may need education about the injured brain.
- Teaching caregivers how to manipulate the environment to ensure the client's safety.
- Teaching the caregivers how to continue to facilitate insight by implementing strategies that the therapist found helpful during treatment.

### Judgment

Judgment is the ability to discriminate between and evaluate different options. Judgment, like many other higher-level cognitive skills, is not an isolated skill. Judgment also involves cognitive flexibility, problem solving, shifting attention, and thinking. Additionally, coming to a conclusion includes the skill of decision-making.

To assess judgment, present the client with a problem and ask the client to weigh the available choices and form a decision. Problems can be simple, moderate, or complex. For example, "You would like to visit with both your friends and your parents. Your friends and your parents are only available to visit you at the hospital on Wednesday evening at 6:00 PM. You prefer to visit with your family separate from your friends. What choices do you have? What would you decide to do and why?" Evaluate the client's thought process in comparing and discriminating ideas. Prompt the client with alternatives if needed (e.g., If you choose your family, what effect do you think this would have on your friends? If you choose your friends, are there alternative ways to visit with your family? What if you needed to see your family on Wednesday night because they were bringing you a new pair of shoes for therapy?).

The skill of judgment can be described in terms of:

- *Complexity of judgment*: The type of judgments that the client is able to make (simple, moderate, complex). The ICF does not break down decisions into simple, moderate, and complex. A client may have no impairment related to simple judgments (weighing one simple situation to another), yet have severe impairment related to complex judgments (weighing multiple complex situations). Consequently, therapists should clarify the type of judgment after the code if possible (e.g., b1645.2, simple judgment)
- *Client's comprehensiveness*: How well the client can consider and discriminate all of the options, e.g., client has no difficulty considering and discriminating all of the options for a simple situation (b1645.0).
- *Related cognitive functions*: Other things that impair the client's ability to make judgments. Score these using other ICF codes (e.g., difficulty sustaining attention, shifting attention, or solving problems).

Clients who have difficulty weighing options and making decisions (judgment) can be taught the following strategy. The environment should be free of distractions, as much as possible, to promote concentration and attention to thinking. It can be helpful for the client to write the question or problem at the top of a piece of paper. Ask the client to brainstorm possible ideas and solutions and write them on paper without evaluating them. After the client has exhausted his/her ideas, go back and evaluate each brainstormed idea individually and make notations after each suggestion. Once all of the suggestions are considered, evaluate the set of ideas and choose the best option. The client will often benefit from asking another person who has the client's best interests at heart to offer suggestions and ideas for the list and to assist with weighing the options and coming to a decision. This would not be an adaptation because asking for advice in making a judgment is a typical and usual process.

If adequate judgment cannot be developed, the therapist can explore adaptations that require the client to seek assistance when making decisions. Guardianship may be a possibility if the client's lack of judgment is a danger to the client or others.

### Problem Solving

Problem solving, like the other functions described in this section, is not an isolated skill. It is the integration of many skills that form the client's ability to solve problems. The skills include attention, ability to devise and initiate a plan, ability to process information and feedback about effectiveness of the solution and need for revision, good impulse control, ability to organize and categorize, mental flexibility, and reasoning (Zoltan, 2007).

A client who has difficulty solving problems will most likely be thinking concretely instead of abstractly, appear impulsive with the task, exhibit confusion as to where to begin and how to solve the problem, and/or have trouble learning from mistakes and successes. Therefore, problem solving is more than just the ability to solve a cognitive problem such as "What would I do if...?" It also involves the client's ability to generalize newly learned skills to other tasks.

If there seems to be a deficit in problem-solving skills, the therapist can best assess the skill through clinical observation. The therapist presents the client with a problem and observes the client's ability to solve it. This includes:

- The client's ability to acknowledge that the problem is indeed a problem. Some clients may not see something as a problem even though the therapist sees it as a problem. This could be due to the client's coping mechanisms or personality. Therefore, the therapist should pose several questions and problems and look for patterns of response. Examples of questions: What would you do if you were driving on a two-lane country back road with no intersecting streets and someone was driving very fast and very close to the back of your car? What would you do if someone was knocking on your door and you didn't know who it was? What would you do if you were lost?

- The ability of the client to fully appreciate and understand the complexity of the problem. Is the client able to see the problem from multiple perspectives? Does the client appreciate all of the elements of the problem?

- The ability of the client to identify solutions to the problem. Is the client able to effectively consider personal or community barriers related to solving the problem? Is the client able to compare this problem to past learning experiences and use insights gained earlier?

A client's problem-solving skills can also be assessed via an action task. For example:

- Use the game Parquet. Chose a simple block design of four or six pieces. Show the design to the client and ask the client to replicate it. Observe how the client solves the problem. Is it thoughtful (studies the picture, organizes the blocks needed, refers to the picture after placing each block) or disorganized (quickly grabs block pieces, doesn't refer to the picture of the design, says that he is done when the block design is incorrect, does not refer to the picture upon completion to check his work, etc.).

- Observe the client's behavior with a complex functional task that requires problem solving, such as setting up the position of his wheelchair for new transfer surface (e.g., transferring from a wheelchair to a recumbent bike). Does the client take his time to think through the problem in a sequential manner or does he appear impulsive, not contemplating or recognizing the problem components of the task?

Once deficits in problem solving have been identified, the therapist must determine a baseline of functioning. Problem-solving functions can be measured in terms of:

- *Descriptors*: poor, fair, good, excellent.
- *Complexity of the problem*: The type of problems the client is able to solve (simple, moderate, complex). The ICF does not break down problems into simple, moderate, and complex. A client may have no impairment related to simple problem solving, yet have severe impairment related to complex problem solving. Therapists should clarify the type of problem solving after the code, if possible (e.g., b1646.2, simple problem solving)
- *Percentage*: e.g., Client is able to problem solve for simple tasks 35% of the time (b1646.3, simple problem solving).
- *Type and extent of cueing*: e.g., client requires occasional verbal cues to problem solve for complex tasks (b1646.1, complex problem solving).
- *Dysfunction related to task*: e.g., client requires supervision at all times when in a community environment secondary to poor problem-solving skills related to safety (b1646.4).

Once a baseline of functioning is determined, the therapist facilitates the development or restoration of problem-solving skills primarily through the use of functional activities that are going to be part of the client's lifestyle after discharge. These may include leisure planning, driving directions, dealing with kid's schedules that overlap, developing a college course schedule that works around other responsibilities, etc. Once functional activities have been identified, the therapist:

- Challenges the client with problem-solving tasks and provides the appropriate cueing to facilitate acknowledgement of a problem, the appreciation and understanding of the problem, and the ability to identify effective solutions. Tasks should be graduated from simple to complex. Cueing is often done in the form of leading questions, such as "What do you think would happen if you don't ask for directions?" and general verbal cues to refocus the client on the problem-solving

process, such as "Did you check the picture of the design to make sure it is right?"

- Provides the client with immediate feedback about his/her performance. Don't wait until the client is finished with the process and then go back and correct it. Feedback is given during the task. If a client is moving on to the next step in the process without fully completing the first step, the therapist stops the client and provides cueing to assist the client in completion of the first step of the task. For example, the therapist makes up an activity schedule that reflects conflicts among the kids' schedules. If the client acknowledges that the mock activity schedule shows a problem but fails to acknowledge the total complexity of the problem, such as failing to take into account feelings of the children, the therapist should halt the client before she attempts to go on to identifying solutions. The therapist might review the whole scope of the problem again because "I think we might be missing something." The therapist would then pose leading questions to help the client identify the parts of the problem that she missed.
- Teaches the client basic activity analysis skills, especially how to break down and look at the individual parts of the activity. For example, ask the client to look at the components of taking a two-hour drive — transferring into the car, having someone load the wheelchair into the car trunk, putting on the seatbelt, performing weight shifts in the car every 30 minutes, opening, reading, and closing a map, etc. The development of analytical skills will help the client with problem-solving functions.

If the client is unable to demonstrate adequate problem-solving skills, the therapist shifts his/her focus from a development or restorative approach to an adaptive approach. Adaptations for problem-solving skills include:

- Providing instructions on how to solve common problems, such as juggling children's sports schedules.
- Provide worksheets for common planning needs, including checklists of necessary supplies and steps to complete a task.
- Educate the client's caregivers about the client's problems in this area and teach them how to cue

the client to facilitate further development of problem-solving skills.

- Teach the client to recheck his/her work at least two times before finalizing a solution.

- Tell the client that it is appropriate to ask for help with problem-solving tasks from people that s/he trusts. Receiving help is not an "easy way out," but rather a compensatory strategy to minimize complications.

### Cross References

In *Recreational Therapy for Specific Diagnoses and Conditions, First Edition*, ICF code b164 Higher-Level Cognitive Functions is listed in 21 chapters: Attention-Deficit/Hyperactivity Disorder, Autism Spectrum Disorder, Borderline Personality Disorder, Burns, Cerebral Palsy, Cerebrovascular Accident, Feeding and Eating Disorders, Fibromyalgia and Juvenile Fibromyalgia, Gambling Disorder, Generalized Anxiety Disorder, Hearing Loss, Intellectual Disability, Major Depressive Disorder, Multiple Sclerosis, Neurocognitive Disorders, Post-Traumatic Stress Disorder, Schizophrenia Spectrum and Other Psychotic Disorders, Spina Bifida, Spinal Cord Injury, Substance-Related Disorders, and Traumatic Brain Injury.

In *Recreational Therapy Basics, Techniques, and Interventions, First Edition*, treatment for ICF code b164 Higher-Level Cognitive Functions is discussed in 10 chapters: Activity and Task Analysis, Education and Counseling, Participation, Stress, Adaptive Sports, Anger Management, Errorless Learning, Montessori Method, Social Skills Training, and Therapeutic Thematic Arts Programming.

### b167 Mental Functions of Language

Specific mental functions of recognizing and using signs, symbols, and other components of language.

Inclusions: functions of reception and decryption of spoken, written, or other forms of language such as sign language; functions of expression of spoken, written, or other forms of language; integrative language functions, spoken and written, such as involved in receptive, expressive, Broca's, Wernicke's, and conduction aphasia

Exclusions: attention functions (b140); memory functions (b144); perceptual functions (b156); thought functions (b160); higher-level cognitive functions (b164); calculation functions (b172); mental functions

of complex movements (b176); b2 Sensory Functions and Pain; b3 Voice and Speech Functions

- *b1670 Reception of Language*
  Specific mental functions of decoding messages in spoken, written, or other forms, such as sign language, to obtain their meaning.

  o *b16700 Reception of Spoken Language*
  Mental functions of decoding spoken messages to obtain their meaning.

  o *b16701 Reception of Written Language*
  Mental functions of decoding written messages to obtain their meaning.

  o *b16702 Reception of Sign Language*
  Mental functions of decoding messages in languages that use signs made by hands and other movements, in order to obtain their meaning.

  o *b16708 Reception of Language, Other Specified*
  o *b16709 Reception of Language, Unspecified*
- *b1671 Expression of Language*
  Specific mental functions necessary to produce meaningful messages in spoken, written, signed, or other forms of language.

  o *b16710 Expression of Spoken Language*
  Mental functions necessary to produce meaningful spoken messages.

  o *b16711 Expression of Written Language*
  Mental functions necessary to produce meaningful written messages.

  o *b16712 Expression of Sign Language*
  Mental functions necessary to produce meaningful messages in languages that use signs made by hands and other movements.

  o *b16718 Expression of Language, Other Specified*
  o *b16719 Expression of Language, Unspecified*
- *b1672 Integrative Language Functions*
  Mental functions that organize semantic and symbolic meaning, grammatical structure, and ideas for the production of messages in spoken, written, or other forms of language.

- *b1678 Mental Functions of Language, Other Specified*
- *b1679 Mental Function of Language, Unspecified*

The codes in this section relate to the reception, expression, and integration of language functions for communication.

Difficulty with reception of spoken, written, or sign language can be due to a variety of things, such as lack of knowledge, difficulty learning, and hand dysfunction. If the cause of difficulty is knowledge or learning, the therapist would use the codes listed in Activities and Participation d1 Learning and Applying Knowledge. If the cause of difficulty is related to hand dysfunction, the therapist would refer to specific hand functions in s7302 Structure of Hand. If the cause of difficulty is related to mental impairments, the therapist would use the mental function codes in this section. Common causes of mental function impairments related to language include damage to the language areas of the brain from stroke, traumatic brain injury, and developmental disability. Language impairments are typically divided into the two main categories of reception of language and expression of language. Some common speech and language impairments include:

*Aphasia (receptive and expressive language impairment):* Receptive aphasia is difficulty understanding spoken language. Expressive aphasia is difficulty expressing verbal language. If a person has both receptive and expressive aphasia it is called global aphasia. In global aphasia, severe deficits are found in all language processes, including speech production, auditory comprehension, reading, and writing. Further delineations of language impairments include fluent and non-fluent aphasia (definitions from *Idyll Arbor's Therapy Dictionary*, burlingame, 2001). In fluent aphasia (also called Wernicke's aphasia), the person's speech is fluent. It has a natural grammatical flow, but there are paraphasic errors, which are words that may be unrelated to the current topic or unintelligible. Auditory comprehension, reading comprehension, and writing comprehension are impaired. In non-fluent aphasia (also called Broca's aphasia), speech is effortful and halting. Auditory comprehension is relatively good but not perfect. Reading comprehension is better than written output.

*Dysarthria (expressive language impairment):* Dysarthria is a loss of function in the muscles used for speech and voice production making it difficult to understand even though all other language and comprehension skills are intact. This is typically characterized by low voice volume with fast and/or slurred speech. This is coded with b3 Voice and Speech Functions.

*Word finding (expressive language impairment):* Difficulty retrieving words in conversation.

### Receptive Language Techniques

To assess a client's receptive language skills, challenge the client with a receptive language task and observe the results. Problems with hearing must be ruled out if asking a question verbally. Document the observations in terms of:

- *Type of deficit*: e.g., client exhibits receptive aphasia (b16700.2), but little expressive aphasia (16710.1). Specific language disorders are also coded using the ICD-10.
- *Extent of impairment*: e.g., client exhibits moderate reception of language impairment (b16700.2).
- *Percent of impairment*: e.g., appears to understand approximately 40% of one-step verbal commands (b16700.3).
- *Type and extent of cueing*: e.g., requires moderate gestural cues to increase receptive language abilities from baseline of 75% (b16700.2).
- *Dysfunction related to task*: e.g., requires moderate gestural cues from friends in social conversation secondary to extremely poor receptive language skills (b16700.4).

When working with clients who have receptive language problems, (1) limit the number of words or signs used in a communication to decrease complexity of communication, (2) limit the number of directions given at one time and gradually increase as appropriate, (3) utilize a variety of cueing techniques to ascertain the types of cues that are most helpful for the client, (4) provide hand over hand assistance with verbal action words. As the client's skills improve, increase the number of words and complexity of the communication while decreasing the cueing and assistance.

If a client has global aphasia, the use of pictures and demonstrative and gestural cues are helpful for communication. Clients with global aphasia who are in the recovery phase should be briefly re-assessed daily for positive changes so the therapist can build on any new skill.

Also see Activities and Participation d3 Communication for information on application of language in activities.

### Expressive Language Techniques

To assess a client's expressive language skills, challenge and observe the client in communication. Document the observations in terms of:

- *Type of deficit*: e.g., client exhibits moderate global aphasia (b16700.2), but little expressive aphasia (16710.2). Specific language disorders are also coded using the ICD-10.
- Extent *of impairment*: client exhibits severe expression of language impairment (b16710.3)
- *Percent of impairment*: e.g., exhibits word-finding problems in 25% of verbal conversations (b16710.2).
- *Type and extent of cueing*: e.g., requires moderate verbal cues to incorporate compensatory strategies for expression of language impairments in social conversation, resulting in a continuation of a mild impairment (b16710.1).
- *Dysfunction related to task*: e.g., requires moderate verbal cues when requesting assistance from store employee secondary to word-finding difficulty, resulting from a moderate impairment (b16710.2).

To enhance a client's expressive language functions a variety of techniques can be employed. Clients who have difficulty expressing needs through one form of language will often seek another form of communication, such as pointing instead of finding the correct word. This is a good compensatory strategy, but it does not encourage neuroplasticity to promote recovery if language impairments are caused by a brain injury. Consequently, clients with expressive language difficulties who are in the recovery stage should be encouraged to vocalize, write, and read. Therapists need to provide clients with increased time to communicate, provide praise, and acknowledge frustration. Common sounds, words, and signs are repetitively drilled to promote recovery. Alternative communication techniques to use with language production, such as pointing, gesturing, demonstrating, writing, and drawing, are taught to decrease the client's frustration and increase successful communication.

If a client has word finding problems, provide cues to enhance word finding, such as it starts with the letter R or it is the color of your shirt. The goal is for the client to identify the correct word or sign and then produce it. Saying the word that the client is trying to express will minimize frustration and increase speed of communication, but it will not enhance neuroplasticity in the recovery phase.

### Integrative Language Techniques

Integrative language functions include the ability to organize the meaning of words and combination of words (semantics) or symbols, and/or grammatically structure words and ideas to produce spoken, written, or other forms of language. This code would be scored as an impairment if the client was able to produce words effectively, but the combination of words made no sense. In adults this is most often seen in psychiatric disorders such as schizophrenia. It is called linguistic disorganization, or, less formally, word salad. Children may be scored with this code if they incorrectly use plural forms or verb tenses or if they use incorrect word order, leave out words, or use a limited number of complex sentences, such as those that contain prepositional clauses.

Recreational therapists do not usually plan treatment for impairments in this code. They can assist the care plans set up by other members of the treatment team, which might include something like challenging the client to coordinate word cards to make a sentence. For example, having separate word cards of "blue," "she," "likes," "necklace," and "the" and then ask the client to arrange the cards in order to make a grammatically correct sentence ("She likes the blue necklace.").

Other ways the therapist can help the client is by allowing sufficient time for the client to think through what s/he wants to say and modeling better grammatical structure.

If integrative language functions cannot be resolved, the therapist can develop compensatory strategies related to leisure engagement. This might consist of premade sentences that can be shared with others (e.g., "I would like to go shopping for jewelry supplies." "I want to make jewelry today." "I need_____") and teaching the client alternative methods for communicating thoughts, ideas, and needs through the use of gestures and demonstrations.

*Cross References*

In *Recreational Therapy for Specific Diagnoses and Conditions, First Edition*, ICF code b167 Mental Functions of Language is listed in 10 chapters: Attention-Deficit/Hyperactivity Disorder, Autism Spectrum Disorder, Cerebrovascular Accident, Fibromyalgia and Juvenile Fibromyalgia, Hearing Loss, Multiple Sclerosis, Neurocognitive Disorders, Schizophrenia Spectrum and Other Psychotic Disorders, Spina Bifida, and Traumatic Brain Injury.

In *Recreational Therapy Basics, Techniques, and Interventions, First Edition*, treatment for ICF code b167 Mental Functions of Language is discussed in five chapters: Stress, Group Psychotherapy Techniques, Montessori Method, Social Skills Training, and Therapeutic Thematic Arts Programming.

## b172 Calculation Functions

Specific mental functions of determination, approximation, and manipulation of mathematical symbols and processes.

Inclusions: functions of addition, subtraction, and other simple mathematical calculations; functions of complex mathematical operations

Exclusions: attention functions (b140); memory functions (b144); thought functions (b160); higher-level cognitive functions (b164); mental functions of language (b167)

- *b1720 Simple Calculation*
  Mental functions of computing with numbers, such as addition, subtraction, multiplication, and division.

- *b1721 Complex Calculation*
  Mental functions of translating word problems into arithmetic procedures, translating mathematical formulas into arithmetic procedures, and other complex manipulations involving numbers.

- *b1728 Calculation Functions, Other Specified*
- *b1729 Calculation Functions, Unspecified*

Number processing is different from calculation. Number processing includes the recognition and comprehension of numbers in verbal or written form. Calculation is the identification and understanding of arithmetic symbols (e.g., +, -, x) and words (e.g., plus, divide, difference), as well as the ability to

recall and apply arithmetic facts to mathematical problems.

Calculation is an important life skill as it is needed to balance a checkbook, figure out pay, add up prices of items at a store to stay within a budget, cook and bake from a recipe, figure out taxes, and figure out a schedule, just to name a few.

Difficulty with calculation functions can be a consequence of knowledge and learning or mental dysfunction. If the problem lies in knowledge and learning, refer to d172 Calculating. If the difficulty is due to mental impairment, such as brain injury, then calculation functions in this section would be the appropriate place to document it. The mental function impairment of having difficulty with calculations is referred to as acalculia.

Assess a client's ability to recognize written numbers, spoken or signed numbers, and numbers written in the form of words. Assess the client's ability to identify both symbolic and written out arithmetic symbols, such as +, addition, -, subtraction. Assess the client when performing simple calculations, such as 2+6, eight subtracted from twelve, and complex calculation functions, such as balancing three checkbook transactions.

Document outcomes in terms of:

- *Extent of impairment*: e.g., client has moderate difficulty with simple calculations (b1720.2)
- *Percent of impairment*: e.g., 50% of checkbook math correct (b1720.3)
- *Type and extent of cueing*: e.g., client independent with addition of double digits, moderate cueing required to multiply single digits. When a client requires varying levels of cueing, the therapist has two ways to score the ICF code: score the average (b1720.1) or use the lowest score (b1720.2). Choosing the lowest score is often best, as it doesn't reflect a higher level of functioning.
- *Dysfunction related to task*: e.g., client requires moderate assistance for purchasing art supplies secondary to moderate difficulty with simple calculations (b1720.2).

To enhance number or calculation functions, begin at the client's baseline of functioning and use repetitive number or calculation tasks at and slightly above the client's level of functioning. Problems should be directly related to life activities that are common for the client, such as adding up price tags.

If number or calculation functions do not improve sufficiently for daily living, evaluate the need for adaptive devices, such as a calculator. Note that calculators are a common tool used by most of the population. If a client has difficulty using a calculator because s/he doesn't understand how to work through the calculation process, these codes should be used to document that difficulty. Step-by-step instructions for performing calculations can be provided. Identification of someone to assist the client with calculations may be needed. The individual could also speak the calculation question to a smart phone (e.g., "Siri, how much is $14.25 plus $52.14.") to find out the answer.

### Cross References

In *Recreational Therapy for Specific Diagnoses and Conditions, First Edition*, ICF code b172 Calculation Functions is listed in five chapters: Attention-Deficit/Hyperactivity Disorder, Fibromyalgia and Juvenile Fibromyalgia, Multiple Sclerosis, Neurocognitive Disorders, and Spina Bifida.

In *Recreational Therapy Basics, Techniques, and Interventions, First Edition*, treatment for ICF code b172 Calculation Functions is discussed in one chapter: Stress.

### b176 Mental Functions of Sequencing Complex Movements

Specific mental functions of sequencing and coordinating complex, purposeful movements.

Inclusions: impairments such as in ideation, ideomotor, dressing, oculomotor, and speech apraxia

Exclusions: psychomotor functions (b147); higher-level cognitive functions (b164); b7 Neuromusculoskeletal and Movement-Related Functions

Sequencing complex movement is a function required in almost every kind of activity from walking to talking to watching a tennis match. Apraxia is the complete inability to sequence certain movements even though there is no loss of motor power, sensation, or coordination. Dyspraxia is the partial loss of the ability to sequence certain movements even though there is no loss of motor power, sensation, or coordination. In other words, the client has the motor power, sensation, and coordination necessary to perform movement, but lacks the ability

to perform these movements due to impaired neurological connections. Apraxia and dyspraxia may be acquired, for example from traumatic brain injury, stroke, or Parkinson's disease, or due to a delay or failure in normal neurological development.

### Types of Apraxia/Dyspraxia

Common types of apraxia/dyspraxia are explained below (Devinsky & D'Esposito, 2003; Galvez-Jimenez & Tuite, 2011; National Institute of Neurological Disorders and Stroke, 2015; Petreska et al., 2007; Zoltan, 2007):

- *Apraxic agraphia/dysgraphia*: Motor writing is impaired but non-motor writing (e.g., typing) is not impaired.
- *Buccofacial or orofacial apraxia/dyspraxia*: Difficulty carrying out movements of the face on command.
- *Conceptual apraxia/dyspraxia*: Impairment in ability to understand the relationships between objects and their specific actions. Inability to use tools. Clients with conceptual apraxia are able to function better if the activity takes place in context, such as engaging in gardening activities in a garden or greenhouse instead of at a table in the therapy room.
- *Conduction apraxia/dyspraxia*: The client has greater impairment of movement when s/he is required to imitate than when s/he is responding to commands.
- *Constructional apraxia/dyspraxia*: Impairment in ability to produce designs in two or three dimensions through copying, drawing, or constructing.
- *Developmental apraxia/dyspraxia*: Disorders affecting the initiation, organization, and performance of actions in children.
- *Disassociation apraxia/dyspraxia*: Unable to make meaningful movements to verbal commands but able to imitate the therapist's movements or use an object.
- *Dressing apraxia/dyspraxia*: Inability to perform dressing tasks.
- *Dyssynchronous apraxia/dyspraxia*: Inability to combine simultaneous preprogrammed movements.
- *Eyelid opening apraxia/dyspraxia*: Difficulty in initiating the act of eyelid opening.

- *Gait apraxia/dyspraxia*: Impaired ability to execute highly practiced, coordinated movements of the legs required for walking.
- *Gaze apraxia*: Difficulty directing gaze.
- *Ideational apraxia/dyspraxia*: Loss of ability to conceptualize, plan, and execute the complex sequence of motor actions involving the use of tools or objects in everyday life. The client is unable to plan movement related to an object because s/he has lost the perception of the object's purpose. The client doesn't know what to do.
- *Ideomotor apraxia/dyspraxia*: Difficulty with goal-directed movement. The client knows what to do, but does not know how to do it.
- *Limb-kinetic apraxia/dyspraxia*: Loss of hand and finger dexterity due to inability to connect or isolate individual movements.
- *Mirror apraxia/dyspraxia*: Deficit in reaching to objects presented in a mirror.
- *Oculomotor (or visuomotor) apraxia/dyspraxia*: Difficulty in controlling eye movement.
- *Oral apraxia/dyspraxia*: Difficulty in forming and organizing intelligible words.
- *Orienting apraxia/dyspraxia*: Difficulty in orienting one's body with reference to other objects.
- *Speech or verbal apraxia/dyspraxia*: Difficulty planning and coordinating movements necessary for speech.

Assessing problems in sequencing complex movement involves the whole treatment team, but the recreational and occupational therapists are especially important in the assessment because they work with clients when the clients are performing complex tasks. Some simple ways for the recreational therapist to test for problems with sequencing complex movements are

- Asking the client to write out a list of activities that s/he used to like. If the client has difficulty writing, or even holding the pen, then apraxia may be present.
- Asking the client to pantomime an activity that s/he has done in the past using a specific piece of equipment, such as a pair of scissors. If the client is not able to make the arm and hand movements to pretend that s/he has the equipment and to pantomime through the actions of using the equipment, then ideomotor apraxia may be present. The therapist should expect fairly crisp and clear movements from the client during this test. If these movements are "fuzzy," out of order, or inappropriate, further testing for dyspraxia is indicated.
- Placing in front of the client a variety of common pieces of equipment used in leisure activities. Ask the client to pick up an item and pantomime using it. Clients who are not able to pick up the items, and who don't have limb weakness or paralysis, may have limb-kinetic apraxia. Clients who incorrectly pantomime the use of items may have conceptual or ideomotor apraxia.
- Asking a client to blow bubbles after demonstrating how to do it. If the client cannot blow bubbles, there is a chance that s/he has buccofacial apraxia.
- Another test to differentiate buccofacial apraxia from dyspraxia is to ask the client to lick his/her lips. If the client can lick his/her lips upon command, s/he probably does not have buccofacial apraxia. If the client does not lick his/her lips on command, place something sweet and sticky, such as jam or honey, on the person's tongue. Then let the client know that you are going to put some jam on his/her lips but *do not* ask the client to do anything with it. If the client licks the jam off his/her lips without your asking him/her to do so, and the person could not lick his/her lips earlier on command, then the client probably has apraxia. If the client does not automatically lick the jam off without you instructing him/her to, then the person probably has dysarthria (Zoltan, 1996).

If the therapist suspects that the client may have apraxia, engage the client in one-on-one activity with the therapist to determine the client's ability to physically complete daily tasks, such as preparing a meal, preparing for and going on a walk, or going shopping. If the client is not able to be independent in these activities but still performs relatively well in other therapy groups, the discharge location or date may need to be adjusted. The therapist works with the client in a one-on-one situation so that the client's performance is not impacted by watching others perform the same task.

Clients with developmental apraxia of speech may also have problems with fine hand use and acting out behavior. The therapist will want to observe the client's functional level of fine hand use and document the client's coping techniques or impairments as the client engages in activity.

The treatment for lack of function in sequencing complex movements usually involves treating the cause of the apraxia, if it is known. Developmental apraxia of speech is the type of apraxia that most commonly has a separate treatment, usually led by the speech pathologist. For the other types of apraxia, the therapist is looking for adaptations that will help reduce the number of problems the apraxia causes. The adaptations depend on the kind of apraxia the client has. Specific treatment directions for different types of apraxia are listed below.

### Buccofacial Apraxia/Dyspraxia

The speech pathologist will probably be responsible for designing the treatment for buccofacial apraxia. The recreational therapist should be aware that the client will not be able to, or have limited ability to, perform actions with the lips and face on command. Visual cues may be more effective.

### Conceptual Apraxia/Dyspraxia

Clients with conceptual apraxia are able to function better if the activity takes place in context, such as engaging in gardening activities in a garden or greenhouse instead of at a table in the therapy room.

### Constructional Apraxia/Dyspraxia

The type of impairment seen in constructional apraxia tends to be different depending on the side of the brain that is affected. For clients with damage to the right hemisphere of the brain, the impairments tend to be related to placing the object in the correct location in space, duplicating an object with correct proportions and perspective, and analyzing the relationship between parts. Clients with right hemisphere impairment do not seem to benefit from having a model close by or having part of the picture already drawn in for them to complete. In fact, Zoltan (1996) indicates that presenting the client with a partially completed construction only confuses the client more, decreasing functional ability.

For clients with damage to the left hemisphere of the brain the impairments tend to be related to initiating and planning the correct sequence of actions needed to reconstruct an object. It is not uncommon for clients with damage to the left hemisphere to also have visual neglect, which can have an added impact on the client's ability to reconstruct an object. Clients with left hemisphere impairments tend to benefit from having the model close by, benefit from having a portion of the drawing started for them, and improve with practice.

If the recreational therapist finds that a client has constructional apraxia during leisure activities, such as arts and crafts projects, the therapist should also consider exploring the client's potential impairment related to meal preparation, dressing correctly for the activity and weather, and other activities that involve self-care in preparing for or engaging in activity.

### Developmental Apraxia/Dyspraxia of Speech

Clients have difficulty communicating. It is not uncommon to see young children with developmental apraxia of speech act out by pushing, hitting, kicking, and otherwise disrupting other children's play. This behavior is thought to be a result of stress and frustration at not being able to communicate ideas, needs, and feelings. As children enter middle school, coping responses to impaired communication caused by apraxia often include being passive or shy and often answering questions with, "I don't know." Clients with developmental apraxia of speech often have decreased functional ability when they are under stress. Age-appropriate stress reduction skill training is often an important part of recreational therapy intervention and should be part of the client's Individualized Education Plan (IEP).

Clients with developmental apraxia of speech often improve to the point of having basic, functional communication skills after frequent and long-term speech therapy. This usually means two to three times a week for at least two years. The recreational therapist will want to use the same techniques suggested by the speech pathologist. Often the client will be able to get the intent of his/her message across even though the sentence structure, words, and pronunciation are incorrect. The recreational therapist should repeat the client's sentence while role modeling the correct form. For example, "Yes, I agree that the kitten looks funny as it chases the string."

Clients with developmental apraxia of speech often have a good vocabulary but are not able to find the words to pronounce. Sign language and picture boards are good methods of increasing the client's ability to communicate.

### Ideomotor Apraxia/Dyspraxia

Clients can often perform a motor planning task if the therapist does not use a verbal command. For example, if the therapist is playing checkers with a client, the client will be able to move a checker piece without cueing. If the therapist cues the client to move the checker piece, the client often becomes confused and will not be able to execute the task. If the client is distracted and is not taking his/her turn, it is far more effective if the therapist cues the client by pointing to the checkerboard instead of using a verbal cue.

There are two forms of ideomotor apraxia (Zoltan, 1996).

The first form occurs when there is damage to the portion of the brain that stores visuokinesthetic motor information. If there is damage to this portion of the brain, the client is unlikely to self-correct performance because s/he does not recognize impairment in performance. The therapist can see that a client has this type of ideomotor impairment when s/he observes that the client is not noticing a problem with his/her performance. This type of impairment increases the therapist's need to structure the environment for increased safety when the client is learning a new activity.

The second type of ideomotor apraxia is when the client has the ability to identify problems with his/her motor performance. Clients with this kind of ideomotor apraxia often improve with practice during therapy and activity. Visual cues or physical cues, such as prompting, manipulation, or hand-over-hand, may increase client performance. Verbal cues tend to have little positive impact and may cause the client's performance to worsen. Ideomotor apraxia may be either unilateral or bilateral.

### Limb-Kinetic Apraxia/Dyspraxia

Leisure planning for clients with limb-kinetic apraxia will probably need to include activities that allow the assistance of others, as this type of apraxia has the greatest impact on the ability to be independent. "The presence of limb apraxia, more than any other type of neuropsychological disorder, correlates with the level of caregiver assistance required six months after stroke" (Koski, Iacoboni, & Mazziotta, 2002).

### Oculomotor Apraxia/Dyspraxia

As would be expected with the inability to control the visual senses, clients with oculomotor apraxia have trouble with reading skills. Social skills may also be delayed, as the client tends to miss subtle gestures and facial expressions. This lack of sensory information in social situations makes it harder for the person to correctly interpret what is going on. Treatment includes helping the client enhance his/her other sensory inputs allowing a fuller understanding of his/her environment.

### Verbal Apraxia/Dyspraxia

Clients with verbal apraxia tend to be far better at understanding language than communicating and using language. This impairment of language often overlaps other impairments including being able to read, write, and use math. The therapist will want to observe the client's actual skills for integration and activity skills related to reading restaurant menus, determining how much money is needed to go swimming at the community pool, keeping a bowling score, etc.

### Compensatory Strategies

Recreational therapists may also assist the client and family in designing compensatory strategies as needed to improve leisure and community participation, such as typing instead of handwriting for apraxic agraphia or adapting fine motor movements to gross motor movement for limb-kinetic apraxia.

### Cross References

In *Recreational Therapy for Specific Diagnoses and Conditions, First Edition*, ICF code b176 Mental Functions of Sequencing Complex Movements is listed in five chapters: Attention-Deficit/Hyperactivity Disorder, Fibromyalgia and Juvenile Fibromyalgia, Multiple Sclerosis, Neurocognitive Disorders, and Spina Bifida.

In *Recreational Therapy Basics, Techniques, and Interventions, First Edition*, there are no references for b176 Mental Functions of Sequencing Complex Movements.

## b180 Experience of Self and Time Functions

Specific mental functions related to the awareness of one's identity, one's body, one's position in the reality of one's environment and of time.

Inclusions: functions of experience of self, body image, and time

- *b1800 Experience of Self*
  Specific mental functions of being aware of one's own identity and one's position in the reality of the environment around oneself.

  Inclusion: impairments such as depersonalization and derealization

- *b1801 Body Image*
  Specific mental functions related to the representation and awareness of one's body.

  Inclusions: impairments such as phantom limb and feeling too fat or too thin

- *b1802 Experience of Time*
  Specific mental functions of the subjective experiences related to the length and passage of time.

  Inclusions: impairments such as jamais vu and déjà vu

- *b1808 Experience of Self and Time Functions, Other Specified*
- *b1809 Experience of Self and Time Functions, Unspecified*

The discussion of this code is divided into three sections because each subheading presents significantly different issues for the recreational therapist.

### Experience of Self

Like orientation to person, experience of self includes a person's awareness of his/her identity. At the most basic level, it requires awareness of self as a separate entity. Experience of self also includes an additional awareness of one's position in the environment. This code includes the impairments of depersonalization, the feeling that the body or the personal self is strange and unreal, and derealization, the perception of objects in the external world as strange and unreal.

Questions that can be asked to determine depersonalization include: "Do you or have you ever felt detached, unattached, or divorced from yourself?" "Did you ever act in so strange a way you considered the possibility that you might be two different people?" "Are you always certain who you are?" "Did you ever feel like you were outside yourself, apart from your body, watching what you were doing?" (Zuckerman, 2000, p. 52).

Questions that can be asked to determine derealization include: "Did you ever get so involved in a daydream that you couldn't tell if it were real or not?" "Did you ever feel that things around you in the world were very strange, remote, unreal, or changing?" "Do things seem natural and real to you, or does it seem like things are make-believe?" "Do things or objects ever seem to be alive?" (Zuckerman, 2000, p. 53).

Causes of depersonalization and derealization include neurological disorders such as epilepsy, migraine, brain tumors, cerebrovascular disease, cerebral trauma, encephalitis, dementia, and Huntington's disease. It can also be caused by toxic and metabolic disorders such as hypoglycemia, hyperparathyroidism, carbon monoxide poisoning, hyperventilation, and hypothyroidism. Psychological causes include idiopathic mental disorders such as schizophrenia, depressive disorders, manic episodes, conversion disorder, anxiety disorders, obsessive-compulsive disorder, personality disorders, and phobic-anxiety depersonalization syndrome. In normally healthy persons it may be caused by exhaustion; boredom; sensory deprivation; emotional shock; and substance use including alcohol, barbiturates, benzodiazepine, marijuana, and any other hallucinogenic substance (Sadock & Sadock, 2003).

Documentation of the condition should include:

- *Number, length, persistence of episode*: e.g., client felt objects were unreal in three separate episodes lasting one to three hours each.
- *Strength of the feeling*: e.g., client expressed concern about not being able to feel like part of the group due to fatigue associated with chemotherapy treatment.

Scoring the extent of impairment a person has with B1800 Experience of Self is challenging. The ICF qualifiers are divided by percent (e.g., moderate impairment = 50-95%). Therapists might find success in scoring these codes by determining the percentage of time in a day the person experiences depersonalization and derealization. For example, if a person states that she experiences this all the time, then it would be a complete impairment (b1800.4).

Approximately 50% of people with depersonalization and/or derealization are believed to have long-lasting conditions (Sadock & Sadock, 2003).

Treatment starts with treating the underlying disorder causing depersonalization or derealization. A full psychiatric evaluation is needed. There may be particular triggers of the behavior, such as fear or anxiety, that can be addressed by recreational therapists in the clinic setting. Recreational therapists can also assist clients in carrying over these strategies and identifying new strategies as appropriate in real life settings.

Clients may need supports, particularly in community settings, to assist as needed when episodes of depersonalization and/or derealization occur. For example, if the client is at a store and experiences depersonalization when paying for an item, the client may need assistance to finish the transaction.

### Body Image

Body image covers the specific mental functions that allow the client to conceive a representation and awareness of his/her body. This includes body image distortions that are common in anorexia and bulimia, such as feeling too fat or too thin. It can also be coded for sensations of a phantom limb after an amputation.

Impairments in body image are identified through verbalizations and behavior of a client. Some examples: "I fell when I tried to get out of bed because I thought my leg was still there. I could have sworn my leg was still there." A 90-pound girl who is 16 years old says, "I am so fat it makes me sick to my stomach to look at myself."

Measurement of body image distortion is typically described with:

- *Descriptors*: such as healthy, unhealthy, distorted, aware, and unaware.
- *Severity*: e.g., client's body image is distorted; client believes that she is grossly obese at 5' 2" and 75 pounds. Scoring the extent of impairment a person has is challenging. The percentage method of scoring ICF qualifiers will not work. Therapists might find success in scoring these codes using the alternative descriptive words (low, medium, high) to document how much the distortion is affecting the client. For example, if this client is refusing to eat because of her body image distortion, then it would be a severe impairment (b1801.3).

Treatment for this code relies mainly on cognitive retraining. The goal is to present enough experiences and examples to change the way the client thinks about the situation. For example, a client who tries to use an amputated limb needs many experiences with having the limb not there before he will understand not to rely on it. These need to be done safely. A client with anorexia needs many examples of healthy bodies, including medical information about nutrition and the need for some fat to be healthy. Miller and Jake (2001) have many examples of recreational therapy techniques to use in *Eating Disorders: Providing Effective Recreational Therapy Intervention*. There is also a chapter on Feeding and Eating Disorders in *Recreational Therapy for Specific Diagnoses and Conditions*.

One important consideration for therapists dealing with eating disorders is that the client will not be able to process well cognitively until s/he is stabilized medically.

### Experience of Time

b1140 Orientation to Time is an awareness of the day, date, month, and year. This is different from b1802 Experience of Time, which includes déjà vu (the illusion of having already experienced something actually being experienced for the first time) and jamais vu (false feeling of unfamiliarity with a real situation that a person has experienced).

Both of these impairments fall under the classification of paramnesia, which is the falsification of memory by distortion of recall. A feeling of déjà vu once in a while in a normal, healthy person is not considered an impairment. Disturbances in memory can be caused by a variety of neurological impairments, substance use, and medical conditions.

Documentation of the specific impairment and its occurrence is noted in the client's medical chart, as in "Client reports feelings of déjà vu almost daily."

Scoring the extent of impairment is challenging. Therapists might find success in scoring these codes by determining the percentage of activates during the day where the person is dysfunctional because of déjà vu and/or jamais vu. For example, if a person states that déjà vu and/or jamais vu keeps him from doing 90% of the activities he wants to do, then it would be a severe impairment (b1802.3).

There are no specific treatment recommendations for either déjà vu or jamais vu. Therapists should treat the underlying condition that is causing the memory disturbance.

## Cross References

In *Recreational Therapy for Specific Diagnoses and Conditions, First Edition*, ICF code b180 Experience of Self and Time Functions is listed in 13 chapters: Attention-Deficit/Hyperactivity Disorder, Borderline Personality Disorder, Burns, Feeding and Eating Disorders, Fibromyalgia and Juvenile Fibromyalgia, Generalized Anxiety Disorder, Intellectual Disability, Major Depressive Disorder, Multiple Sclerosis, Neurocognitive Disorders, Osteoporosis, Post-Traumatic Stress Disorder, and Spina Bifida.

In *Recreational Therapy Basics, Techniques, and Interventions, First Edition*, treatment for ICF code b180 Experience of Self and Time Functions is discussed in 15 chapters: Education and Counseling, Parameters and Precautions, Psychoneuroimmunology, Stress, Adaptive Sports, Adventure Therapy, Bibliotherapy, Cognitive Behavioral Counseling, Mind-Body Interventions, Montessori Method, Physical Activity, Reality Orientation, Reminiscence, Social Skills Training, and Therapeutic Thematic Arts Programming.

### b189 Specific Mental Functions, Other Specified or Unspecified

Any other Specific Mental Function, whether specified or unspecified, not mentioned in the previous categories is scored under this code. Therapists make a notation of the impairment to the right of the scored code.

### b198 Mental Functions, Other Specified

Any other specified Mental Function not mentioned in the previous categories is scored under this code. Therapists make a notation of the impairment to the right of the scored code.

### b199 Mental Functions, Unspecified

Any other unspecified Mental Function not mentioned in the previous categories is scored under this code. Therapists make a notation of the impairment to the right of the scored code.

## References

Atkinson, H. H., Rosano, C., Simonsick, E. M., Williamson, J. D., Davis, C., Ambrosius, W. T., Rapp, S. R., Cesari, M., Newman, A. B., Harris, T. B., Rubin, S. M., Yaffe, K., Satterfield, S., & Kritchevsky, S. (2007). Cognitive function, gait speed decline, and comorbidities: The health, aging and body composition study. *Journal of Gerontology, 62A*(8), 844-850.

Barco, P. P., Crosson, B., Bolesta, M. M., Werts, D., & Stout, R. (1991). Training awareness and compensation in post acute head injury rehabilitation. In Kreutzer, J. S. & Wehman, P. H. *Cognitive rehabilitation for persons with traumatic brain injury*. Bisbee, AZ: Imaginart Press.

Bernstein, D., Clarke-Stewart, A., Penner, L. A., & Roy, E. J. (2007). *Psychology*. Cengage Learning.

burlingame, j. (2001). *Idyll Arbor's therapy dictionary*, (2nd ed.). Ravensdale, WA: Idyll Arbor, Inc.

burlingame, j. & Blaschko, T. (2010). *Assessment tools for recreational therapy and related fields, fourth edition*. Ravensdale, WA: Idyll Arbor.

Davis, C. L., Tomporowski, P. D., Boyle, C. A., Waller, J. L., Miller, P. H., Naglieri, J. A., & Gregoski, M. (2007). Effects of aerobic exercise on overweight children's cognitive functioning. *Research Quarterly in Exercise Sport, 78*(5), 510-519.

Devinsky, O. & D'Esposito, M. (2003). *Neurology of cognitive and behavioral disorders*. Oxford University Press.

Edwards, D. F., Hahn, M., Baum, C., & Dromerick, A. W. (2006). The impact of mild stroke on meaningful activity and life satisfaction. *Journal of Stroke and Cerebrovascular Diseases, 15*(4), 151-157.

Farlex Partner Medical Dictionary. (2012). *Stupor*. Retrieved from http://medical-dictionary.thefreedictionary.com/stupor.

Fisher, M., Holland, C., Subramaniam, K., & Vinogradov, S. (2010). Neuroplasticity-based cognitive training in schizophrenia: An interim report on the effects 6 months later. *Schizophrenia Bulletin, 36*(4), 869-879.

Gale Encyclopedia of Medicine. (2008). *Delirium*. Retrieved from http://medical-dictionary.thefreedictionary.com/delirium.

Galvez-Jimenez, N. & Tuite, P. (2011). *Uncommon causes of movement disorders*. Cambridge University Press.

Halligan, P. W. (2006). Awareness and knowing: Implications for rehabilitation. *Neuropsychological Rehabilitation, 16*(4), 456-473.

Hockenbury, D. H. & Hockenbury, S. E. (2008). *Psychology*. Macmillan.

Horgan, O. & MacLachlan, M. (2004). Psychosocial adjustment to lower-limb amputation: A review. *Disability and Rehabilitation, 26*(14), 837-850.

Inzitari, M., Di Carlo, A., Baldereschi, M., Maggi, S., Pracucci, G., Scafato, E., Farchi, G., Inzitari, D. (2006). Risk and predictors of motor performance decline in a normally-functioning population-based sample of elderly subjects: The Italian longitudinal study on aging. *Journal of American Geriatrics Society 54*:318-324.

Koski, L., Iacoboni, M. & Mazziotta, J.C. (2002). Deconstructing apraxia: Understanding disorders of intentional movement after stroke. *Current Opinion in Psychiatry, 15*(1), 71-77.

Lautenschlager, N. T., Cox, K. L., Flicker, L., Foster, J. K., van Bockxmeer, F. M., Xiao, J., Greenop, K. R., & Almeida, O. P. (2008). Effect of physical activity on cognition function in older adults at risk for Alzheimer disease. *The Journal of the American Medical Association, 300*(9), 1027-1037.

Littlewood, R. (2004). Possession states. *Psychiatry, 3*(8), 8-10.

Majerus, S., Gill-Thwaites, H., Andrews, K., Laureys, S. (2005). Behavioral evaluation of consciousness in severe brain damage. *Prog Brain Res. 150*:397-413.

McCabe, P., Lippert, C., Weiser, M., Hilditch, M., Hartridge, C., & Villamere, J. (2007). Community reintegration following acquired brain injury. *Brain Injury, 21*(2), 231-257.

Miller, D. & Jake. L. (2001). *Eating disorders: Providing effective recreational therapy intervention.* Ravensdale, WA: Idyll Arbor.

Nathan, A. & Mirviss, S. (1998) *Therapy techniques using the creative arts.* Ravensdale, WA: Idyll Arbor.

National Institute of Neurological Disorders and Stroke. (2015). NINDS apraxia information page. Retrieved from http://www.ninds.nih.gov/disorders/apraxia/apraxia.htm

Nys, G. M. S., van Zandvoort, M. J. E., van der Worp, H. B., de Haan, E. H. F., de Kort, P. L. M., Jansen, B. P. W., & Kappelle, L. J. (2006). Early cognitive impairment predicts long-term depressive symptoms and quality of life after stroke. *Journal of the Neurological Sciences, 247*(2), 149-156.

O'Sullivan, S. & Schmitz, T. (1988). *Physical rehabilitation: Assessment and treatment.* Philadelphia, PA: F. A. Davis Company.

Petreska, B., Adriani, M., Blanke, O., & Billard, A. G. (2007). Apraxia: A review. In C. von Hofsten & K. Rosander (Eds.). *Progress in Brain Research*, vol. 164.

Potter, D. & Keeling, D. (2005). Effects of moderate exercise and circadian rhythms on human memory. *Journal of Sport and Exercise Psychology, 27*, 117-125.

Sadock, B. & Sadock, V. (2003). *Kaplan & Sadock's synopsis of psychiatry, 9th edition.* Philadelphia, PA: Lippincott Williams & Wilkins.

Segen's Medical Dictionary. (2012a). *Fugue state.* Retrieved from http://medical-dictionary.thefreedictionary.com/fugue+state.

Segen's Medical Dictionary. (2012b). *Trance state.* Retrieved from http://medical-dictionary.thefreedictionary.com/trance+state.

Vance, D. E. & Crowe, M. (2006). A proposed model of neuroplasticity and cognitive reserve in older adults. *Activities, Adaptation, and Aging, 30*(3), 61-79.

Zoltan, B. (1996). *Vision, perception, and cognition, 3rd edition.* Thorofare, NJ: Slack Incorporated.

Zoltan, B. (2007). *Vision, perception, and cognition, 4th edition.* Thorofare, NJ: Slack Incorporated.

Zuckerman, E. (2000). *Clinician's thesaurus, fifth edition.* New York: Guilford Publications.

# Chapter 2 Sensory Functions and Pain

This chapter is about the functions of the senses, seeing, hearing, tasting, and so on, as well as the sensation of pain.

*Sample Scoring of Sensory Functions and Pain*

- A client who had a stroke has resultant left neglect (b2101 Visual Field Functions). This means that he does not acknowledge the left half of his visual field (complete impairment = 4). The complete scoring would look like this: b2101.4.
- A child with juvenile rheumatoid arthritis complains of pain throughout all of her joints (b28016 Pain in Joints, complete impairment = 4). The complete scoring would look like this: b28016.4.

Sensory functions and pain have a direct relationship with health, functioning, and quality of life. For example, taste and smell, the things that make food enjoyable, have been found to deteriorate with age and older adulthood diseases such as Parkinson's and Alzheimer's. This results in decreased food intake, decreased interest in food, and decreased variety in the types of food eaten, causing macronutrient and micronutrient deficiencies (Ahmed & Haboubi, 2010). Individuals who undergo chemotherapy have also been found to have decreased or altered senses of taste and smell resulting in malnutrition, weight loss, and prolonged morbidity of chemotherapy-induced adverse effects (Steinbach et al., 2009).

For other senses, a study of 2956 older adults with hearing impairments showed significantly poorer health-related quality of life compared to those without hearing impairments (Chia et al., 2007).

In regards to pain, a meta-analysis of the literature on neuropathic pain found that it has a negative impact on physical functioning, emotional functioning (particularly affecting depression and anxiety), sleep, role and social functioning, and quality of life. Jensen et al. (2007) recommended that health-related quality of life be assessed regularly in patients with neuropathic pain to identify whether treatments that reduce pain also have additional benefits for quality of life.

Physical pain can also be a response to emotional pain. Consequently, a thorough review of underlying variables should always be included in an assessment. For example, in a study of 2360 adolescents aged 12-15, frequency and number of reported pains were positively related to levels of internalizing and externalizing problems (Larson & Sund, 2007).

Pain has also been found to impair engagement in life activities. For example, a focus group study of 33 individuals of various ages with rheumatoid arthritis found that pain affected everyday life activity and was a barrier to engagement in valued life activities (Ahlstrand et al., 2012).

*Assessment of Sensory Functions and Pain*

Assessment depends on the sense that is being tested. Refer to each of the codes in this chapter.

*Treatment of Sensory Functions and Pain*

Treatment also depends on the sense that is being tested. Refer to each of the codes in this chapter.

*Evidence Review*

Reviews of several studies are provided below to highlight evidence-based practice related to sensory functions and pain. This is only a sample of the evidence; further review of the literature may be needed to identify evidence-based practice interventions that address a particular deficit/concern.

Field, Diego, and Hernandez-Reif (2010) reviewed the literature on preterm infant massage. Infant massage involves moderate pressure stroking (tactile sensation) and flexion/extension of the upper and lower extremities (kinesthetic stimulation). On average, the massage was delivered for 10-15 minutes two to three times a day for 5-10 days. Findings indicated that the massage increased weight gain and decreased hospital days, saving approximately $10,000 per infant.

Body Function Theory (BFT), described as a "body experience approach to leisure" by Banhidi and Zintl (2015), is utilized in recreational therapy practice. It seeks to stimulate a person's five senses towards pleasure. This originated in the 1700s when "medical spas and thermal baths were a leisure-based therapeutic treatment prescribed by medical doctors so that wealthy people could experience leisure, under the false image of medial authority [because] leisure was still considered to be a form of waste or sloth contributing to societal ills…" (p. 69). The authors conclude that stimulation of the senses in a specific therapeutic manner can effect a person's perception of pleasure through all of the senses and thus contribute to quality of life and health.

Forty-six youths aged eight to 18 that utilized cochlear implants for hearing impairments participated in a one-week residential camp (Devine, Piatt, & Dawson, 2015). The camp consisted of traditional camp activities, such as swimming, crafts, hiking, and drama. The camp experience was designed to help participants learn skills that could be generalized to their home, school, and community life. The skills included: how to use spoken language more effectively, how to advocate for themselves in social settings, and how to care for their assistive hearing technology. Findings indicated that social acceptance and health-related quality of life scores were higher at post-camp and 10-week follow-up compared to pre-camp scores. A correlation between social acceptance and health-related quality of life was also found at post-camp and follow-up. The authors note that the correlation might be a consequence of "friendships built, social supports developed, and opportunities to engage in recreation with others who had similar abilities (including camp counselors) and experience a form of normalcy during camp" (p. 307). The authors recommend that individuals who use assistive listening devices for hearing impairments "be provided with opportunities to socially interact and develop bonds that can contribute to perceptions of social acceptance and an increased quality of life through recreation" (p. 307).

A secondary analysis of data from the National Longitudinal Transition Study-2 (n = 11,270) found that high community travel scores (using public transportation, arranging airplane or train trips, independently traveling to places outside the home) in youth with visual impairments predict post-school employment (Cmar, 2015). The author recommends that "Professionals can support students in gaining these vital skills by providing community experiences, positive role models, and verbal encouragement … [and that] [r]esearch-based predictors of

employment should be considered by planning transition services for adolescents with visual impairments" (p. 95).

There is strong evidence that pain-reducing treatment increases the quality of life for clients. The following studies are some of the findings that support the efficacy of recreational therapy modalities for the treatment of pain.

Guzman et al. (2006) conducted a review of 10 randomized studies of adults with at least three months of low back pain. The studies treated the pain in multi-disciplinary rehabilitation programs with a total of 1964 clients. Findings indicated that subjects who participated in an intensive multidisciplinary biopsychosocial rehabilitation program with a functional restoration approach had improved function (strong evidence) and reduced pain (moderate evidence) when compared with non-multidisciplinary treatments. Less intensive psychophysical treatments did not improve pain, function, or vocational readiness when compared to non-multidisciplinary therapy.

Stanos et al. (2007) outline the roles, responsibilities, and outcomes of a multidisciplinary approach to pain management in a rehabilitation setting. Recreational therapists are identified as prominent team players in identifying interests, addressing leisure barriers, leading activities to promote mental and physical health, teaching clients how to use strategies learned from other disciplines, such as correct biomechanics, pacing, relaxation techniques, in social and community functions, increasing social awareness, and promoting community integration. The recreational therapy treatments reduced stress, fear, and depression while fostering self-efficacy and confidence. Tai Chi, a common recreational therapy intervention, was also identified as an effective mind-body technique for pain management resulting in increased physical, mental, social, and emotional health; decreased anxiety; decreased pain perception; and increased flexibility. Incorporation of the mind and body in Tai Chi also helps to reprogram the nervous system, improve coordination, and reduce abnormal motor patterns.

Tomas-Carus et al. (2007) conducted a study of 34 females with fibromyalgia. Participants were divided into two groups: a 12-week aquatic exercise group that met in warm water for 60 minutes, three times a week and a control group that continued with their usual leisure activities. Those who participated in the exercise group showed less body pain and role emotional problems. They also showed improved physical function, general health perception, vitality, social function, mental health, balance, and stair climbing ability. At the end of the 12-week aquatic exercise program, the participants in the exercise group were instructed NOT to engage in exercise training for the following 12 weeks to determine if the gains would be maintained or lost. After the "detraining" period, the individuals in the exercise group continued to maintain a reduction in body pain and emotional problems. All other areas of gains were lost or reduced. The authors recommend continued engagement in physical activity to preserve gains.

Vonadies (2010) reviewed the literature related to guided imagery and pain. The literature indicates that guided imagery positively impacts the human immune system, reduces psychological perception of pain, improves mood, reduces symptoms of anxiety and depression, and reduces abdominal pain, chronic pain, post-operative pain, cancer pain, and burn pain. The authors provide a guided imagery protocol for recreational therapists to use with individuals experiencing pain.

Other studies show improved balance and proprioception as a result of recreational therapy interventions. Here are some examples.

Fong et al. (2012) conducted a study of 66 participants (42 adolescents and 24 adults — half Tae Kwon Do [TKD] practitioners and half non-TKD practitioners). They measured baseline sway velocity of the non-dominant leg, along with somatosensory, vestibular, and visual ratios. Adolescents who did not practice TKD showed significantly lower vestibular ratio than TKD adolescents and adults. TKD appears to speed up the development of postural control and vestibular function in adolescents. Consequently, the authors recommend that clinicians consider the use of TKD exercise as a therapeutic intervention for young people with balance or vestibular dysfunction.

Goldshtrom et al. (2011) conducted a study of children aged six to nine living in a group residential facility. Twenty-three children participated in an eight-week Rhythmex (rhythmic exercise) program, two to three times a week for five minutes. A control group consisting of 14 children did not participate in the program. Results indicated that the children who

participated in the program improved an average of 12 months on the *Visual-Motor Integration* scores from pre- to post-intervention compared to the control group. Aggressive behavior also significantly improved compared to the control group.

Lee et al. (2010) conducted a study of nine older adults (65+) without severe physical and cognitive impairment. The participants were from an adult day care program. In the study they engaged in the Dancing Heart Program, which consists of improvisational dance, personal story telling of the participants' past, and intergenerational dance performances with children. The program was held once a week for 90 minutes for eight months. Findings indicated the Dancing Heart Program helped improve physical and cognitive functioning, particularly flexibility, circulation, energy, balance, thinking, learning new things, remembering, coordination, strength, and endurance. It also decreased fear of falling and helped increase social interaction.

### Cross References

In *Recreational Therapy for Specific Diagnoses and Conditions, First Edition*, ICF code b2 Sensory Functions and Pain and its subcategories are listed in 29 chapters: Amputation and Prosthesis, Autism Spectrum Disorder, Back Disorders and Back Pain, Burns, Cancer, Cerebral Palsy, Cerebrovascular Accident, Chronic Obstructive Pulmonary Disease, Diabetes Mellitus, Epilepsy, Fibromyalgia and Juvenile Fibromyalgia, Guillain-Barré Syndrome, Hearing Loss, Heart Disease, Intellectual Disability, Major Depressive Disorder, Multiple Sclerosis, Osteoarthritis, Osteoporosis, Parkinson's Disease, Post-Traumatic Stress Disorder, Rheumatoid Arthritis, Sickle Cell Disease, Spina Bifida, Spinal Cord Injury, Substance-Related Disorders, Total Joint Replacement, Traumatic Brain Injury, and Visual Impairments and Blindness.

In *Recreational Therapy Basics, Techniques, and Interventions, First Edition*, treatment for ICF code b2 Sensory Functions and Pain and its subcategories are discussed in 17 chapters: Activity and Task Analysis, Body Mechanics and Ergonomics, Consequences of Inactivity, Parameters and Precautions, Psychoneuroimmunology, Stress, Activity Pattern Development, Adaptive Sports, Animal Assisted Therapy, Aquatic Therapy, Assertiveness Training, Balance Training, Cognitive Behavioral Counseling, Leisure Education and Counseling,

Mind-Body Interventions, Physical Activity, and Sensory Interventions.

## *Seeing and Related Functions (b210 - b229)*

### *b210 Seeing Functions*

Sensory functions relating to sensing the presence of light and sensing the form, size, shape, and color of the visual stimuli.

Inclusions: visual acuity functions; visual field functions; quality of vision; functions of sensing light and color, visual acuity of distant and near vision, monocular and binocular vision; visual picture quality; impairments such as myopia, hypermetropia, astigmatism, hemianopsia, color-blindness, tunnel vision, central and peripheral scotoma, diplopia, night blindness, and impaired adaptability to light

Exclusions: perceptual functions (b156)

- *b2100 Visual Acuity Functions*
  Seeing functions of sensing form and contour, both binocular and monocular, for both distant and near vision.

  o *b21000 Binocular Acuity of Distant Vision*
  Seeing functions of sensing size, form, and contour, using both eyes, for objects distant from the eye.

  o *b21001 Monocular Acuity of Distant Vision*
  Seeing functions of sensing size, form, and contour, using either right or left eye alone, for objects distant from the eye.

  o *b21002 Binocular Acuity of Near Vision*
  Seeing functions of sensing size, form, and contour, using both eyes, for objects close to the eye.

  o *b21003 Monocular Acuity of Near Vision*
  Seeing functions of sensing size, form, and contour, using either right or left eye alone, for objects close to the eye.

  o *b21008 Visual Acuity Functions, Other Specified*
  o *b21009 Visual Acuity Functions, Unspecified*
- *b2101 Visual Field Functions*
  Seeing functions related to the entire area that can be seen with fixation of gaze.

Inclusions: impairments such as in scotoma, tunnel vision, anopsia

- *b2102 Quality of Vision*
  Seeing functions involving light sensitivity, color vision, contrast sensitivity, and the overall quality of the picture.

  o *b21020 Light Sensitivity*
  Seeing functions of sensing a minimum amount of light (light minimum), and the minimum difference in intensity (light difference).

  Inclusions: functions of dark adaptation; impairments such as night blindness (hyposensitivity to light) and photophobia (hypersensitivity to light)

  o *b21021 Color Vision*
  Seeing functions of differentiating and matching colors.

  o *b21022 Contrast Sensitivity*
  Seeing functions of separating figure from ground, involving the minimum amount of luminance required.

  o *b21023 Visual Picture Quality*
  Seeing functions involving the quality of the picture.

  Inclusions: impairments such as in seeing stray lights, affected picture quality (floaters or webbing), picture distortion, and seeing stars or flashes

  o *b21028 Quality of Vision, Other Specified*
  o *b21029 Quality of Vision, Unspecified*
- *b2108 Seeing Functions, Other Specified*
- *b2109 Seeing Functions, Unspecified*

Recreational therapists must be aware of difficulties that clients have in seeing functions and how they affect participation in life activities. Visual impairments can be due to genetics (e.g., astigmatism), injury to the visual center of the brain (e.g., stroke, traumatic brain injury, multiple sclerosis), injury to the structures of the eye (e.g., damage to the retina), and the normal aging process. Impairments that affect seeing functions include cataract, macular degeneration, and diabetic retinopathy. Therapists need to be aware of visual functions as they affect normal activity. If an impairment is noted, the therapist scores the extent of the visual impairment along with the related Activities and Participation categories that are affected by the visual impairment, such as d166 Reading.

The three subheadings of b210 Seeing Functions each have their own evaluation, treatment, and adaptation techniques, as described below.

### Visual Acuity

Common conditions that affect a person's ability to see at far and near distances include:

- *Myopia* (near sightedness): A person is able to see things up close but has difficulty seeing things that are at a distance.
- *Hyperopia* (far sightedness): A person is able to see things at a distance but has difficulty seeing things that are close.
- *Astigmatism*: In the normal, healthy eye, light rays from an object enter the eye and converge to create a clear picture. In astigmatism, the light rays that enter the eye do not converge at a single point because of cornea or lens distortion or the shape of the eyeball. The rays may focus correctly in one direction, but they do not focus in other directions at the same time resulting in a blurry picture.
- *Amblyopia* (lazy eye): There is a decreased acuity of vision, also referred to as a dimness of vision, in one eye. No physical defect or disease accounts for the impairment. Most people have a dominant eye. In amblyopia the non-dominant eye has become so much less dominant that the brain-eye connection has weakened enough to result in less visual acuity.
- *Diplopia* (double vision): This is usually the result of decreased range of motion in one eye although it may also be related to amblyopia or physical damage to one eye.
- *Depth perception problems*: The client has difficulty determining the distance of objects by using binocular vision.
- *Total blindness*: No sight.
- *Legally blind*: Visual acuity of less than 6/60 or 20/200 or visual field restriction of 20° or less.
- *Glaucoma*: A disease of the eye that increases intraocular fluid pressure. If left untreated, the optic disk becomes damaged, the eyeball can harden, and partial to complete loss of vision can occur, starting with a loss of peripheral vision.

- *Macular degeneration*: Damage to the macula of the retina that causes blindness in the center of the visual field. It is caused by several different diseases. In severe cases complete loss of vision may occur in the macular region.

Visual acuity is evaluated by measuring how clearly a person is able to see at various distances. burlingame (2001) says, "Visual acuity is measured by stating '20/__,' with the value placed in the blank space representing how far/close a person must be to an object to perceive it as clearly as a person with normal vision would at 20 feet. In other words, if a client had a visual acuity of 20/200, the client could see clearly at 20 feet what most people can see clearly at 200 feet" (p 312). The definition for legal blindness of "6/60" is a measure of near vision that means the person can see as well at six feet as a normal person can see at 60 feet.

The therapist scores the extent of the visual acuity impairment as it affects the client's ability to participate in activities using the terms no, mild, moderate, severe, and complete with corresponding impairment scores of 0, 1, 2, 3, or 4. Moderate impairment of binocular acuity of near vision would be scored b21002.2. It is possible to have a different score for different activities, with the activity noted to the right of the score. In addition to the extent of impairment, a therapist will score the Activities and Participation codes that are affected by visual acuity impairments and make additional notes in their own documentation that describe compensatory techniques, equipment, and/or assistance needed. An example might be "Secondary to myopia, client wears prescription lenses at all times in community settings to clearly see signage."

Treatment for myopia, hyperopia, astigmatism, and legal blindness generally requires prescription lenses, although laser surgery is becoming a popular option. If a person has amblyopia, the strong eye may be patched for periods of time to strengthen the lazy eye.

If double vision (diplopia) is a problem, clients are often instructed to alternate which eye wears the patch so that they wear the patch on the right eye one day and then the left eye the next day. This eliminates one of the two images, but it adds a new problem of not having depth perception. Range of motion exercises for the eye along with the use of the alternating patch may resolve the problem. If the problem does not resolve, the client is referred to an ophthalmologist for further evaluation and recommendations. Diplopia is typically caused by damage to the brain due to traumatic brain injury, stroke, or multiple sclerosis.

If depth perception is a problem, the client will have difficulty determining the distance of objects, posing a challenge to reaching out and accurately grasping an object, judging the distance of traffic, and walking up and down stairs. People who have depth perception problems can often learn how to correctly judge the distance of objects, but it requires practice. The therapist should provide a sufficient number of situations for the client to feel comfortable in a real-world situation on his/her own.

Glaucoma is treated with eye drops that helps to decrease the pressure of the eye or with surgery to create a bleb, seen as a lump above the iris, that helps in draining the aqueous humors in the eye and, thereby, reducing the pressure.

Therapists who have clients with any of these conditions need to encourage their clients to follow the appropriate procedures. This ranges from coming up with strategies to keep glasses from being lost to devising ways to make sure the client wears a patch at appropriate times and takes eye drops as required. Other adaptations that might be required include large print books, larger calendars, special screen settings on computers to allow larger font sizes, and larger signage. For some situations the client can carry a magnifier, ranging from eyeglasses to a closed circuit television system, to help with activities.

If a person is legally blind or totally blind, the person is taught how to use other senses (e.g., listening for the clicking noise at the traffic light and the sound of the traffic to sense when the light has changed, reading Braille), adaptations (e.g., pinning socks together before throwing them in the wash; keeping one dollar bills flat, folding five dollar bills in half, and folding ten dollar bills in quarters), assistance from others (e.g., seeing eye dog, spouse), technology (e.g., talking watch, computer program that reads aloud), and mobility equipment for safety (e.g., walking stick).

### Visual Field Functions

Common visual field impairments include:

- *Visual neglect*: A lack of awareness of one side of the environment, also known as hemianopsia.

Left neglect is very common in individuals who have a right cerebrovascular accident (CVA). The person neglects the left side of his/her environment from the midline over. Symptoms include bumping into things on the left and lack of awareness of items that are on the left side of the table. Seeing functions in the both eyes are usually intact, but the brain is incapable of processing information from the left half of both visual fields. It is not an eye problem. Unlike other kinds of visual function problems, a person with visual neglect can't see objects in the left half of his/her visual field *and* she also loses the awareness that there is *anything on* the left side of his/her body. Neglect can be very dangerous. A client with neglect doesn't have the proper brain function to realize that there may be a car coming down the road from the left when attempting to cross the street. It is also difficult to use environmental cues: When walking down a hallway, a client who has left neglect will have no awareness of what is on the left side of the hall. On the return trip, the client will report that there is nothing familiar about the hallway because he didn't see the left side of the hallway on the way there and can't see the original right side of the hallway, which he was watching on the first trip, on the way back.

- *Field loss*: A person's visual field is described as the total area that the person is able to see without moving his/her eye. "The normal monocular field of vision is approximately 60° upward, 60° inward, 70-75° downward, and 100-110° outward" (Zoltan, 1996, p 33). Field loss is actually loss of visual function in a certain visual field quadrant of the eye. Each eye is divided into four quadrants, upper and lower, left and right. Field loss is often the result of brain injury. Some of the terms used are

  o Homonymous hemianopsia: loss of the outer half of the visual field from one eye and the inner half of the visual field of the other eye. See visual neglect, above.

  o Circumferential blindness: No vision around the circumference of each eye's visual field.

  o Bitemporal hemianopsia: Loss of the outer vision of both eyes.

o   Homonymous inferior quadrantanopsia: loss of vision in right or left lower quadrant of both eyes.

- *Visual spatial inattention*: Visual neglect of particular quadrant(s) of the eye. It is inattention due to a brain dysfunction, rather than a vision loss due to damage of the eye.

When evaluating visual field function, the therapist will score the visual field function code based on the percentage of field loss. Homonymous hemianopsia, because it is loss of half the field of view would be scored b2101.3. The therapist also documents the type of visual field loss, amount of assistance needed, the client's ability to utilize compensatory strategies, and safety concerns related to visual field problems along with recommended safety precautions. In addition to the extent of impairment, a therapist will score the Activities and Participation codes that are affected by visual field loss.

Visual field defects may resolve with neuroplasticity, although in many cases they do not. Recreational therapists do not provide treatment for visual field defects, but they do provide many important adaptations.

In cases of visual neglect, clients are taught how to compensate for neglect by turning their head to the neglected side to scan the neglected side of the environment. Visual cues, often referred to as anchors, can be helpful. These are brightly colored lines that are placed on the far side of the neglected environment as a visual cue so that the client knows when s/he has turned his/her head far enough to see the neglected environment. Two ways to provide cues are to stick a piece of red tape along the neglected side of the computer monitor frame or place a neon colored ruler on the neglected side of a book page.

In addition to an anchor, the therapist uses multimodal cues to prompt the client to turn his/her head to the neglected side. This may include verbal cues such as "Do you see the pen? Keep turning your head to the left until you see the pen," gestural cues such as pointing to the left side of the client's neglected environment, or auditory cues such as tapping on the left side of the table to cue the client to turn his/her head to the neglected left side.

The ultimate goal is for the client to independently scan the neglected environment using a consistent rhythmic approach. This is accomplished while walking when the client turns his head to the left to scan the neglected left side of the environment with every other step taken. While reading, the client routinely turns her head to the left to scan the neglected left side after reaching the right side of the page.

If the client is unable to independently compensate for visual neglect, precautions must be taken to ensure the safety of the client. Such adaptations and precautions include the use of mirrors. Placing mirrors on the unaffected visual side can cue the client to look towards the neglected side or, at the very least, provide a reflection of the neglected environment in the unaffected visual field. For example, placing a mirror on the opposite wall directly across from the bathroom door alerts a client who is walking down the hallway to a bathroom door on the person's neglected side.

Another technique is to use bicycle mirrors. Place a pair of prescription or non-prescription glasses on the client and clip a bicycle mirror to the outer edge of the frame of the glasses on the unaffected side. Play around with the positioning of the bicycle mirror so that when the client looks straight ahead s/he sees a reflection of the neglected side in the unaffected visual field. This way when a client with left neglect looks straight ahead, he sees the right side of the environment and a reflection of the left side of his environment. There are no studies on the effectiveness of mirrors and left neglect but they are commonly used in rehabilitation facilities as a technique for accommodation. Mirrors are not helpful for all clients, especially those who are unable to identify that the reflection is of the opposite side.

Teaching clients how to compensate for field loss and visual-spatial inattention is the same as visual neglect. The client needs to learn how to move his/her head into a position that allows him/her to see in the area of field loss. Mirrors, however, are not usually used. Since the client only needs to compensate for a small piece of visual field loss or inattention, the use of mirrors can become confusing, bothersome, and ineffective.

### Quality of Vision

Quality of vision can be affected by night blindness (hyposensitivity — decreased sensitivity to light making it difficult to see when it is dark), photophobia (hypersensitivity — increased sensitivity to daylight making it difficult to see during the day), color blindness (partial or total inability to distinguish certain colors, usually red from green, or a total inability to see colors), floaters, stray lights, and seeing stars or flashes. Hypersensitivity that requires the client to wear sunglasses for comfort when outside might be scored as a moderate impairment b21020.2.

Documentation of quality of vision is usually done by another member of the treatment team, but the recreational therapist may be one of the first to notice changes in vision that show up during activities. In many cases early detection and reporting to the rest of the team can limit the amount of damage that occurs.

The recreational therapist will document Activities and Participation codes that are affected by visual impairments and make additional notes in their own documentation, including the specific quality of vision dysfunction (e.g., client has floater that distracts him when reading), the extent that the impairment interferes with specific activities (e.g., difficulty seeing the card rack causes a moderate impairment with card playing), compensatory strategies taught and implemented (e.g., client educated about adaptations for night blindness), effectiveness of compensatory strategies (e.g., client independently matched and coordinated an outfit using clothing labels that have the color of the piece of clothing written on the clothing label), and amount of assistance required to function in particular situations (e.g., requires moderate assistance to read menu in a dark restaurant).

Treatment may be performed in part by the therapist, but it is more likely that the therapist will be responsible for appropriate adaptations, as discussed below.

People who have night blindness should avoid driving at night and have adequate lighting in the home when it becomes dark. Bright nightlights can be especially helpful if s/he needs to get up in the middle of the night. If nightlights are not sufficient, turning on a table lamp before getting out of bed during the night may be an adaptation that is necessary for safety. It is normal for people, as they get older, to require more light to see because the retina gets thicker. Therapists working with older adults should be sure that they provide adequate lighting in their environment for all of their activities,

especially ones requiring fine visual discrimination, such as reading.

If photophobia is present, the person benefits from wearing protective sunglasses and staying out of direct sunlight. The therapist needs to make sure that eye shades, such as caps, and sunglasses are available and used as appropriate.

Depending on the colors that are indistinguishable, people who are colorblind will need to make accommodations. These include pinning matched socks together before putting them in the wash, labeling clothes with the name of their color, and watching for the location of traffic lights to determine which color is lit.

Other treatment and adaptations may be required for contrast sensitivity and overall picture quality. Often practice will improve the client's ability to work around the vision problems. Adaptations include learning to take second and third looks to be sure of what was actually seen and making sure that adequate lighting is always available. Some of the adaptations described for low visual acuity functions (b2100 Visual Acuity Functions) may also be helpful.

See the Visual Impairments and Blindness chapter in the *Recreational Therapy for Specific Diagnoses and Conditions* book for more information.

***Cross References***

In *Recreational Therapy for Specific Diagnoses and Conditions, First Edition*, ICF code b210 Seeing Functions is listed in eight chapters: Cerebral Palsy, Cerebrovascular Accident, Diabetes Mellitus, Epilepsy, Guillain-Barré Syndrome, Multiple Sclerosis, Traumatic Brain Injury, and Visual Impairments and Blindness.

In *Recreational Therapy Basics, Techniques, and Interventions, First Edition*, treatment for ICF code b210 Seeing Functions is discussed in two chapters: Activity and Task Analysis and Balance Training.

### *b215 Functions of Structures Adjoining the Eye*

Functions of structures in and around the eye that facilitate seeing functions.

Inclusions: functions of internal muscles of the eye, eyelid, external muscles of the eye, including voluntary and tracking movements and fixation of the eye, lachrymal glands, accommodation, pupillary reflex; impairments such as in nystagmus, xerophthalmia, and ptosis

Exclusions: seeing functions (b210); b7 Neuromusculoskeletal and Movement-Related Functions

- *b2150 Functions of Internal Muscles of the Eye*
  Functions of the muscles inside the eye, such as the iris, that adjust the shape and size of the pupil and lens of the eye.

  Inclusions: functions of accommodation; pupillar reflex

- *b2151 Functions of the Eyelid*
  Functions of the eyelid, such as the protective reflex.

- *b2152 Functions of External Muscles of the Eye*
  Functions of the muscles that are used to look in different directions, to follow an object as it moves across the visual field, to produce saccadic jumps to catch up with a moving target, and to fix the eye.

  Inclusions: nystagmus; cooperation of both eyes

- *b2153 Functions of Lachrymal Glands*
  Functions of the tear glands and ducts.

- *b2158 Functions of Structures Adjoining the Eye, Other Specified*
- *b2159 Functions of Structure Adjoining the Eye, Unspecified*

Problems with the structures adjoining the eye can cause significant problems for clients. Nystagmus, as well as fixation and tracking problems, can impact many activities including walking and fine motor activities. Eyelid functioning can affect the wetness of the eye and may require eye drops if the eyelid does not blink. If one eyelid does not open, depth perception problems will be present.

Therapists evaluate problems by scoring one of the categories if an impairment is noted. Other common problems that a therapist may note are impairments caused by nystagmus (jumpy vision), fixation and tracking of the eye, and eyelid functioning. Problems with the pupil and iris muscles will be scored here, but they may also cause problems with vision that should be scored in the earlier codes for visual functioning. For example, if the iris is damaged so the pupil has a mild impairment in closing (b2151.1), the client will almost certainly have some photophobia that should be scored with

b21020 Light Sensitivity. The therapist will be mainly responsible for reporting how these functional deficits impact Activities and Participation by using the codes in that section.

Treatment and adaptations will generally be in activities supporting the goals of other team members including encouraging the client to work on strengthening and controlling eye movements through range of motion exercises and using eye drops as appropriate. Adaptations required for Activities and Participation codes should be scored using those codes.

### Cross References

In *Recreational Therapy for Specific Diagnoses and Conditions, First Edition*, ICF code b215 Functions of Structures Adjoining the Eye is listed in two chapters: Rheumatoid Arthritis and Visual Impairments and Blindness.

In *Recreational Therapy Basics, Techniques, and Interventions, First Edition*, there are no references for b215 Functions of Structures Adjoining the Eye.

### b220 Sensations Associated with the Eye and Adjoining Structures

Sensations of tired, dry, and itching eye and related feelings.

Inclusions: feelings of pressure behind the eye, of something in the eye, eye strain, burning in the eye; eye irritation

Exclusion: sensation of pain (b280)

If a client has problems with any of the sensations mentioned above, the therapist scores this code as it relates to the extent of the impairment, such as mild eye irritation (b220.1). Some of these conditions, especially sensations of pressure or burning, may be indications of serious conditions. Sudden onsets should be reported to the medical team immediately.

The therapist usually will not have a direct intervention for these problems. However therapists need to be aware of these problems because they impact participation in activities, such as irritation of the eye that impacts ability to focus on the computer screen for 30 minutes as required for writing a letter. Therapists will be responsible for making sure ongoing treatment is carried out during recreational therapy groups and activities.

Adaptations required for Activities and Participation codes should be scored using those codes.

### Cross References

In *Recreational Therapy for Specific Diagnoses and Conditions, First Edition*, there are no references for ICF code b220 Sensations Associated with the Eye and Adjoining Structures.

In *Recreational Therapy Basics, Techniques, and Interventions, First Edition*, there are no references for ICF code b220 Sensations Associated with the Eye and Adjoining Structures.

### b229 Seeing and Related Functions, Other Specified and Unspecified

Any other seeing or related functions, whether specified or unspecified, not mentioned in the previous categories are scored under this code. Therapists make a notation of the problem to the right of the scored code.

## Hearing and Vestibular Functions (b230 - b249)

### b230 Hearing Functions

Sensory functions relating to sensing the presence of sounds and discriminating the location, pitch, loudness, and quality of sounds.

Inclusions: functions of hearing, auditory discrimination, localization of sound source, lateralization of sound, speech discrimination; impairments such as deafness, hearing impairment, and hearing loss

Exclusions: perceptual functions (b156) and mental functions of language (b167)

- *b2300 Sound Detection*
  Sensory functions relating to sensing the presence of sounds.

- *b2301 Sound Discrimination*
  Sensory functions relating to sensing the presence of sound involving the differentiation of ground and binaural synthesis, separation, and blending.

- *b2302 Localization of Sound Source*
  Sensory functions relating to determining the location of the source of sound.

- *b2303 Lateralization of Sound*
  Sensory functions relating to determining whether the sound is coming from the right or left side.

- *b2304 Speech Discrimination*
  Sensory functions relating to determining spoken language and distinguishing it from other sounds.

- *b2308 Hearing Functions, Other Specified*
- *b2309 Hearing Functions, Unspecified*

If hearing functions are impaired, the person should receive further evaluation from relevant health professionals, such as an ear, nose, and throat physician or an audiologist, to determine the specific problems and interventions needed.

It is possible that the therapist may become aware of hearing problems before the rest of the treatment team, especially those related to activities such as localization or lateralization of sound. If the therapist notes a problem, s/he should request a referral as needed for further evaluation. Any issues related to Activities and Participation should be documented using those codes. Examples include d350 Conversation, d115 Listening, and d7600 Parent-Child Relationships.

Recreational therapists do not treat hearing impairments, but they may be responsible for helping the client learn how to use adaptive hearing equipment in real-life settings.

Hearing impairments can be a safety concern because the client will not be able to hear warning sounds or activity cues, such as smoke detectors, doorbells, or oven timers. The client may need to be instructed in the use of adaptive equipment, such as a flashing light on the telephone, flashing light by the door to signal a ringing doorbell, and timers that produce a vibration instead of a sound. Clients who are deaf or significantly hearing impaired might benefit from learning sign language along with exploration of other forms of communication, such as augmentative communication devices, verbalizations, writing, gesturing, body language, and TTY for using the telephone.

### Cross References

In *Recreational Therapy for Specific Diagnoses and Conditions, First Edition*, ICF code b230 Hearing Functions is listed in two chapters: Cerebral Palsy and Hearing Loss.

In *Recreational Therapy Basics, Techniques, and Interventions, First Edition*, there are no references for ICF code b230 Hearing Functions.

### b235 Vestibular Functions

Sensory functions of the inner ear related to position, balance, and movement.

Inclusions: functions of position and positional sense; functions of balance of the body and movement

Exclusion: sensation associated with hearing and vestibular functions (b240)

- *b2350 Vestibular Function of Position*
  Sensory functions of the inner ear related to determining the position of the body.

- *b2351 Vestibular Function of Balance*
  Sensory functions of the inner ear related to determining the balance of the body.

- *b2352 Vestibular Function of Determination of Movement*
  Sensory functions of the inner ear related to determining movement of the body, including its direction and speed.

- *b2358 Vestibular Functions, Other Specified*
- *b2359 Vestibular Functions, Unspecified*

Vestibular impairments may be deduced by a therapist by ruling out other problems that can cause difficulty with positioning, balance, and movement, such as brain injury, loss of strength, impaired flexibility, and impaired motor planning. However, vestibular impairments are best determined by specific testing and evaluation of the inner ear. Consequently, the health professional who confirms a vestibular problem would most likely be the one to score these codes. A moderate balance impairment, with balance affecting about 30% of normal activities, would be scored as b2351.2. Therapists are more likely to use codes in the Activities and Participation Chapters that are affected by vestibular impairments, such as d4602 Moving Around outside the Home and Other Buildings or d415 Maintaining a Body Position.

Additional notes related to vestibular impairments that therapists may make in their documentation include the extent that it interferes with specific activities and compensatory strategies taught and implemented. For example, "Vestibular problems with balance cause a moderate impairment with walking. Client educated about safety precautions to decrease risk of falls from vestibular balance problems."

Vestibular impairments may or may not be able to be corrected. Much of the treatment will be medical, but the therapist is involved in providing activities that help in the retraining of stability, position, and balance. Often vestibular problems are only a part of balance issues. The therapist can provide valuable exercises that help other parts of the problem such as strength and proprioception from nerve pathways besides the inner ear.

If vestibular problems remain, therapists prescribe equipment and adaptations to minimize risk of injury. Two books that describe treatment for balance problems are Best-Martini and Jones-DiGenova (2014), *Exercises for Frail Elders* and Rose (2010) *FallProof! A Comprehensive Balance and Mobility Training Program*.

### Cross References

In *Recreational Therapy for Specific Diagnoses and Conditions, First Edition*, ICF code b235 Vestibular Functions is listed in seven chapters: Cerebral Palsy, Cerebrovascular Accident, Guillain-Barré Syndrome, Hearing Loss, Osteoarthritis, Osteoporosis, and Substance-Related Disorders.

In *Recreational Therapy Basics, Techniques, and Interventions, First Edition*, treatment for ICF code b235 Vestibular Functions is discussed in four chapters: Body Mechanics and Ergonomics, Aquatic Therapy, Balance Training, and Mind-Body Interventions.

### b240 Sensations Associated with Hearing and Vestibular Functions

Sensations of dizziness, falling, tinnitus, and vertigo.

Inclusions: sensations of ringing in ears, irritation in ear, aural pressure, nausea associated with dizziness or vertigo

Exclusions: vestibular functions (b235); sensation of pain (b280)

- *b2400 Ringing in Ears or Tinnitus*
  Sensation of low-pitched rushing, hissing, or ringing in the ear.

- *b2401 Dizziness*
  Sensation of motion involving either oneself or one's environment; sensation of rotating, swaying, or tilting.

- *b2402 Sensation of Falling*
  Sensation of losing one's grip and falling.

- *b2403 Nausea Associated with Dizziness or Vertigo*
  Sensation of wanting to vomit that arises from dizziness or vertigo.

- *b2404 Irritation in the Ear*
  Sensation of itching or other similar sensations in the ear.

- *b2405 Aural Pressure*
  Sensation of pressure in the ear.

- *b2408 Sensations Associated with Hearing and Vestibular Function, Other Specified*
- *b2409 Sensations Associated with Hearing and Vestibular Function, Unspecified*

The recreational therapist may make notations about specific sensation impairment, such as ringing in the ears or nausea during long car rides, to the extent that it interferes with specific activities. A mild impairment in hearing caused by tinnitus would be scored b2400.1. Activities and Participation codes that are affected by any of the impairments, such as d9200 Play, d640 Doing Housework, or d4553 Jumping, should also be scored.

The therapist inquires about some, but not all, of these sensations. It is more common for therapists to rely on the client to tell the therapist about feeling such sensations and only inquire about these sensations when they are suspected by observed actions, such as loss of balance, pressing on the ear, or doubling over.

Sometimes the impairments are correctable with pharmacology. The therapist documents the extent of correction observed in real-life situations.

Compensatory strategies may be taught and implemented. Documentation should include the effectiveness of compensatory strategies and amount of assistance required to minimize problems with these sensations.

If impairments persist, therapists assist the client in identifying adaptations to minimize risk of injury and maximize functional performance. Examples include avoiding activities that stimulate sensation impairment, such as riding in a car for a prolonged period of time, increasing attention to or asking another's opinion about a sound or noise if the client is unable to hear it correctly due to ringing in the ears.

***Cross References***

In *Recreational Therapy for Specific Diagnoses and Conditions, First Edition*, ICF code b240 Sensations Associated with Hearing and Vestibular Functions is listed in two chapters: Cerebrovascular Accident (Stroke) and Hearing Loss.

In *Recreational Therapy Basics, Techniques, and Interventions, First Edition*, there are no references for ICF code b240 Sensations Associated with Hearing and Vestibular Functions.

### b249 Hearing and Vestibular Functions, Other Specified and Unspecified

Any other Hearing and Vestibular Functions, whether specified or unspecified, not mentioned in the previous categories is scored under this code. Therapists make a notation of the impairment to the right of the scored code.

## Additional Sensory Functions (b250 - b279)

### b250 Taste Function

Sensory functions of sensing qualities of bitterness, sweetness, sourness, and saltiness.

Inclusions: gustatory functions; impairments such as ageusia and hypogeusia

There are four broad classifications of taste including sweet, sour, bitter, and salty. Each taste is sensed by receptors on a particular portion of the tongue. The taste buds on the tongue transmit their information to the medial temporal lobe. The combination of the signals from these receptors form part of what we call taste. The rest of what we call taste is made up of a combination of other senses including the sense of smell, touch, vision, and hearing. This code deals only with the part that comes directly from the mouth.

To evaluate, the therapist notes how impaired the client's sense of taste is. A complete loss of the sense of taste would be scored as b250.4. In addition to noting the extent of the impairment, therapists may make additional notes about taste impairments such as level of assistance required to adapt to any impairments, for example, "Client is independent in identifying expiration dates on food items."

Recreational therapists are more likely to score issues with taste in the Activities and Participation code d120 Other Purposeful Sensing, which is intentionally using the sense of taste to experience stimuli. Documentation should also include impact on activity, as in "Client reports loss of pleasure in eating secondary to taste function impairment. Consequently, client has been consuming fewer calories and has lost 20 pounds within the last month."

Recreational therapists do not provide treatment for problems with taste.

They do provide adaptations. People who have taste impairments are instructed to be alert to food expiration dates and food labels. For example, a client may be eating a salty food without realizing it by taste when client should not eat salty foods because of high blood pressure. The recreational therapist can help with these adaptations by showing the client how to read sodium levels on food packages and explaining other ways besides taste to identify foods the may not be edible, such as checking expiration dates and paying attention to the temperature of foods.

### Cross References

In *Recreational Therapy for Specific Diagnoses and Conditions, First Edition*, there are no references for ICF code b250 Taste Function.

In *Recreational Therapy Basics, Techniques, and Interventions, First Edition*, there are no references for ICF code b250 Taste Function.

### b255 Smell Function

Sensory functions of sensing odors and smells.

Inclusions: olfactory functions; impairments such as anosmia or hyposmia

It is estimated that people can discriminate among 10,000 different odors (Sadock & Sadock, 2003). Once an odor enters the nose it stimulates communication to the olfactory bulb in the brain where it is interpreted.

Recreational therapists generally do not score this code. They are more likely to score the Activities and Participation code d120 Other Purposeful

Sensing, which is intentionally using the sense of smell to experience stimuli.

Recreational therapists note specific problems, such as inability to identify the smell of smoke, level of assistance required for compensatory strategies, and impact on activity. For example, "Client reports loss of interest in cooking secondary to smell impairments. Consequently, client has been eating packaged heat-up meals that are not meeting her nutrition needs."

Treatment of problems with the sense of smell is usually the responsibility of other members of the medical team. The recreational therapist is responsible for teaching adaptations that will keep the client safe in the home and community.

Adaptations provided by recreational therapists include ways to compensate for smell deficits. People who are unable to smell or have difficulty discriminating odors need to take additional precautions for safety, such as smoke detectors, and be alert to dangerous situations that are normally discovered by smell. They should not, for example, leave food unattended on the stovetop and should have a gas heater checked regularly for leaks.

### Cross References

In *Recreational Therapy for Specific Diagnoses and Conditions, First Edition*, ICF code b255 Smell Function is listed in one chapter: Parkinson's Disease.

In *Recreational Therapy Basics, Techniques, and Interventions, First Edition*, there are no references for ICF code b255 Smell Function.

### b260 Proprioceptive Function

Sensory functions of sensing the relative position of body parts.

Inclusions: functions of statesthesia and kinesthesia

Exclusions: vestibular functions (b235); sensations related to muscles and movement functions (b780)

Proprioceptive functioning is the ability to identify where a limb is in space without vision. It includes both position (statesthesia) and movement (kinesthesia). To evaluate statesthesia, the client should close his/her eyes and the therapist should slowly move one of the client's limbs, such as slowly moving the right arm from client's lap out laterally. Ask the client to describe where the limb is located. To evaluate kinesthesia, ask the client to close his/her eyes and then passively and slowly move a client's limb into a different position. Ask the client to describe what movements the therapist made with the limb.

Although the function of proprioception is coded as an isolated skill in this chapter, the function of proprioception is required for many skills requiring physical movement including d450 Walking, d420 Transferring Oneself, and d4554 Swimming. Impairments in functioning in other areas should be noted using the relevant codes.

The therapist assesses the extent of the proprioceptive impairment, including specific proprioceptive impairments, the extent that it interferes with specific activities, compensatory strategies taught and implemented, effectiveness of compensatory strategies, and amount of assistance required to minimize proprioceptive problems. The code may be scored based on its effect on other activities with a moderate impairment scored as b260.2 and a note on the activities affected.

Recreational therapy treatment for problems with proprioception involves providing practice with positioning and movement in real-life situations. As noted in the Fong et al. (2012) study, clients can improve their abilities related to movement and positioning.

If proprioception impairments do not fully resolve, clients are taught how to compensate for the deficits by using the sense of vision.

### Cross References

In *Recreational Therapy for Specific Diagnoses and Conditions, First Edition*, ICF code b260 Proprioceptive Function is listed in five chapters: Cerebral Palsy, Cerebrovascular Accident, Chronic Obstructive Pulmonary Disease, Spina Bifida, and Spinal Cord Injury.

In *Recreational Therapy Basics, Techniques, and Interventions, First Edition*, treatment for ICF code b260 Proprioceptive Function is discussed in three chapters: Activity and Task Analysis, Aquatic Therapy, and Physical Activity.

### b265 Touch Function

Sensory functions of sensing surfaces and their texture or quality.

Inclusions: functions of touching, feeling of touch; impairments such as numbness, anesthesia, tingling, paresthesia, and hyperesthesia

Exclusions: sensory functions related to temperature and other stimuli (b270)

Therapists score this code if there is touch function impairment. This is different from the Activities and Participation code d120 Other Purposeful Sensing, which is intentionally using the sense of touch to experience stimuli. It is unclear why there is an overlap in the inclusions for b265 Touch Function and b2702 Sensitivity to Pressure. We suggest that the therapist be aware of the overlap and score functions where the client has functional difficulties sensing a surface or an object using this code. Dysfunctions in sensing passive touch should be scored with codes included in b2702 Sensitivity to Pressure.

Therapists commonly evaluate sensation of light touch and stereognosis as it pertains to the client's ability to perform life tasks, such as identifying a house key when standing outside the house at night and experiencing pleasure from light touch in intimacy.

To evaluate light touch the therapist asks the client to close his/her eyes. The therapist then gently touches the client with various items, such as a cotton ball or a Q-tip and asks the client to tell the therapist what the object feels like. To evaluate stereognosis, the therapist asks the client to close his/her eyes and places a common item like a hairbrush or key in the client's hand. The client is asked to identify the item by touch.

Documentation should include the type and extent of the touch impairment. Numbness reducing the sense of touch by 60% would be scored as b265.3. The therapist should document the specific touch impairment (e.g., light touch absent in the right upper extremity), the extent that it interferes with specific activities (e.g., poor stereognosis impairs client's ability to identify the light switch in the dark), compensatory strategies taught and implemented (e.g., client educated about using night lights to compensate for stereognosis), effectiveness of compensatory strategies (e.g., client able to independently find his house key on his key ring in the dark by using a keychain light), and amount of assistance required to minimize touch problems. Related

Activities and Participation codes that are affected by touch impairment, such as d770 Intimate Relationships, should also be scored.

Recreational therapists do not provide treatment for impairments with touch functions, but they may be asked to evaluate the effectiveness of treatment in real-life situations.

If touch functions continue to be impaired after treatment, compensatory strategies are taught to minimize injury and maximize safety, such as using visual skills to evaluate the texture of something if the client is unable to identify it by feel.

### Cross References

In *Recreational Therapy for Specific Diagnoses and Conditions, First Edition*, ICF code b265 Touch Function is listed in six chapters: Amputation and Prosthesis, Cerebral Palsy, Diabetes Mellitus, Fibromyalgia and Juvenile Fibromyalgia, Guillain-Barré Syndrome, and Spina Bifida.

In *Recreational Therapy Basics, Techniques, and Interventions, First Edition*, there are no references for ICF code b265 Touch Function.

## b270 Sensory Functions Related to Temperature and Other Stimuli

Sensory functions of sensing temperature, vibration, pressure, and noxious stimulus.

Inclusions: functions of being sensitive to temperature, vibration, shaking or oscillation, superficial pressure, deep pressure, burning sensation, or a noxious stimulus

Exclusions: touch functions (b265); sensation of pain (b280)

- *b2700 Sensitivity to Temperature*
  Sensory functions of sensing cold and heat.

- *b2701 Sensitivity to Vibration*
  Sensory functions of sensing shaking or oscillation.

- *b2702 Sensitivity to Pressure*
  Sensory functions of sensing pressure against or on the skin.

  Inclusions: impairments such as sensitivity to touch, numbness, hypoesthesia, hyperesthesia, paresthesia, and tingling

- *b2703 Sensitivity to a Noxious Stimulus*
  Sensory functions of sensing painful or uncomfortable sensations.

  Inclusions: impairments such as hypalgesia, hyperpathia, allodynia, analgesia, and as in anesthesia dolorosa

- *b2708 Sensory Functions Related to Temperature and Other Stimuli, Other Specified*
- *b2709 Sensory Functions Related to Temperature and Other Stimuli, Unspecified*

### Temperature

Sensation of temperature is important for safety. If adaptations for loss of temperature sensation are not implemented, the client could experience burns, frostbite, or heat stroke. Bodily processes can also be affected by temperature and have detrimental effects, such as extreme heat increasing blood pressure.

The inability to sense outside temperatures is a common problem in complete spinal cord injury. A person who has a complete spinal cord injury will not have sensation below the level of impairment. Additionally, many people with complete spinal cord injuries do not sweat below the level of injury, so the client may sweat profusely above the level of injury on hot days in an attempt to cool the body. Also, people with tetraplegia or high-level paraplegia may not sweat above the injury level as well. This may give the person a false sense of the temperature. For example when a client is wet from sweating, a cool breeze may indicate to the person that it is getting cooler outside when the temperature of the day has not gotten cooler or the person may think it is hotter out than it really is due to the profuse sweating.

Therapists score this code if there is temperature sensation impairment. This is different from the Activities and Participation code d120 Other Purposeful Sensing, which is intentionally using temperature sensing to experience stimuli.

Therapists evaluate a client's ability to distinguish temperatures on the skin and in his/her environment.

To distinguish temperatures on specific skin surfaces, such as on lower extremities with a client who has paralysis in the legs, use a warm and a cold item. Alternate place the warm and cold items in different locations on the skin and ask the client to tell you if s/he feels something warm or cold. For a warm and cold item, the therapist can use the corner of a cold washcloth and another washcloth that was warmed in the microwave or capped test tubes filled with warm and cold water.

To evaluate the client's ability to sense temperature in the environment, open a window or door or go outside for a minute and ask the client to describe the temperature.

In addition to scoring the extent of the temperature impairment and related Activities and Participation codes that are affected by the impairment, such as d630 Preparing Meals or d5404 Choosing Appropriate Clothing, the therapist may make additional notes related to temperature functions. These notes include the specific temperature impairment (e.g., no sensation of temperature from the waist down), the extent that it interferes with specific activities (e.g., Client reports desire to sit on the beach for prolonged periods of time after discharge. Prolonged sun exposure without full temperature sensation increases client's risk for heat stroke.), and the amount of assistance required to minimize temperature problems (e.g., requires moderate cues to utilize other senses to assess temperature of items prior to taking action).

Treatment for impairments in temperature sensing is outside the scope of practice for recreational therapists, but they will provide adaptations.

People who have difficulty determining temperature changes on the skin or in the environment need to learn how to rely on other senses to compensate for the loss. Hearing adaptations include listening to the weather station on the radio or television. Visual adaptations include looking at others to see how they are dressed for the day and making sure the light is off on the electric stove to indicate that it is cool. Clients should routinely take precautionary measures when they are unsure, such as using a potholder if the pot may still be hot and not carrying a hot casserole dish on the lap to be able to propel a wheelchair and carry the dish at the same time. People who have a complete spinal cord injury are to also avoid more than one hour of exposure to outside temperatures above 90°F. If a client complains of feeling ill and has had prolonged exposure to high outdoor temperatures, move the client into a cooler environment and utilize cooling techniques, such as air conditioning or cool towels on the forehead, around the neck, and under the arms. Symptoms should subside within 30-60 minutes. If a person with a spinal cord injury

anticipates having to be outdoors on a hot and humid day, precautions should be taken to keep the core body temperature down. These include drinking lots of cool water, wearing a hat, staying in the shade, wetting a towel and placing it around the neck, and wearing loose clothing that breathes.

The therapist should document compensatory strategies taught and implemented (e.g., Client instructed to wear a 45+ sun block, sit in the shade under a beach umbrella, wear a brimmed hat, and drink cool water when sitting on the beach for prolonged period of time to decrease risk of heat stroke and sunburn), and effectiveness of compensatory strategies (e.g., client able to sit outside in the sun using techniques to decrease effects of unrecognized heat for one hour without adverse effects).

### Other Stimuli

Sensitivity to vibration and pressure are involved in reacting to things in the environment that touch the client. It would include the ability to sense when someone is touching the client on the shoulder to get the client's attention and the ability of the client to realize when s/he has bumped into something that s/he doesn't see. There are numerous disabilities that cause touch function impairments including spinal cord injury and diabetic neuropathy.

Being able to sense noxious stimuli (b2703 Sensitivity to a Noxious Stimulus) is one of the most important ways we avoid serious injuries. Not being able to feel pain can lead to serious risks for clients in that they can continue with actions that are causing serious injury and not realize that they have a condition that requires immediate medical attention.

This is the section we suggest you use to document the inability to sense pain. The related code, b280 Sensation of Pain, is used to record pain that the client experiences. If there are indications that the inability to sense pain is an issue, the therapist should also look at b280 Sensation of Pain for more information about the client's experiences with pain.

To evaluate the extent of impairment, the therapist can provide a set of stimuli to various areas of the skin. These should include light touch, vibration, and potentially painful stimuli, such as a pinprick, to evaluate how well the client can sense the stimuli.

Documentation should include the type and extent of the touch impairment and related Activities and Participation codes that are affected by touch impairment, such as d770 Intimate Relationships and d6500 Making and Repairing Clothes. The therapist should cover the specific touch impairment (e.g., light touch absent in the right upper extremity), the extent that it interferes with specific activities (e.g., lack of pain receptors in leg puts client at risk for injury when in the rose garden), and amount of assistance required to minimize touch problems (e.g., requires moderate cues to scan full environment to identify location of outside touch, such as when someone taps the client on the back to get his attention).

Recreational therapists monitor the success of treatment for impairments in sensing other stimuli, as provided by other team members.

If touch functions continue to be impaired after treatment, compensatory strategies are taught to minimize injury and maximize safety. Examples include weight shifts to decrease decubitus ulcers and using visual skills to scan the body for injuries. The therapist documents the compensatory strategies taught and implemented and the effectiveness of compensatory strategies.

### Cross References

In *Recreational Therapy for Specific Diagnoses and Conditions, First Edition*, ICF code b270 Sensory Functions Related to Temperature and Other Stimuli is listed in seven chapters: Amputation and Prosthesis, Diabetes Mellitus, Fibromyalgia and Juvenile Fibromyalgia, Heart Disease, Intellectual Disability, Multiple Sclerosis, and Parkinson's Disease.

In *Recreational Therapy Basics, Techniques, and Interventions, First Edition*, treatment for ICF code b270 Sensory Functions Related to Temperature and Other Stimuli is discussed in one chapter: Sensory Interventions.

### b279 Additional Sensory Functions, Other Specified and Unspecified

Additional Sensory Functions, whether specified or unspecified, not mentioned in the previous categories are scored under this code. Therapists make a notation of the impairment to the right of the scored code.

## Pain (b280 - b289)

### b280 Sensation of Pain

Sensation of unpleasant feeling indicating potential or actual damage to some body structure.

Inclusions: sensations of generalized or localized pain, in one or more body part, pain in a dermatome, stabbing pain, burning pain, dull pain, aching pain; impairments such as myalgia, analgesia, and hyperalgesia

- *b2800 Generalized Pain*
  Sensation of unpleasant feeling indicating potential or actual damage to some body structure felt all over, or throughout the body.

- *b2801 Pain in Body Part*
  Sensation of unpleasant feeling indicating potential or actual damage to some body structure felt in a specific part, or parts, of the body.

  o *b28010 Pain in Head and Neck*
    Sensation of unpleasant feeling indicating potential or actual damage to some body structure felt in the head and neck.

  o *b28011 Pain in Chest*
    Sensation of unpleasant feeling indicating potential for actual damage to some body structure felt in the chest.

  o *b28012 Pain in Stomach or Abdomen*
    Sensation of unpleasant feeling indicating potential or actual damage to some body structure felt in the stomach or abdomen.

    Inclusions: pain in the pelvic region

  o *b28013 Pain in Back*
    Sensation of unpleasant feeling indicating potential or actual damage to some body structure felt in the back.

    Inclusions: pain in the trunk; low backache

  o *b28014 Pain in Upper Limb*
    Sensation of unpleasant feeling indicating potential or actual damage to some body structure felt in either one or both upper limbs, including hands.

  o *b28015 Pain in Lower Limb*
    Sensation of unpleasant feeling indicating potential or actual damage to some body

structure felt in either one or both lower limbs, including feet.

  o  *b28016 Pain in Joints*
Sensation of unpleasant feeling indicating potential or actual damage to some body structure felt in one or more joints, including small and big joints.

      Inclusions: pain in the hip; pain in the shoulder

  o  *b28018 Pain in Body Part, Other Specified*
  o  *b28019 Pain in Body Part, Unspecified*
- *b2802 Pain in Multiple Body Parts*
Unpleasant sensation indicating potential or actual damage to some body structure located in several body parts.

- *b2803 Radiating Pain in a Dermatome*
Unpleasant sensation indicating potential or actual damage to some body structure located in areas of skin served by the same nerve root.

- *b2804 Radiating Pain in a Segment or Region*
Unpleasant sensation indicating potential or actual damage to some body structure located in areas of skin in different body parts not served by the same nerve root.

This set of codes relates to pain in the body. The manifestation of physical pain can result from a traumatic or non-traumatic injury or occur as a secondary disability from another health problem, such as back pain from poor posture and improper weight bearing and shifting on the affected leg caused by years of compensating for a bad knee. The health problem can also be a result of a congenital disability, the aging process, and other disabilities that commonly have associated body pain, such as fibromyalgia.

Physical pain is described as acute or chronic.

- *Acute pain* is described as having a short duration and is usually from a known cause such as an injury or an acute illness. Recovery is usually expected from acute pain.
- *Chronic pain* is described as a persistent pain of long duration (at least several months). It is an expected or unexpected long-term pain including pain that is a symptom of a chronic progressive disease or pain that persists after the expected healing period. It often results in a severely de-

creased activity level and, as a result, a disability. Some chronic pain has a source that cannot be identified. Other chronic pain has an identified source, but treatment has not yet succeeded (and may never succeed) in relieving the pain.

In addition to the physical origins of pain, psychogenic pain can originate from psychological stressors. Stressors that are suppressed may manifest in pain. It is difficult to tell whether a pain is psychogenic only, psychogenic pain in conjunction with physical pain, or physical pain with an, as yet, unidentified cause. Pain that does not appear to have a physical source should not automatically be described as psychogenic pain. The pain sensors themselves can go awry causing impaired pain sensations without another kind of physical origin.

Therapists score the extent of the pain. Moderate pain in the lower back would be scored b28013.2. Determining the extent of pain is described below. They then score the related Activities and Participation codes that are affected by physical pain, such as d2401 Handling Stress, d4105 Bending, d4154 Maintaining a Standing Position, d4300 Lifting, d450 Walking, d4552 Running, d540 Dressing, and d6506 Taking Care of Animals.

If possible, the source of the pain is identified though testing and scans. The team assesses the location of the pain, the severity of the pain, the duration of the pain, and related activities that cause or exacerbate the current pain. Therapists ask the client how long s/he has been experiencing the pain and what methods and interventions have been employed in the past to help manage the pain.

Pain can be very difficult to measure because it is subjective and people's pain tolerance varies. Pain tolerance is often affected by mood, personality, and circumstance. A common way to measure pain is to ask the client to rate his/her pain on a scale of zero to ten. Zero equals no pain; a one equals mild pain that doesn't interfere with activities. Five equals moderate pain that interferes with activities but is not disabling. Ten equals the severest pain imaginable. It is disabling and the client is unable to function. The Body Functions qualifier could be the pain score divided by two, with a pain scale of 10 scored as b280.4.

Another common way to measure pain is through face pictures. This is especially useful with children, when there is reduced mental capacity, and when there is a language barrier. There are eleven faces. Each face corresponds with the numbers zero through ten. For example, a happy face is the number zero and a face drawn with eyes wide open. Pain ratings of ten are shown by an anguished expression. The client is asked to point to the face that best represents how s/he is currently experiencing pain.

For more detailed analysis of the pain, a pain map may be drawn. A pain map is an anatomical chart of the front and back of the body. The client makes an 'x' in areas where pain is experienced. Next to each area, the client charts the dates when pain is experienced, pain descriptors (e.g., burning, throbbing), pain intensity (zero through ten), interference with life activities (e.g., unable to drive the kids to school in the morning), what increases the pain, and what seems to decrease the pain. Clients are usually asked to do a pain map each day for several days, using a new pain map form for each day or for parts of a day if there is a lot of variation throughout the day. This helps the therapist to identify patterns of pain and possible interventions to help manage pain. It also helps the client to become more aware of his/her pain. In some instances, however, an increased awareness to pain can backfire. Increased attention and focus on pain can increase the intensity and duration of pain.

To document the pain, the therapist describes the pain rating scales used, pain levels and patterns identified, locations of pain, pain triggers, pain descriptors, level of assistance the client needs to implement pain management interventions, and the extent that pain interferes with specific activities. In addition to scoring the pain functions impairment, the therapist also scores related Activities and Participation codes that are affected by the pain.

In analyzing preferred activities, therapists ask the client to rate his/her pain prior to the start of the activity, during the activity, and after the activity to help determine a pain pattern and note progression or regression of pain. Activities can be modified to reduce the level of pain they cause. Other documentation includes education about manifestation of pain in the body, pain management interventions tried, and effectiveness of pain management interventions.

Treatment for pain will vary depending on the root cause, if it can be identified, the experience of the client in dealing with the pain, and the extent that psychological issues are involved. See the specific

diagnosis that is causing the pain for treatment direction.

For recreational therapists adaptations for pain are similar to treatment. Treatment is designed to relieve pain. Adaptations help the client live with pain that cannot be eliminated. In addition to pharmacology, common interventions include adaptation of activities, improving psychological processes, using the power of distraction, and relaxation training.

### Cross References

In *Recreational Therapy for Specific Diagnoses and Conditions, First Edition*, ICF code b280 Sensation of Pain is listed in 21 chapters: Amputation and Prosthesis, Autism Spectrum Disorder, Back Disorders and Back Pain, Burns, Cancer, Cerebral Palsy, Diabetes Mellitus, Fibromyalgia and Juvenile Fibromyalgia, Guillain-Barré Syndrome, Heart Disease, Major Depressive Disorder, Multiple Sclerosis, Osteoarthritis, Osteoporosis, Parkinson's Disease, Post-Traumatic Stress Disorder, Rheumatoid Arthritis, Sickle Cell Disease, Spina Bifida, Spinal Cord Injury, and Total Joint Replacement.

In *Recreational Therapy Basics, Techniques, and Interventions, First Edition*, treatment for ICF code b280 Sensation of Pain is discussed in 12 chapters: Consequences of Inactivity, Stress, Activity Pattern Development, Adaptive Sports, Animal Assisted Therapy, Aquatic Therapy, Assertiveness Training, Cognitive Behavioral Counseling, Leisure Education and Counseling, Neuro-Developmental Treatment, Physical Activity, and Sensory Interventions.

## b289 Sensation of Pain, Other Specified or Unspecified

Additional Sensations of Pain, whether specified or unspecified, not mentioned in the previous categories are scored under this code. Therapists make a notation of the impairment to the right of the scored code.

## b298 Sensory Functions and Pain, Other Specified

## b299 Sensory Functions and Pain, Unspecified

Additional impairments related to Sensory Functions and Pain, whether specified or unspecified, not mentioned in the previous categories are scored under this code. Therapists make a notation of the impairment to the right of the scored code.

## References

Ahmed, T. & Haboubi, N. (2010). Assessment and management of nutrition in older people and its importance to health. *Clinical Interventions in Aging, 5*, 207-216.

Ahlstrand, I., Bjork, M., Thyberg, I., Borsbo, B., & Falkmer, T. (2012). Pain and daily activities in rheumatoid arthritis. *Disability and Rehabilitation, 34*(15), 1245.

Banhidi, M. & Zintl, K. (2015). Body functions theory: A European-based therapeutic recreation facilitation technique. *World Leisure Journal, 57*(1), 69-71.

Best-Martini, E. & Jones-DiGenova, K. (2014). *Exercises for Frail Elders* (2nd ed.). Champaign, IL: Human Kinetics.

burlingame, j. (2001). *Idyll Arbor's therapy dictionary* (2nd ed.). Ravensdale, WA: Idyll Arbor, Inc.

Chia, E., Wang, J., Rochtchina, E., Cumming, R., Newall, P., & Mitchell, P. (2007). Hearing impairment and health-related quality of life: The Blue Mountains hearing study. *Ear and Hearing, 28*(2), 187-195.

Cmar, J. L. (2015). Orientation and mobility skills and outcome expectations as predictors of employment for young adults with visual impairments. *Journal of Visual Impairment and Blindness, 109*(2), 95.

Devine, M. A., Piatt, J., & Dawson, S. L. (2015). The role of a disability-specific camps in promoting social acceptance and quality of life for youth with hearing impairments. *Therapeutic Recreation Journal, 49*(4), 293-309.

Field, T., Diego, M., & Hernandez-Reif, M. (2010). Preterm infant massage therapy research: A review. *Infant Behavior and Development, 33*, 115-124.

Fong, S., Fu, S., & Ng, G. (2012). Tae kwon do training speeds up the development of balance and sensory functions in young adolescents. *Journal of Science and Medicine in Sport, 15*(1), 64.

Goldshtrom, Y., Korman, D., Goldshtrom, I., & Bendavid, J. (2011). The effect of rhythmic exercises on cognition and behavior of maltreated children: A pilot study. *Journal of Bodywork and Movement Therapies, 15*(3), 326-334.

Guzman, J., Esmail, R., Karjalainen, K., Malmivaara, A., Irvin, E., & Bombardier, C., (2006). Multidisciplinary bio-psycho-social rehabilitation for chronic low-back pain. The Cochrane Library.

Jensen, M. P., Chodroff, M. J., & Dworkin, R. H. (2007). The impact of neuropathic pain on health-related quality of life. *Neurology, 68*(15), 1178-1182.

Larsson, B. & Sund, A. M. (2007). Emotional/behavioural, social correlates and one-year predictors of frequent pains among early adolescents: Influences of pain characteristics. *European Journal of Pain, 11*, 57-65.

Lee, Y., Tabourne, C. E. S., & Harris, J. E. (2010). Effects of dancing heart program (DHP) as therapeutic recreation intervention on risk of falling among community dwelling elders. *Annual in Therapeutic Recreation, 18*, 157-163.

Rose, D. (2010) *FallProof! A Comprehensive Balance and Mobility Training Program* (2nd ed.). Champaign, IL: Human Kinetics.

Sadock, B. & Sadock, V. (2003). *Kaplan & Sadock's synopsis of psychiatry, 9th edition*. Philadelphia, PA: Lippincott Williams & Wilkins.

Stanos, S. P., McLean, J., & Rader, L. (2007). Physical medicine rehabilitation approach to pain. *Anesthesiology Clinics, 25*, 721-759.

Steinbach, S., Hummel, T., Bohner, C., Berktold, S., Hundt, W., Kriner, M., Heinrich, P., Sommer, H., Prechtl, A., Schmidt, B., Bauerfeind, I., Seck, K., Jacobs, V. R., Schmalfeldt, B., & Harbeck, N. (2009). Qualitative and quantitative assessment of taste and smell changes in patients undergoing chemotherapy for breast cancer or gynecologic malignancies. *American Society of Clinical Oncology, 27*(11), 1899-1905.

Tomas-Carus, P., Hakkinen, A., Gusi, N., Alejo, L., Hakkinen, K., & Ortega-Alonso, A. (2007). Aquatic training and detraining on fitness and quality of life in fibromyalgia. *Medicine and Science in Sports and Exercise, 39*(7), 1044-1050.

Vonadies, V. (2010). Guided imagery as a therapeutic recreation modality to reduce pain. *Annual in Therapeutic Recreation, 18*, 164-174.

Zoltan, B. (1996). *Vision, perception, and cognition: A manual for the evaluation and treatment of the neurologically impaired adult*. Thorofare, NJ: Slack.

# Chapter 3 Voice and Speech Functions

This chapter is about the functions of producing sounds and speech.

*Sample Scoring of Voice and Speech Functions*

- A client who had a stroke has resultant dysarthria (b320 Articulation Functions). His speech is about 50% intelligible (severe impairment = 3). The complete scoring would look like this: b320.3.
- A six-month-old child babbles, coos, and gurgles (b3401 Making a Range of Sounds) only 25% of the time expected during sensory stimulation (75% of time does not respond, severe impairment = 3). The complete scoring would look like this: b3401.3.

The concepts of language and speech are often thought of as being the same. However, they are quite different. Language, as in b167 Mental Functions of Language, is a method of expression or communication, which may or may not be vocal. Speech, as in b3 Voice and Speech Functions, on the other hand, is the use of the voice for talking, singing, and other sounds.

Common causes of voice and speech function impairments include hearing impairments, developmental disability, cleft lip, cleft palate, cerebral palsy, traumatic brain injury, multiple sclerosis, Alzheimer's disease, Parkinson's disease, cerebrovascular accident, brain tumor, injury to muscles needed for speech, medication side effects, amyotrophic lateral sclerosis, throat or tongue cancer, surgical removal of the tongue or voice box, and selective mutism, where a child chooses or pretends not to be able to talk in certain settings. Selective mutism may indicate an emotional or psychiatric disturbance in the child possibly caused by child abuse.

Voice and speech functions can greatly impact leisure and community engagement, health, and quality of life. Hence, it receives considerable attention in recreational therapy practice. For example, 21 adolescents with a history of pre-school speech-language impairments were evaluated for psychosocial impairments (Snowling et al., 2006). Those whose speech impairments resolved over time had good psychosocial outcomes. Those who had unresolved expressive language difficulties had an increased incidence of attention problems. Those who had unresolved receptive and expressive impairments had an increased incidence of social difficulties. Those with receptive and expressive impairments along with a low IQ had an increased incidence of both attention and social difficulties.

A systematic review of the literature found that speech impairments in childhood may be associated with activity limitations and participation restrictions in learning to read and reading, learning to write and writing, focusing attention, thinking, calculating, communicating, mobility, self-care, relating to persons in authority, relationships with friends and peers, parent-child relationships, sibling relationships, school education, and acquiring, keeping and terminating a job (McCormack et al., 2009).

A study of 1,174 children aged eight to twelve with cerebral palsy found that speech difficulties reduced the mean score for relationships with parents (Dickinson et al., 2007). A longitudinal study of 244 twenty-five year olds who had a history of speech impairment found they had poorer outcomes in communication, cognition, academics, educational attainment, and occupational status (Johnson, Beitchman, & Brownlie, 2010). As a final example, a study of adults with Parkinson's disease with speech impairments (an intelligibility impairment at varying levels) reported significantly less satisfaction with their number of social activities. Severity of speech impairment affected social network composition and the study subjects participated in fewer leisure activities with lower frequency (Brown, Rowley, & Brown, 2012).

*Assessment of Voice and Speech Functions*

The ear, nose, and throat specialist and the speech-language pathologist are the primary allied health professionals who evaluate, diagnosis, and treat voice and speech impairments. Recreational therapists assess voice and speech function in the context of leisure and community activities predominately through observation.

*Treatment of Voice and Speech Functions*

In addition to an ear, nose, and throat specialist, the speech-language pathologist is the primary allied health professional to evaluate, diagnosis, and treat voice and speech impairments. Depending on the specific voice and speech impairment, recommendations are made for surgery (e.g., repair of cleft palate), medications (e.g., for psychiatric problem), counseling (e.g., for abuse, coping, and adjustment), specialized equipment (e.g., hearing aids, augmentative communication device), or therapy interventions (e.g., strengthening facial muscles, learning how to slow down the rate of speech, tailored learning environment for children who are deaf, and learning American Sign Language).

Recreational therapists incorporate recommended speech equipment and techniques into treatment plans to facilitate the development of voice and speech functions in various leisure and community tasks. Consequently, recreational therapists are familiar with common voice and speech impairments, equipment, and techniques to be able to accurately describe impairments when they are observed and effectively facilitate voice and speech skills.

Recreational therapists assess the impact of the impairment on leisure and community activities and create a treatment plan that addresses the issues. For example, the therapist may educate a swim instructor on how to best accommodate a child with a stuttering problem, teach the client alternative communication techniques that are specific to interacting with his/her peer group, facilitate the development of self-esteem through identification of the client's strengths and opportunities for peer recognition of strengths to balance feelings of self-consciousness related to speech difficulties, identify other forms of communication to more accurately reflect the meaning of the message such as the use of body language, the environment, writing, facial expressions, eye contact, etc.

Recreational therapists document voice and speech impairments as they relate to participation in specific life activities. Documentation related to speech and voice functions includes the specific impairment, techniques used to enhance voice and speech production, use of equipment or techniques in real-life settings (e.g., able to effectively communicate with peers at school utilizing an augmentative communication device with minimal assistance),

ability to use compensatory strategies (e.g., able to sign 50 words independently), and impact of impairment on life tasks (e.g., client reports that dysarthria is a major hindrance to forming social relationships).

*Evidence Review*

Several studies highlight evidence-based practice related to voice and speech functions. Other studies are available for specific client situations.

Dattilo et al. (2008) conducted an online focus group discussing leisure with eight adults with cerebral palsy who used augmentative communication devices. The following benefits of leisure and community recreation emerged: improved physical and mental health, enjoyment, increased independence, enhanced social connections, and education of society. Identified barriers to leisure participation included: personal, social, communication, technology, financial, accessibility, safety, transportation, and personal care attendants. Identified supports to help them overcome barriers included: personal, social, family, personal care attendants, augmentative communication devices, and other assistive technologies.

Parr (2007) conducted an in-depth study of 20 adults with severe aphasia post stroke and found evidence of social exclusion at three different levels:

- *Infrastructural exclusion*: limitations on access to employment; income; services for health, housing, education, and leisure; communications media; information and communication technology; information; the location of resources and services; the nature of the place.
- *Interpersonal exclusion*: limitations on association with groups and places in society, family, neighbors, friends, workmates, people of similar age or gender or culture or religion. Feeling excluded because they are no longer part of a group to which they once belonged, or because they belong to a group that they have always perceived as being excluded.
- *Personal exclusion*: alienation; isolation; lack of identity; low self-esteem; passivity; dependence; bewilderment; fear; anger; apathy; low aspirations; hopelessness.

The author advocates that treatment "for managing long-term consequences of aphasia to be expanded, intervention being offered at relevant periods as the individual's life when aphasia unfolds, and barriers to participation rise up.... Therapists should expand beyond traditional confines towards collaboration with a constellation of health, welfare, employment, education, and leisure services" (p. 120). He also recommends the promotion of social inclusion training including support for communication, opportunities and accessibility to social inclusion, respect and acknowledgement of communication challenges, and attention given to the environment to optimize social inclusion.

Brady et al. (2011) conducted in-depth interviews with 24 adults with varying degrees of stroke-related dysarthria. Dysarthria at all degrees — mild to severe — was found to significantly impact social participation and sense of identity. Social participation was impacted by the communication impairment, the reaction of others to the impairment, changed circumstances, and the person's deliberate strategies to avoid and restrict social interactions. Identity was impacted by change in speech and how other's perceived the individual. The authors concluded that "the degree of intelligibility does not necessarily reflect the psychosocial impacts of dysarthria and should be taken into consideration in referral for treatment and intervention planning. Future work should address the development and evaluation of the effectiveness of interventions designed to address the psychosocial impacts of dysarthria" (p. 185).

### Cross References

In *Recreational Therapy for Specific Diagnoses and Conditions, First Edition*, ICF code b3 Voice and Speech Functions and its subcategories are listed in eight chapters: Autism Spectrum Disorder, Cerebral Palsy, Guillain-Barré Syndrome, Hearing Loss, Multiple Sclerosis, Neurocognitive Disorders, Parkinson's Disease, and Schizophrenia Spectrum and Other Psychotic Disorders.

In *Recreational Therapy Basics, Techniques, and Interventions, First Edition*, treatment for ICF code b3 Voice and Speech Functions and its subcategories are discussed in two chapters: Constraint-Induced Movement Therapy and Neuro-Developmental Treatment.

### b310 Voice Functions

Functions of the production of various sounds by the passage of air through the larynx.

Inclusions: functions of production and quality of voice; functions of phonation, pitch, loudness, and other qualities of voice; impairments such as aphonia, dysphonia, hoarseness, hypernasality, and hyponasality

Exclusions: mental functions of language (b167); articulation functions (b320)

- *b3100 Production of Voice*
  Functions of the production of sound made through coordination of the larynx and surrounding muscles with the respiratory system.

  Inclusions: functions of phonation, loudness; impairment of aphonia

- *b3101 Quality of Voice*
  Functions of the production or characteristics of voice including pitch, resonance, and other features.

  Inclusions: functions of high or low pitch; impairments such as hypernasality, hyponasality, dysphonia, hoarseness, or harshness

- *b3108 Voice Functions, Other Specified*
- *b3109 Voice Functions, Unspecified*

Speech-language pathologists will typically be the primary healthcare professional to evaluate deficits and score voice functions. The recreational therapist evaluates how the problem affects the client's participation in leisure and community activities.

The recreational therapist incorporates recommended techniques from the speech-language pathologist. In some cases the techniques that work in the clinical setting with the speech-language pathologist do not work in a leisure or community setting and the recreational therapist must adapt the techniques to fit the situation and report the concerns to the speech-language pathologist.

Treatment interventions will vary depending on the specific impairment and level of dysfunction. For example, if a client's voice volume is too low, verbal cueing may be utilized to prompt the client to "yell" as if the person was on the other side of the room. Recreational therapists are also aware of, and address, the secondary complications of voice function impairments. For example, production of speech may cause difficulties in social communication, and quality of voice impairments may affect social acceptance. In addition to the ICF codes noted in this chapter, secondary problems need to be recorded with Activities and Participation codes and treated using those codes.

If a client is unable to speak (aphonia) or the quality of voice is poor enough that others can't understand the client, adaptations such as American Sign Language may be taught along with other forms of direct and indirect communication, including writing, gesturing, body language, and eye contact.

### Cross References

In *Recreational Therapy for Specific Diagnoses and Conditions, First Edition*, ICF code b310 Voice Functions is listed in two chapters: Guillain-Barré Syndrome and Hearing Loss.

In *Recreational Therapy Basics, Techniques, and Interventions, First Edition*, there are no references for ICF code b310 Voice Functions.

### b320 Articulation Functions

Functions of the production of speech sounds.

Inclusions: functions of enunciation, articulation of phonemes; spastic, ataxic, flaccid dysarthria; anarthria

Exclusions: mental functions of language (b167); voice functions (b310)

Articulation functions can be described as difficulty forming sounds and stringing sounds together. Common articulation problems include substituting one sound for another, such as wabbit for rabbit, omitting a sound, such as han for hand, and distorting a sound, such as ship for sip or incorrect enunciation of phoneme blends such as 'bl' or 'th.'

Speech-language pathologists will typically be the primary healthcare professional to evaluate deficits and score articulation functions. The recreational therapist evaluates how the problem affects the client's participation in leisure and community activities. Documentation should include any Body Structure deficits that underlie the articulation deficits.

Treatment interventions will vary depending on the specific impairment and level of dysfunction. However, there are several intervention techniques that are commonly employed to improve articulation. One involves over-pronunciation of each syllable in a word with a decreased rate of speaking. The therapist can verbally cue the client to slow down the speech

rate by asking the client to tap his/her finger on the table in tempo to the syllables, as in "He... went... to... the... kit... chen... to... get... a... bowl ... of... spa... ghet... ti."

Other techniques involve speech drills that work on specific problem areas, such as saying a set of 12 words that begin with the phoneme blend 'bl' three times each. Facial and mouth exercises may be used to improve muscular control, strength, and range of motion. All interventions that are incorporated into the recreational therapy treatment plan are checked with the speech-language pathologist to ensure consistency of approaches and techniques. In some cases recommended techniques that work in the clinic setting with the speech-language pathologist do not work in a leisure or community setting and the recreational therapist must adapt the techniques to fit the situation. Adaptations are then reported to the speech-language pathologist.

Adaptations for articulation functions are similar to those used in b310 Voice Functions. Since many articulation problems are caused by damage to the central nervous system, such as stroke, there may be added complications in the utilization of compensatory techniques, including difficulty gesturing due to paralysis. To optimize effectiveness, all impairments must be considered when designing compensatory strategies.

### Cross References

In *Recreational Therapy for Specific Diagnoses and Conditions, First Edition*, ICF code b320 Articulation Functions is listed in three chapters: Guillain-Barré Syndrome, Hearing Loss, and Multiple Sclerosis.

In *Recreational Therapy Basics, Techniques, and Interventions, First Edition*, treatment for ICF code b320 Articulation Functions is discussed in one chapter: Neuro-Developmental Treatment.

### b330 Fluency and Rhythm of Speech Functions

Functions of the production of flow and tempo of speech.

Inclusions: functions of fluency, rhythm, speed, and melody of speech; prosody and intonation; impairments such as stuttering, stammering, cluttering, bradylalia, and tachylalia

Exclusions: mental functions of language (b167); voice functions (b310); articulation functions (b320)

- *b3300 Fluency of Speech*
  Functions of the production of smooth, uninterrupted flow of speech.

  Inclusions: functions of smooth connection of speech; impairments such as stuttering, stammering, cluttering, dysfluency, repetition of sounds, words, or parts of words, and irregular breaks in speech

- *b3301 Rhythm of Speech*
  Functions of the modulated, tempo, and stress patterns in speech.

  Inclusions: impairments such as stereotypic or repetitive speech cadence

- *b3302 Speed of Speech*
  Functions of the rate of speech production.

  Inclusions: impairments such as bradylalia and tachylalia

- *b3303 Melody of Speech*
  Functions of modulation of pitch patterns in speech.

  Inclusions: prosody of speech, intonation, melody of speech; impairments such as monotone speech

- *b3308 Fluency and Rhythm of Speech Functions, Other Specified*
- *b3309 Fluency and Rhythm of Speech Functions, Unspecified*

Voice and speech are more than just words. The tone, flow, pitch, and melody of the voice also convey much of the message. People want to express feelings of love in a sweet and quiet way, but they also want to express anger in a quick and explosive manner or express business competence in a way that sounds to the point. The differences are referred to globally as the fluency and rhythm of speech. When problems occur in this area, messages may not be clear because the tone doesn't match the meaning of the words. The message may be misinterpreted by the receiver or be a disappointment to the sender when it doesn't sound the way the person intends it to sound.

Other members of the healthcare team, usually the speech-language pathologist, will be doing much of the evaluation of deficits in fluency and rhythm of speech. The recreational therapist evaluates how the deficits affect participation in life activities.

Issues such as stammering can cause marked reluctance to participate in normal activities because the client may be embarrassed about the inability to speak clearly. In other instances, the person may not be aware of his/her abnormal speech patterns. For example, someone in the manic phase of bipolar disorder may not be aware that his speech is rapid and pressured (tachylalia). The amount of awareness that the client has is an important part of the evaluation.

Treatment involves finding ways to improve fluency and rhythm. Fluency and rhythm impairments are commonly made worse by stress and anxiety. So when there are impairments, therapists should first consider ways that stress can be minimized or eliminated including teaching deep breathing, planning and organizing ahead of time, and practicing events that produce anxiety.

When the client is not aware that there is a deficit, education may be necessary. Tape recordings and videotaping will help the client to see how his/her speech patterns are different.

In some cases, such as stammering, the client may not be able to completely control the problem, so adaptations may be required. The therapist can educate the client about other forms of communication to assist with conveying messages effectively including the role of body language, dress, and environment. Utilization of alternative modes of communication should also be encouraged as appropriate. These might include written reports in lieu of or in addition to verbal reports, using PowerPoint presentations and videos, and using e-mail or texting instead of talking on the phone. Relying totally on alternative forms of communication should not be encouraged unless it is absolutely necessary.

Adaptations in the environment are often necessary, too. Educating peers and people in places of authority, such as teachers, employers, and parents, about the impairment and how they can best assist the person in communicating should also be part of the treatment plan to facilitate further skill development and effective communication. Some possibilities are allowing the person extra time to convey a thought, providing cueing if needed, reiterating points that are clear, and asking for clarification of points that are unclear.

In *Recreational Therapy for Specific Diagnoses and Conditions, First Edition*, ICF code b330 Fluency and Rhythm of Speech Functions is listed in four chapters: Hearing Loss, Multiple Sclerosis, Neurocognitive Disorders, and Schizophrenia Spectrum and Other Psychotic Disorders.

In *Recreational Therapy Basics, Techniques, and Interventions, First Edition*, treatment for ICF code b330 Fluency and Rhythm of Speech Functions is discussed in one chapter: Neuro-Developmental Treatment.

## b340 Alternative Vocalization Functions

Functions of the production of other manners of vocalization.

Inclusions: functions of the production of notes and range of sounds, such as in singing, chanting, babbling, and humming; crying aloud and screaming

Exclusions: mental functions of language (b167); voice functions (b310); articulation functions (b320); fluency and rhythm of speech functions (b330)

- *b3400 Production of Notes*
  Functions of production of musical vocal sounds.

  Inclusions: sustaining, modulating, and terminating productions of single or connected vocalizations with variation in pitch such as in singing, humming, and chanting

- *b3401 Making a Range of Sounds*
  Functions of production of a variety of vocalizations.

  Inclusions: functions babbling in children

- *b3408 Alternative Vocalization Functions, Other Specified*
- *b3409 Alternative Vocalization Functions, Unspecified*

Deficits in alternate vocalization functions may not be noticed in a formal evaluation by the treatment team. They tend to show up more in activities than in diagnostic situations. Evaluation involves observations of the client in many situations, watching for appropriate alternative vocalizations. Checking the client's ability to sing is one possibility, but the other types of vocalization or lack of them will probably be more important for most treatment situations. For infants, deficits in babbling behavior can be one of the first indications of a psychological problem, such as autism. The recreational therapist is aware of the range of normal functions and notes when a client is outside the norms.

Documentation includes observations of the client with detailed notes about the situation. For example, "b3401.3: Sarah, who is three years old, fell off the swing and badly skinned her knee, but seemed to be fighting against making any crying sound." This is the kind of deficit that may point toward problems other than voice and speech functions, but documenting this deficit is part of the evidence necessary to figure out underlying impairments or issues impacting behavior.

In treatment, the recreational therapist incorporates recommended techniques from voice and speech specialists. Treatment interventions will vary depending on the specific impairment and level of dysfunction. Common interventions to promote alternative vocalizations include addressing underlying issues (e.g., issues of abuse that conditioned a child not to scream), providing sensory stimulation (e.g., tickling the infant and providing bright colored toys and mirrors to promote babbling), and playing games and engaging in recreational activities that promote alternative vocalizations (e.g., a game of echoing sounds to promote the development of sound ranges, singing and humming to music, playing games that encourage the child to scream such as being "it" in the game hide-and-seek and having to say "ready or not here I come").

If an individual is unable to sing, chant, babble, hum, cry, or scream, adaptations to express communicative needs can be explored, as appropriate. Some examples: A person could mouth words to a song to still participate in the singing experience. Running the index finger from the corner of the eye to the check could signal crying as represented by tears falling.

In *Recreational Therapy for Specific Diagnoses and Conditions, First Edition*, ICF code b340 Alternative Vocalization Functions is listed in one chapter: Autism Spectrum Disorder.

In *Recreational Therapy Basics, Techniques, and Interventions, First Edition*, there are no references for ICF code b340 Alternative Vocalization Functions.

*b398 Voice and Speech Functions, Other Specified*

*b399 Voice and Speech Functions, Unspecified*

*References*

Brady, M. C., Clark, A. M., Dickson, S., Paton, G., & Barbour, R. S. (2011). The impact of stroke-related dysarthria on social participation and implications for rehabilitation. *Disability and Rehabilitation, 33*(3), 178-186.

Brown, A., Rowley, D. T., & Brown, B. (2012). Social participation and speech impairment in Parkinson's disease. *International Motor Speech Conference*, Santa Rosa, CA.

Dattilo, J., Estrella, G., Estrella, L. J., Light, J., McNaughton, D., & Seabury, M. (2008). "I have chosen to live life abundantly": Perceptions of leisure by adults who use augmentative and alternative communication. *Augmentative and Alternative Communication, 24*(1), 16-28.

Dickinson, H. O., Parkinson, K. N., Ravens-Sieberer, U., Schirripa, G., Thyen, U., Arnaud, C., Beckung, E., Fauconnier, J., McManus, V., Michelsen, S. I., Parkes, J., & Colver, A. (2007). Self-reported quality of life for 8-12 year-old children with cerebral palsy: A cross-sectional European study. *The Lancet, 369*, 2171-2178.

Johnson, C. J., Beitchman, J. H., & Brownlie, E. B. (2010). Twenty-year follow-up of children with and without speech-language impairments: Family, educational, occupation, and quality of life outcomes. *American Journal of Speech-Language Pathology, 19*(1), 51-65.

McCormack, J., McLeod, S., McAllister, L., & Harrison, L. J. (2009). A systematic review of the association between childhood speech impairment and participation across the lifespan. *International Journal of Speech-Language Pathology, 11*(2), 155-170.

Parr, S. (2007). Living with severe aphasia: Tracking social exclusion. *Aphasiology, 21*(1), 98-123.

Snowling, M. J., Bishop, D. V. M., Stothard, S. E., Chipchase, B., & Kaplan, C. (2006). Psychosocial outcomes at 15 years of children with a preschool history of speech-language impairment. *Journal of Child Psychology and Psychiatry, 47*(8), 759-765.

# Chapter 4 Functions of the Cardiovascular, Hematological, Immunological, and Respiratory Systems

This chapter is about the functions involved in the cardiovascular system (functions of the heart and blood vessels), the hematological and immunological systems (functions of blood production and immunity), and the respiratory system (functions of respiration and exercise tolerance).

*Sample Scoring of Functions of the Cardiovascular, Hematological, Immunological, and Respiratory Systems*

- As per consensus of the treatment team, participating in 30 minutes of continuous light physical activity (b4550 General Physical Endurance) is a realistic goal for the client given her current health condition. At this time, she is only able to sustain 10 minutes of continuous light physical activity (approximately 33% of the goal; moderate impairment). The complete scoring would look like this: b4550.2.
- A client fatigues easily (b4552 Fatigability) and consequently has severely limited his engagement in leisure and community activities — saving his energy for "required" daily activities only. He reports feeling fatigued at least 70% of his waking hours (severe impairment). His decreased leisure and community activity level is creating a downward spiral of deconditioning and significantly impacting his quality of life. The complete scoring would look like this: b4552.3.

General physical endurance, aerobic capacity, and fatigability can significantly limit or enhance ability to participate in leisure and community tasks, as well as ability to engage in regular leisure time physical activity. Many illnesses and conditions can negatively impact exercise tolerance functions. These include physical disabilities, such as high-level spinal cord injury or multiple sclerosis, psychiatric conditions, such as depression, surgery, general deconditioning from chronic health conditions, inactivity, obesity, respiratory impairments including asthma and chronic obstructive pulmonary disease, and any other condition impacting mobility and movement.

When a client's ability to engage in leisure and community tasks or leisure time physical activity is compromised due to such dysfunction, health and quality of life are negatively affected. For example, inactive lifestyles lead to a downward spiral of deconditioning and impairment of multiple physiological and psychological systems, diminished self-concept, greater dependence on others for daily living needs, and reduced ability for normal societal interactions. Engagement in physical activity produces upward spirals that increase oxygen consumption and anaerobic threshold; decrease heart rate, blood pressure, and perceived exertion; improve ability to tolerate physical stress; reduce risk of heart disease, diabetes, hypertension, colon cancer, and obesity; improve blood lipid and lipoprotein profile;

help maintain bone density, muscles, and joints; increase muscular strength and endurance; improve ability for locomotion; increase flexibility; promote psychological well-being; and improve self-image, sleep quality, stress management, and self-efficacy (Durstine et al., 2000, p 208).

In 2008/2009 data utilized to set the Healthy People 2020 objectives, 56% of adults with a disability engaged in no leisure time physical activity, compared to 36.2% of adults with no disability. Only 18.4% of adolescents met current aerobic physical activity requirements (U.S. Dept of Health and Human Services [USDHHS], 2008; Boslaugh & Andresen, 2006). Current USDHHS physical activity recommendations include:

- *Children and adolescents*: 60 minutes of daily moderate to vigorous physical activity, with at least three of those days including vigorous, muscle strengthening activity and bone strengthening activity. These impact activities, such as running, are required to promote bone growth.
- *Adults*: a minimum of 150 minutes of moderate intensity aerobic activity a week with the goal of moving towards 300 minutes of moderate intensity aerobic activity a week. There should be at least two days a week of muscle strengthening activity. Adults can also opt for 150 minutes of vigorous aerobic activity a week instead of 300

minutes of moderate aerobic activity a week, as they each provide about equal benefits.

Interestingly, a recent study found that even "spending more time in light-intensity activity than sedentary time... has an inverse linear relationship with a number of cardiometabolic biomarkers" (Hamilton et al. 2008, p. 294). Consequently, regular movement, regardless of its intensity level, can also have a positive effect on health.

For individuals with disabilities, recommended physical activity guidelines might be contraindicated or above their ability level. Consequently, physical activity recommendations for individuals with disabilities must be individually tailored and take a systematic approach to optimize engagement by addressing not only functional ability but also person-environment facilitators and barriers. When addressing physical activity with people who have disabilities, it is recommended that therapists utilize the ICF "to identify various combinations of factors that increase or decrease participation in physical activity.... Broad recommendations to engage in rehabilitative exercise or become more physically active are likely to fail without a systematic framework for identifying key problem areas. Understanding the impairment(s), activity limitation(s) and participation restriction(s), within the context of person-environment factors, is the first step towards developing more precise, tailored programs that will have a greater likelihood of success" (Rimmer, 2006, p. 1094)

### Assessment of Functions of the Cardiovascular, Hematological, Immunological, and Respiratory Systems

Recreational therapists assess and monitor cardiovascular, hematological, and respiratory systems via vital signs (heart rate, respiration, oxygen saturation level, and blood pressure) and follow related precautions and parameters in therapy sessions. Vital signs may also be assessed in community recreation programs in response to injury, such as a blow to the head during a sporting event, an unforeseen health event, such as fainting, or to ensure the safety of a participant such as assessing blood pressure when a client with a T1 complete spinal cord injury appears to be going into autonomic dysreflexia. In regards to the immunological system, recreational therapists assess the environment and make adjustments to meet client's allergy and immune system needs. Responses to activity and environment are recorded. These will include vital signs and other observations.

While recreational therapists do not score the majority of codes in this chapter, they are responsible for the client's safety in sessions and for providing an appropriate treatment plan. Recreational therapists do score b455 Exercise Tolerance Functions.

### Treatment of Functions of the Cardiovascular, Hematological, Immunological, and Respiratory Systems

Recreational therapists choose and implement treatment interventions aimed at controlling or improving the cardiovascular, hematological, immunological, and respiratory systems by choosing interventions based on the needs of the client. For example, relaxation training and stress management interventions may be used to lower blood pressure and respiration, physical activity may be utilized to enhance exercise tolerance functions, and interventions aimed at improving mood and positive emotions may be used to boost the immune system.

### Evidence Review

The studies provided below highlight evidence-based practice related to cardiovascular, hematological, immunological, and respiratory systems. A full review of the literature will identify more evidence-based practice interventions that reflect of the needs and characteristics of any particular client.

Harkins (2008) reviewed research over the last 10 years related to the benefits of humor and laughter. Findings indicated that the utilization of humor as an intervention increased cardiovascular functioning, increased immune functions, decreased pain, decreased anxiety and stress, improved quality of life and life satisfaction, decreased depression, enhanced mood, decreased disruptive behaviors, and improved sense of resilience. Recommendations include educating clients about benefits of humor, encouraging exploration of personal life to find opportunities for laughter and humor, using humor in reminiscence groups to foster bonding, using humor in cognitive stimulation sessions to improve memory storage because people remember humorous material better than non-humorous material, and implementation of laughter during yoga and in other groups and clubs.

Rainforth et al. (2007) reviewed 107 studies on stress reduction and blood pressure. Particular stress reduction techniques included biofeedback, relaxation-assisted biofeedback, progressive muscle relaxation, stress management training, and a Transcendental Meditation (TM) program. The only technique found to be effective for blood pressure reduction was the TM program. TM was found to modulate cardiovascular disease risk factors, anxiety and psychological health, smoking and alcohol abuse, need for anti-hypertensive medications, myocardial ischemia, and carotid atherosclerosis. A systematic review and meta-analysis of the TM program found that after an eight-year follow up (on average) individuals with high blood pressure who engaged in TM had a 23% lower rate of mortality from all causes and 30% lower rate of mortality from cardiovascular disease. TM is thought to facilitate "more coherent and integrated functioning of the nervous system [to] facilitate adaptive physiologic responses to stress, thereby helping to prevent negative physiologic consequences such as hypertension and cardiovascular disease" (p. 527).

Individuals with a *Mini-Mental State Exam* score below 25 are commonly excluded from physical rehabilitation programs because they have difficulties following simple directions. Heyn, Johnson, and Kramer (2008) did a meta-analysis of 41 studies that disputed this assumption, finding that participation in exercise programs, including recreational therapy exercise programs, resulted in similar strength and endurance outcomes regardless of the scores on the *Mini-Mental State Exam*. Consequently they say, "there is a need to evaluate best rehabilitation practice protocols and reconsider current geriatric healthcare policy and practice such that cognitively impaired older individuals should be provided with physical rehabilitation as a standard of care practice as well as with opportunities to participate in community-based exercise training programs with the aim to improve physical health" (p. 408).

### Cross References

In *Recreational Therapy for Specific Diagnoses and Conditions, First Edition*, ICF code b4 Functions of the Cardiovascular, Hematological, Immunological, and Respiratory Systems and its subcategories are listed in 30 chapters: Amputation and Prosthesis, Back Disorders and Back Pain, Borderline Personality Disorder, Burns, Cancer, Cerebral Palsy, Cere-

brovascular Accident, Chronic Obstructive Pulmonary Disease, Diabetes Mellitus, Epilepsy, Feeding and Eating Disorders, Fibromyalgia and Juvenile Fibromyalgia, Generalized Anxiety Disorder, Guillain-Barré Syndrome, Heart Disease, Intellectual Disability, Multiple Sclerosis, Neurocognitive Disorders, Obesity, Osteoarthritis, Osteoporosis, Parkinson's Disease, Rheumatoid Arthritis, Sickle Cell Disease, Spina Bifida, Spinal Cord Injury, Substance-Related Disorders, Total Joint Replacement, Traumatic Brain Injury, and Visual Impairments and Blindness.

In *Recreational Therapy Basics, Techniques, and Interventions, First Edition*, treatment for ICF code b4 Functions of the Cardiovascular, Hematological, Immunological, and Respiratory Systems and its subcategories are discussed in 20 chapters: Activity and Task Analysis, Body Mechanics and Ergonomics, Consequences of Inactivity, Parameters and Precautions, Psychoneuroimmunology, Stress, Activity Pattern Development, Adaptive Sports, Adventure Therapy, Animal Assisted Therapy, Aquatic Therapy, Behavior Strategies and Interventions, Bibliotherapy, Cognitive Behavioral Counseling, Energy Conservation Techniques, Group Psychotherapy Techniques, Mind-Body Interventions, Neuro-Developmental Treatment, Physical Activity, and Walking and Gait Training.

## Functions of the Cardiovascular System (b410 - b429)

### b410 Heart Functions

Functions of pumping the blood in adequate or required amounts and pressure throughout the body.

Inclusions: functions of heart rate, rhythm, and output; contraction force of ventricular muscles; functions of heart valves; pumping the blood through the pulmonary circuit; dynamics of circulation to the heart; impairments such as tachycardia, bradycardia, and irregular heart beat and as in heart failure, cardiomyopathy, myocarditis, and coronary insufficiency

Exclusions: blood vessel functions (b415); blood pressure functions (b420); exercise tolerance functions (b455)

- *b4100 Heart Rate*
  Functions related to the number of times the heart contracts every minute.

Inclusions: impairments such as rates that are too fast (tachycardia) or too slow (bradycardia)

- *b4101 Heart Rhythm*
  Functions related to the regularity of the beating of the heart.

  Inclusions: impairments such as arrhythmias

- *b4102 Contraction Force of Ventricular Muscles*
  Functions related to the amount of blood pumped by the ventricular muscle during every beat.

  Inclusions: impairments such as in diminished cardiac output

- *b4103 Blood Supply to the Heart*
  Functions related to the volume of blood available to the heart muscle.

  Inclusion: impairments such as coronary ischemia

- *b4108 Heart Functions, Other Specified*
- *b4109 Heart Function, Unspecified*

This section covers all of the functions of the heart and its responsibility for circulating blood throughout the body. Any interruption in the function of the heart is immediately life threatening. Recreational therapists should know how to do cardiopulmonary resuscitation as part of their practice. Malfunctions may or may not be life threatening, but the onset of a malfunction, such as tachycardia, is a significant event that the recreational therapist must know how to handle.

Recreational therapists will not likely score heart function codes, but they must recognize and handle emergency conditions related to heart function.

During treatment recreational therapists monitor heart rate in therapy sessions when clients have

- Cardiac precautions or parameters.
- Specific exercise tolerance issues or goals that need to be monitored to denote current functioning status. Possible goals include the length of time client is able to maintain target heart rate during aerobic exercise or the heart rate response to a particular form, length, and intensity of exercise.
- Heart rate as an indicator of response. Heart rate is monitored to ascertain the effect of relaxation training or response to anxiety-producing stimuli.

- Obtaining baseline status to determine alternate approaches when feelings of discomfort are reported by a client or suspected by the therapist. One possibility is a client report of feeling lightheaded during a community integration session.

When monitoring a client's heart rate, the recreational therapist may feel a change or note a concern with the regularity, speed, or strength of the client's pulse. The therapist records and documents heart rates in discipline documentation, as well as alerting other health professionals to immediate concerns. For example, the therapist may be taking a client's resting heart rate prior to physical activity and note that the pulse is rapid and irregular. The client does not appear to be in distress. The therapist immediately takes the client back to the nursing station, does not leave the client unattended, and verbally alerts the client's primary nurse to the finding to seek confirmation of the problem and determine needed interventions.

In general, treatment of a heart function problem is outside the scope of recreational therapy practice. However, it is not uncommon for recreational therapists to implement a treatment plan in which heart rate is an indicator. The therapist may also be the member of the treatment team that monitors heart rate for the reasons reviewed previously. Recreational therapists may also teach clients how to find and monitor heart rate, as well as how to best respond to heart rate changes in a community setting, such as decreasing the intensity of exercise to lower heart rate or calling an emergency response unit.

Adaptations may be required for the client to ensure that physical activity is within safe limits for the client's condition. It may be possible to change the intensity of the activity through the use of adaptive equipment or activity modifications, for example. Close evaluation of the activities that the client plans to engage in after therapy is essential for clients with cardiac problems to decrease risk of injury or death. For example, a client who has had a triple bypass tells the recreational therapist that he plans to go for long walks on the beach every day after he is discharged. Walking on sand, as well as walking in heat, increases stress on the heart, so this may not be a good goal. Clients may not always understand the level of effort required by some activities, so it is important for the therapist to take a close look at the client's planned activity pattern after discharge and make recommendations.

The chapter on Parameters and Precautions in *Recreational Therapy Basics, Techniques, and Interventions* covers how to monitor vital signs.

### Cross References

In *Recreational Therapy for Specific Diagnoses and Conditions, First Edition*, ICF code b410 Heart Functions is listed in 10 chapters: Chronic Obstructive Pulmonary Disease, Diabetes Mellitus, Feeding and Eating Disorders, Generalized Anxiety Disorder, Guillain-Barré Syndrome, Heart Disease, Obesity, Osteoarthritis, Osteoporosis, and Sickle Cell Disease.

In *Recreational Therapy Basics, Techniques, and Interventions, First Edition*, treatment for ICF code b410 Heart Functions is discussed in seven chapters: Parameters and Precautions, Adaptive Sports, Animal Assisted Therapy, Cognitive Behavioral Counseling, Energy Conservation Techniques, Mind-Body Interventions, and Physical Activity.

### b415 Blood Vessel Functions

Functions of transporting blood throughout the body.

Inclusions: functions of arteries, capillaries, and veins; vasomotor function; functions of pulmonary arteries, capillaries, and veins; functions of valves of veins; impairments such as in blockage or constriction of arteries; atherosclerosis, arteriosclerosis, thromboembolism, and varicose veins

Exclusions: heart functions (b410); blood pressure functions (b420); hematological system functions (b430); exercise tolerance functions (b455)

- *b4150 Functions of Arteries*
  Functions related to blood flow in the arteries.

  Inclusions: impairments such as arterial dilation; arterial constriction such as in intermittent claudication

- *b4151 Functions of Capillaries*
  Functions related to blood flow in the capillaries.

- *b4152 Functions of Veins*
  Functions related to blood flow in the veins, and the functions of valves of veins.

  Inclusions: impairments such as venous dilation; venous constriction; insufficient closing of valves as in varicose veins

- *b4158 Blood Vessel Functions, Other Specified*
- *b4159 Blood Vessel Functions, Unspecified*

This section covers all of the functions of the blood vessels, which are responsible for circulating blood throughout the body. As with heart functions, some are immediately life threatening and others are not. Recreational therapists will not likely score ICF codes for blood vessel functions.

During treatment recreational therapists may note the existence of a problem and take subsequent actions, such as alerting the primary physician. One example is Raynaud's phenomenon. During an episode, the fingers and/or toes can become white or deep blue due to blood vessel constriction. If the vessels in the hands or feet remain constricted until circulation is completely cut off, the fingers or toes will become deformed or gangrene may set in. Similarly, the therapist needs to be aware of other indications of deficits in blood vessel functions such as the onset of numbness or pain.

Documentation depends on the incident. The most important aspect of the documentation is that the rest of the medical team knows about the incident. In a community recreation setting, it may be the responsibility of the therapist to make sure that medical care is provided for the client.

Treatment is outside the scope of recreational therapy practice.

Adaptations may be required for the client to ensure that the amount of exercise or the type of exercise is within safe limits for the client's condition.

### Cross References

In *Recreational Therapy for Specific Diagnoses and Conditions, First Edition*, ICF code b415 Blood Vessel Functions is listed in seven chapters: Chronic Obstructive Pulmonary Disease, Diabetes Mellitus, Guillain-Barré Syndrome, Heart Disease, Obesity, Spinal Cord Injury, and Total Joint Replacement.

In *Recreational Therapy Basics, Techniques, and Interventions, First Edition*, there are no references for ICF code b415 Blood Vessel Functions.

### b420 Blood Pressure Functions

Functions of maintaining the pressure of blood within the arteries.

Inclusions: functions of maintenance of blood pressure; increased and decreased blood pressure;

impairments such as in hypotension, hypertension, and postural hypotension

Exclusions: heart functions (b410); blood vessel functions (b415); exercise tolerance functions (b455)

- *b4200 Increased Blood Pressure*
  Functions related to a rise in systolic or diastolic blood pressure above normal for the age.

- *b4201 Decreased Blood Pressure*
  Functions related to a fall in systolic or diastolic blood pressure below normal for the age.

- *b4202 Maintenance of Blood Pressure*
  Functions related to maintaining an appropriate blood pressure in response to changes in the body.

- *b4208 Blood Pressure Functions, Other Specified*
- *b4209 Blood Pressure Functions, Unspecified*
  Recreational therapists are not likely to score ICF codes for b420 Blood Pressure Functions, however recreational therapists do monitor and record blood pressure when (1) clients have cardiac precautions or parameters; (2) specific exercise tolerance issues or goals need to be monitored to denote current functioning status, such as the blood pressure response to a particular form, length, and intensity of exercise or response to movement into and out of different positions such as squatting to standing or sitting to standing; (3) blood pressure is an indicator of response, for example a response to stress or activity or a response to removal of an external stimulus during an episode of autonomic dysreflexia; and (4) obtaining baseline status to determine the next approach when feelings of discomfort are reported by a client or suspected by the therapist, such as when the client reports feeling lightheaded during community integration session or the client becomes pale.

Blood pressure readings taken by the recreational therapist are recorded in the medical record. Any reading that is abnormal, outside of parameters, or causes immediate concern is immediately reported to the appropriate health professional to determine the next intervention.

In general, medical management, such as prescription of medication, for blood pressure functions is outside the scope of practice for recreational therapists. However it is not uncommon for recreational therapists to implement a treatment plan:

- That assists in blood pressure control, such as physician-cleared physical activity for weight loss to decrease blood pressure, relaxation training, or positional changes in therapy sessions to assist in resolving postural hypotension in a client who has been lying in bed for a prolonged period of time.
- In which blood pressure is an indicator of response to an activity.
- To monitor blood pressure for the reasons mentioned previously.

Recreational therapists may also teach clients how to monitor blood pressure with automatic blood pressure cuffs in community settings and how to best respond to blood pressure changes during a community activity. Possible training could include changing intensity of physical activity, implementing relaxation techniques, searching for annoying external stimuli if in autonomic dysreflexia, or being assertive enough to call for an emergency response unit.

Adaptations may be required for the client with hypertension or cardiac precautions and parameters to ensure that physical activity is within safe limits for the client's condition, as well as to prevent fainting or falling episodes with clients who are subject to hypotension. These may include changing the intensity of the activity through the use of adaptive equipment or activity modifications. Close evaluation of the activities that the client plans to engage in after therapy is essential for clients with cardiac problems to decrease risk of complications, injury, or death.

### *Cross References*

In *Recreational Therapy for Specific Diagnoses and Conditions, First Edition*, ICF code b420 Blood Pressure Functions is listed in 10 chapters: Chronic Obstructive Pulmonary Disease, Diabetes Mellitus, Feeding and Eating Disorders, Guillain-Barré Syndrome, Heart Disease, Multiple Sclerosis, Obesity, Osteoarthritis, Parkinson's Disease, and Spinal Cord Injury.

In *Recreational Therapy Basics, Techniques, and Interventions, First Edition*, treatment for ICF code b420 Blood Pressure Functions is discussed in six chapters: Parameters and Precautions, Activity Pattern Development, Adaptive Sports, Animal Assisted Therapy, Mind-Body Interventions, and Physical Activity.

*b429 Functions of the Cardiovascular System, Other Specified and Unspecified*

## *Functions of the Hematological and Immunological Systems (b430 - b439)*

### *b430 Hematological System Functions*

Functions of blood production, oxygen, and metabolite carriage, and clotting.

Inclusions: functions of the production of blood and bone marrow; oxygen-carrying functions of blood; blood-related functions of spleen; metabolite-carrying functions of blood; clotting; impairments such as in anemia, hemophilia, and other clotting dysfunctions

Exclusions: functions of the cardiovascular system (b410 - b429); immunological system functions (b435); exercise tolerance functions (b455)

- *b4300 Production of Blood*
  Functions related to the production of blood and all its constituents

- *b4301 Oxygen-Carrying Functions of the Blood*
  Functions related to the blood's capacity to carry oxygen throughout the body.

- *b4302 Metabolite-Carrying Functions of the Blood*
  Functions related to the blood's capacity to carry metabolites throughout the body.

- *b4303 Clotting Functions*
  Functions related to the coagulation of blood, such as at a site of injury.

- *b4308 Hematological System Functions, Other Specified*

- *b4309 Hematological System Functions, Unspecified*

These functions have to do with the production of blood and the circulation of blood throughout the body. Recreational therapists are not likely to score ICF codes for b430 Hematological System Functions.

However, recreational therapists are aware of, plan for, address, and problem solve for problems associated with production, oxygen, metabolite carrying, and clotting so they can respond appropriately in therapy sessions. For example, problems with blood production, oxygen carrying, or metabolite carrying will have significant effects on energy levels and require monitoring of oxygen saturation levels in therapy sessions. Issues with clotting functions caused by hemophilia or clotting agents such as Coumadin may require special precautions to decrease risk of bleeding or bruising during activities.

One important issue with these functions is the level of oxygen in the blood. Oxygen saturation levels are monitored when working with clients who have poor blood oxygen levels, such as chronic obstructive pulmonary disease, as well as clients who are on oxygen therapy. Monitoring oxygen saturation levels provides immediate feedback about the client's activity tolerance, need or lack of need for further oxygen, and effectiveness of oxygen intake techniques when oxygen saturation levels fall below set parameters. Changes in activity, such as taking slow and deep breaths through the nose to increase oxygen saturation levels, may be required periodically during activities.

Adaptations may need to be made so that the amount of effort and safety of the activity is appropriate for the client's condition.

### *Cross References*

In *Recreational Therapy for Specific Diagnoses and Conditions, First Edition*, ICF code b430 Hematological System Functions is listed in five chapters: Chronic Obstructive Pulmonary Disease, Multiple Sclerosis, Rheumatoid Arthritis, Sickle Cell Disease, and Total Joint Replacement.

In *Recreational Therapy Basics, Techniques, and Interventions, First Edition*, treatment for ICF code b430 Hematological System Functions is discussed in one chapter: Aquatic Therapy.

### *b435 Immunological System Functions*

Functions of the body related to protection against foreign substances, including infections, by specific and non-specific immune responses.

Inclusions: immune response (specific and non-specific); hypersensitivity reactions; functions of lymphatic vessels and nodes; functions of cell-mediated immunity, antibody-mediated immunity; response to immunization; impairments such as in autoimmunity, allergic reactions, lymphadenitis, and lymphedema

Exclusions: hematological system functions (b430)

- *b4350 Immune Response*
  Functions of the body's response to sensitization to foreign substances, including infections.

  o *b43500 Specific Immune Response*
    Functions of the body's response of sensitization to a specific foreign substance.

  o *b43501 Non-Specific Immune Response*
    Functions of the body's general response of sensitization to foreign substances, including infections.

  o *b43508 Immune Response, Other Specified*
  o *b43509 Immune Response, Unspecified*

- *b4351 Hypersensitivity Reactions*
  Functions of the body's response of increased sensitization to foreign substances, such as in sensitivities to different antigens.

  Inclusions: impairments such as hypersensitivities or allergies

  Exclusion: tolerance to food (b5153)

- *b4352 Functions of the Lymphatic Vessels*
  Functions related to vascular channels that transport lymph.

- *b4353 Functions of Lymph Nodes*
  Functions related to glands along the course of lymphatic vessels.

- *b4358 Immunological System Functions, Other Specified*

- *b4359 Immunological System Functions, Unspecified*

These functions have to do with the immune system, both in the blood and in the lymph system. When it is working properly, the immune system is responsible for fighting infections. Problems with the immune system cause allergies and autoimmune diseases. Allergies, especially food allergies, can be life threatening. The therapist needs to know about any restrictions on the client's activities caused by deficits in these areas.

While recreational therapists do not evaluate these functions, they need to understand the limitations of clients who have deficits in any of these functions.

Treatment of underlying disorders is outside the therapist's scope of practice. However, discomfort caused by some of the deficits in this area, especially those caused by autoimmune diseases, such as the

pain associated with fibromyalgia, may be alleviated by gentle exercise and/or passive and active stretching. Recreational therapists can develop these programs and monitor their effects.

Adaptations need to be made so that the amount of effort and safety of the activity is appropriate for the client's condition. If there are deficits in the disease-fighting abilities of the client's immune system, the therapist needs to maintain careful control of the environment the client is exposed to. Strict isolation is a possibility. The therapist also needs to know about any allergies, including food allergies, so that s/he can make sure the client isn't exposed to dangerous allergens.

### Cross References

In *Recreational Therapy for Specific Diagnoses and Conditions, First Edition*, ICF code b435 Immunological System Functions is listed in four chapters: Amputation and Prosthesis, Cancer, Chronic Obstructive Pulmonary Disease, and Sickle Cell Disease.

In *Recreational Therapy Basics, Techniques, and Interventions, First Edition*, treatment for ICF code b435 Immunological System Functions is discussed in three chapters: Psychoneuroimmunology, Bibliotherapy, and Physical Activity.

### b439 Functions of the Hematological and Immunological Systems, Other Specified and Unspecified

### Functions of the Respiratory System (b440 - b449)

### b440 Respiration Functions

Functions of inhaling air into the lungs, the exchange of gases between air and blood, and exhaling air.

Inclusions: functions of respiration rate, rhythm, and depth; impairments such as apnea, hyperventilation, irregular respiration, paradoxical respiration, and bronchial spasm, and as in pulmonary emphysema

Exclusions: respiratory muscle functions (b445); additional respiratory functions (b450); exercise tolerance functions (b455)

- *b4400 Respiration Rate*
  Functions related to the number of breaths taken per minute.

Inclusions: impairments such as rates that are too fast (tachypnea) or too slow (bradypnea)

- *b4401 Respiratory Rhythm*
  Functions related to the periodicity and regularity of breathing.

  Inclusions: impairments such as irregular breathing

- *b4402 Depth of Respiration*
  Functions related to the volume and expansion of the lungs during breathing.

  Inclusions: impairments such as superficial or shallow respiration

- *b4408 Respiration Functions, Other Specified*
- *b4409 Respiration Functions, Unspecified*

These functions have to do with the way air gets into the body, getting oxygen into the blood, and carbon dioxide out of the blood. Deficits in these functions may be life threatening. They certainly will have an effect on the client's ability to participate in activities, even ones with minimal physical demands.

While recreational therapists do not evaluate these functions, they need to understand the limitations of clients who have deficits. If one of these functions is the cause of deficits in exercise tolerance, the treatment needs to be written in this section rather than in b455 Exercise Tolerance Functions.

One important issue with these functions is the level of oxygen in the blood. Recreational therapists need to know how to monitor oxygen saturation levels. Recreational therapists may also need to monitor respiration during activity in particular client groups that are at risk for, or have, respiration impairments, such as chronic obstructive pulmonary disease or asthma or if the client is in the recovery stage after heart surgery. Techniques to monitor these functions are described in detail in Parameters and Precautions in *Recreational Therapy Basics, Techniques, and Interventions*.

Recreational therapists can work with the rest of the medical team to provide therapy under this section. See the treatment for exercise tolerance functions for more ideas on general programming. Some specific diagnoses that the therapist may treat that are covered in this section include asthma and bronchial spasms, hyperventilation, especially if it is caused by psychological issues, and expansion of the lungs. Working on expansion of the lungs involves

finding ways to get the client to take deeper breaths. Simple activities, such as contests where the client is using a straw to blow a ping-pong ball across a table, can be used to increase lung function in a way that reduces the emphasis on "therapy" and is more likely to elicit the client's compliance.

Sometimes there is no effective treatment for the condition. Adaptations need to be made so that the required amount of effort is appropriate for the client's condition.

### Cross References

In *Recreational Therapy for Specific Diagnoses and Conditions, First Edition*, ICF code b440 Respiration Functions is listed in 13 chapters: Cancer, Cerebral Palsy, Chronic Obstructive Pulmonary Disease, Generalized Anxiety Disorder, Guillain-Barré Syndrome, Multiple Sclerosis, Obesity, Osteoarthritis, Osteoporosis, Sickle Cell Disease, Spina Bifida, Spinal Cord Injury, and Substance-Related Disorders.

In *Recreational Therapy Basics, Techniques, and Interventions, First Edition*, treatment for ICF code b440 Respiration Functions is discussed in three chapters: Parameters and Precautions, Energy Conservation Techniques, and Physical Activity.

### b445 Respiratory Muscle Functions

Functions of the muscles involved in breathing.

Inclusions: functions of thoracic respiratory muscles; functions of the diaphragm; functions of accessory respiratory muscles

Exclusions: respiration functions (b440); additional respiratory functions (b450); exercise tolerance functions (b455)

- *b4450 Functions of the Thoracic Respiratory Muscles*
  Functions of the thoracic muscles involved in breathing.

- *b4451 Functions of the Diaphragm*
  Functions of the diaphragm as involved in breathing.

- *b4452 Functions of Accessory Respiratory Muscles*
  Functions of the additional muscles involved in breathing.

- *b4458 Respiratory Muscle Functions, Other Specified*
- *b4459 Respiratory Muscle Functions, Unspecified*

These functions have to do with the muscles used to get air into and out of the body. Deficits in these functions are often the result of damage to the nerves that control the muscles, for example from spinal cord injury or ALS. The problems will be written in two places: where the damage to the nerves is discussed and here where the deficits resulting from the nerve damage are described. Other deficits in the functions of the respiratory muscles may be caused by damage to the muscles themselves.

These problems may be life threatening. They certainly will have an effect on the client's ability to participate in activities, even ones with minimal physical demands.

Recreational therapists need to understand the limitations of clients who have these deficits. If one of these functions is the cause of deficits in exercise tolerance, the treatment needs to be written in this section rather than in b455 Exercise Tolerance Functions.

As with everything related to respiration and blood circulation, the level of oxygen in the blood is an important issue, as well as heart rate, blood pressure, and respiration.

Recreational therapists can work with the rest of the medical team to provide therapy under this section. See the treatment for exercise tolerance functions for more ideas on general programming.

Sometimes there is no effective treatment for the condition. Adaptations need to be made so that the required amount of effort is appropriate for the client's condition.

### Cross References

In *Recreational Therapy for Specific Diagnoses and Conditions, First Edition*, ICF code b445 Respiratory Muscle Functions is listed in six chapters: Cerebral Palsy, Chronic Obstructive Pulmonary Disease, Guillain-Barré Syndrome, Multiple Sclerosis, Obesity, and Spinal Cord Injury.

In *Recreational Therapy Basics, Techniques, and Interventions, First Edition*, there are no references for ICF code b445 Respiratory Muscle Functions.

### b449 Functions of the Respiratory System, Other Specified and Unspecified

## Additional Functions and Sensations of the Cardiovascular and Respiratory Systems (b450 - b469)

### b450 Additional Respiratory Functions

Additional functions related to breathing, such as coughing, sneezing, and yawning.

Inclusions: functions of blowing, whistling, and mouth breathing

Recreational therapists are not likely to score b450 Additional Respiratory Functions, however if additional respiratory functions such as excessive yawning, coughing, sneezing, difficulty blowing, or mouth breathing, are observed in therapy sessions, it is documented and brought to the attention of the medical team for evaluation.

Recreational therapists can work with the rest of the treatment team to provide therapy under this section. Some of the therapy will be building skills. Other parts will be extinguishing inappropriate behaviors.

### Cross References

In *Recreational Therapy for Specific Diagnoses and Conditions, First Edition*, ICF code b450 Additional Respiratory Functions is listed in three chapters: Cerebral Palsy, Chronic Obstructive Pulmonary Disease, and Spinal Cord Injury.

In *Recreational Therapy Basics, Techniques, and Interventions, First Edition*, there are no references for ICF code b450 Additional Respiratory Functions.

### b455 Exercise Tolerance Functions

Functions related to respiratory and cardiovascular capacity as required for enduring physical exertion.

Inclusions: functions of physical endurance, aerobic capacity, stamina, and fatigability

Exclusions: functions of the cardiovascular system (b410 - b429); hematological system functions (b430); respiration functions (b440); respiratory muscle functions (b445); additional respiratory functions (b450)

- *b4550 General Physical Endurance*
  Functions related to the general level of tolerance of physical exercise or stamina.

- *b4551 Aerobic Capacity*
  Functions related to the extent to which a person can exercise without getting out of breath.

- *b4552 Fatigability*
  Functions related to susceptibility to fatigue, at any level of exertion.

- *b4558 Exercise Tolerance Functions, Other Specified*

- *b4559 Exercise Tolerance Functions, Unspecified*

Recreational therapists frequently address exercise tolerance functions for rehabilitation and health promotion. Healthy People 2010 recommends that healthy adults participate in at least 30 minutes of moderate physical activity five times a week to maintain health. The recommendations for children and teenagers are 60 minutes of moderate physical leisure activity five times a week to maintain health. The amount of time, intensity, and frequency of exercise for people who have health issues will vary depending on the person's limitations and abilities.

This section is used to document impairments in exercise tolerance that are not caused by other conditions. Many of the ideas presented here can be used for deficits documented in other parts of this chapter. The recreational therapist should check other sections to make sure they understand what is causing the deficit and only document in b455 Exercise Tolerance Functions if there is no other known cause for a lack of exercise tolerance. Given the average level of exercise for people in Western civilizations, this is likely to be a heavily used code.

Exercise functions are measured by frequency (how often the client engages in the specific activity), time (amount of time the client is able to engage in the specific activity), and intensity (mild, moderate, vigorous). Vital signs are used as a measure to assess and evaluate a client's functioning in each of the measures described.

Prior to establishing exercise tolerance goals, therapists are fully aware of and document any medical complications that could compromise optimal exercise tolerance functions.

The therapist makes the following notations during activities:

- Amount of time engaged in cardiovascular activity.
- The intensity of the cardiovascular activity.
- The client's ability to self-monitor vital signs and outward signs of fatigue.
- The client's ability to adapt exercises within the program to meet needs, including range restrictions and intensity alterations.
- The client's ability to perform the exercises correctly and safely.
- The client's reaction to participation in the exercise program.
- Vital sign measurements.

In addition to the above notations, recreational therapists can also score the ICF code **b455 Exercise Tolerance Functions**. The extent of impairment will be determined by identifying what is deemed an appropriate normative goal for the client. For example, if a client is able to participate in 10 minutes of light physical activity, where it is expected that 30 minutes of light physical activity would be the normative goal given the client's health situation, then the person would be assessed as having a 66% impairment because he is able to engage in 10 minutes out of 30 minutes (b4550.3).

Treatment and adaptations for deficits in exercise tolerance are a large topic. They are covered in detail in the companion volume, *Recreational Therapy Basics, Techniques, and Interventions,* in the chapter on Physical Activity.

***Cross References***

In *Recreational Therapy for Specific Diagnoses and Conditions, First Edition*, ICF code **b455 Exercise Tolerance Functions** is listed in 27 chapters: Amputation and Prosthesis, Back Disorders and Back Pain, Borderline Personality Disorder, Burns, Cancer, Cerebral Palsy, Cerebrovascular Accident, Chronic Obstructive Pulmonary Disease, Diabetes Mellitus, Epilepsy, Feeding and Eating Disorders, Fibromyalgia and Juvenile Fibromyalgia, Guillain-Barré Syndrome, Heart Disease, Intellectual Disability, Multiple Sclerosis, Neurocognitive Disorders, Obesity, Osteoarthritis, Osteoporosis, Parkinson's Disease, Rheumatoid Arthritis, Sickle Cell Disease, Spina Bifida, Total Joint Replacement, Traumatic Brain Injury, and Visual Impairments and Blindness.

In *Recreational Therapy Basics, Techniques, and Interventions, First Edition*, treatment for ICF code b455 Exercise Tolerance Functions is discussed in 14 chapters: Body Mechanics and Ergonomics, Consequences of Inactivity, Parameters and Precautions, Activity Pattern Development, Adventure Therapy, Animal Assisted Therapy, Aquatic Therapy, Behavior Strategies and Interventions, Cognitive Behavioral Counseling, Energy Conservation Techniques, Group Psychotherapy Techniques, Leisure Education and Counseling, Mind-Body Interventions, and Physical Activity.

### b460 Sensations Associated with Cardiovascular and Respiratory Functions

Sensations such as missing a heart beat, palpitation, and shortness of breath.

Inclusions: sensations of tightness of chest, feelings of irregular beat, dyspnea, air hunger, choking, gagging, and wheezing

Exclusions: sensation of pain (b280)

These functions cover some of the other cardiorespiratory conditions that can affect a client. Many of them are serious sensations that should not be ignored. The therapist should be aware of these symptoms and plan any treatment in a way that takes them into account.

If these symptoms have been noted and precautions have been outlined for a client, the therapist must be careful not to exceed any recommended levels of activity or violate any of the other precautions. Sometimes the therapist will be the first to hear reports of these sensations. Most of them are serious enough that the therapist should stop any physical activity and call for appropriate medical assistance.

Adaptations can be made in activities to allow the client to monitor his/her own sensations and adjust the level of activity as required to maintain appropriate functioning. The therapist should watch for signs that self-monitoring is not being done appropriately, especially when a client thinks s/he needs to "tough it out." Monitoring by the therapist is appropriate when the client is unable to do it. Activities can be adapted to meet a client's needs.

### Cross References

In *Recreational Therapy for Specific Diagnoses and Conditions, First Edition*, ICF code b460 Sensations Associated with Cardiovascular and Respiratory Functions is listed in one chapter: Heart Disease.

In *Recreational Therapy Basics, Techniques, and Interventions, First Edition*, there are no references for ICF code b460 Sensations Associated with Cardiovascular and Respiratory Functions.

### b469 Additional Functions and Sensations of the Cardiovascular and Respiratory Systems, Other Specified and Unspecified

### b498 Functions of the Cardiovascular, Hematological, Immunological, and Respiratory Systems, Other Specified

### b499 Functions of the Cardiovascular, Hematological, Immunological, and Respiratory Systems, Unspecified

### References
Boslaugh, S. E. & Andresen, E. M. (2006). Correlates of physical activity for adults with disability. *Preventing Chronic Disease, 3*(3), A78.
Durstine, J. L., Painter, P., Franklin, B. A., Morgan, D., Pitetti, K. H., & Roberts, S. O. (2000). Physical activity for the chronically ill and disabled. *Sports Medicine, 30*(3), 207-219.
Hamilton, M. T., Healy, G. N., Dunstan, D. W., Zderic, T. W., & Owen, N. (2008). Too little exercise and too much sitting: Inactivity physiology and the need for new recommendations on sedentary behavior. *Current Cardiovascular Risk Reports, 2*, 292-298.
Harkins, L. E. (2008). Literature analysis of humor therapy research. *American Journal of Recreation Therapy, 8*(4), 35-47.
Heyn, P. C., Johnson, K. E., & Kramer, A. F. (2008). Endurance and strength training outcomes on cognitively impaired and cognitively intact older adults: A meta-analysis. *Journal of Nutritional Health and Aging, 12*(6), 401-409.
Rainforth, M. V., Schneider, R. H., Nidich, S. I., Gaylord-King, C., Salerno, J. W., & Anderson, J. W. (2007). Stress reduction programs in patients with elevated blood pressure: A systematic review and meta-analysis. *Current Hypertension Reports, 9*(6), 520-528.
Rimmer, J. H. (2006). Use of the ICF in identifying factors that impact participation in physical activity/rehabilitation among people with disabilities. *Disability and Rehabilitation, 28*(17), 1087-1095.
U.S. Department of Health and Human Services. (2008). *Physical activity guidelines for Americans.* Accessed via website http://www.health.gov/PAGuidelines/guidelines/default.aspx.

# Chapter 5 Functions of the Digestive, Metabolic, and Endocrine Systems

This chapter is about the functions of ingestion, digestion, and elimination, as well as functions involved in metabolism and endocrine glands.

*Sample Scoring of Functions of the Digestive, Metabolic, and Endocrine Systems*

- A 12-year-old boy with spina bifida has episodes of fecal incontinence (b5253 Fecal Continence) approximately four times a week. He has about nine bowel movements a week. This equates to a ration of 4:9 or about 44% of the time (moderate impairment = 2). As a result, he is limiting his engagement with friends. The complete scoring would look like this: b5253.2.
- A 54-year-old male is obese (obesity class 3) (b530 Weight Maintenance Functions, complete impairment = 4). He has uncontrolled type 2 diabetes and had a right below-knee amputation. The complete scoring for weight maintenance would look like this: b530.4.
- An 18-year-old female sustained a complete T6 spinal cord injury. Consequently, her body doesn't rid itself of excess heat effectively because there is no sweating below injury level (b5501 Maintenance of Body Temperature). On hot days, she becomes overwhelmed by the heat and quickly exhibits signs of heat stroke (complete impairment = 4). In an effort to stay cool, she has been staying inside with the air conditioning on and rarely goes outside. The complete scoring would look like this: b5501.4.

Digestive, metabolic, and endocrine functions can significantly impact leisure and community functioning. These negatively affect health, quality of life, and social participation. Consequently, a team approach, including recreational therapy, is necessary to address the systemic issues. For example, difficulty with fecal incontinence in adolescents and adults with spinal cord injury is associated with depression, anxiety, and significant impairments in quality of life (Hocevar & Gray, 2008). Difficulties with digestive functions post stroke that result in eating smaller pieces or the need for only soft food can result in avoiding social activities out of concern for eating safely and properly. The client may fear vomiting or be embarrassed by cutting food into small pieces (Medin et al., 2010).

Obesity results in increased mortality, cardiovascular disease, obesity-related cancer, type 2 diabetes, physical impairment, psychological and social impairments, poorer quality of life, and economic burden on the healthcare system (Dixon, 2010). Likewise, individuals who are underweight due to an eating disorder or underlying disease process, such as cancer, that impacts body weight and appetite also have health and quality of life challenges. For example, individuals who are anorexic are at risk for premature death due to the impact on multiple organ systems along with having an impaired quality of life (Mitchell & Crow, 2006).

Some diagnoses may result in difficulties with core body temperature regulation, causing dysfunction. For example, individuals with multiple sclerosis overheat easily. Cooling the core body temperature of a person who has multiple sclerosis has been found to decrease fatigue and symptom flares (Kos et al., 2008). Individuals with a spinal cord injury can have difficulty regulating core body temperature due to the inability to lose excess heat by sweating (Karlsson, 2006).

## Assessment of Functions of the Digestive, Metabolic, and Endocrine Systems

Difficulty with digestive, metabolic, and endocrine functions are identified through chart review, client verbalizations and interviews, reports from others, observation, and the therapist's knowledge of clinical disability. Problems may also be identified through specific tests, such as BMI calculations and swallowing exams by speech-language pathologists.

## Treatment of Functions of the Digestive, Metabolic, and Endocrine Systems

Recreational therapists know that fecal incontinence and digestive functions can impair leisure and community participation. They strive to reduce difficulties related to these functions when they affect healthy participation in leisure and community activities. The interventions may include bowel management planning, managing fecal and digestive accidents, coping strategies, problem solving, family training, community integration training, and leisure education and counseling.

For individuals who are obese, recreational therapists take a systematic approach aimed at decreasing sedentary behavior and increasing engagement in personally meaningful leisure time physical activity within the client's parameters and precautions. The goal is promotion of active living with weight reduction, resolution of obesity-related disabling conditions, such as type 2 diabetes, and improved quality of life. Recreational therapists also work toward healthy dietary habits in leisure and community activities to promote caloric control and healthy eating without compromising engagement and activity enjoyment. Underlying psychological issues contributing to or resulting from weight gain are addressed, along with development or restoration of activity skills, family training, community integration, leisure education and counseling, and resource education related to physical activity and active living.

For individuals who are underweight, gradually stepped-up caloric consumption is encouraged. Underlying psychological, emotional, environmental, and social issues affecting caloric consumption are addressed, along with behavior change interventions. For those who are underweight due to an eating disorder, common recreational therapy interventions revolve around self-worth, stress management, reducing perfectionism and control, eliminating body image disturbances, reducing compulsive exercise, providing leisure education, and increasing social functioning (Miller & Jake, 2001).

Lastly, recreational therapists are aware of disabilities resulting in core body temperature dysfunction, implement safety precautions in therapy sessions, and provide education and training on how to plan ahead and manage core body temperature issue in leisure and community tasks to reduce risks, such as heat stroke and fatigue.

### Evidence Review

Several studies are provided below to highlight evidence-based practice related to digestive, metabolic, and endocrine systems functions. This is only a sample of the evidence. A thorough review of the literature is needed to identify evidence-based practice interventions that reflect the needs of a particular client.

Jakes et al. (2003) conducted a cross-sectional analysis of 15,515 adults in Norfolk (UK). They used television-watching hours as an indicator for sedentary behavior. They found that low participation in vigorous recreation and increased hours of television were associated with obesity, high blood pressure, and high plasma lipids. Individuals who participated in at least one hour of vigorous recreation a week and watched fewer than two hours of television a day had lower BMIs and diastolic blood pressures compared to those who participated in no vigorous recreation and watched four or more hours of television a day. In the compendium of energy cost, television is equivalent to "reclining" and has lower energy expenditure than other sedentary activities, such as sewing, playing board games, reading, or writing. For children, the literature indicated that television watching resulted in a lower metabolic rate than when at rest. The data suggests that reducing television watching by one hour could result in risk reduction of coronary heart disease by 2.5% and stroke by 4%. Interventions aimed at decreasing television time and increasing engagement in vigorous recreation to at least one time a week are recommended to decrease weight and cardiovascular disease risk.

Porter, Shank, and Iwasaki (2012) conducted a survey of 26 adults with type 2 diabetes regarding leisure time physical activity (LTPA) and extent of meaning experienced during LTPA. Findings indicated that more time was spent in LTPA when the meaning of the LTPA increased. Meaning was enhanced when participants experienced a sense of connection or belonging with individuals and groups or a sense of connection or belonging within the self. Attributes that made a difference included increased positive interactions with individuals and groups, a sense of increasing self-identity, control or power over oneself and things, competence and mastery, positive emotions of escalation, positive emotions of well-being, hope, optimism, and continued growth and development. The authors speculate that "systematically structured leisure counseling, provided by a recreational therapist early in the disease process, aimed at identifying, exploring, and enhancing the experience of such personal meanings in LTPA may prove helpful in diabetes management" (p. 204).

Schaffner and Buchanan (2008) evaluated the effectiveness of an outpatient day treatment program for 77 women diagnosed with eating disorders. They used an integrative approach based on evidence-based treatments and other interventions based on client needs including individual therapy, family therapy, and group therapy covering skills, general processes, meal processes, and experiences related to food. The treatment team consisted of dieticians, psychologists, social workers, a psychiatrist, a marriage and family therapist, a recreational therapist, and a professional counselor. Post treatment (average 12.8 weeks), clients reported a significant reduction in the eating disorder and depressive and anxiety symptoms, along with a significant increase in weight.

Taylor et al. (2012) conducted a convenience study of 10 children aged 10-18 diagnosed with type 1 diabetes and 11 parents. The group attended a one-week residential family camp operated by a recreational therapist. In the camp both the children and parents participated in traditional camp activities and both formal and informal diabetes education. Data were gathered pre- and post-camp and three months after the camp. Findings indicated increased perception of autonomy support from parents and a decrease in HbA1c levels.

### Cross References

In *Recreational Therapy for Specific Diagnoses and Conditions, First Edition*, ICF code b5 Functions of the Digestive, Metabolic, and Endocrine Systems and its subcategories are listed in 19 chapters: Back Disorders and Back Pain, Cerebral Palsy, Cerebrovascular Accident, Chronic Obstructive Pulmonary Disease, Diabetes Mellitus, Epilepsy, Feeding and Eating Disorders, Fibromyalgia and Juvenile Fibromyalgia, Generalized Anxiety Disorder, Guillain-Barré Syndrome, Intellectual Disability, Major Depressive Disorder, Multiple Sclerosis, Obesity, Parkinson's Disease, Rheumatoid Arthritis, Sickle Cell Disease, Spina Bifida, and Spinal Cord Injury.

In *Recreational Therapy Basics, Techniques, and Interventions, First Edition*, treatment for ICF code b5 Functions of the Digestive, Metabolic, and Endocrine Systems and its subcategories are discussed in five chapters: Parameters and Precautions, Psychoneuroimmunology, Stress, Adaptive Sports, and Physical Activity.

## Functions Related to the Digestive System (b510 - b539)

### b510 Ingestion Functions

Functions related to taking in and manipulating solids or liquids through the mouth into the body.

Inclusions: functions of sucking, chewing, and biting, manipulating food in the mouth, salvation, swallowing, burping, regurgitation, spitting, and vomiting; impairments such as dysphagia, aspiration of food, aerophagia, excessive salvation, drooling, and insufficient salivation

Exclusions: sensations associate with digestive system (b535)

- *b5100 Sucking*
  Functions of drawing into the mouth by a suction force produced by movements of the cheeks, lips, and tongue.

- *b5101 Biting*
  Functions of cutting into, piercing, or tearing off food with the front teeth.

- *b5102 Chewing*
  Functions of crushing, grinding, and masticating food with the back teeth (e.g., molars)

- *b5103 Manipulation of Food in the Mouth*
  Functions of moving food around the mouth with the teeth and tongue.

- *b5104 Salivation*
  Function of the production of saliva within the mouth.

- *b5105 Swallowing*
  Functions of clearing the food and drink through the oral cavity, pharynx, and esophagus into the stomach at an appropriate rate and speed.

  Inclusions: oral, pharyngeal, or esophageal dysphagia; impairments in esophageal passage of food

  o *b51050 Oral Swallowing*
    Function of clearing the food and drink through the oral cavity at an appropriate rate and speed.

o    *b51051 Pharyngeal Swallowing*
     Function of clearing the food and drink through the pharynx at an appropriate rate and speed.

o    *b51052 Esophageal Swallowing*
     Function of clearing the food and drink through the esophagus at an appropriate rate and speed.

o    *b51058 Swallowing, Other Specified*
o    *b51059 Swallowing, Unspecified*
•    *b5106 Regurgitation and Vomiting*
     Functions of moving food or liquid in the reverse direction to ingestion, from stomach to esophagus to mouth and out.

•    *b5108 Ingestion Functions, Other Specified*
•    *b5109 Ingestion Functions, Unspecified*

It is not anticipated that recreational therapists will score ingestion functions. If a client has ingestion function impairments, it will most likely be the speech-language pathologist or the ear, nose, and throat specialist who will score the extent of the client's impairment in these areas. Recreational therapists, however, need to be aware of ingestion impairments and address the impact that ingestion functions have on activity participation and the client's ability to follow correct swallowing techniques and adhere to diet levels in a real-life environment.

Ingestions functions can be impaired as a result of brain injury, such as a cerebrovascular accident that impairs muscular functions related to swallowing, mouth impairments, such as missing teeth, damage to the esophagus, as from burns, and surgery, such as a wired jaw.

A common problem resulting from cerebrovascular accident or traumatic brain injury is dysphagia. Dysphagia is defined as difficulty swallowing due to impaired neurological functions that control ingestion functions or due to some obstruction of the esophagus such as an esophageal tumor. Obstructions generally allow swallowing liquids. Impaired neurological function may prevent swallowing both solids and liquids. If a client has difficulty swallowing, s/he could choke or aspirate food and liquids causing harm or injury.

The speech-language pathologist evaluates the client's ingestion functions through a swallowing study that allows the therapist to see how the client bites, chews, manipulates, and swallows food. The results of the study will indicate to the therapist the type of diet the client should follow. There are four common food levels (pureed, mechanical soft, chopped, and regular) and four common fluid consistencies (one called thin and three with varying levels of thickness).

•    *Pureed foods* are blenderized.
•    *Mechanical soft* foods are those that require little or no chewing such as mashed potatoes, short flat noodles, and cooked carrots.
•    *Chopped diet* consists of foods that require some, but not rigorous chewing, such as cubed chicken, chopped lasagna, and chopped string beans.
•    *Regular diet* has no food texture restrictions.
•    *Thin liquids* include water, ice tea, coffee, and lemonade.
•    *Thick liquid* diet means that thin liquids need to be thickened. Thick liquids are those with significant solid material in the liquid. They come in three consistencies (UPMC, 2014). Nectar-thick liquids are easily pourable and are comparable to apricot nectar or thicker cream soups. Honey-thick liquids are slightly thicker, are less pourable, and drizzle from a cup or bowl. Pudding-thick liquids hold their own shape. They are not pourable and are usually eaten with a spoon. A product called Thick It is commonly used to thicken thin liquids. As per the product's label, a certain amount of the Thick It powder is stirred into the thin liquid to make it the desired consistency.

In addition to determining the diet level, the speech-language pathologist will recommend specific swallowing techniques to decrease risk of aspiration such as thorough chewing, tucking in the chin, and swallowing twice.

People who do not have dysphagia, but who do have other difficulties with chewing and swallowing, such as missing teeth, burned esophagus, or wired jaw, will also have specific recommendations. Individuals who are missing moderate numbers of teeth may have difficulty chewing and manipulating food resulting in the recommendation of eating mechanical soft and chopped foods. Certain foods may irritate a burned esophagus and, depending on the extent of damage to the esophagus, a feeding tube may be needed. A person who has a wired jaw will typically be allowed to eat small amounts of pureed foods and thin liquids through a straw.

Therapists document the type of diet the client is following, causes of swallowing impairments, ability of the client to adhere to special diet in real-life settings, ability of the client to follow swallowing techniques in real-life settings, and any other restrictions or adaptations that are required by impairments in functioning.

Treatment is aimed at restoring functions discussed in this section. Progression to a regular diet and thin liquids is possible in many cases with the aid of a speech-language pathologist.

For treatment and adaptations, the recreational therapist needs to be aware of diet levels (both food and liquid) and recommended swallowing techniques for several reasons:

- To know what a client is allowed and not allowed to have during a therapy session. The therapist needs to know if there are restrictions when the client asks for a glass of water, wants to eat a cookie that was made in the therapy kitchen, or wants to order a specific food or liquid in the community.

- To problem solve for the impact that diet levels have on activity participation. For example, the client may refuse to engage in community socializing activities because food and drink are often available and the client does not want to use thickener in front of his peers.

- To reinforce proper food choice in a real-life community environment. The therapist needs to teach the client what items on the menu are considered mechanical soft.

- To reinforce proper swallowing techniques in a real-life community environment, such as using swallowing techniques at a restaurant.

Adaptations seek to normalize to the greatest extent possible the client's experience of eating. Other adaptations include working with the client to deal with emotional issues resulting from difficulty in eating and working with family and friends to explain how they can help the client eat appropriately.

### Cross References

In *Recreational Therapy for Specific Diagnoses and Conditions, First Edition*, ICF code b510 Ingestion Functions is listed in eight chapters: Cerebral Palsy, Chronic Obstructive Pulmonary Disease, Feeding and Eating Disorders, Fibromyalgia and Juvenile Fibromyalgia, Guillain-Barré Syndrome, Multiple Sclerosis, Parkinson's Disease, and Rheumatoid Arthritis.

In *Recreational Therapy Basics, Techniques, and Interventions, First Edition*, treatment for ICF code b510 Ingestion Functions is discussed in one chapter: Parameters and Precautions.

### b515 Digestive Functions

Functions of transporting food through the gastrointestinal tract, breakdown of food, and absorption of nutrients.

Inclusions: functions of transport of food through the stomach, peristalsis; breakdown of food, enzyme production, and action in stomach and intestines; absorption of nutrients and tolerance to food; impairments such as in hyperacidity of stomach, malabsorption, intolerance to food, hypermotility of intestines, intestinal paralysis, intestinal obstruction, and decreased bile production

Exclusions: ingestion functions (b510); assimilation functions (b520); defecation functions (b525); sensations associated with the digestive system (b535)

- *b5150 Transport of Food through Stomach and Intestines*
  Peristalsis and related functions that mechanically move food through stomach and intestines.

- *b5151 Breakdown of Food*
  Functions of mechanically reducing food to smaller particles in the gastrointestinal tract.

- *b5152 Absorption of Nutrients*
  Functions of passing food and drink nutrients into the bloodstream from along the intestines.

- *b5153 Tolerance to Food*
  Functions of accepting suitable food and drink for digestion and rejecting what is unsuitable.

  Inclusions: impairments such as hypersensitivities, gluten intolerance

- *b5158 Digestive Functions, Other Specified*
- *b5159 Digestive Functions, Unspecified*

Recreational therapists are not likely to score ICF codes included in b515 Digestive Functions. If a person has difficulty digesting foods and liquids, the person would be referred to a gastroenterologist for further evaluation and documentation of the extent of digestive function impairments. Recommendations from the gastroenterologist are followed by the healthcare team such as avoidance of certain foods or total restriction of food types.

Documentation for the recreational therapist is generally limited to noting how well the client follows dietary restrictions in the community.

Adaptations or particular skills may be required, such as assertiveness in refusing to eat harmful foods. Treatment for these adaptations may be better described using Activities and Participation codes related to social interactions.

### Cross References

In *Recreational Therapy for Specific Diagnoses and Conditions, First Edition*, ICF code b515 Digestive Functions is listed in five chapters: Feeding and Eating Disorders, Guillain-Barré Syndrome, Parkinson's Disease, Sickle Cell Disease, and Spina Bifida.

In *Recreational Therapy Basics, Techniques, and Interventions, First Edition*, there are no references for ICF code b515 Digestive Functions.

### b520 Assimilation Functions

Functions by which nutrients are converted into components of the living body.

Inclusions: functions of storage of nutrients in the body

Exclusions: digestive functions (b515); defecation functions (b525); weight maintenance functions (b530); general metabolic functions (b540)

Scoring or addressing impairments of assimilation functions is not within the scope of recreational therapy practice.

As with other functions in this chapter, the recreational therapist may need to teach skills required for appropriate adaptations caused by deficits in assimilation of food.

### Cross References

In *Recreational Therapy for Specific Diagnoses and Conditions, First Edition*, there are no references for ICF code b520 Assimilation Functions.

In *Recreational Therapy Basics, Techniques, and Interventions, First Edition*, there are no references for ICF code b520 Assimilation Functions.

### b525 Defecation Functions

Functions of elimination of wastes and undigested food as feces and related functions.

Inclusions: functions of elimination, fecal consistency, frequency of defecation; fecal continence, flatulence; impairments such as constipation, diarrhea, watery stool, and anal sphincter incompetence or incontinence

Exclusions: digestive functions (b515); assimilation functions (b520); sensations associated with the digestive system (b535)

- *b5250 Elimination of Feces*
  Functions of the elimination of waste from the rectum, including the functions of contraction of the abdominal muscles in doing so.

- *b5251 Fecal Consistency*
  Consistency of feces such as hard, firm, soft, or watery.

- *b5252 Frequency of Defecation*
  Functions involved in the frequency of defecation.

- *b5253 Fecal Continence*
  Functions involved in voluntary control over the elimination function.

- *b5254 Flatulence*
  Functions involved in the expulsion of excessive amounts of air or gases from the intestines.

- *b5258 Defecation Functions, Other Specified*
- *b5259 Defecation Functions, Unspecified*

Defecation functions are traditionally monitored and scored by nursing staff, so it is not anticipated that recreational therapists will score defecation function codes. Recreational therapists may document defecation functions as they impact a client's ability to participate in activities, such as "Client had three episodes of fecal incontinence during one hour afternoon session" or "Excessive flatulence is a severe hindrance to social activity participation."

Recreational therapists need to be aware of defecation functions that pose a health threat and monitor the client appropriately. Examples include proper hydration for a client with diarrhea or checking with nursing staff prior to going out of the hospital for community integration training to make sure that a client at risk for autonomic dysreflexia isn't having any bowel issues, such as impacted bowels. Recreational therapists may also monitor defecation functions to assist with tracking the amount of food consumed for clients diagnosed with an eating disorder. If working with toddlers who are potty training, frequency of bowel movements are routinely tracked since holding bowel movements can become habitual in children who don't want to stop playing and come inside to use the bathroom or who have had a painful bowel movement and hold bowels to avoid a repeat of the painful feeling.

Defecation functions are managed through medication, diet, behavior modification, and adaptive devices. Undergarments may be worn for fecal incontinence that is not yet controlled.

Recreational therapists who conduct community integration training need to be aware of the defecation impairments of their clients to adequately prepare for possible situations. This may include a change of clothes, wipes, plastic bags, and room spray, especially for those who are easily embarrassed. The therapist should always have a cell phone to call emergency services for problems like a client going into autonomic dysreflexia.

Some impairments in defecation functions require an ostomy as a temporary or permanent solution to an intestinal or anus malformation or disease. An ostomy is a surgical procedure that, in a sense, disconnects the intestinal tract at a place that is predetermined and pulls the end of the intestine to the surface of the abdomen. An artificial opening is created on the abdomen and the intestine is pulled through. The portion of the intestine that exits the abdomen is called the stoma. It is red to pink and looks raw, although it is not painful because intestinal tissue does not have pain receptors. A pouch-like bag is attached around the stoma to collect bowel waste. As fecal material passes through the intestines, the body absorbs much of the liquid from the digesting food and the fecal material becomes firmer as it travels through the tract. Consequently, the location of the ostomy will determine the consistency of the fecal material, which will vary from firm to soft, pasty, or liquid-like. If an ostomy is at the jejunum of the small intestine, it is called a jejunostomy. If the ostomy is at the ileum of the small intestine, it is called an ileostomy. If the ostomy is done to the large intestine, it is called a colostomy. Fecal material that is excreted in a liquid-like form creates a high risk for skin breakdown and subsequent infections. The

pouch-like bag is changed and replaced routinely throughout the day.

Psychosocial adjustment to having an ostomy can be difficult. Tight clothing is contraindicated so that the pouch does not become constricted. Activities that cause rubbing or pressure against the pouch are also contraindicated so precautions must be taken to avoid activities like contact sports. Odor and leaking can become a hindrance to socialization and forming intimate relationships because of embarrassment, fear of rejection, and humiliation. In the American culture defecation functions are often seen as dirty. It is something that is not talked about and is done in private. Having an ostomy confronts the individual with challenges throughout the day. They can include leaks, odors, hindrances to activity, or simply awareness of its position and the need to guard it against contact from a child jumping on the lap or a person sliding over too closely on a bench seat. Consequently, some clients eventually hate the ostomy and either consciously or unconsciously begin to neglect its care. This exacerbates problems when the pouch becomes over filled and leaks or increased fecal material results in stronger odor. The increase in problems often strengthens the client's neglect of its care, making matters increasingly worse. These ideas for treatment will make the situation better:

- Recreational therapy's role in caring for an ostomy focuses primarily on psychosocial adjustment and integrating its care into real-life settings.
- The recreational therapist and primary nurse often collaborate to problem solve for leaking issues related to specific activity movements.
- Self-esteem is promoted by providing activities and experiences that result in success and highlight the person's strengths. Identifying a person's strengths and developing ongoing opportunities that highlight the person's strengths will continually foster good self-esteem and minimize the effect of the ostomy.
- Recreational therapists reinforce needed care for the ostomy and educate the person as needed about the role that defecation functions play in health.

*Cross References*

In *Recreational Therapy for Specific Diagnoses and Conditions, First Edition*, ICF code b525 Defecation Functions is listed in seven chapters: Cerebral Palsy, Cerebrovascular Accident, Fibromyalgia and Juvenile Fibromyalgia, Guillain-Barré Syndrome, Multiple Sclerosis, Parkinson's Disease, and Spina Bifida.

In *Recreational Therapy Basics, Techniques, and Interventions, First Edition*, there are no references for ICF code b525 Defecation Functions.

### b530 Weight Maintenance Functions

Functions of maintaining appropriate body weight, including weight gain in the developmental period.

Inclusions: functions of maintenance of acceptable Body Mass Index (BMI); impairments such as underweight, cachexia, wasting, overweight, emaciation, and such as in primary and secondary obesity

Exclusions: assimilation functions (b520); general metabolic functions (b540); endocrine gland functions (b555)

It is unlikely that recreational therapists will score this code. It is more likely that recreational therapists will score the related Activities and Participation code d5701 Managing Diet and Fitness.

*Cross References*

In *Recreational Therapy for Specific Diagnoses and Conditions, First Edition*, ICF code b530 Weight Maintenance Functions is listed in eight chapters: Back Disorders and Back Pain, Cerebral Palsy, Diabetes Mellitus, Feeding and Eating Disorders, Intellectual Disability, Major Depressive Disorder, Obesity, and Spina Bifida.

In *Recreational Therapy Basics, Techniques, and Interventions, First Edition*, treatment for ICF code b530 Weight Maintenance Functions is discussed in two chapters: Adaptive Sports and Physical Activity.

### b535 Sensations Associated with the Digestive System

Sensations arising from eating, drinking, and related digestive functions.

Inclusions: sensations of nausea, feeling bloated, and the feeling of abdominal cramps, fullness of stomach, globus feeling, spasm of stomach, gas in stomach, and heartburn

Exclusions: sensation of pain (b280); ingestion functions (b510); digestive functions (b515); defecation functions (b525)

- *b5350 Sensation of Nausea*
  Sensation of needing to vomit.

- *b5351 Feeling Bloated*
  Sensation of distension of the stomach or abdomen.

- *b5352 Sensation of Abdominal Cramps*
  Sensation of spasmodic or painful muscular contractions of the smooth muscles of the gastrointestinal tract.

- *b5358 Sensations Associated with the Digestive System, Other Specified*
- *b5359 Sensations Associate with the Digestive System, Unspecified*

Nursing is the healthcare discipline that traditionally monitors and scores sensations associated with digestive functions. However, recreational therapists may document sensations associated with digestive functions if they affect a client's ability to participate in activities. Examples include a client who complains of severe heartburn or abdominal cramping after lunch affecting his ability to participate in therapy or a client who is three months pregnant and reports vomiting twice a day after meals. Other causes of nausea, bloating, and cramping after food ingestion include food poisoning, food intolerance, and excessive food intake. Problems like these should be reported to the rest of the healthcare team.

Treatment interventions will vary depending on the cause of the problem.

Recreational therapists report impairments to appropriate health professionals and are prepared to handle vomiting in a community environment by having a spill kit to clean up vomit, bags for vomiting, wipes, and pair of hospital scrubs or other clothes in case a change of clothes is needed.

*Cross References*

In *Recreational Therapy for Specific Diagnoses and Conditions, First Edition*, ICF code b535 Sensations Associated with the Digestive System is listed in two chapters: Feeding and Eating Disorders and Generalized Anxiety Disorder.

In *Recreational Therapy Basics, Techniques, and Interventions, First Edition*, there are no references for ICF code b535 Sensations Associated with the Digestive System.

### b539 Functions Related to the Digestive System, Other Specified and Unspecified

## Functions Related to Metabolism and the Endocrine System (b540 - b559)

### b540 General Metabolic Functions

Functions of regulation of essential components of the body such as carbohydrates, proteins, and fats, the conversion of one to another, and their breakdown into energy.

Inclusions: functions of metabolism, basal metabolic rate, metabolism of carbohydrate, protein, and fat, catabolism, anabolism, energy production in the body; increase or decrease in metabolic rate

Exclusions: assimilation functions (b520); weight maintenance functions (b530); water, mineral, and electrolyte balance functions (b545); thermoregulatory functions (b550); endocrine glands functions (b555)

- b5400 Basal Metabolic Rate
  Functions involved in oxygen consumption of the body at specified conditions of rest and temperature.

  Inclusions: increase or decrease in basic metabolic rate; impairments such as in hyperthyroidism and hypothyroidism

- b5401 Carbohydrate Metabolism
  Functions involved in the process by which carbohydrates in the diet are stored and broken down into glucose and subsequently into carbon dioxide and water.

- b5402 Protein Metabolism
  Functions involved in the process by which proteins in the diet are converted to amino acids and broken down further in the body.

- b5403 Fat Metabolism
  Functions involved in the process by which fat in the diet is stored and broken down in the body.

- b5408 General Metabolic Functions, Other Specified
- b5409 General Metabolic Functions, Unspecified

Recreational therapists are not likely to score ICF codes in b540 General Metabolic Functions. However, recreational therapists are aware of metabolic impairments and their impact on activity. For example, if it is known that the client has a problem metabolizing fat, specific recommendations may be prescribed by the client's physician that need to be incorporated into activity. If the physician wishes to limit the amount of fats in the client's diet, the therapist must address issues surrounding food choices in a real-life setting. If the physician wants to increase physical activity to assist with fat metabolism, the therapist looks for physical leisure interests to assist with increasing physical activity.

Recreational therapists document the specific impairment (e.g., impairment with carbohydrate metabolism resulting from diabetes) and their association with activity (e.g., goal is to increase moderate physical leisure activity to five times a week for 30 minutes to assist with managing diabetes).

Treatment and adaptations involve the ongoing coordination of efforts with the rest of the treatment team to change the client's level of activity and recreational choices so they are appropriate for the deficits the client has.

### Cross References

In *Recreational Therapy for Specific Diagnoses and Conditions, First Edition*, ICF code b540 General Metabolic Functions is listed in three chapters: Diabetes Mellitus, Feeding and Eating Disorders, and Obesity.

In *Recreational Therapy Basics, Techniques, and Interventions, First Edition*, treatment for ICF code b540 General Metabolic Functions is discussed in two chapters: Parameters and Precautions and Physical Activity.

### b545 Water, Mineral, and Electrolyte Balance Functions

Functions of the regulation of water, mineral, and electrolytes in the body.

Inclusions: functions of water balance; balance of minerals such as calcium, zinc, and iron, and balance of electrolytes such as sodium and potassium;

impairments such as in water retention, dehydration, hypercalcemia, hypocalcemia, iron deficiency, hypernatremia, hyponatremia, hyperkalemia, and hypokalemia

Exclusions: hematological system functions (b430); general metabolic functions (b540); endocrine gland functions (b555)

- *b5450 Water Balance*
  Functions involved in maintaining the level or amount of water in the body.

  Inclusions: impairments such as in dehydration and rehydration

  o *b54500 Water Retention*
    Functions involved in keeping water in the body.

  o *b54501 Maintenance of Water Balance*
    Functions involved in maintaining the optimal amount of water in the body.

  o *b54508 Water Balance Functions, Other Specified*

  o *b54509 Water Balance Functions, Unspecified*

- *b5451 Mineral Balance*
  Functions involved in maintaining equilibrium between intake, storage, utilization, and excretion of minerals in the body.

- *b5452 Electrolyte Balance*
  Functions involved in maintaining equilibrium between intake, storage, utilization, and excretion of electrolytes in the body.

- *b5458 Water, Mineral, and Electrolyte Balance Functions, Other Specified*

- *b5459 Water, Mineral, and Electrolyte Balance Functions, Unspecified*

Recreational therapists are not likely to score ICF codes in b545 Water, Mineral, and Electrolyte Balance Functions. However, recreational therapists must be familiar with signs of dehydration, such as pruned lips, reduced tears, dry mouth, and reduced urination, and causes of dehydration, such as prolonged vomiting, diarrhea, lack of fluid intake, intense exercise, and hot conditions. Dehydration can be fatal, especially in infants and young children, who dehydrate faster than adults. If dehydration is left untreated, seizures, coma, and death may occur.

Therapists must offer clients appropriate fluids when increased activity is causing loss of fluids. For example, physical activity increases metabolic rate, increased metabolic rate increases fluid loss through sweat, and the body sweats to reduce internal body heat that is generated through activity. Appropriate fluids must be available during activities and the therapist must make sure that the clients drink the fluids as appropriate and learn to monitor their own fluid needs. If serious dehydration is believed to be present, the therapist brings it to the immediate attention of the client's primary nurse for further evaluation and treatment.

Similarly, the therapist must be aware of electrolyte balance during strenuous activities. Working with the dietary and nursing staff, the recreational therapist can provide fluids, such as sports drinks, that will replace electrolytes during activities. For some clients, use of fluids with electrolytes will need to be monitored and charted.

Mineral balance impairments can present as psychiatric conditions. Two common examples are

- *Hypercalcemia* (excessive calcium in the blood): causes apathy, muscle weakness, delirium, and personality and cognitive changes.
- *Hypocalcemia* (decreased calcium): causes delirium and personality changes, seizures, and intracranial pressure in the brain.

Therapists should not be quick to suggest a client has a psychiatric condition, especially one that has an unexpected onset, prior to a physician ruling out underlying conditions and seeking evaluation from a psychiatrist, psychologist, or neuropsychologist.

### Cross References

In *Recreational Therapy for Specific Diagnoses and Conditions, First Edition*, ICF code b545 Water, Mineral, and Electrolyte Balance Functions is listed in three chapters: Diabetes Mellitus, Epilepsy, and Feeding and Eating Disorders.

In *Recreational Therapy Basics, Techniques, and Interventions, First Edition*, treatment for ICF code b545 Water, Mineral, and Electrolyte Balance Functions is discussed in one chapter: Parameters and Precautions.

### b550 Thermoregulatory Functions

Functions of the regulation of body temperature.

Inclusions: functions of maintenance of body temperature; impairments such as hypothermia, hyperthermia

Exclusions: general metabolic functions (b540); endocrine gland functions (b555)

- *b5500 Body Temperature*
  Functions involved in regulating the core temperature of the body.

  Inclusions: impairments such as hyperthermia or hypothermia

- *b5501 Maintenance of Body Temperature*
  Functions involved in maintaining optimal body temperature as environmental temperature changes.

  Inclusions: tolerance to heat or cold

- *b5508 Thermoregulatory Functions, Other Specified*
- *b5509 Thermoregulatory Functions, Unspecified*
  Recreational therapists are not likely to score ICF Codes under b550 Thermoregulatory Functions. However, recreational therapists assess and monitor body temperature in some situations, such as a client who complains of feeling feverish on an outing. They monitor thermoregulatory behaviors that can affect core body temperature. For example, to keep core body temperature cool on a hot day, clients should dress in light cotton clothes, take a cold bottle of water, wear a hat, and sit in the shade when possible.

On community outings the therapist is responsible for being sure that all clients are appropriately dressed for the prevailing conditions. Many of these issues are covered in Activities and Participation codes.

### Cross References

In *Recreational Therapy for Specific Diagnoses and Conditions, First Edition*, ICF code b550 Thermoregulatory Functions is listed in five chapters: Epilepsy, Feeding and Eating Disorders, Fibromyalgia and Juvenile Fibromyalgia, Rheumatoid Arthritis, and Spinal Cord Injury.

In *Recreational Therapy Basics, Techniques, and Interventions, First Edition*, treatment for ICF code b550 Thermoregulatory Functions is discussed in one chapter: Parameters and Precautions.

### b555 Endocrine Gland Functions

Functions of production and regulation of hormonal levels in the body, including cyclical changes.

Inclusions: functions of hormonal balance; hyperpituitarism, hypopituitarism, hyperthyroidism, hypothyroidism, hyperadrenalism, hypoadrenalism, hyperparathyroidism, hypoparathyroidism, hypergonadism, hypogonadism

Exclusions: general metabolic functions (b540); water, mineral, and electrolyte balance functions (b545); thermoregulatory functions (b550); sexual functions (b640); menstruation functions (b650)

Recreational therapists will not likely score b555 Endocrine Gland Functions. Recreational therapists are aware, however, that endocrine gland impairments can affect behavior, mood, energy level, sleep problems, mental functions, psychological stability, and growth. The endocrine system is so important to body functions that almost any psychological or physiological problem could be caused by an endocrine dysfunction. Recreational therapists document the impairment using other ICF codes specific to the type of impairment. When it is appropriate, the other members of the medical team will order testing of the endocrine system to score this ICF code.

An example of how endocrine dysfunction affects multiple areas of health is provided through the descriptions of hyperthyroidism and hypothyroidism, two common endocrine gland impairments:

- *Hyperthyroidism*: Feelings of fatigue and general weakness, insomnia, unexplained weight loss, heart palpitations, increased perspiration, agitated behavior, feelings of anxiousness. In severe cases the client can present with memory impairments, orientation impairments, manic excitement, delusions, and hallucinations.
- *Hypothyroidism*: Feeling mentally slow, unexplained weight gain, thin and dry hair that comes out easily when combing and brushing, cold intolerance, reduced hearing, a deeper voice sound, loss of the lateral eyebrow. In severe cases the client can present with paranoia, hallucinations, and depression.

Clients who are suspected of having deficits in endocrine gland functions are evaluated for underlying endocrine function impairments as part of the process for ruling out underlying medical conditions. A referral to a psychologist, psychiatrist, or neuropsychologist may also be made to rule out psychiatric conditions. Endocrine function impairments are predominately treated with medication and monitored by an endocrinologist. Adaptations may be required to take into account the presenting symptoms.

### Cross References

In *Recreational Therapy for Specific Diagnoses and Conditions, First Edition*, there are no references for ICF code b555 Endocrine Gland Functions.

In *Recreational Therapy Basics, Techniques, and Interventions, First Edition*, there are no references for ICF code b555 Endocrine Gland Functions.

## b569 Functions Related to Metabolism and the Endocrine System, Other Specified and Unspecified

## b598 Functions of the Digestive, Metabolic, and Endocrine Systems, Other Specified

## b599 Functions of the Digestive, Metabolic, and Endocrine Systems, Unspecified

### References

Dixon, J. B. (2010). The effect of obesity on health outcomes. *Molecular and Cellular Endocrinology, 316*(2), 104-108.

Hocevar, B. & Gray, M. (2008). Intestinal diversion (colostomy or ileostomy) in patients with severe bowel dysfunction following spinal cord injury. *J Wound Ostomy Continence Nursing, 35*(2), 159-166.

Medin, J., Larson, J., von Arbin, M., Wredling, R., Tham, K. (2010). Striving for control in eating situations after stroke. *Scandinavian Journal of Caring Sciences, 24*, 772-780.

Jakes, R. W., Day, N. E., Khaw, K. T., Luben, R., Oakes, S., Welch, A., Bingham, S., & Wareham, N. J. (2003). Television viewing and low participation in vigorous recreation are independently associated with obesity and markers of cardiovascular risk: EPIC-Norfolk population-based study. *European Journal of Clinical Nutrition, 57*, 1089-1096.

Kos, D., Kerckhofs, E., Nagels, G., D'hooghe, M. B., Ilsbroukx, S. (2008). Origin of fatigue in multiple sclerosis: Review of the literature. *The American Society of Neurorehabilitation, 22*(1), 91-100.

Karlsson, A. K. (2006). Autonomic dysfunction in spinal cord injury: Clinical presentation of symptoms and signs. *Progress in Brain Research, 152*, 1-8.

Miller, D. & Jake, L. (2001). *Eating disorders: Providing effective recreational therapy interventions*. Ravensdale, WA: Idyll Arbor, Inc.

Mitchell, J. & Crow, S. (2006). Medical complications of anorexia nervosa and bulimia nervosa. *Current Option in Psychiatry, 19*(4), 438-443.

Porter, H. R., Shank, J., & Iwasaki, Y. (2012). Promoting a collaborative approach with recreational therapy to improve physical activity engagement in type 2 diabetes. *Therapeutic Recreation Journal, XLVI*(3), 204-219.

Schaffner, A. & Buchanan, L. P. (2008). Integrating evidence-based treatments with individual needs in an outpatient facility for eating disorders. *Eating Disorders, 16*, 378-392.

Taylor, J., Piatt, J., Hill, E., & Malcolm, T. (2012). Diabetes camps and self-determination theory: Controlling glycemic level in youth with type 1 diabetes. *Annual in Therapeutic Recreation, 20*, 46-58.

UPMC. (2014). Thickened Liquids: Nectar-Thick. Accessed via website www.upmc.com/patients-visitors/education/nutrition/pages/thickened-liquids-nectar-thick.aspx.

# Chapter 6 Genitourinary and Reproductive Functions

This chapter is about the functions of urination and the reproductive functions, including sexual and procreative functions.

*Sample Scoring of Genitourinary and Reproductive Functions Codes*

- A young male client who sustained a complete spinal cord injury tells you he is worried about leading a fulfilling life. He is single and concerned about his ability to have intercourse because he is unable to achieve an erection (b6703 Genital Functions, 4 = complete impairment). He fears this will hinder his ability to find a life partner and that he will be alone for the rest of his life. The complete scoring would look like this: b6703.4.
- An adult female client who has multiple sclerosis (MS) shares with you that her relationship with her husband is not what it used to be. Her husband is interested in sex, but she is not. She tells you that about 50% of the time "it doesn't feel the same" due to sensation problems related to the MS (b6708 Sensations Associated with Genital and Reproductive Functions, Other Specified, severe difficulty = 3). As a result, she is unable to become sexually aroused (b6400 Functions of Sexual Arousal Phase, severe difficulty = 3). The complete scoring for both codes would look like this: b6708.3, b6400.3.

When difficulties arise in bladder and sexual functions, engagement in leisure, community, and social life can be significantly impacted causing major shifts in quality of life and health.

For example, 1,705 older adult males with urinary incontinence were compared to older adult males who were urinary continent (Kwong et al., 2010). The researchers found that the older adult males who were urinary incontinent had lower quality of life scores and poorer self-perceived general health compared to the older adult males who were continent.

Landefeld et al. (2008) report that urinary and fecal incontinence can cause feelings of shame and embarrassment, physical discomfort, disruption to daily lives, stress in relationships, low productivity at work, job difficulties, arrangement of daily activities by bathroom location, avoidance of activities that provoke incontinence, anxiety about "accidents," depression, social isolation, social exclusion, financial challenges, reduction of community interactions, sexual activity limitations, and greater amounts of informal and formal caregiving possibly affecting family relationships. The total economic cost is about $20 billion in the United States.

Individuals who have a disability related to reproductive functions may face physical, mental, behavioral, psychological, emotional, social, communication, and spiritual changes. All of these have the potential to affect sexual functioning and relationships. Although research specific to the health benefits of sexual activity is scarce, Bullough and Bullough (1994) notes that "[what] is important is to recognize that pleasurable experiences are essential to health, to the quality of life, and to the quality of relationships. The more we enjoy ourselves and each other, and the more gratified and fulfilled we feel, the more energy we have not only to realize our own dreams but to nurture and support the dreams of the people we love" (p. 464).

## Assessment of Genitourinary and Reproductive Functions

Recreational therapists may learn of incontinence or sexual difficulties through review of the client's medical chart, direct questioning, or observation of behaviors followed by exploration of the issue. Since incontinence and sexuality are commonly private matters, the client may not immediately disclose his/her concerns. The therapist may need to initiate and explore these issues delicately.

Knowledge of risk factors helps identify clients who may have difficulties or challenges. Risk factors for incontinence in adults include (1) physical status (e.g., age, sex, obesity, limited physical activity), (2) genetic factors (e.g., family history), (3) neuropsychiatric conditions (e.g., multiple sclerosis, spinal cord injury, dementia, depression, stroke, diabetic neuropathy), (4) trauma (e.g., childbirth, prostatectomy, radiation), and (5) associated causalities (e.g., diarrhea, inflammatory bowel disease, irritable bowel syndrome, menopause, smoking, constipation).

Fewer than half of incontinent adults report their symptoms during healthcare visits due to social stigma, discomfort disclosing symptoms, limited knowledge about potential benefits of intervention, competing demands and time limits during the healthcare visit, and lack of directness by the care provider (Landefeld et al., 2008). The last two concerns are within the control of the therapist. S/he should take the opportunity to ask. In regards to adult sexuality, it is recommended that therapists broach the subject of sexual activity with all clients in appropriate ways. Sexual activity encompasses many domains. Therefore anyone being seen for a health-related condition has the possibility of experiencing sexual difficulties (Taylor & Davis, 2007).

### Treatment of Genitourinary and Reproductive Functions

Incontinence and sexual functioning can be related to one or many factors, consequently treatment of incontinence or sexual functioning can range from simple to complex. From a behavioral and lifestyle approach, there are particular issues that can reduce incontinence risk. These include achieving a healthy body weight, increasing physical activity, adhering to a healthy diet, stopping smoking, limiting high-impact recreational activities, training pelvic floor muscles, and managing comorbid conditions.

For sexual functioning, Taylor and Davis (2007) recommend using the extended PLISSIT model (Ex-PLISSIT). The Ex-PLISSIT model is an extension of the PLISSIT model (P = permission giving, LI = limited information, SS = specific suggestions, IT = intensive therapy). The "extended" component is that the therapist seeks permission before each component in the model, not just the first time the subject is discussed. It also encourages the therapist and client to "reflect and review" at each component in the model to better understand the perspective of the client, to make sure all questions and concerns have been addressed, and to provide information and strategies that meet the needs of the client. Recreational therapists commonly complete the first three components of the PLISSIT model and make referrals as needed for the last component. More details of the model are discussed in the Sexual Well Being chapter of *Recreational Therapy Basics, Techniques, and Interventions* (Porter, 2016).

### Evidence Review

Reviews of several studies are provided below to highlight evidence-based practice related to genitourinary and reproductive functions. This is only a sample of the evidence; a thorough review of the literature may be needed to identify evidence-based practice interventions that reflect the needs of a specific client.

Matevosyan (2009) conducted a review of 84 studies related to reproductive health in women with serious mental illness. Women who have serious mental illness were found to have more lifetime sex partners, low contraceptive use, higher rates of unwanted pregnancies, and high risk for sexually transmitted infections. The literature also showed consumption of psychotropic agents during pregnancy and breastfeeding, menstrual dysfunction, unwanted pregnancies and abortion, perinatal and neonatal distress, sexual dysfunction, parenting difficulties and loss of custody, sexual abuse, and barriers to gynecological care. It is recommended that sex education be part of psychosocial rehabilitation programs.

Fletcher et al. (2009) conducted a review of 60 articles related to multiple sclerosis (MS) and sexuality. Sexual dysfunction (SD) in clients with MS ranges from 50-73% in men and 45-70% in women. SD substantially impacts quality of life and is frequently underdiagnosed. Most common complaints from males with MS are erectile dysfunction, reduced libido, and anorgasmia. In women, sensory genital dysfunction, difficulty achieving orgasm, decreased vaginal lubrication, and reduced libido were most frequent. Cognitive dysfunction affects 45-65% of people with MS and compromises sexual function. Spasticity, tremors, fatigue, bowel and bladder dysfunction, and adverse effects associated with medication also impact sexual functioning. Other factors causing SD include psychological, emotional, social, and cultural aspects of having a chronic disability, including negative self-image, mood dysregulation, body-image changes, fear of rejection, and community difficulties.

Lindau et al. (2007) obtained a nationally representative sample of 3,005 community dwelling older adults age 57-85. They found that sexual activity declines with age, women report less sexual activity than men, and, of those who are sexually activity, about half report at least one sexual problem.

Problems frequently identified by women were low desire, poor vaginal lubrication, and inability to climax. Men frequently identified erectile difficulties. Those who reported subjective health status as poor were less likely to be sexually active and more likely to report sexual difficulties. Only 38% of men and 22% of women reported discussing sexual activity questions or difficulties with their physicians.

Shamliyan et al. (2008) conducted a review of the literature and identified 96 randomized, controlled trials related to non-surgical treatment of urinary incontinence in women. Findings indicated that pelvic floor muscle training and bladder training were moderately helpful in resolving incontinence. Anticholinergic drugs, oxybutynin, totlerodine, and duloxetine were also helpful.

Bower (2008) surveyed 156 children across 10 countries (6-17 years of age) who reported having difficulties with incontinence. Boys reported lower quality of life scores than girls. Both boys and girls reported lower self-esteem, independence, and mental health. They also felt that their parents were annoyed by their bladder incontinence problems.

Wiegerink et al. (2006) conducted a literature review on sexual activity and cerebral palsy (CP). Findings in the 14 papers they found indicate that adolescents and young adults with CP were less socially and sexually active compared to peers, and dating was often delayed and less frequent. Issues related to psychological maladjustment, poor self-efficacy, low sexual self-esteem, overprotection, and negative attitudes of others may also impair social and sexual relationships.

### Cross References

In *Recreational Therapy for Specific Diagnoses and Conditions, First Edition*, ICF code b6 Genitourinary and Reproductive Functions and its subcategories are listed in 15 chapters: Back Disorders and Back Pain, Cancer, Cerebral Palsy, Cerebrovascular Accident, Diabetes Mellitus, Feeding and Eating Disorders, Fibromyalgia and Juvenile Fibromyalgia, Guillain-Barré Syndrome, Heart Disease, Multiple Sclerosis, Neurocognitive Disorders, Parkinson's Disease, Rheumatoid Arthritis, Sickle Cell Disease, and Spina Bifida.

In *Recreational Therapy Basics, Techniques, and Interventions, First Edition*, treatment for ICF code b6 Genitourinary and Reproductive Functions and its subcategories are discussed in three chapters:

Psychoneuroimmunology, Stress, and Sexual Well-Being.

## Urinary Functions (b610 - b639)

### b610 Urinary Excretory Functions

Functions of filtration and collection of the urine.

Inclusions: functions of urinary filtration, collection of urine; impairments such as in renal insufficiency, anuria, oliguria, hydronephrosis, hypotonic urinary bladder, and ureteric obstruction

Exclusions: urination functions (b620)

- *b6100 Filtration of Urine*
  Functions of filtration of urine by the kidneys.

- *b6101 Collection of Urine*
  Functions of collection and storage of urine by the ureters and bladder.

- *b6108 Urinary Excretory Functions, Other Specified*
- *b6109 Urinary Excretory Functions, Unspecified*
  It is not within the scope of recreational therapy practice to score urinary excretory functions. If a person has difficulty with filtration of urine or collection of urine, the person is referred to a urologist (a physician who specializes in the urinary system) and appropriate treatment is prescribed. Recreational therapists do treat urination functions, as seen in the next set of codes.

### Cross References

In *Recreational Therapy for Specific Diagnoses and Conditions, First Edition*, ICF code b610 Urinary Excretory Functions is listed in three chapters: Diabetes Mellitus, Multiple Sclerosis, and Sickle Cell Disease.

In *Recreational Therapy Basics, Techniques, and Interventions, First Edition*, there are no references for ICF code b610 Urinary Excretory Functions.

### b620 Urination Functions

Functions of discharge of urine from the urinary bladder.

Inclusions: functions of urination, frequency of urination, urinary continence; impairments such as in stress, urge, reflex, overflow, continuous incontinence, dribbling, automatic bladder, polyuria, urinary retention, and urinary urgency

Exclusions: urinary excretory functions (b610); sensations associated with urinary functions (b630)

- *b6200 Urination*
  Functions of voiding the urinary bladder.

  Inclusions: impairments such as in urine retention

- *b6201 Frequency of Urination*
  Functions involved in the number of times urination occurs.

- *b6202 Urinary Continence*
  Functions of control over urination.

  Inclusions: impairments such as in stress, urge, reflex, continuous, and mixed incontinence

- *b6208 Urination Functions, Other Specified*
- *b6209 Urination Functions, Unspecified*

Nursing staff are the primary health professionals who monitor and record urination functions. However, recreational therapists may also score these components. Difficulty with urination functions can be caused by:

- Neurological damage, which may be caused by cerebrovascular accident, traumatic brain injury, spinal cord injury, or diabetes.
- Congenital malformations.
- Urinary tract infections.
- Bladder cancer.
- Intoxication.
- Seizures.
- Extreme fear or anxiety.
- Medication, which may include psychotherapy drugs and medications that have the primary purpose or secondary effect of increasing urination or retaining urine.

Other conditions that affect frequency of urination and urinary continence outside of physiological processes include:

- *Cognitive impairments*: Inability to respond appropriately to the signal of a full bladder resulting in frequent episodes of urinary incontinence throughout the day.
- *Lack of mobility*: Inability to get to a commode, toilet, or urinal, which may result in urinary incontinence or decreased frequency of urination due to limited assistance with urination.

- *Communication impairments*: Leading to difficulty in ascertaining the location of a bathroom.

In young children, urinary incontinence is frequent. Approximately 82% of two year olds, 49% of three year olds, 26% of four year olds, and 7% of five year olds have episodes of urinary incontinence on a regular basis (Sadock & Sadock, 2003). "Psychosocial issues [that] precipitate some cases of enuresis [include]… the birth of a sibling, hospitalization between the ages of two and four, the start of school, the breakup of a family because of divorce or death, and a move to a new domicile" (Sadock & Sadock, 2003, p 1257).

Urinary continence is important for several reasons:

- Urinary incontinence causes odors that can impede socialization.
- Urinary incontinence can negatively affect self-esteem.
- Urinary incontinence can limit a person's community activities because the person fears going out of the home and having a bladder accident. This may contribute to secondary conditions, such as muscle atrophy and deconditioning of the cardiopulmonary system.
- Urinary incontinence increases risk for skin breakdown, especially when skin remains wet for prolonged periods of time. See b8 Functions of the Skin and Related Structures for more information about skin breakdown.

Recreational therapists teach clients how to manage urinary functions in real-life settings and assist clients in problem solving for specific life tasks that are common to their lifestyle. Examples include flying on an airplane, taking long road trips, self-catheterizing in a public bathroom, going to the beach, and locating bathrooms at the mall. Recreational therapists may consult with nurses or occupational therapists for problems like positioning in a wheelchair to self-catheterize in a public bathroom or difficulty holding Texas catheter in place.

Treatment for urinary functions may include medication, behavioral modification (e.g., positive rewards for young children), changes in toileting routine, use of materials to increase a child's awareness of being wet, urinary collection devices, such as an indwelling catheter, a Texas catheter, or a urinal, and devices to assist with releasing the bladder, such as straight catheterizing.

Recreational therapists document the specific urinary function impairment, frequency of impairment, specific life activities that are affected by the urinary function impairment, specific adaptations and recommendations, treatment and outcomes, and level of assistance.

Some specific adaptations that have been found to be helpful with urinary functions are provided below.

- If a client is having difficulty closing the bathroom stall door: When propelling a wheelchair into a bathroom stall, hook one end of a bungee cord to some place on the stall door. Hook the other end to some other place in the bathroom, such as the toilet paper holder, wheelchair, or side bar on the stall. Another idea is to use a dressing stick (a stick with a hook on the end of it) to grab the bottom of the stall door to pull it closed. A small dressing stick could be kept in a backpack.
- If there is a possibility that a client may have a bladder accident in the community: Clients who have problems with urinary incontinence, should pack an extra change of clothes, cleanup supplies, and a Ziploc bag to hold wet clothes in case of a bladder accident.

### *Indwelling Catheter*

An indwelling catheter is a flexible plastic tube that is placed into the urethra. At the end of the tube is a urine collection bag. The bag must be placed below the client's knees for best drainage. Otherwise, the urine may back up in the tube. Urine may also back up in the tube if the bag becomes full and is not emptied. Urine that backs up into the bladder can cause infection and damage to the elasticity of the bladder. The bag is strapped onto the lower leg or hooked onto the bottom of a wheelchair. Clients should not walk holding onto the collection bag or hang it on a walker because it is not low enough for good flow. Indwelling catheters are used for the short term. Long-term use of an indwelling catheter is not recommended due to high risk of infections since any foreign item that enters the body puts a person at risk for infection.

### *Straight Catheterizing*

Straight catheterizing is the insertion of a thin plastic tube into the urethra to stimulate the bladder to release the urine being held in the bladder. The inability to release urine from the bladder is a common problem in spinal cord injuries. Clients are initially taught (if able) to do this independently from a slightly elevated supine position in bed. The tube is packaged in individually sealed wraps for sterility and is opened only when the client is ready to use it. A gel is placed on the tip of the tube for ease of insertion. Once the bladder is stimulated, the urine will release through the tube. The collection device at the end of the tube can be varied. Once the client becomes more comfortable with the technique, it behooves the client to learn how to straight catheterize from a seated position (if possible). The ability to lie down to straight catheterize is unrealistic in many real-life situations.

The recreational therapist working in a rehabilitation setting is typically the person who initiates the conversation with nursing about the client's readiness to learn how to straight catheterize from a sitting position. This is done in preparation for community integration training. The therapist and nurse discuss the client's performance. When ready, the ability to straight catheterize in a public bathroom is set as a community integration goal, such as "Client to straight catheterize in a public bathroom at modified independence secondary to increased time and assistive devices." The following is a list of ideas to assist a client in straight catheterizing from a seated position in a bathroom:

- Make cathing packs. Put everything that is needed for one cathing session into a plastic grocery bag, fold it over, and put it into a backpack. The backpack can be hung on the back of a wheelchair. It is good to take a few extra packs just in case the client intentionally or unintentionally stays out later than anticipated or the client consumes more fluids than usual and needs to catheterize more often. The more fluids consumed, the more often the need to catheterize. With normal fluid intake, people self-catheterize every four to six hours.
- When straight catheterizing in a public bathroom, take out a cathing pack from the backpack and hook one of the plastic bag handles onto the wheelchair. Let the other end of the bag hang

open. Open pants or raise skirt (loose clothing makes it easier). Get into a slightly reclined sitting position and then reach into the bag to retrieve supplies. Use one hand to insert the tube and the other to guide the end of the tube over the toilet.

- If a client is having difficulty keeping his/her pants flap open wide enough when self-catheterizing in a reclined sitting position, use a bungee cord with rubber tips on the hooks. Hook one end to the inside of the pants flap and hook the other end somewhere on the wheelchair to provide tension. Using a bungee cord will free up both hands for catheterizing.
- If a client is unable to catheterize from a reclined sitting position, discuss issues related to finding places to lie down and catheterize in typical community settings.

### Texas Catheter

A Texas catheter is an external urine collection system. A condom-like device is placed onto the penis and a special tape is wrapped around the top of the device. At the base of the device is a thin plastic flexible tube that feeds into a urine collection bag that it strapped to the lower leg. The use of a Texas catheter is less likely to cause infection since it is an external, rather than an internal, collection device. However, it does have limitations. At times the tape can become loose and leak and some people find the device bothersome and uncomfortable. Texas catheters are also used by people who lack access to bathrooms, including truck drivers or a person who is on a long airplane flight and lacks mobility to get to the airplane bathroom or is limited in his ability to use the bathroom because of its small size.

### Urinal

A urinal is an external plastic collection device that is held over the penis to collect urine. Males can use a variety of collection devices outside of the medical-style urinal. For example, a plastic bottle with a good leak-proof lid can be kept in a backpack for urination. The use of a bottle can be helpful when the client is unable to access a bathroom. Once the bottle is used, the urine can be disposed of immediately or the bottle can be put back into the backpack to be emptied later. If the person prefers to empty the bottle later, a sock can be pulled over the bottle to mask the contents of the bottle.

### Sanitary Pads for Urination

For women, sanitary pads that are specifically designed to hold urine can be helpful for urinary incontinence. They may also be used for situations when the client is unable to access a bathroom, such as a long car ride where finding an accessible bathroom is difficult. Consciously allowing oneself to urinate using a pad can be uncomfortable. Clients may find it helpful to use the pad in a safe environment first to decrease anxiety and worry about its effectiveness.

### Cross References

In *Recreational Therapy for Specific Diagnoses and Conditions, First Edition*, ICF code b620 Urination Functions is listed in eight chapters: Cerebral Palsy, Cerebrovascular Accident, Guillain-Barré Syndrome, Multiple Sclerosis, Neurocognitive Disorders, Parkinson's Disease, Sickle Cell Disease, and Spina Bifida.

In *Recreational Therapy Basics, Techniques, and Interventions, First Edition*, there are no references for ICF code b620 Urination Functions.

## b630 Sensations Associated with Urinary Functions

Sensations arising from voiding and related urinary functions.

Inclusions: sensations of incomplete voiding or urine, feeling of fullness of bladder

Exclusions: sensations of pain (b280); urination functions (b620)

Recreational therapists are responsible for documenting sensations associated with urinary functions and reporting information to the treatment team. The sensations may be a symptom of some dysfunction in urination functions, which would be treated under code b620 Urination Functions. Other possibilities include treatment for pain or stress that would be coordinated with other members of the treatment team.

### Cross References

In *Recreational Therapy for Specific Diagnoses and Conditions, First Edition*, ICF code b630 Sensations Associated with Urinary Functions is listed in one chapter: Multiple Sclerosis.

In *Recreational Therapy Basics, Techniques, and Interventions, First Edition*, there are no references for ICF code b630 Sensations Associated with Urinary Functions.

### b639 Urinary Functions, Other Specified and Unspecified

## Genital and Reproductive Functions (b640 - b679)

### b640 Sexual Functions

Mental and physical functions related to the sexual act, including the arousal, preparatory, orgasmic, and resolution stages.

Inclusions: functions of the sexual arousal, preparatory, orgasmic, and resolution phase; functions related to sexual interest, performance, penile erection, clitoral erection, vaginal lubrication, ejaculation, orgasm; impairments such as impotence, frigidity, vaginismus, premature ejaculation, priapism, and delayed ejaculation

Exclusions: procreation functions (b660); sensations associated with genital and reproductive functions (b670)

- *b6400 Functions of Sexual Arousal Phase*
  Functions of sexual interest and excitement.

- *b6401 Functions of Sexual Preparatory Phase*
  Functions of engaging in sexual intercourse.

- *b6402 Functions of Orgasmic Phase*
  Functions of reaching orgasm.

- *b6403 Functions of Sexual Resolution Phase*
  Functions of satisfaction after orgasm and accompanying relaxation.

  Inclusions: impairments such as dissatisfaction with orgasm

- *b6408 Sexual Functions, Other Specified*
- *b6409 Sexual Functions, Unspecified*

Sexual functioning is not a therapist-observed behavior. Consequently assessment of functioning is based on client report and scored appropriately by the recreational therapist.

Talking about sexual functioning can be uncomfortable for many clients. Some may find it embarrassing or inappropriate, while others may have questions they are apprehensive to ask due to the sensitive nature of the topic. Consequently, clients may bring up issues related to sexuality in indirect ways, such as making sexual jokes or statements like "No one is ever going to want to date me." Indirect statements, including jokes, provide the therapist with an opportunity to broach the subject.

It is important to understand which part of sexual function the client is concerned about. For clients with a condition that changes their appearance or functioning like burns or spinal cord injury, it may be the sexual arousal phase. They may be worried that no one will ever be interested in them sexually again. A man who has had an operation for prostate cancer may need information about achieving an erection. For others, such as a client who had a heart attack, the concern may be whether s/he will be able to perform sexually during the orgasmic phase.

Functional issues related to sexuality are documented here. Related relationship issues are documented using d770 Intimate Relationships or one of the other relationship codes. Concerns with sexuality will usually have both components.

The manner in which the therapist approaches the subject will vary depending on the client. However, it is always done with respect and sincerity (e.g., "In addition to the goals that we set for your stay here I was wondering if you would like information on issues related to sexuality. It is common for people to have questions about sexuality after having heart surgery. Would you like to talk about it with me or someone else on your team?"). Notice in the example provided that the therapist "normalizes" sexuality by saying that "many people have questions." This helps to lessen client anxiety. Other comments that can help to lessen anxiety include those that validate how the client is feeling, such as, "I know this must be an awkward conversation that you probably didn't expect to have." or "I sense that this topic makes you uncomfortable. Would you like to change the subject? Just know that if you change your mind, we can talk about it or, if you prefer, I can give you some information in a sealed envelop that you can read on your own."

A transdisciplinary approach is commonly used when addressing issues of sexuality in a healthcare setting. It may include a physician to clear the client for engagement in sexual activity or give him/her a prescription for medication, physical therapy to address issues related to positioning, occupational therapy to address issues related to dressing and undressing, nursing to address adaptive devices, recreational therapy to address issues related to dating and socializing, and psychology to address issues related to self-esteem and confidence.

Although attention to sexual health is gaining more recognition in healthcare, a clear protocol on how to address these issues is not always available. Consequently, many issues are addressed by the team member who initiates the conversation or the team member the client confides his/her concerns to. Due to the strong focus on participation in real-life activities and the unique therapeutic relationship that is built, recreational therapists are often key professionals in addressing sexual health. Recreational therapists consult other health disciplines when needed for further recommendations, such as discussing with the client's physical therapist how to work around a client's movement limitations for sexual positioning.

Due to the sensitivity of the topic, many clients want assurance that the discussion is not documented or spoken about with other people. The therapist should inform the client that s/he will not discuss the specifics of the conversation with others. However, if specific questions need to be answered, such as clearance from the physician to engage in sexual activity, the therapist will need to divulge the client's name. If it is determined that further information is needed or that the client could benefit from additional conversations with other staff, the therapist will check with the client prior to making these arrangements. The therapist also informs the client that documentation will reflect the specific information provided, but the details of the conversation will not be part of the medical chart.

The therapist documents the specific education provided and the client's ability to apply the information learned. For example, "Client educated about sexual positions that will not aggravate back pain. Client able to recall information independently." Documentation may also include referrals, for example "Client agreed to talk with nursing about sexual devices for impotence. Primary nurse scheduled to meet with client this evening." Evaluation of techniques and equipment comes from the client and must be documented as such. For example, "Client reports that sexual position recommendations did not aggravate back pain." or "Client reports that suction device was effective for achieving erection."

Some of the common problems and general adaptations for sexual functioning are provided below.

### *Male Issues*

*Concern: Unable to Initiate or Maintain Erection*
Recommendations:

- *Stuffing*: Manually placing the flaccid penis into the vagina to promote hardness and erection.
- *External vacuum pumps with ring*: Placing a tubular suction device over the penis draws blood into the penis that promotes erection. Once erect, a ring is placed at the base of the penis to maintain the erection. The ring should not be worn for an extended period of time due to the risk of tissue death from lack of freshly oxygenated blood. Many healthcare settings have sample devices and can instruct the client on how to obtain the device.
- *Penile injections*: This is a direct injection of a chemical substance into the penis for erection. Encourage the client to speak with a urologist for more information on substances available.
- *Penile implants*: There are several different types of implants that are placed permanently into the penis for manual erection. There can be some complications with skin breakthrough with use. Encourage the client to speak with a urologist for more information.
- *Medication*: including Viagra and Cialis.

*Concern: Unable to Ejaculate*
Recommendations: There are three ways to retrieve sperm.

- *Electroejaculation*: Achieved through the use of a rectal probe. This is done at a medical facility.
- *Vibro massage*: Use of an external vibrator on the penis. Can be done at home.
- *Chemical stimulation*: Injection of a substance. This is done at a medical facility.

### *Female Issues*

*Concern: Decreased Lubrication*
Recommendations:

- Encourage the client to have her partner check her lubrication prior to intercourse.
- Encourage the use of a water-based lubricant such as KY Jelly. Do not use oil or Vaseline.

They will not dissolve and will increase risks for infections.

*Concern: Pregnancy*
Recommendations:

- There are various issues to take into consideration when planning a child. Pregnancy can affect sensation, skin breakdown, dysreflexia, spasticity, balance, etc. It is important for the client to discuss these issues with her physician or OB-Gyn so as to fully understand the implications and precautions specific to the situation.

*Concern: Birth Control*
Recommendation:

- Any type of devices inserted into the vagina for birth control should be thoroughly checked by both the client and his/her partner to ensure proper positioning for effectiveness. If the client has decreased sensation or physical limitations, there is a chance that it may be positioned incorrectly rendering the birth control product ineffective.
- Oral contraceptives are to be approved by the physician, as well as the OB-Gyn.
- Use a variety of birth control methods to decrease risks of pregnancy.

### Both Male and Female Issues

*Concern: Decreased Sensation*
Recommendations:

- Decreased sensation directly affects the ability to reach orgasm, lubricate, and/or erect. Refer to the section on each of the individual concerns for recommendations.
- Other erogenous zones may be present after a neurological injury. They are known to "move." For example, prior an injury the genital may have been a sensitive area and now the neck may be a sensitive area.

*Concern: Unable to Reach Orgasm*
Recommendations:

- There are two basic types of orgasms: reflexive from sensation to the body part and psychogenic through thoughts and fantasies.
- If an orgasm cannot be reached, encourage the client to think about what "sex" truly means to him/her. Does it need to include an orgasm? Is intimacy itself the valued outcome? Encourage the client to talk about this with his/her partner.

*Concern: Bowel and Bladder*
Recommendations: Clients who have neurological impairments may have bowel and bladder accidents during sexual activity due to muscle contraction and relaxation. There are several ways to decrease the chances of this happening.

- Empty the bowel and bladder prior to sexual activity.
- Place towels on the bed to catch the urine or bowel so that it is easy to clean up and resume activity.
- Place a urinal next to the bed.

*Concern: Physical Mobility*
Recommendations:

- Chose positions that are most comfortable for the individual and couple.
- Chose positions that do not break specific precautions or parameters set by other health professionals.
- Be aware of the required balance and strength for each position and make safe decisions.
- Experiment with various positions.

*Concern: Communication*
Recommendations:

- Encourage the client to discuss needs with his/her partner prior to sexual activity to decrease anxiety, as well as the anxiety of the partner. Discuss what may happen and how you would like to deal with it.
- Encourage both partners to discuss their views about sexual expression including intimacy versus intercourse and orgasm.

### Cross References

In *Recreational Therapy for Specific Diagnoses and Conditions, First Edition*, ICF code b640 Sexual Functions is listed in eight chapters: Back Disorders and Back Pain, Cancer, Cerebrovascular Accident, Heart Disease, Multiple Sclerosis, Parkinson's Disease, Rheumatoid Arthritis, and Spina Bifida.

In *Recreational Therapy Basics, Techniques, and Interventions, First Edition*, treatment for ICF code b640 Sexual Functions is discussed in one chapter: Sexual Well-Being.

### b650 Menstruation Functions

Functions associated with the menstrual cycle, including regularity of menstruation and discharge of menstrual fluids.

Inclusions: functions of regularity and interval of menstruation, extent of menstrual bleeding, menarche, menopause; impairments such as primary and secondary amenorrhea, menorrhagia, polymenorrhea, and retrograde menstruation, and in premenstrual tension

Exclusions: sexual functions (b640); procreation functions (b660); sensations associated with genital and reproductive functions (b670); sensation of pain (b280)

- *b6500 Regularity of Menstrual Cycle*
  Functions involved in the regularity of the menstrual cycle.

  Inclusions: too frequent or too few occurrences of menstruation

- *b6501 Interval between Menstruation*
  Functions relating to the length of time between two menstrual cycles.

- *b6502 Extent of Menstrual Bleeding*
  Functions involved in the quantity of menstrual flow.

  Inclusions: too little menstrual flow (hypomenorrhea); too much menstrual flow (menorrhagia, hypermenorrhea)

- *b6508 Menstruation Functions, Other Specified*
- *b6509 Menstruation Functions, Unspecified*
  Menstrual functions are addressed primarily by the client's gynecologist. However, various members of the treatment team play roles in managing menstruation issues. For example, the recreational therapist may help the client problem solve for menstrual care in a community setting, including positioning and changing sanitary napkins or tampons. If difficulty with menstrual care is due to physical impairments, the occupational therapist may make recommendations for adaptive equipment or techniques that can also be carried over into the community setting for recreational therapists to further assess. Recreational therapists are not anticipated to score the codes in this section, but discipline-specific documentation should reflect these functions, interventions provided, and an assessment of the client's functioning in menstrual care as appropriate.

#### Cross References

In *Recreational Therapy for Specific Diagnoses and Conditions, First Edition*, ICF code b650 Menstruation Functions is listed in two chapters: Feeding and Eating Disorders and Fibromyalgia and Juvenile Fibromyalgia.

In *Recreational Therapy Basics, Techniques, and Interventions, First Edition*, there are no references for ICF code b650 Menstruation Functions.

### b660 Procreation Functions

Functions associated with fertility, pregnancy, childbirth, and lactation.

Inclusions: function of male fertility and female fertility, pregnancy and childbirth, and lactation; impairments such as azoospermia, oligozoospermia, galactorrhea, agalactorrhea, alactation, and such as in subfertility, sterility, spontaneous abortions, ectopic pregnancy, miscarriage, small fetus, hydramnios and premature childbirth, and delayed childbirth

Exclusions: sexual functions (b640); menstruation functions (b650)

- *b6600 Functions Related to Fertility*
  Functions related to the ability to produce gametes for procreation.

  Inclusion: impairments such as in subfertility and sterility

  Exclusion: sexual functions (b640)

- *b6601 Functions Related to Pregnancy*
  Functions involved in becoming pregnant and being pregnant.

- *b6602 Functions Related to Childbirth*
  Functions involved during childbirth.

- *b6603 Lactation*
  Functions involved in producing milk and making it available to the child.

- *b6608 Procreation Functions, Other Specified*
- *b6609 Procreation Functions, Unspecified*
  Functions related to childbirth are commonly addressed by obstetricians. It is not within the scope of recreational therapy to score the codes in this section. However, recreational therapists may, in

some settings, address related issues and assist the client in problem solving for barriers, such as problem solving with a client who has a spinal cord injury on how to breastfeed a child in a community setting. Notations about the specific problems, interventions, and evaluation of the client's skills are written, as appropriate, in discipline-specific documentation.

### Cross References

In *Recreational Therapy for Specific Diagnoses and Conditions, First Edition*, ICF code b660 Procreation Functions is listed in one chapter: Feeding and Eating Disorders.

In *Recreational Therapy for Specific Diagnoses and Conditions, First Edition*, there are no references for ICF code b660 Procreation Functions.

## b670 Sensations Associated with Genital and Reproductive Functions

Sensations arising from sexual arousal, intercourse, menstruation, and related genital or reproductive functions.

Inclusions: sensations of dyspareunia, dysmenorrhea, hot flushes during menopause and night sweats during menopause

Exclusions: sensation of pain (b280); sensations associated with urinary functions (b630); sexual functions (b640); menstruation functions (b650); procreation functions (b660)

- *b6700 Discomfort Associated with Sexual Intercourse*
  Sensations associated with sexual arousal, preparation, intercourse, orgasm, and resolution.

- *b6701 Discomfort Associated with the Menstrual Cycle*
  Sensations involved with menstruation, including pre- and post-menstrual phases.

- *b6702 Discomfort Associated with Menopause*
  Sensations associated with cessation of the menstrual cycle.

  Inclusions: hot flushes and night sweats during menopause

- *b6708 Sensations Associated with Genital and Reproductive Functions, Other Specified*
- *b6709 Sensations Associated with Genital and Reproductive Functions, Unspecified*

Sensations associated with genital and reproductive functions are not commonly scored by recreational therapists. They are more likely to use ICF codes in b640 Sexual Functions. Recreational therapists are responsible for documenting sensations if they are described by clients during treatment sessions. The therapist reports the information to the treatment team. The sensations may be a symptom of some dysfunction, which would be coded under the appropriate function. Other possibilities include treatment for pain or stress that would be coordinated with other members of the treatment team.

### Cross References

In *Recreational Therapy for Specific Diagnoses and Conditions, First Edition*, there are no references for ICF code b670 Sensations Associated with Genital and Reproductive Functions.

In *Recreational Therapy Basics, Techniques, and Interventions, First Edition*, treatment for ICF code b670 Sensations Associated with Genital and Reproductive Functions is discussed in one chapter: Sexual Well-Being.

## b679 Genital and Reproductive Functions, Other Specified and Unspecified

## b698 Genitourinary and Reproductive Functions, Other Specified

## b699 Genitourinary and Reproductive Functions, Unspecified

### References

Bower, W. F. (2008). Self-reported effect of childhood incontinence on quality of life. *Journal of Wound, Ostomy & Continence Nursing, 35*(6), 617-621.
Bullough, V. L. (1994). *Human sexuality: An encyclopedia.* New York: Garland Publishing, Inc.
Fletcher, S. G., Castro-Borrero, W., Remington, G., Treadaway, K., Lemack, G. E., & Frohman, E. M. (2009). Sexual dysfunction in patients with multiple sclerosis: A multidisciplinary approach to evaluation and management. *Nature Clinical Practice Urology, 6*(2), 96-107.
Kwong, P. W., Cumming, R. G., Chan, L., Seibel, M. J., Naganathan, V., Creasey, H., LeCouteur, D., Waite, L. M., Sambrook, P. N., & Handelsman, D. (2010). Urinary incontinence and quality of life among older community-

dwelling Australian men: the CHAMP study. *Age and Aging, 39*, 349-354.

Landefeld, C. S., Bowers, B. J., Feld, A. D., Hartmann, K. E., Hoffman, E., Ingber, M. J., Kling, J. T., McDougal, W. S., Nelson, H., Orav, E. J., Pignone, M., Richardson, L. H., Rohrbaugh, R. M., Siebens, H. C., & Trock, B. J. (2008). National institutes of health state-of-the-science conference statement: Prevention of fecal and urinary incontinence in adults. *Annals of Internal Medicine, 148*, 449-458.

Lindau, S. T., Schumm, L. P., Laumann, E. O., Levinson, W., O'Muircheataigh, C. A., & Waite, L. J. (2007). A study of sexuality and health among older adults in the United States. *New England Journal of Medicine, 357*, 762-774.

Matevosyan, N. R. (2009). Reproductive health in women with serious mental illness: A review. *Sexuality & Disability, 27*, 109-118.

Porter, H. (2016). *Recreational therapy basics, techniques, and interventions*. Enumclaw, WA: Idyll Arbor.

Sadock, B. & Sadock, V. (2003). *Kaplan & Sadock's synopsis of psychiatry, 9th edition*. Philadelphia, PA: Lippincott Williams & Wilkins.

Shamliyan, T. A., Kane, R. L., Wyman, J., & Wilt, T. J. (2008). Systematic review: Randomized, controlled trials of nonsurgical treatments for urinary incontinence in women. *Annals of Internal Medicine, 148*, 459-473.

Taylor, B. & Davis, S. (2007). The extended PLISSIT model for addressing sexual wellbeing of individuals with an acquired disability or chronic illness. *Sexuality and Disability, 25*, 135-139.

Wiegerink, D. Roebroeck, M. E., Donkervoort, M., Stam, H. J., & Cohen-Kettenis, P. T. (2006). Social and sexual relationships of adolescents and young adults with cerebral palsy: A review. *Clinical Rehabilitation, 20*, 1023-1031.

# Chapter 7 Neuromusculoskeletal and Movement-Related Functions

This chapter is about the functions of movement and mobility, including functions of joints, bones, reflexes, and muscles.

*Sample Scoring for Neuromusculoskeletal and Movement Related Functions*

- Overall, a client has a reduction of 60% (severe impairment = 3) in muscle power (b730 Muscle Power Functions). The correct scoring would look like this: b730.3.
- A client has a 25% impairment (moderate impairment = 2) with hand-eye coordination (b7602 Coordination of Voluntary Movements). The correct scoring would look like this: b7602.2.

Gait patterns, voluntary and involuntary movement, balance, mobility of bones and joints, and the endurance, strength, and tone of muscle are basic functions that support body movement. Individuals may have difficulty with these neuromusculoskeletal and movement functions due to illness, disease, disability, or the normal aging process (von Bonsdorff & Rantanen, 2011). When a person has difficulty with these basic functions, participation in activities can be significantly hindered and have detrimental effects on health and quality of life. For example, a two-year study of 6,841 older adults living in the community found that limitations in physical functioning predicted impairment in cooking, shopping, and performing housework (Seidel, Brayne, & Jagger, 2011). Difficulties in performing these activities of living can also yield further problems. For example, a study of 594,267 adults with chronic physical and/or psychiatric disabilities found that difficulties performing functional activities, such as shopping, leisure, going to school, or taking care of the house, were a significant predictor of suicide (Kaplan et al., 2007).

## Assessment for Neuromusculoskeletal and Movement Related Functions

Refer to the specific code for assessment information.

## Treatment for Neuromusculoskeletal and Movement Related Functions

Refer to the specific code for treatment information.

## Evidence Review

Reviews of several studies are provided below to highlight evidence-based practice related to neuromusculoskeletal and movement related functions. This is only a sample of the evidence. A thorough review of the literature is needed to identify evidence-based practice interventions that reflect the needs and characteristics of a particular client.

McColgin, Driver, and Goggin (2009) provide recommendations for evaluation and treatment of balance in older adults. Therapists should first collect subjective information about the client including medical problems, home and community environment, participation in physical activity, past injuries, and current limitations. This information helps characterize the problem and determine assessment needs. Second, objective data is obtained through standardized testing such as the *Maximum Step Length Assessment*, *Rapid Step Test*, and *Senior Fitness Test*. Third, an assessment is made based on the subjective and objective data to determine needs and baseline data. Fourth, a plan is established to reduce risk of falling, including engagement in a structured program such as Matter of Balance or Fallproof! (Rose, 2010) or unstructured, independent exercises. The article provides specific examples of balance exercises, such as single-leg stand, eight-foot balance beam walk, forward step up/step down, and treadmill walk.

Goldberg et al. (2009) describe the integrative musculoskeletal rehabilitative services provided to U.S. military service members. The authors note that "the complex nature of combat wounded and polytrauma patients requires an integrated and interdisciplinary team that is innovative, adaptable, and focused on the needs of the patient" (p. 781). Services provided include primary care, physical therapy, occupational therapy, vestibular therapy, gait analysis, prosthetics, recreational therapy, and chiropractic care. The article "presents a description of the model and the experiences of our musculo-skeletal rehabilitation team [in the] hope that [it] will assist other centers and add to the small but emerging literature on this topic" (p. 781). In regards to recreational therapy, as part of the interdisciplinary team, RT conducts an assessment and establishes a treatment plan in collaboration with other rehabilitation team members. Common short-term goals include concentration, attention, memory, problem solving, critical thinking, communication skills, safety awareness, judgment, strength, endurance, fine and gross motor function, balance and propriocep-tion, independent community mobility, performance of ADLs, social skills and interaction, confidence, self-esteem, adjustment to disability, body image, reduction of withdrawal, knowledge and use of adaptive equipment, and community resource development. Common long-term goals include leisure-related skills, attitudes, and knowledge of an appropriate leisure lifestyle and demonstrating leisure independence and personal enjoyment through participation in appropriate leisure opportunities. Available leisure opportunities include snow skiing, snowboarding, dog-sledding, snowmobiling, waterskiing, surfing, stand-up paddle boarding, kayaking, whitewater rafting, sailing, fly fishing, deep sea fishing, boating, horseback riding, golf, rock climbing, mountaineering, camping, cycling, swimming, scuba, wheelchair sports, Paralympic sports, and community re-entry activities such as going to restaurants, movies, shops, zoos, libraries, and parks. "Recreational therapy is unique in the sense that it becomes the clinic and the modality…. It can clarify for the patient the fact that there is much life and fun beyond rehab and that opportunities are boundless" (p. 791).

Clark et al. (2010) described how impaired standing balance affects ability to perform functional tasks and increases risk of falling. The authors compared a laboratory-grade force platform (FP) to the Wii Balance Board (WBB). Thirty participants performed single and double leg standing balance tests on the FP and WBB at two different times. "[F]indings suggest that the WBB is a valid tool for assessing standing balance. Given that the WBB is portable, widely available, and a fraction of the cost of an FP, it could provide the average clinician with a

standing balance assessment tool suitable for the clinical setting" (p. 307). The authors additionally note that the instant feedback provided by Wii Fit games has the potential to enhance motivation levels and consequently has been integrated into rehabilita-tion programs of neurologically impaired clients with balance deficits.

Kuster, Knauth, and Langhof (2007) conducted a study of 87 children 10 to 19 years old who were being treated for obesity in a children's rehabilitation center. Recreational therapy interventions included endurance training (one hour twice a week), swim-ming and aquatic games (45 minutes twice a week), team sports (90 minutes once a week), early morning exercises (30 minutes twice a week), postural gymnastics (45 minutes once a week), aqua fitness (45 minutes once a week), hiking in mountainous terrain (two to three hours once or twice a week), and leisure-time activity excursions in the community, which required easy hiking to get there. Participants engaged in the program for four to six weeks. Following the program, body weight, BMI, over-weight proportions, systolic blood pressure, choles-terol, triglycerides, blood sugar, basal insulin, HOMA, leptin, TSH, Te, fT3, and T4 all decreased. Endurance capacity, motor skills, and strength improved. The authors note the importance of recreational therapists who work with this population to "emphasize active recreation opportunities in leisure education sessions, implement interesting and sustaining fitness programs… and provide… information about nutrition choices during free time…. During inpatient therapy, the undesirable developments in metabolism can be stopped and reversed" (p. 47).

### Cross References

In *Recreational Therapy for Specific Diagnoses and Conditions, First Edition*, ICF code b7 Neuro-musculoskeletal and Movement-Related Functions and its subcategories are listed in 25 chapters: Amputation and Prosthesis, Back Disorders and Back Pain, Burns, Cancer, Cerebral Palsy, Cerebrovascular Accident, Chronic Obstructive Pulmonary Disease, Epilepsy, Feeding and Eating Disorders, Fibromyal-gia and Juvenile Fibromyalgia, Generalized Anxiety Disorder, Guillain-Barré Syndrome, Heart Disease, Intellectual Disability, Multiple Sclerosis, Obesity, Osteoarthritis, Osteoporosis, Parkinson's Disease, Post-Traumatic Stress Disorder, Rheumatoid

Arthritis, Spina Bifida, Spinal Cord Injury, Total Joint Replacement, and Traumatic Brain Injury.

In *Recreational Therapy Basics, Techniques, and Interventions, First Edition*, treatment for ICF code b7 Neuromusculoskeletal and Movement-Related Functions and its subcategories are discussed in 17 chapters: Activity and Task Analysis, Body Mechanics and Ergonomics, Consequences of Inactivity, Parameters and Precautions, Psychoneuroimmunology, Activity Pattern Development, Adaptive Sports, Animal Assisted Therapy, Aquatic Therapy, Balance Training, Constraint-Induced Movement Therapy, Energy Conservation Techniques, Mind-Body Interventions, Motor Learning and Training Strategies, Neuro-Developmental Treatment, Physical Activity, and Walking and Gait Training.

## Functions of the Joints and Bones (b710 - b729)

### b710 Mobility of Joint Functions

Functions of the range and ease of movement of a joint.

Inclusions: functions of mobility of single or several joints, vertebral, shoulder, elbow, wrist, hip, knee, ankle, small joints of hands and feet; mobility of joints generalized; impairments such as in hypermobility of joints, frozen joints, frozen shoulder, arthritis

Exclusions: stability of joints (b715); control of voluntary movement functions (b760)

- *b7100 Mobility of a Single Joint*
  Functions of the range and ease of movement of one joint.

- *b7101 Mobility of Several Joints*
  Functions of the range and ease of movement of more than one joint.

- *b7102 Mobility of Joints Generalized*
  Functions of the range and ease of movement of joints throughout the body.

- *b7108 Mobility of Joint Functions, Other Specified*
- *b7109 Mobility of Joint Functions, Unspecified*

Limited joint mobility affects the range of motion of a joint. There are two major types of range of motion, active range of motion (AROM) and passive range of motion (PROM). AROM refers to the client's ability to voluntarily move a joint by his/her own efforts. PROM refers to a joint that is moved by another person. With AROM, the client would move his/her own arm. With PROM the client lacks voluntary control over the mobility of a joint but it can be moved by the therapist, as when the therapist stretches a client's paralyzed fingers after activity to prevent development of contractures.

There are several causes for deficits with mobility in joints. They may be caused by damage to the joint. Some examples of disease-caused damage are osteoarthritis, rheumatoid arthritis, and cancers. Trauma, such as fractures and sprains can also limit joint mobility. Surgery on a joint, such as in total hip replacement, may require the client to limit mobility of the joint. Contractures, a tightening or loss of the elasticity of skin, fascia, muscle, or joint capsule, also cause a loss of range of motion. Muscle tissue tightness that causes a noticeable change in ability is usually considered to be a mild contracture.

It is also important to note that when muscle tissue has little or no movement for a period of time the tissue shortens in length. A shortening of muscle tissue length causes an overall reduction in the client's ability to move the nearby joints through their normal range of motion. It is common for pain to accompany a reduction in muscle length, which, in turn, causes the client to "guard" the muscle, further reducing movement.

Muscles become less resilient with age. As one ages the length of time that it takes a muscle and its related joints to stiffen decreases. It is not unusual for someone in his/her fifties and beyond to be stiff after sleeping. By the time someone is in their seventies, a good night's sleep can cause the individual to be stiff to the point of causing mobility problems for the first ten to twenty minutes. An impairment of a client's range of motion is a common secondary diagnosis for clients in treatment.

When assessing joint mobility, recreational therapists are concerned about how it impacts performance during life activities and recreation, such as the ability to reach shelves in the grocery store or to play a sport. Precautions will vary depending on the cause of the joint mobility dysfunction and can be obtained from the treating physician. ROM parameters and restrictions can be found in the medical chart in an acute care or rehab setting or can be requested from the primary treating physician. Joint protection interventions may be indicated for clients with conditions, such as rheumatoid arthritis, that respond negatively to repetitive ROM tasks.

If joint mobility is acutely restricted because of a medical condition, such as hip or knee replacement or rheumatoid arthritis, specific abilities or precautions will be written in the medical chart for the recreational therapist to incorporate into treatment. For the recreational therapist working in a community setting, it is important to have a full awareness of a client's joint mobility impairments so that the client is not challenged above his/her level, resulting in injury.

Traditionally recreational therapists measure joint mobility function in a broad fashion to reflect the effect that it has on activity. Once the recreational therapist is aware of all the client's joint mobility precautions and restrictions, the common recreational therapy assessment includes the therapist asking the client to appropriately move his/her joints independently through active ranges.

Documentation usually discusses the limitations the joint mobility impairment places on life activities. For example, if a client has limited shoulder joint mobility and it impairs his ability to do a 360° golf swing, the therapist may document, "Client able to perform a 180° back to front golf swing. Limited shoulder joint mobility impairs client's ability to achieve a full 360° golf swing." If a client has impaired knee flexion making it difficult to squat down to garden, the therapist may document, "Recommend client garden from a seated position rather than a squatting position due to impaired knee flexion, which hinders balance and safety."

Recreational therapists, although trained to assess joint mobility grossly through observation, will most likely defer to other disciplines that are more formally trained to measure ROM for scoring the ICF codes in this section. In some cases recreational therapists may measure joint mobility using a goniometer, especially in a rehabilitation center where the recreational therapist has been cross-trained by other professionals. A goniometer is a two-armed instrument that is jointed in the center by a pin. The pin is placed over the center of the joint where the motion occurs, such as on the side of the knee. One instrument arm is held in line with the stationary body segment and the other arm is moved (opened) along with the motion of the body segment. When the joint is fully in extension or flexion,

whichever is being measured, the indicator shows the number of degrees the segment has moved. The documentation is made in a specific format, determined by the facility, to record the range of motion in the joints measured.

Treatment for joint mobility impairments will vary depending on the reason. For example, a client who has a total hip replacement will have hip range of motion restrictions for several months after surgery to allow the prosthetic joint to stabilize. Range of motion restrictions will also vary for people with rheumatoid arthritis depending on the stage of the disease. Therefore therapists must fully understand the nature of the joint mobility dysfunction, whether protective to avoid joint instability or inflammation or restrictive, as from contractures that prevent full joint mobility. It depends on the client's specific diagnosis.

While keeping within parameters set by a diagnosis, recreational therapists encourage AROM to increase available range while employing joint protection techniques as appropriate. Activities are redesigned within (and slightly above, if appropriate) available ranges. Adaptive equipment is prescribed as necessary to maximize independence and task performance.

Mild contractures can usually be reduced with moderate and frequent activity combined with relaxation that leads to a reduction in stress and muscle guarding. Activities such as playing with a pet, fixing a meal, gardening, and other enjoyable activities help reduce muscle tightness.

If a client has joint mobility restrictions, proper precautions and adaptations must be taken to reduce injury and ensure safety. People who need to protect their joints need to be educated about joint protection techniques. Joint protection refers to the use of larger joints to do the work of small joints to limit repetitive small joint range of motion and unnecessary workload. One example is to use a universal cuff to hold a paintbrush so that the wrist and arm are doing most of the work and finger movement in minimized. Another example is the use of lightweight gardening equipment to minimize joint stress and encourage work of larger muscles and joints to perform the task. Joint protection does not mean that joints should not be ranged or bear weight. Secondary complications may arise if joints are not ranged. Key concepts of joint protection mean the client should:

- Respect joint pain as a signal to stop an activity.

- Avoid positions of deformity. For example, press water from a sponge rather than squeezing, hold stirring spoons so that the bowl of the spoon is on the ulnar side of the hand and avoid turning the wrist inwards.

- Avoid pressure that pushes the finger and wrist joints in an ulnar direction. For example, turn handles or lids in the direction of the radius even if this means using the non-dominant hand.

- Avoid external and internal deforming forces, such as the strong pinch and grasp that are typically required for knitting or hammering.

- Use each joint in its most stable anatomical and functional plane. For example, avoid twisting the knees when standing up by standing up first and then turning.

- Use the strongest and largest joints available for the job because proximal joints are stronger than distal joints, and their use protects the weaker distal ones. For example, carry a pocketbook over the forearm instead of in the hand, carry heavy items by putting a hand and forearm flat underneath and steadying the object with the other hand.

- Use correct patterns of motion based on body mechanics and ergonomics.

- Avoid holding one position for an undue length of time.

- Avoid starting an activity that cannot be stopped if it proves to be beyond the client's capability.

### Cross References

In *Recreational Therapy for Specific Diagnoses and Conditions, First Edition*, ICF code b710 Mobility of Joint Functions is listed in 13 chapters: Amputation and Prosthesis, Back Disorders and Back Pain, Cerebrovascular Accident, Chronic Obstructive Pulmonary Disease, Intellectual Disability, Multiple Sclerosis, Osteoarthritis, Osteoporosis, Parkinson's Disease, Rheumatoid Arthritis, Spinal Cord Injury, Total Joint Replacement, and Traumatic Brain Injury.

In *Recreational Therapy Basics, Techniques, and Interventions, First Edition*, treatment for ICF code b710 Mobility of Joint Functions is discussed in seven chapters: Activity and Task Analysis, Consequences of Inactivity, Adaptive Sports, Aquatic Therapy, Mind-Body Interventions, Motor Learning and Training Strategies, and Neuro-Developmental Treatment.

## b715 Stability of Joint Functions

Functions of the maintenance of structural integrity of the joints.

Inclusions: functions of the stability of a single joint, several joints, and joints generalized; impairments such as in unstable shoulder joint, dislocation of a joint, dislocation of shoulder and hip

Exclusions: mobility of joint functions (b710)

- *b7150 Stability of a Single Joint*
  Functions of the maintenance of structural integrity of one joint.

- *b7151 Stability of Several Joints*
  Functions of the maintenance of structural integrity of more than one joint.

- *b7152 Stability of Joints Generalized*
  Functions of the maintenance of structural integrity of joints throughout the body.

- *b7158 Stability of Joint Functions, Other Specified*

- *b7159 Stability of Joint Functions, Unspecified*
  Recreational therapists do not treat unstable joints, nor assess the extent of their impairment. However they need to be aware of unstable joints and any precautions or parameters that must be followed to ensure that further injury does not occur.

The recreational therapist may need to adapt activities for the client when there are deficits in joint stability. For example, a client with a shoulder dislocation may be required to wear a protective harness to prevent the arm from being raised above the head. Activities that require raising the arms will need to be modified or adaptive equipment may be required, such as a grabber to reach objects on a high shelf.

Joint instability may be caused by activities, such as playing a sport. If recreational therapists suspect joint instability from an injury during activity sessions, as evidenced by pain or misalignment, medical attention should be sought immediately.

### Cross References

In *Recreational Therapy for Specific Diagnoses and Conditions, First Edition*, ICF code b715 Stability of Joint Functions is listed in two chapters: Rheumatoid Arthritis and Total Joint Replacement.

In *Recreational Therapy Basics, Techniques, and Interventions, First Edition*, treatment for ICF code b715 Stability of Joint Functions is discussed in two chapters: Aquatic Therapy and Balance Training.

### b720 Mobility of Bone Functions

Functions of the range and ease of movement of the scapula, pelvis, carpal, and tarsal bones.

Inclusions: impairments such as frozen scapula and frozen pelvis

Exclusions: mobility of joints functions (b710)

- *b7200 Mobility of the Scapula*
  Functions of the range and ease of movement of the scapula.

  Inclusions: impairments such as protraction, retraction, laterorotation, and medial rotation of the scapula

- *b7201 Mobility of the Pelvis*
  Functions of the range and ease of movement of the pelvis.

  Inclusion: rotation of the pelvis

- *b7202 Mobility of Carpal Bones*
  Functions of the range and ease of movement of the carpal bones.

- *b7203 Mobility of Tarsal Bones*
  Functions of the range and ease of movement of the tarsal bones.

- *b7208 Mobility of Bone Functions, Other Specified*
- *b7209 Mobility of Bone Functions, Unspecified*
  Recreational therapists do not treat mobility of bone functions, nor score the ICF codes in this section, but they are aware of bone mobility impairments as communicated through medical documentation by other health professionals. If mobility of a bone is impaired, recreational therapists follow specific precautions and parameters required for the client. Many of the causes and treatments for deficits in mobility of bones are similar to the causes and treatments for deficits in b710 Mobility of Joint Functions. Review that section for more information. Activity adaptations to accommodate bone mobility impairments are made as appropriate.

### Cross References

In *Recreational Therapy for Specific Diagnoses and Conditions, First Edition*, ICF code b720

Mobility of Bone Functions is listed in one chapter: Osteoporosis.

In *Recreational Therapy Basics, Techniques, and Interventions, First Edition*, there are no references for ICF code b720 Mobility of Bone Functions.

### b729 Functions of the Joints and Bones, Other Specified and Unspecified

## Muscle Functions (b730 - b749)

### b730 Muscle Power Functions

Functions related to the force generated by the contraction of a muscle or muscle groups.

Inclusions: functions associated with the power of specific muscles and muscle groups, muscles of one limb, one side of the body, the lower half of the body, all limbs, the trunk and the body as a whole; impairments such as weakness of small muscles in feet and hands, muscle paresis, muscle paralysis, monoplegia, hemiplegia, paraplegia, quadriplegia, and akinetic mutism

Exclusions: functions of structures adjoining the eye (b215); muscle tone functions (b735); muscle endurance functions (b740)

- *b7300 Power of Isolated Muscles and Muscle Groups*
  Functions related to the force generated by the contraction of specific and isolated muscles and muscle groups.

  Inclusions: impairments such as weakness of small muscles of feet and hands

- *b7301 Power of Muscles of One Limb*
  Functions related to the force generated by the contraction of the muscles and muscle groups of one arm or leg.

  Inclusions: impairments such as monoparesis and monoplegia

- *b7302 Power of Muscles of One Side of the Body*
  Functions related to the force generated by the contraction of the muscles and muscle groups found on the left or right side of the body.

  Inclusions: impairments such as hemiparesis and hemiplegia

- *b7303 Power of Muscles in Lower Half of the Body*
  Functions related to the force generated by the contraction of the muscle groups found in the lower half of the body.

  Inclusions: impairments such as paraparesis and paraplegia

- *b7304 Power of Muscles of All Limbs*
  Functions related to the force generated by the contraction of muscles and muscle groups of all four limbs

  Inclusions: impairments such as tetraparesis and tetraplegia

- *b7305 Power of Muscles of the Trunk*
  Functions related to the force generated by the contraction of muscles and muscle groups in the trunk.

- *b7306 Power of All Muscles of the Body*
  Functions related to the force generated by the contraction of all muscles and muscle groups of the body.

  Inclusions: impairments such as akinetic mutism

- *b7308 Muscle Power Functions, Other Specified*
- *b7309 Muscle Power Functions, Unspecified*

Muscle power (commonly called muscle strength) can be affected by many things including neurological impairment, such as hemiplegia from a stroke, deconditioning from inactivity or chronic disease, lack of sleep, lack of proper nutrition, and diseases that attack the muscles. Muscle power functions may also be restricted due to specific health conditions or injuries, such as weight lifting restrictions after having a heart attack or a bone or muscle injury. Refer to specific diagnoses for more information on how to address muscle power dysfunction as it relates to a specific diagnosis.

In general, muscle power refers to the degree of muscle power when movement is resisted with objects or gravity. Common ways to measure muscle power include:

- *Subjective strength test*: Ask the client to perform specific actions and observe the client's performance. For example, ask the client to hold your hand and then instruct the client to hold onto your hand tightly and not let go when you try to pull your hand away.

- *Weights*: Ask the client to perform a familiar strength task that has a specific weight. Record the amount of weight the client is able to manipulate and the number of repetitions s/he is able to perform prior to fatigue.

- *Manual muscle evaluation* (MME): The MME is a classification of strength that allows therapists to rate a client's strength along a scale. The specific techniques used by a therapist to arrive at the classification may vary. See Table 4 for a possible method of scoring.

**Table 4: Manual Muscle Evaluation — Strength**

**Complete range of motion against gravity with full resistance**
Grade: 100%, 5, Normal (N)
**Complete range of motion against gravity with some resistance**
Grade: 75%, 4, Good (G)
**Complete range of motion against gravity**
Grade: 50%, 3, Fair (F)
**Complete range of motion with gravity eliminated**
Grade: 25%, 2, Poor (P)
**Evidence of contractility**
Grade: 10%, 1, Trace (T)
**No evidence of contractility**
Grade: 0%, 0, Zero (0)

If spasm or contracture exists, place Spasm (S) or Contracture (C) after the grade of a movement incomplete for this reason.

From burlingame (2001), used with permission.

Recreational therapists commonly document muscle power dysfunction by describing the specific impairment, clarifying muscle power abilities and limitations, and documenting the impact of muscle power dysfunction as it relates to specific activities. For example, "The client has muscular dystrophy. He is able to lift a maximum of five pounds in right hand with an MME grade of P. He can swing one-pound hammer using right upper extremity for two minutes prior to muscle fatigue.

Scoring the extent of muscle power impairment in ICF codes requires a technique for determining the percentage of impairment. Therapists might score these codes based on client report. For example, if a client states that he has 40% of the strength he used to have in his legs, then the therapist would score b7303 Power of Muscles in Lower Half of the Body as a severe impairment (b7303.3). The therapist could also use strength-testing equipment, such as a hand dynamometer, that measures hand strength, or a pinch strength gauge meter. Normative data is commonly available to which the client's reading could be compared to determine the extent of impairment.

Therapeutic interventions to improve muscle power functions will vary depending on the cause of the impairment. Impairment related to neurological dysfunction, such as that caused by a stroke, respond best to neuroplasticity interventions along with general strength training. People with muscle power impairment from deconditioning respond best to general strength training alone. General strength training includes the use of graduated tasks of weight and repetition, gradually increasing the weight of the item and/or the number of times the item is used in a given period of time. Other interventions may include assisting with sleep quality and quantity (see b134 Sleep Functions for common interventions) and nutritional intake. When disease affects muscle strength, the interventions are disease specific.

Adaptations for muscle power impairments include the redesign of activity components to meet muscle power restrictions or abilities. Lightweight adaptive equipment may also be prescribed to meet the client's abilities.

### Cross References

In *Recreational Therapy for Specific Diagnoses and Conditions, First Edition*, ICF code b730 Muscle Power Functions is listed in 20 chapters: Amputation and Prosthesis, Back Disorders and Back Pain, Burns, Cancer, Cerebral Palsy, Cerebrovascular Accident, Chronic Obstructive Pulmonary Disease, Feeding and Eating Disorders, Guillain-Barré Syndrome, Heart Disease, Intellectual Disability, Multiple Sclerosis, Obesity, Osteoarthritis, Osteoporosis, Parkinson's Disease, Rheumatoid Arthritis, Spina Bifida, Total Joint Replacement, and Traumatic Brain Injury.

In *Recreational Therapy Basics, Techniques, and Interventions, First Edition*, treatment for ICF code b730 Muscle Power Functions is discussed in nine chapters: Activity and Task Analysis, Consequences of Inactivity, Adaptive Sports, Aquatic Therapy, Balance Training, Constraint-Induced Movement Therapy, Energy Conservation Techniques, Mind-

Body Interventions, and Motor Learning and Training Strategies.

### *b735 Muscle Tone Functions*

Functions related to the tension present in the resting muscles and the resistance offered when trying to move the muscles passively.

Inclusions: functions associated with the tension of isolated muscles and muscle groups, muscles of one limb, one side of the body, and the lower half of the body, muscles of all limbs, muscles of the trunk, and all muscles of the body; impairments such as hypotonia, hypertonia, and muscle spasticity

Exclusions: muscle power functions (b730); muscle endurance functions (b740)

- *b7350 Tone of Isolated Muscles and Muscle Groups*
  Functions related to the tension present in the resting isolated muscles and muscle groups and the resistance offered when trying to move those muscles passively.

  Inclusions: impairments such as in focal dystonias, e.g., torticollis

- *b7351 Tone of Muscles of One Limb*
  Functions related to the tension present in the resting muscles and muscle groups in one arm or leg and the resistance offered when trying to move those muscles passively.

  Inclusions: impairments associated with monoparesis and monoplegia

- *b7352 Tone of Muscles of One Side of Body*
  Functions related to the tension present in the resting muscles and muscle groups of the right or left side of the body and the resistance offered when trying to move those muscles passively.

  Inclusions: impairments associated with hemiparesis and hemiplegia

- *b7353 Tone of Muscles in Lower Half of Body*
  Functions related to the tension present in the resting muscles and muscle groups in the lower half of the body and the resistance offered when trying to move those muscles passively.

  Inclusions: impairments associated with paraparesis and paraplegia

- *b7354 Tone of Muscles in All Limbs*
  Functions related to the tension present in the resting muscles and muscle groups in all four limbs and the resistance offered when trying to move those muscles passively.

  Inclusions: impairments associated with tetra-paresis and tetraplegia

- *b7355 Tone of Muscles of Trunk*
  Functions related to the tension present in the resting muscles and muscle groups of the trunk and the resistance offered when trying to move those muscles passively.

- *b7356 Tone of All Muscles of the Body*
  Functions related to the tension present in the resting muscles and muscle groups of the whole body and the resistance offered when trying to move those muscles passively.

  Inclusions: impairments such as in generalized dystonias and Parkinson's disease, or general paresis and paralysis

- *b7358 Muscle Tone Functions, Other Specified*
- *b7359 Muscle Tone Functions, Unspecified*

Muscle tone is the degree of tension or resistance in a muscle at rest and in response to stretch. Muscle tone dysfunction is typically divided into two problems:

- *Flaccidity (or hypotonia)*: a decrease in muscle tone. A diminished resistance to passive movement will be noted, and muscles may feel abnormally soft and flaccid. Diminished deep tendon reflexes also may be noted.
- *Rigidity (or hypertonia)*: an increase in muscle tone causing greater resistance to passive movement. Two types of rigidity may be seen: *lead pipe* and *cogwheel*. Lead pipe rigidity is a uniform, constant resistance felt by the examiner as the extremity is moved through a range of motion. Cogwheel rigidity is considered a combination of the lead pipe type with tremor. It is characterized by a series of brief relaxations or "catches" as the extremity is passively moved.

Muscle tone problems result from brain injury, such as traumatic brain injury or stroke, or neurological impairment, such as spinal cord injury or Parkinson's disease.

Decreased or increased muscle tone can affect activity performance. Therapists begin by observing the state of the client's muscles at rest and when performing activities. Therapists document muscle tone impairments by diagnosis (hypotonic, hypertonic) and location, as well as activities impaired by muscle tone dysfunction. For example, "Increased tone in right upper extremity impairs client's ability to cast a fishing line resulting in the need for moderate assistance with this task." ICF codes under b735 Muscle Tone Functions and the specific Activities and Participation codes under d4 Mobility and d920 Recreation and Leisure would be scored. Recreational therapists will most likely not score the codes for muscle tone functions.

If muscle tone impairments are noted, interventions to maximize function and decrease secondary problems are introduced, as noted here:

- *Flaccidity*: If muscles are hypotonic due to brain impairment, tactile stimulation to the muscle can be helpful to improve tone. Hypotonic muscles due to nerve injury may respond to tactile stimulation only if it is an incomplete injury. Flaccid or hypotonic limbs due to brain injury can be incorporated into functional activities to promote neuroplasticity, while the incorporation of flaccid and hypotonic limbs due to nerve injury into functional activities is helpful to prevent muscle contractures.
- *Rigidity*: Stretching muscles through their range of motion prior to and after activity performance is important to reduce increased tone caused by activity and prevent contractures. In some instances, however, range of motion may be contraindicated, as when working with a tenodesis splint in a client with tetraplegia. Splints may be prescribed to stretch out rigid muscles for prevention or reduction of muscle contractures. Recreational therapists need to be aware of and assist the client as needed to don/doff splints. If rigidity is causing functional problems, pharmacological interventions may be used to decrease muscle rigidity.

Sometimes flaccidity and rigidity occur together because flaccid muscles often experience contractures. Treatment in those cases aims to eliminate the contractures while also using the muscles in a way that increases their tone.

Should muscle tone functions remain unresolved, precautions are taken to ensure client safety, prevent contractures, and improve functional abilities.

### Cross References

In *Recreational Therapy for Specific Diagnoses and Conditions, First Edition*, ICF code b735 Muscle Tone Functions is listed in 14 chapters: Amputation and Prosthesis, Back Disorders and Back Pain, Cerebral Palsy, Cerebrovascular Accident, Guillain-Barré Syndrome, Heart Disease, Intellectual Disability, Multiple Sclerosis, Obesity, Osteoarthritis, Osteoporosis, Spina Bifida, Total Joint Replacement, and Traumatic Brain Injury.

In *Recreational Therapy Basics, Techniques, and Interventions, First Edition*, treatment for ICF code b735 Muscle Tone Functions is discussed in eight chapters: Consequences of Inactivity, Adaptive Sports, Aquatic Therapy, Balance Training, Constraint-Induced Movement Therapy, Mind-Body Interventions, Motor Learning and Training Strategies, and Neuro-Developmental Treatment.

### b740 Muscle Endurance Functions

Functions related to sustaining muscle contraction for the required period of time.

Inclusions: functions associated with sustaining muscle contraction for isolated muscles and muscle groups, and all muscles of the body; impairments such as in myasthenia gravis

Exclusions: exercise tolerance functions (b455); muscle power functions (b730); muscle tone functions (b735)

- *b7400 Endurance of Isolated Muscles*
  Functions related to sustaining muscle contraction of isolated muscles for the required period of time.

- *b7401 Endurance of Muscle Groups*
  Functions related to sustaining muscle contraction of isolated muscle groups for the required period of time.

  Inclusions: impairments associated with monoparesis, monoplegia, hemiparesis and hemiplegia, paraparesis and paraplegia

- *b7402 Endurance of All Muscles of the Body*
  Functions related to sustaining muscle contraction of all muscles of the body for the required period of time.

  Inclusions: impairments associated with tetraparesis, tetraplegia, general paresis, and paralysis

- *b7408 Muscle Endurance Functions, Other Specified*

- *b7409 Muscle Endurance Functions, Unspecified*
  Muscle endurance functions can be affected by neurological impairments, such as stroke, and muscular impairments, such as fibromyalgia, or from deconditioning as a secondary complication related to another health problem.

To assess muscle endurance functions, the therapist presents the client with a muscle endurance task that is within appropriate parameters and precautions for the client. The therapist monitors vital signs as needed. The therapist measures muscle endurance functions in terms of time (e.g., client presents with standing tolerance of 15 minutes), weight (e.g., client able to perform 10 bicep curls with five-pound weight prior to fatigue), and intensity (e.g., low intensity ball toss with eight-ounce ball results in upper extremity muscle endurance of six minutes prior to fatigue).

Scoring the extent of muscle power impairment in ICF codes requires a technique for determining the percentage of impairment. Therapists might score these codes based on client report. For example, if a client states that he has 40% of the endurance he used to have, then the therapist would score b7402 Endurance of All Muscles of the Body as a severe impairment (b7402.3). Otherwise, endurance would need to be tested utilizing a standardized measure and compared the results to normative data to determine the extent of impairment.

Therapists promote muscle endurance through the use of graduated muscle endurance tasks by increasing time, frequency, and/or intensity of the activity.

If muscle endurance does not recover to normal levels or if there are specific muscle endurance precautions, activity adaptations are made. Some examples might be to decrease the weight of objects to decrease muscle workload, redesign an activity to meet compromised muscle endurance, decrease the task speed, decrease the task intensity, decrease the distance, decrease the task time, increase rest periods, explore energy saving techniques, and explore adaptive equipment to assist with managing muscle endurance.

***Cross References***

In *Recreational Therapy for Specific Diagnoses and Conditions, First Edition*, ICF code b740 Muscle Endurance Functions is listed in 13 chapters: Amputation and Prosthesis, Back Disorders and Back Pain, Burns, Cerebrovascular Accident, Guillain-Barré Syndrome, Intellectual Disability, Osteoarthritis, Osteoporosis, Parkinson's Disease, Rheumatoid Arthritis, Spina Bifida, Total Joint Replacement, and Traumatic Brain Injury.

In *Recreational Therapy Basics, Techniques, and Interventions, First Edition*, treatment for ICF code b740 Muscle Endurance Functions is discussed in six chapters: Activity and Task Analysis, Consequences of Inactivity, Aquatic Therapy, Constraint-Induced Movement Therapy, Energy Conservation Techniques, and Motor Learning and Training Strategies.

### b749 Muscle Functions, Other Specified and Unspecified

## Movement Functions (b750 - b789)

### b750 Motor Reflex Functions

Functions of involuntary contraction of muscles automatically induced by specific stimuli.

Inclusions: functions of stretch motor reflex, automatic local joint reflex, reflexes generated by noxious stimuli and other exteroceptive stimuli; withdrawal reflex, biceps reflex, radius reflex, quadriceps reflex, patellar reflex, ankle reflex

- *b7500 Stretch Motor Reflex*
  Functions of involuntary contractions of muscles automatically induced by stretching.

- *b7501 Reflexes Generated by Noxious Stimuli*
  Functions of involuntary contractions of muscles automatically induced by painful or other noxious stimuli.

  Inclusion: withdrawal reflex

- *b7502 Reflexes Generated by Other Exteroceptive Stimuli*
  Functions of involuntary contractions of muscles automatically induced by external stimuli other than noxious stimuli.

- *b7508 Motor Reflex Functions, Other Specified*
- *b7509 Motor Reflex Functions, Unspecified*
  A reflex is a reaction that occurs in response to a stimulus without conscious thought or will. The reflexes covered by this ICF code are a result of nerve impulses that do not even reach the brain. One example is the patellar ("knee jerk") reflex, which is one of the deep tendon reflexes included in b7502 Reflexes Generated by Other Exteroceptive Stimuli. The patellar reflex may be used with a client to assess some kinds of stress. Table 5 shows all of the deep tendon reflexes and the spinal nerve root that is involved. Table 6 provides scoring for deep tendon reflexes. Documentation involves the type of reflex and the numeric rating.

**Table 5: Deep Tendon Reflexes**

| Reflex | Main Spinal Nerve Roots |
|---|---|
| Biceps | C5, C6 |
| Brachioradialis | C6 |
| Triceps | C7 |
| Patellar | L4 |
| Achilles tendon | S1 |

**Table 6: Rating System for Deep Tendon Reflexes**

(Numeric Rating: Description of Function)
4+: brisk, hyperactive, clonus
3+: is more brisk than normal, but does not necessarily indicate a pathologic process, gross functional ability not usually impaired
2+: Normal
1+: Low normal, with slight diminution in response, having minor impact on functional ability
0: no response

From burlingame (2001), p. 261. Used with permission.

Other reflexes occur as a result of the proprioceptors in muscles noticing a stretch, noxious stimuli, and other external stimuli. The recreational therapist will usually not assess a reflex response unless it is being used to track some aspect of the client's state. For example, a pinprick may be used to distinguish between the lowest three levels on the *Rancho Los Amigos Scale*.

In pediatrics, the presence or absence of a reflex is commonly noted to monitor development and impairments. There are three reflexes that probably belong in b750 Motor Reflex Functions. Other primitive reflexes seem to fit better in b755 Involuntary Movement Reaction Functions. They will be discussed there. The three reflexes that seem to represent motor reflex functions are

**Babinski** (birth to four months)
When the lateral side of the sole of the foot is gently scraped with a fingernail, the toes extend.

**Withdrawal reflex** (birth and continues)
When the sole of the foot is gently scratched with a fingernail, flexion of the hip, knee, and foot occur followed by a similar response in the unstimulated foot.

**Palmar grasp** (birth to four months)
When the palm of the hand is gently pressed, the infant's fingers grasp around the object.

Recreational therapists, although noting the presence or absence of reflexes, will most likely not score the codes for motor reflex functions.

There is no specific treatment related to reflexes. Treatment is typically directed at the underlying cause of the reflex deficit.

Some adaptations may be necessary. For example, clients who do not properly respond to noxious stimuli, such as potentially damaging heat, will need to be protected from dangerous situations and learn strategies to avoid injury. See b270 Sensory Functions Related to Temperature and Other Stimuli for some additional ideas.

### Cross References

In *Recreational Therapy for Specific Diagnoses and Conditions, First Edition*, ICF code b750 Motor Reflex Functions is listed in five chapters: Amputation and Prosthesis, Cerebrovascular Accident, Guillain-Barré Syndrome, Spinal Cord Injury, and Substance-Related Disorders.

In *Recreational Therapy Basics, Techniques, and Interventions, First Edition*, there are no references for ICF code b750 Motor Reflex Functions.

### b755 Involuntary Movement Reaction Functions

Functions of involuntary contractions of large muscles or the whole body induced by body position, balance, and threatening stimuli.

Inclusions: functions of postural reactions, righting reactions, body adjustment reactions, balance reactions, supporting reactions, defensive reactions

Exclusion: motor reflex functions (b750)

Involuntary movement reaction functions are movements that the body makes in reaction to a position, such as leaning forward to stand from a sitting position, balance challenges, such as waving the arms during loss of balance in attempt to regain balance, or threatening stimuli, where the person may cover the face or head to protect it from injury. Reaction impairments are often a sign of central nervous system injury.

Some of the most important involuntary movement reaction functions involve maintaining balance, posture, and stability in a variety of situations. Improving or maintaining balance, posture, and stability are underlying, basic functional skills required to participate in everyday activities.

Pediatric practitioners have identified over 70 reflexes and involuntary movement reaction functions in the newborn. The reflexes are discussed in b750 Motor Reflex Functions. The involuntary movement reaction functions that are most important for recreational therapy are shown in Table 7. Postural reactions, also called postural response or gravity reflexes, are shown in Table 8. Locomotor reflexes, which resemble voluntary movements, are shown in Table 9. These involuntary movement reaction functions are distinguished from reflexes because they involve some part of the brain. Reflexes involve only the spinal cord.

### Table 7: Primitive Infant Reflexes

**Doll-eye** (birth to two weeks)
When an infant's head is manually turned, the eyes will stay fixed instead of moving with the head.

**Sucking** (birth to three months)
Activated when the nipple touches the back of the palate.

**Moro** (birth to six months)
When dropping the head a few inches while supporting the infant's back and buttocks, the infant senses a lack of support and immediately abducts the arms at the shoulders with open hands and extended fingers. This is immediately followed by adduction of the arms and flexion of the fingers. Absence of this reflex is concerning as it is a primary indicator of a neurological problem.

**Asymmetric tonic neck** (birth to six months)
When in supine position, turning the infant's head to the right results in extension of the right arm and leg and flexion of the left arm and leg — and vice versa if the infant's head is turned to the left; also referred to as the "fencing position."

**Rooting/search** (birth to 12 months)
When side of mouth or cheek is touched, the infant turns his head towards the side of the mouth or cheek that was touched.

**Plantar grasp** (four to 12 months)
When pressure is applied to the sole of the infant's foot, his toes curl around.

**Symmetric tonic neck** (six to seven months)
When supported in a seated position, simultaneous arm extension and leg flexion occur as a result of extending the head and neck; flexion of the head and neck results in the opposite — arm flexion and leg extension.

**Startle** (7-12 months)
When in supine, tapping on the infant's abdomen results in flexion of the arms and legs. The startle reflex can also be elicited when the infant coughs, sneezes, or hears a loud noise, all of which can cause distress and crying.

Piek, 2006; Pramanik, 2007; Ricci & Kyle, 2008; Schlinger, 1995.

**Table 8: Postural reactions**

**Neck righting** (birth to six months)
Orients the body in relation to the head. Extension of the head through dorsiflexion results in extension of the vertebral column, whereas ventroflexion of the head causes flexion or rounding of the vertebral column. When the infant's head is inclined laterally towards the shoulder it elicits lateral curvature of the

spine with the concavity directed towards the same shoulder.

**Labyrinthine righting** (two to 12 months)
Hold the baby under his arms and stretch out your arms in front of you, tilt the infant forward, backward, or to the side; the infant will move his head and neck in a manner so that the head remains in a vertical position — straight up and down.

**Pull-up reflex** (three to 12 months)
When in a seated position and held by either one or both arms, the infant will attempt to remain upright using a reflexive pull up reaction of the arms.

**Parachute** (four to 12 months)
Parachute-sideways: Protective extension with the arms when tilted to the side in a supported sitting position.
Parachute-forward: Protective extension with the arms when held up in the air and moved forward. The infant reflexively reaches forward to catch himself.
Parachute-backward: Protective extension with the arms when titled backwards.

**Propping** (four to 12 months)
Moving the infant off balance from a sitting position which elicits extension of the arms.

**Body righting** (six to 12 months)
Orients the head in relation to the ground, which is important for voluntary rolling.

**Optical righting** (six to 12 months)
In response to visual stimuli, the infant changes his head position to correct his posture.

Piek, 2006; Pramanik, 2007; Ricci & Kyle, 2008; Schlinger, 1995.

**Table 9: Locomotor reflexes**

**Crawling** (birth to four months)
When in prone position, apply pressure to the sole of the foot, which usually results in a crawling response from all four limbs.

**Stepping/walking** (birth to five months)
When the infant's feet are placed on a flat surface with its body weight forward, the infant will "walk" forward.

**Swimming** (birth to five months)
When the infant is placed over water in a prone position, the swimming reflex is elicited — flexion and extension of arms and legs.

Piek, 2006; Pramanik, 2007; Ricci & Kyle, 2008; Schlinger, 1995.

Therapists assess reaction impairments through observation during activity. If the reaction movement is present, it is said to be positive. If it is not present, it is said to be negative. If the reaction movement is present but not at full intensity, the level of impairment is noted and explained as needed.

For documentation, the specific activity used for observation and its conditions are documented. For example, "During dynamic standing activity of plant care client had moderately impaired righting reactions." ICF scoring for a reaction that is moderately impaired would be b755.2.

Recovery of movement reactions may occur in some cases depending on the cause of the problem. Reaction impairments that are not recovered may cause significant problems with life activities. The impairments may require the use of devices, such as walking devices or extra body protection gear during sporting activities.

### Cross References

In *Recreational Therapy for Specific Diagnoses and Conditions, First Edition*, ICF code b755 Involuntary Movement Reaction Functions is listed in 10 chapters: Amputation and Prosthesis, Cerebrovascular Accident, Intellectual Disability, Multiple Sclerosis, Osteoarthritis, Osteoporosis, Parkinson's Disease, Spina Bifida, Substance-Related Disorders, and Traumatic Brain Injury.

In *Recreational Therapy Basics, Techniques, and Interventions, First Edition*, treatment for ICF code b755 Involuntary Movement Reaction Functions is discussed in six chapters: Activity and Task Analysis, Consequences of Inactivity, Aquatic Therapy, Balance Training, Mind-Body Interventions, and Neuro-Developmental Treatment.

### b760 Control of Voluntary Movement Functions

Functions associated with control over and coordination of voluntary movements.

Inclusions: functions of control of simple voluntary movements and of complex voluntary movements, coordination of voluntary movements, supportive functions of arm or leg, right left motor coordination, eye hand coordination, eye foot coordination; impairments such as control and coordination problems, e.g., dysdiadochokinesia

Exclusions: muscle power functions (b730); involuntary movement functions (b765); gait pattern functions (b770)

- *b7600 Control of Simple Voluntary Movements* Functions associated with control over and coordination of simple or isolated voluntary movements.

- *b7601 Control of Complex Voluntary Movements* Functions associated with control over and coordination of complex voluntary movements.

- *b7602 Coordination of Voluntary Movements* Functions associated with coordination of simple and complex voluntary movements, performing movements in an orderly combination.

  Inclusions: right left coordination, coordination of visually directed movements, such as eye hand coordination and eye foot coordination; impairments such as dysdiadochokinesia

- *b7603 Supportive Functions of Arm or Leg* Functions associated with control over and coordination of voluntary movements by placing weight either on the arms (elbows or hands) or on the legs (knees or feet).

- *b7608 Control of Voluntary Movement Functions, Other Specified*
- *b7609 Control of Voluntary Movement Functions, Unspecified*

This section looks at the four aspects of controlling voluntary movement. The first two codes look at controlling simple and complex movements. The third code looks at coordination of movement, while the fourth code looks at the specific problem of using the arms or legs as supports for voluntary movement.

### Control of Simple and Complex Voluntary Movement

Voluntary movement functions refer to the voluntary control of muscles. An example of a simple voluntary movement would be raising your hand to answer a question. An example of a complex voluntary movement would be positioning yourself into an advanced yoga posture. Voluntary movement functions can be hindered by damage to the brain or nervous system.

Therapists assess voluntary movement disorders by asking the client to perform specific voluntary movements and observing a client's performance of voluntary movements in an activity. Observation of performance in an activity is especially needed when cognitive impairments are present that could hinder the person's ability to understand the performance you are requesting. For example it is important to understand whether the difficulty for a person with a left cerebrovascular accident and resultant receptive aphasia is in processing the spoken request or in actually making the movement.

Voluntary movement disorders that are affected by underlying brain or nervous system problems that have the potential for recovery, such as incomplete spinal cord injury, brain injury, cerebrovascular accident, and Guillain-Barré syndrome, are addressed through the use of neuroplasticity or other retraining interventions.

Voluntary movement disorders, although having a potential for recovery, are not always fully recovered, and some voluntary movement disorders, such as complete spinal cord injury, will not recover. In this situation, the therapist adapts activities so they match the client's abilities. When voluntary movement is restricted, secondary problems can occur such as muscle contractures (b710 Mobility of Joint Functions), joint instability (b715 Stability of Joint Functions), muscle atrophy (affecting b730 Muscle Power Functions and b740 Muscle Endurance Functions), increased or decreased muscle tone (b735 Muscle Tone Functions), and pain (b280 Sensation of Pain).

Therapists document the specific impairment, the specific activity affected, the level of assistance, and any recommendations. Impairment of voluntary function is often documented by the amount of active range of motion. For example, "Voluntary movement of the right upper extremity is impaired resulting in moderately impaired finger/wrist/elbow flexion and extension. Consequently, client is able to perform only 50% of a simple repotting task. Client instructed on how to use right upper extremity as a functional assist for task and is able to incorporate techniques learned with minimal assistance." The *Functional Independence Measure* categories can be used to score the ICF codes.

## Spontaneous Movements

Spontaneous movements are important markers for the health of infants. These voluntary movements are seen in the first 20 weeks of life. Recreational therapists should note the absence or presence of spontaneous movements in their assessment and documentation. Spontaneous movements in early postnatal life include (Kalverboer & Gramsbergen, 2001):

- *Writhing general movements*: Gross movements involving the whole body lasting a few seconds to several minutes. The movements are a variable sequence of extension and flexion of arm, leg, neck, and trunk movements that wax and wane in intensity, force, and speed; have a gradual beginning and end. Movements typically occur at term until about six to nine weeks.

- *Fidgety general movements*: Small circular movements with moderate speed and variable acceleration of neck, trunk, and limbs in all directions. The movements are continual in the awake infant, except during focused attention and fussing or crying. Movements typically occur about six to nine weeks until about 20 weeks.

- *Wiggling-oscillating movements*: Small movements with moderate speed. Movements are irregular, oscillatory, waving-like movements that are most noticeable when arms are partially or fully extended. Movements typically occur at six weeks until about 12-14 weeks.

- *Saccadic movements*: Moderate to large movements with moderate speed. Movements are jerky and in a zigzag fashion that are most noticeable when arms are partially or fully extended. Movements typically occur around six weeks until about 15 weeks.

- *Swiping movements*: Large movements at high speed. Movements are sudden but are fluid/smooth, have a ballistic-like appearance (like bouncing a ball up and down) and are most noticeable in extended arms and sometimes in partially or extended full legs. Movements typically occur around eight weeks until about 20 weeks.

- *Hand-hand manipulation*: Both hands come together in midline and repetitively touch, stroke, or grasp each other. Movements typically occur around 12-15 weeks.

- *Manipulation of clothing*: The fingers on one or both hands repetitively touch, stroke, or grasp an article of clothing. Movements typically occur around 15 weeks.
- *Reaching/touching*: One or both arms reach to an object in one's immediate environment (fingers touch surface of the object). Movements typically occur around 12-18 weeks.
- *Legs lifted, hand-knee contact*: Both legs lift vertically upward, with partial or full extension of the knees; hips slightly tilted upward; one or both hands touching or grasping the knees; sometimes involves anteflexion of the head (thrusts top of head forward). Movements typically occur around 15 weeks.
- *Trunk rotation*: While lying down, pushes soles of feet down on the lying surface, lifts one hip, and rotates. Movement typically occurs around 12-15 weeks.
- *Axial rolling*: Rolls over from supine to prone (back to stomach) started by the head. Movement typically occurs around 18-20 weeks.

### Coordination of Voluntary Movements

Coordination is the ability to execute smooth, accurate, controlled movements. The ability to produce these movements is a complex process that is dependent on a fully intact neuromuscular system. Coordinated movements are characterized by appropriate speed, distance, direction, rhythm, and muscle tension. In addition, they involve appropriate synergist influences, easy reversal between opposing muscle groups, and proximal fixation to allow distal motion or maintenance of a posture. Incoordination and coordination deficit are general terms used to describe abnormal motor function characterized by awkward, extraneous, uneven, or inaccurate movements (O'Sullivan & Schmitz, 1988).

Some of the deficits that affect control of voluntary movement functions include:

- *Asthenia*: Characterized by generalized muscle weakness. Client may also have difficulty initiating voluntary movement, stopping a movement, or changing the force, speed, or direction of a movement.
- *Ataxia*: This is a general term that describes general difficulty with coordination of motor function of the muscles involved with walking. (Also see b770 Gait Pattern Functions.)

- *Dysdiadochokinesia*: Impairment in ability to perform rapid alternating movements, such as rapid alternation between pronation and supination of the forearm. Movements are irregular, with a rapid loss of range and rhythm.
- *Dysmetria*: Impairment in the ability to accurately judge the distance or range of a movement needed to reach an item or goal. If it is an overestimation, it is referred to as *hypermetria*. If it is an underestimation, it is referred to as *hypometria*.
- *Movement decomposition*: Impairment in ability to perform a smooth sequence of movements. Movements are performed in separate single sequential steps rather than as a smooth and integrated movement. For example, if a client is asked to touch her nose with her index finger, she may first extend her index finger, then extend her arm from the shoulder, and then flex her elbow so that her index finger touches her nose.
- *Nystagmus*: Impairment of the oscillatory movement of the eyes resulting in "jumpy" vision making it difficult to fixate. When trying to fixate on a peripheral object, an involuntary drift back to the midline position is observed. See b215 Functions of Structures Adjoining the Eye for more information or to code this impairment. Several deficits related to eye movements are associated with cerebellar lesions.

Recreational therapists do not typically use standardized tests for upper and lower extremity coordination. Clients are usually challenged with a coordination task that directly relates to functional tasks that are part of the client's lifestyle and observations of impairments or abilities are made. For example, coordination impairments result in client being able to swing a bat accurately enough to hit a ball off a tee only 30% of the time (b7602.3, swinging baseball bat). The therapist must be familiar with the appropriate terminology that reflects coordination deficits and be aware of standardized tests that can provide further assessment of suspected problems. Therapists must also be aware of age-specific developmental changes, such as slower reaction times with aging, and disability restrictions that may influence test performance. ICF score should be made relative to expected abilities.

*Supportive Functions of the Arm or Leg*

The voluntary movement of purposively placing weight through the arms (elbows or hands) or legs (knees or feet) is needed for mobility (d410 Changing Basic Body Position, d415 Maintaining a Body Position, d420 Transferring Oneself, d430 Lifting and Carrying Objects, d435 Moving Objects with Lower Extremities, d445 Hand and Arm Use, d450 Walking, d455 Moving Around). Weight bearing through the arms and legs supports the body when performing specific movements, such as leaning one hand on a table to provide upper body support when reaching for a high object or lunging forward with one leg to support the upper body when throwing a baseball. Although these movements in some situations are performed quickly without much forethought, they are under voluntary control. Some clients may intentionally limit the amount of weight they place through the arms or legs due to specific precautions set by the physician, pain, impaired sensation, and psychological issues, such as lacking confidence in their strength. Ruling these out can be helpful in determining if supportive functions are impaired.

This code refers to specific body functions that impair the ability to use arms or legs as supports. This is most commonly caused by brain and nervous system impairments. Some possibilities are brain injury, multiple sclerosis, cerebrovascular accident, Parkinson's disease, pinched nerve in the back that causes legs to buckle at times, and Guillain-Barré syndrome.

Therapists document the specific impairment, the specific activity affected, the level of assistance, and any recommendations. For example, "Requires moderate assistance for throwing a baseball due to moderately impaired supportive function of the left lower extremity" (b7603.2).

Therapists address the supportive functions of arms and legs by assisting the client into a position that incorporates arm and leg support, such as having the client practice using the left arm as a support by placing the client's left hand on a table and having him reach and grasp high items. Continued use of the arm or leg as a support assists with re-teaching the client how to use the arms and legs as supports, as well as developing muscle strength and bone density that is needed for good support.

Therapists seek to resolve voluntary movement dysfunctions by using motor learning and training strategies. Balance techniques can also be used to improve voluntary motor functions, especially the aspects of using the legs appropriately for support. Some of these techniques are aimed at improving strength, but they also improve balance and coordination by repeated use of neural pathways related to movement and coordination. Whether the pathways are damaged from disease or trauma or not functioning because of lack of use, the therapeutic repetition of skills promotes neuroplasticity and restrengthening of functionality, thus assisting the return of previous levels of ability to perform voluntary movement.

If impairments are not resolved or only resolved partially, the therapist teaches the client alternative ways to support the body with different tasks to maximize performance and safety or re-designs activities to maximize independence, safety, and performance. Assistive devices such as walkers and canes may be used to help with balance.

*Cross References*

In *Recreational Therapy for Specific Diagnoses and Conditions, First Edition*, ICF code b760 Control of Voluntary Movement Functions is listed in 10 chapters: Amputation and Prosthesis, Cerebrovascular Accident, Epilepsy, Guillain-Barré Syndrome, Intellectual Disability, Multiple Sclerosis, Parkinson's Disease, Spina Bifida, Substance-Related Disorders, and Traumatic Brain Injury.

In *Recreational Therapy Basics, Techniques, and Interventions, First Edition*, treatment for ICF code b760 Control of Voluntary Movement Functions is discussed in six chapters: Activity and Task Analysis, Consequences of Inactivity, Aquatic Therapy, Constraint-Induced Movement Therapy, Motor Learning and Training Strategies, and Neuro-Developmental Treatment.

### *b765 Involuntary Movement Functions*

Functions of unintentional, non- or semi-purposive involuntary contractions of a muscle or group of muscles.

Inclusions: involuntary contractions of muscles; impairments such as tremors, tics, mannerisms, stereotypies, motor perseveration, chorea, athetosis, vocal tics, dystonic movements, and dyskinesia

Exclusions: control of voluntary movement functions (b760); gait pattern functions (b770)

- *b7650 Involuntary Contractions of Muscles*
  Functions of unintentional, non- or semi-purposive involuntary contractions of a muscle or group of muscles, such as those involved as part of a psychological dysfunction.

  Inclusions: impairments such as choreatic and athetotic movements; sleep-related movement disorders

- *b7651 Tremor*
  Functions of alternating contraction and relaxation of a group of muscles around a joint, resulting in shakiness.

- *b7652 Tics and Mannerisms*
  Functions of repetitive, quasi-purposive, involuntary contractions of a group of muscles.

  Inclusions: impairments such as vocal tics, coprolalia, and bruxism

- *b7653 Stereotypies and Motor Perseveration*
  Functions of spontaneous, non-purposive movements such as repetitively rocking back and forth and nodding the head or wiggling.

- *b7658 Involuntary Movement Functions, Other Specified*
- *b7659 Involuntary Movement Functions, Unspecified*

Involuntary movement functions are primarily caused by lesions in the basal ganglia. Basal ganglia lesions are common in Parkinson's disease, Wilson's disease, and Huntington's disease. Below is a list of common involuntary movement dysfunctions.

- *Athetosis*: Characterized by slow, involuntary, writhing, twisting, "wormlike" movements. Distal upper extremities are primarily affected along with rotary movements of the extremity. Athetosis is a clinical feature of cerebral palsy.
- *Bradykinesia*: Characterized by slowed or decreased movements. This may include decreased arm swing, slow shuffling gait, difficulty initiating or changing direction of movement, lack of facial expression, and difficulty stopping a movement once begun.
- *Chorea*: Characterized by involuntary, rapid, irregular, and jerky movements; also referred to as choreiform movements. This is a clinical feature of Huntington's disease.

- *Choreoathetosis*: A movement disorder with features of both chorea and athetosis.
- *Dystonia*: Characterized by involuntary muscle contraction of the extremities resulting in bizarre twisting movements. A prolonged contraction at the end of a movement is called a *dystonic posture*.
- *Hemiballismus*: Characterized by a sudden, jerky, forceful, wild, flailing motions of the arm and leg of one side of the body.
- *Tremors*: An involuntary oscillatory movement resulting from alternating contractions of opposing muscle groups. Two types of tremors are associated with cerebellar lesions. An *intention or kinetic tremor* occurs during voluntary motion of a limb and tends to increase as the limb nears its extended goal. Intention tremors are diminished or absent at rest. *Postural or static tremors* may be evident by back-and-forth oscillatory movements of the body while the patient maintains a standing posture. They also may be observed as up-and-down oscillatory movements of a limb when it is held against gravity. There are many different types of tremors. burlingame (2001, p. 305) lists some of them:

  o *Action tremor*: Involuntary oscillating and rhythmic movements of the outstretched upper limb during activity.
  o *Coarse tremor*: Slow, rhythmic movements.
  o *Essential tremor*: Inherited tendency to develop a fine tremor, usually after the age of fifty. Also known as a familial tremor.
  o *Fine tremor*: Fast, rhythmic movements.
  o *Intension tremor*: Increase in intensity when the individual attempts a voluntary movement that requires coordination.
  o *Intermittent tremor*: Occurs when voluntary movement is attempted or occurs in hemiplegia.
  o *Motofacient tremor*: In muscle groups of the face.
  o *Passive tremor*: Only seen when the client is at rest.
  o *Persistent tremor*: Present whether the client is resting or attempting activity.
  o *Resting tremor*: Present when the limb is supported and the patient is at rest, as in

Parkinsonism. Resting tremors typically disappear or reduce with voluntary movement and they may increase with emotional stress.

o   *Volitional tremor*: Seen through the entire body during voluntary movement, as in multiple sclerosis.

Additional tremors that are common to Parkinson's disease include a "pill-rolling" movement. It looks like the client is rolling a pill up and down the first two fingers with his/her thumb. Another tremor movement is the pronation and supination of the forearm, as well as tremor of the head.

Involuntary motor functions are assessed through observation during functional activity, at rest, and through equilibrium and non-equilibrium coordination tests. Recreational therapists will most likely not score the extent of involuntary movement impairment, but rather note the type of involuntary movement impairment and its impact on activity engagement (e.g., "Client's ability to paint small details is severely impaired by intension tremor.").

Involuntary motor functions are primarily controlled fully or partially through pharmacology. The therapist redesigns activities to minimize or eliminate interference with motor responses and minimizes chances of harm or injury. This may include removing unnecessary or unsafe items from the work area when poor motor responses could result in task interference. Weighted objects (e.g., weighted utensils) or weighted fabric wrist cuffs can also be helpful in decreasing intension and essential tremors, although fatigue occurs more rapidly.

### Cross References

In *Recreational Therapy for Specific Diagnoses and Conditions, First Edition*, ICF code **b765 Involuntary Movement Functions** is listed in eight chapters: Amputation and Prosthesis, Cerebrovascular Accident, Generalized Anxiety Disorder, Multiple Sclerosis, Osteoporosis, Parkinson's Disease, Spinal Cord Injury, and Substance-Related Disorders.

In *Recreational Therapy Basics, Techniques, and Interventions, First Edition*, treatment for ICF code **b765 Involuntary Movement Functions** is discussed in two chapters: Consequences of Inactivity and Balance Training.

### b770 Gait Pattern Functions

Functions of movement patterns associated with walking, running, or other whole body movements.

Inclusions: walking patterns and running patterns; impairments such as spastic gait, hemiplegia gait, paraplegic gait, asymmetric gait, limping, and stiff gait pattern

Exclusions: muscle power functions (b730); muscle tone functions (b735); control of voluntary movement functions (b760); involuntary movement functions (b765)

Although physical therapists are the primary healthcare professionals to evaluate and prescribe treatment interventions related to walking and moving, all healthcare professionals must be familiar with gait cycle terminology and approaches to treatment so that strategies and equipment can be carried over into everyday functional, community and/or leisure-based tasks. Gait patterns are important as part of **d450 - d469 Walking and Moving**. See Walking and Gait Training in *Recreational Therapy for Specific Diagnoses and Conditions* for specific information on the gait cycle, normal gait pattern, and abnormal gait patterns.

On the unit the physical therapist may measure the client's stride length and cadence through a simple test called the *Fifty-Foot Walk Test*. Because walking in a hospital setting is often less complex than walking in the community a client's functional level could be different in the two settings. The recreational therapist may want to use the *Fifty-Foot Walk Test* with clients in a community setting to determine if the client (1) has a significant difference in skill between the unit and the community, (2) is able to walk efficiently, (3) is at an increased risk of falling, or (4) has difficulty dividing attention well enough to walk and pay attention to other stimulation at the same time (b1402 Dividing Attention).

In addition to the stride length and cadence information from the *Fifty-Foot Walk Test* there are other methods to describe and measure a client's functional ability. ICF codes that can be scored based on this information include this code and codes under d4 Mobility. Recreational therapists who are typically addressing walking and moving in a functional environment measure walking and moving by the following:

- *Distance*: How far did the client walk? Distance is easily measured in the community by re-walking the distance when the client is resting. Therapists should know the length of their stride so they can make good estimates of distances. If the therapist knows his/her stride length, all s/he needs to do is walk the same distance as the client and multiply the number of strides times the stride length. If the therapist took 100 normal stride steps and has a 2.5-foot stride, the client walked approximately 250'. With practice, the therapist will become adept at "eyeing" a distance and being able to approximate the number of feet walked by the client.

- *Surface*: What type of surface did the client move across? Depending upon the situation, the therapist can provide broad descriptions, such as "uneven community surfaces" or specific descriptions, such as grass, gravel, cobblestone, inclines, etc. For example, if the client displayed different needs for walking on grass as compared to cobblestone, then distinctions must be drawn in the documentation. If the client's performance was consistent throughout the evaluation, then the therapist may opt to broadly describe the surface. It is always a good idea to err on the side of over-description rather than under-description, especially if specific surfaces are deemed important to the client or rehab team for the client's reentry into the community.

- *Amount of assistance*: What type of assistance and how much assistance did the client require? This is typically described using the FIM scale that indicates the degree of assistance needed. Also include detailed information on the amount of supervision required for safety, the type of device (if any) used by the client, and amount and type of cueing.

- *Type and extent of cuing*: e.g., verbal cues, gestural cues, demonstrative cues, tactile cues; minimal, moderate, maximum.

- *Time*: The length of time the client walked.

- *Description of environment*: Environmental factors can influence a client's walking ability. For example, if the environment is noisy it might distract the client from focusing on technique resulting in the need for increased assistance. If the environment is crowded, the client's balance skills will be challenged more, resulting in the

need for a device that provides more stability, such as needing to use a walker instead of single point cane.

- *Abnormal gait patterns observed*: See Walking and Gait Training in *Recreational Therapy for Specific Diagnoses and Conditions* for specific information on abnormal gait patterns, such as antalgic gait, arthogenic gait, ataxic gait, dystrophic gait, festinating gait, footdrop gait, gastrocnemius-soleus gait, and hemiplegic gait.

The recreational therapist will most likely not score Gait Pattern Functions. However, all of forementioned descriptors, as appropriate, will be reflected in documentation. Examples:

- Client walked approximately 150' on outdoor uneven surfaces in quiet setting with a rolling walker and minimal assistance for right knee buckling.

- Client walked approximately 50' in 15 minutes over grassy surface with a single point cane and close supervision secondary to need for max verbal and tactile cues to decrease walking speed.

- Client walked approximately 45' on cobblestone, 25' on gravel, and 60' on slightly uneven concrete without an assistive device at modified independence secondary to increased time. Client independent in initiating rest break.

- Client exhibits a hemiplegic gait and requires moderate verbal cues to slow down and concentrate on right heel strike.

- Client is dependent to don/doff right ankle foot orthosis.

Treatment for functional problems with gait patterns has many aspects. They include strength, endurance, flexibility, and several balance issues. Most of these are covered in other sections of the ICF. Activities and Participation d4 Mobility has additional information on mobility treatment.

Adaptations for problems with gait patterns include making sure that the client has as many visual cues as possible, teaching the use of assistive devices such as canes, and using other mobility devices, such as wheelchairs and banana carts, when the client needs to move faster or through more obstacles than his/her abilities allow.

*Cross References*

In *Recreational Therapy for Specific Diagnoses and Conditions, First Edition*, ICF code b770 Gait Pattern Functions is listed in seven chapters: Amputation and Prosthesis, Cerebrovascular Accident, Multiple Sclerosis, Osteoporosis, Parkinson's Disease, Substance-Related Disorders, and Total Joint Replacement.

In *Recreational Therapy Basics, Techniques, and Interventions, First Edition*, treatment for ICF code b770 Gait Pattern Functions is discussed in five chapters: Consequences of Inactivity, Aquatic Therapy, Balance Training, Energy Conservation Techniques, and Neuro-Developmental Treatment.

## b780 Sensations Related to Muscles and Movement Functions

Sensations associated with the muscles or muscle groups of the body and their movement.

Inclusions: sensations of muscle stiffness and tightness of muscles, muscle spasm or constriction, and heaviness of muscles

Exclusion: sensation of pain (b280)

- *b7800 Sensation of Muscle Stiffness*
  Sensation of tightness or stiffness of muscles.

- *b7801 Sensation of Muscle Spasm*
  Sensation of involuntary contraction of a muscle or a group of muscles.

- *b7808 Sensations Related to Muscles and Movement Functions, Other Specified*
- *b7809 Sensations Related to Muscles and Movement Functions, Unspecified*

Muscle stiffness can be due to a variety of disorders, muscle shortening when in prolonged rest, and general deconditioning. Muscle spasms can be caused by a lack of potassium or from a neurological injury that impairs muscle nerve innervation.

Muscle stiffness and spasm are assessed through observation of dysfunction, assessing a limited range of motion, and direct questioning of the client. Muscle spasm, like muscle stiffness, is assessed through direct observation of involuntary muscle contractions in activity and at rest, as well as direct questioning of the client.

Recreational therapists will most likely not score this code. Therapists document the specific impairment noted and the related cause, if known, as well as the extent of impairment that it causes with specific activities.

Muscle stiffness and spasms are treated according to the origin of the problem. This may include the use of pharmacology and exercise.

Muscle stiffness and spasms that are not able to be controlled can result in increased chances of injury or harm to the client, such as increased risk for falls. Precautions should be taken to reduce falls. The therapist should also provide adaptations for activities that are affected by impairments, such as adding extra time for stretching during the morning routine.

*Cross References*

In *Recreational Therapy for Specific Diagnoses and Conditions, First Edition*, ICF code b780 Sensations Related to Muscles and Movement Functions is listed in eight chapters: Amputation and Prosthesis, Back Disorders and Back Pain, Cerebrovascular Accident, Fibromyalgia and Juvenile Fibromyalgia, Parkinson's Disease, Rheumatoid Arthritis, Spinal Cord Injury, and Substance-Related Disorders.

In *Recreational Therapy Basics, Techniques, and Interventions, First Edition*, treatment for ICF code b780 Sensations Related to Muscles and Movement Functions is discussed in two chapters: Consequences of Inactivity and Aquatic Therapy.

## b789 Movement Functions, Other Specified and Unspecified

## b798 Neuromusculoskeletal and Movement-Related Functions, Other Specified

## b799 Neuromusculoskeletal and Movement-Related Functions, Unspecified

*References*

burlingame, j. (2001). *Idyll Arbor's therapy dictionary*, 2nd ed. Ravensdale, WA: Idyll Arbor, Inc.

Clark, R. A., Bryant, A. L., Pua, Y., McCrory, P., Bennell, K., & Hunt, M. (2010). Validity and reliability of the Nintendo Wii balance board for assessment of standing balance. *Gait and Posture, 31*, 307-310.

Goldberg, K. F., Green, B., Moore, J., Wyatt, M., Boulanger, L., Belnap, B., Harsch, P., & Donaldson, D. S. (2009). Integrated musculoskeletal rehabilitation care at a comprehensive combat and complex casualty care program. *Journal of Manipulative and Physiological Therapeutics, 32*(9), 781-791.

Kalverboer, A. F. & Gramsbergen, A. A. (2001). *Handbook of brain and behavior in human development*. New York: Springer.

Kaplan, M. S., McFarland, B. H., Huguet, N., & Newsom, J. T. (2007). Physical illness, functional limitations, and suicide risk: A population-based study. *American Journal of Orthopsychiatry, 77*(1), 56-60.

Kuster, M., Knauth, B., & Langhof, H. (2007). Effects of inpatient rehabilitation on the metabolic system and physical capacity of obese children and adolescents. *American Journal of Recreation Therapy, 1*, 40-48.

McColgin, C., Driver, S., & Goggin, N. (2009). Devising a balance program to reduce the risk of falls in older adults. *PALAESTRA, 24*(3), 38-42.

O'Sullivan, S. & Schmitz, T. (1988). *Physical rehabilitation: Assessment and treatment*. Philadelphia, PA: F. A. Davis Company.

Patla, A. (1997). Understanding the roles of vision in the control of human locomotion. *Gait and Posture, 5*, 54-69.

Piek, J. P. (2006). *Infant motor development, volume 10*. Champaign, IL: Human Kinetics.

Pramanik, D. (2007). *Principles of physiology*. New York: Academic Publishers.

Ricci, S. S. & Kyle, T. (2008). *Maternity and pediatric nursing*. Philadelphia, PA: Lippincott Williams & Wilkins

Rose, D. (2010) *FallProof! A Comprehensive Balance and Mobility Training Program* (2nd ed.). Champaign, IL: Human Kinetics.

Schlinger, H. D. (1995). *A behavior analytic view of child development*. New York: Springer.

Seidel, D., Brayne, C., & Jagger, C. (2011). Limitations in physical functioning among older people as a predictor of subsequent disability in instrumental activities of daily living. *Age and Ageing, 40*, 463-469.

von Bonsdorff, M. B. & Rantanen, T. (2011). Progression of functional limitations in relation to physical activity: A life course approach. *Eur Rev Aging Phys Act, 8*, 23-30.

# Chapter 8 Functions of the Skin and Related Structures

This chapter is about the functions of skin, nails, and hair.

*Sample Scoring for Functions of the Skin and Related Structures*

- An older adult has very thin skin which easily tears and bleeds (b810 Protective Functions of the Skin). This is of particular concern because the client is on blood thinners. Consequently, the recreational therapist pays careful attention to the safety needs of the client during activities to decrease bumps, scraps, and injury to her skin. Given the integrity of the skin, such precautions are followed at all times by all staff as this is a complete skin impairment (complete impairment = 4). The correct scoring would look like this: b810.4.
- A client undergoing drug and alcohol treatment complains that he feels the sensation of spiders crawling up and down his arms (b840 Sensation Related to the Skin) all day, every day (complete impairment = 4). The correct scoring would look like this: b840.4.

Recreational therapists understand the protective and restorative functions of the skin and related sensations as they pertain to skin care within real-life activity. This is particularly important because:

- Clients who have impaired sensation need to protect their skin. For example, a client with a complete spinal cord injury who loses sensation below the waist must be diligent in performing weight shifts, keeping skin clean and dry, and performing routine skin inspections to prevent decubitus ulcers from forming.
- Clients who have peripheral neuropathy from diabetes need to conduct daily inspections of the feet for development of ulcers.
- Clients who are taking blood-thinning medications require careful protection of the skin from injury because medication decreases clotting, therefore skin openings will continue to bleed rather than clot.
- Clients who are taking medications that increase the skin's sensitivity to light require more protection from sunlight than is normally required.
- Clients who have compromised immune systems need to prevent skin openings that provide an opportunity for bacteria to enter the bloodstream.
- Clients who have an infectious disease that can be spread via bodily fluids may put others at risk if the blood from a skin opening is touched by another person who also has a skin opening for the infected blood to enter.
- Clients who have skin damage may require special care in activities. For example, a client with severe burns needs to be protected from

activities that could cause physical contact and related pain. A client with an extremity amputation requires routine and diligent inspection of the skin on the stump during prosthetic training to assess the fit of the prosthetic, prosthetic tolerance, and skin tolerance to friction.

The skin and related structures, which includes hair and nails, impact both activity participation and quality of life. For example, a review of 31 studies found that pressure ulcers impact not only physical functioning. They also have an impact on social functioning, psychological health, general health, relationships, and finances (Gorecki et al., 2009). A literature review by Lemieux, Maunsell, and Provencher (2008) found that hair loss in women undergoing chemotherapy for breast cancer is distressing, traumatizing, can lead to refusal of chemotherapy, and can negatively affect body image.

Recreational therapists incorporate team-oriented treatment techniques into therapy sessions, such as increasing hand activity in sessions to decrease fingernail biting. They also plan and implement interventions in the context of leisure and community activities to maximize participation and prevent secondary complications. Examples include weight shifts during community activities and drying the skin thoroughly after swimming. Recreational therapists also address issues tied to skin and related structures. Examples include dealing with self-esteem issues related to hair loss, self-consciousness issues related to bloody nails that are repeatedly bitten too short, and incorporating weight shifts into activities so they don't disrupt social conversation.

### Assessment of Functions of the Skin and Related Structures

Some skin and related structure issues are typically present with specific disabilities, illnesses, and medications. Recreational therapists note these concerns. They also obtain information about the client's skin and related structures through a review of the medical chart, observation, and discussion. Issues and concerns are noted and incorporated appropriately into the client's treatment plan.

### Treatment of Functions of the Skin and Related Structures

Treatment of skin and related structures will vary depending on the specific issue. Clients who need to perform weight shifts are taught how to integrate weight shifts into real life activity. They are also taught reminder strategies, such as an alarm on their phone.

Clients are taught how to keep skin clean and dry during specific recreation and community activities to prevent skin breakdown, Some examples include thoroughly drying the residual limb after swimming before donning the prosthetic, keeping dry when propelling a wheelchair in the rain by using a poncho and clip on umbrella, performing routine skin inspections and taking added precautions to protect skin during recreation activities.

Recreational therapists also remind clients about choosing appropriate footwear related to recreation activities to prevent foot ulceration if the person has diabetes. The shoes should not put pressure on the foot, particular the toes and heel.

Recreational therapists take precautions if the person is prone to skin tears (fragile skin) or is at risk of bleeding due to blood thinning medications. This includes making sure that the skin is not subjected to any type of shearing, as from sliding across a bench, that work surfaces are smooth and free of sharp corners and edges, and that supplies and equipment do not pose risk of harm.

If an individual is sensitive to sunlight, the therapist employs precautionary measures, such as keeping the skin covered, walking in shaded areas, and applying sunscreen.

If a client has an infectious disease or a compromised immune system, precautions are taken to decrease risk of skin openings.

If the client has issues related to hair, such as loss of hair due to chemotherapy, thinning hair, or hair needing to be pinned up during sports, appropriate interventions are chosen. These may include teaching the client how to don a hair scarf, pull hair up in a rubber band, or tuck hair into a swim cap for sports participation.

In regards to nails, therapists teach client how to care for nails, such as filing and polishing, particularly when the activity is viewed as recreational. If a client has problems related to nails, such as excessive nail biting, the therapist assists the client in identifying triggers, such as stress, and seeks to reduce or minimize triggers. Other techniques include developing coping skills or applying aversive reminders, such as preventing nail biting by applying a bad-tasting product onto the fingernails.

### Evidence Review

Reviews of several studies are provided below to highlight evidence-based practice related to functions of the skin and related structures. This is only a sample of the evidence. A thorough review of the literature is needed to identify evidence-based practice interventions that reflect the needs and characteristics of a particular client.

Leite and Faro (2006) conducted a study of 35 adults who had paraplegia at the T6 level or below for one to three years. They found that pressure ulcers occurred less frequently among individuals with active leisure lifestyles. They concluded that leisure activities are significant in pressure ulcer prevention.

McCaffrey (2006) conducted an in-depth exploratory study that consisted of focus group discussions and individual interviews with children who had cancer, their parents, hospital professionals, and hospital teachers. Sixteen major stressors were identified by the children: hair loss, procedures, needles, nasogastric tubes, lumbar punctures, bone marrow tests, chemotherapy, loss of control, long hospital stays, relapses, fear of dying, other children dying, check-up results, cannot be with friends, and infections. The children also indicated that the major stressors had the following effects: lack of self-esteem, ignorance of others, cumulative drug effects, miserable, tired, sad, lethargic, depressed, more mature than friends, weight loss, lifelong maintenance, unable to do sports, no school — too sick, isolation, and hospital is a shock. Coping mechanisms for the children included watching television and movies, food from home, wearing a hat to cover hair loss, painting, listening to music, stories for entertainment, and massage. Stressors, effects of stressors, and coping mechanisms of parents and hospital professionals were also identified in the study.

Armstrong et al. (2007) conducted a randomized controlled trial of 225 adults with diabetes at high risk for ulceration. "Patients that ulcerated had a temperature difference that was 4.8 times greater at the site of ulceration in the week before ulceration" (p. 1042). Although this article did not discuss this, recreational therapists can teach clients with diabetes how to keep feet cooler to decrease risk of bacteria growth and foot ulcer development. For example, high periods of physical activity, high environmental temperatures, stress, anxiety, and sock or footwear choices can all contribute to increased foot temperature. Recreational therapists can provide education on how to reduce these risks and problem solve for high-heat situations in leisure and community activities such as choosing cotton socks, changing socks regularly, and airing out feet.

### Cross References

In *Recreational Therapy for Specific Diagnoses and Conditions, First Edition*, ICF code b8 Functions of the Skin and Related Structures and its subcategories are listed in seven chapters: Amputation and Prosthesis, Burns, Cerebral Palsy, Chronic Obstructive Pulmonary Disease, Guillain-Barré Syndrome, Multiple Sclerosis, and Parkinson's Disease.

In *Recreational Therapy Basics, Techniques, and Interventions, First Edition*, treatment for ICF code b8 Functions of the Skin and Related Structures and its subcategories are discussed in one chapter: Psychoneuroimmunology.

## Functions of the Skin (b810 - b849)

### b810 Protective Functions of the Skin

Functions of the skin for protecting the body from physical, chemical, and biological threats.

Inclusions: functions of protecting against the sun and other radiation, photosensitivity, pigmentation, quality of skin; insulting function of skin, callus formation, hardening; impairments such as broken skin, ulcers, bedsores, and thinning skin

Exclusions: repair functions of skin (b820); other functions of the skin (b830)

Recreational therapists are not likely to score b810 Protective Functions of the Skin. However, they do document specific skin problems, such as a decubitus ulcer on the buttock, the specific care that is required during activity, such as weight shifts every 20 minutes, the client's ability to perform and problem solve for such care, special precautions taken by the therapist to ensure skin protection and optimal conditions for skin repair, and coordination with other members of the healthcare team. For example "Client instructed on importance of thoroughly drying skin after swimming to prevent conditions that contribute to the development of decubitus ulcers. Client able to verbally repeat information independently, however was only 75% effective in drying skin completely after swimming due to limited mobility. Plan is to contact client's occupational therapist to problem solve for adaptive devices to maximize ability to dry skin thoroughly after swimming."

In addition to the issues discussed, therapists also document any noted skin changes and action taken. Some examples: "When changing in the pool locker room, therapist noted a 1" by 2" reddened area on client's left hip. Primary nurse notified." "When checking residual limb after walking, an abnormal reddened area was evident. For duration of community integration session, prosthetic was removed and wheelchair was utilized for mobility. Upon return, therapist notified nursing for skin care and physical therapy to reassess prosthetic fit and appropriateness of prosthetic adjustments."

Many diagnoses have specific skin care issues. Recreational therapists should be familiar with them.

### Cross References

In *Recreational Therapy for Specific Diagnoses and Conditions, First Edition*, ICF code b810 Protective Functions of the Skin is listed in four chapters: Chronic Obstructive Pulmonary Disease, Multiple Sclerosis, Pressure Ulcers, and Sickle Cell Disease.

In *Recreational Therapy Basics, Techniques, and Interventions, First Edition*, there are no references for ICF code b810 Protective Functions of the Skin.

### b820 Repair Functions of the Skin

Functions of the skin for repairing breaks and other damage to the skin.

Inclusions: functions of scab formation, healing, scarring; bruising and keloid formation

Exclusions: protective functions of the skin (b810); other functions of the skin (b830)

Recreational therapists are not likely to score b820 Repair Functions of the Skin. However, when there is an issue with this code, repair functions of the skin can be enhanced through therapeutic interventions, which recreational therapists carry over into their sessions. These interventions may include

- *Bandaging*: cover with gauze and medical tape.
- *Antibiotics*: topical, oral, or intravenous.
- *Protection*: Guard against agents that further injure the skin or diminish healing capacity. For example, remove pressure from the area of skin breakdown; avoid activities that could break fragile, healing skin.

Recreational therapists document the specific interventions they use to prevent further injury to compromised skin as well as promote the healing process. For example, if a client has an early stage decubitus ulcer on top of the left knee from crossing his legs, the therapist may document: "Client required minimal verbal cues to protect ulcer on top of left knee during activity."

### Cross References

In *Recreational Therapy for Specific Diagnoses and Conditions, First Edition*, ICF code b820 Repair Functions of the Skin is listed in four chapters: Cerebral Palsy, Chronic Obstructive Pulmonary Disease, Pressure Ulcers, and Sickle Cell Disease.

In *Recreational Therapy Basics, Techniques, and Interventions, First Edition*, there are no references for ICF code b820 Repair Functions of the Skin.

### b830 Other Functions of the Skin

Functions of the skin other than protection and repair, such as cooling and sweat secretion.

Inclusions: functions of sweating, glandular functions of the skin, and resulting body odor

Exclusions: protective functions of the skin (b810); repair functions of skin (b820)

Recreational therapists are not likely to score b830 Other Functions of the Skin. However, recreational therapists know about these functions and incorporate them into therapy sessions and documentation. For example, the skin functions as a cooling agent by sweating to decrease internal heat. Internal heat, however, may not always be fully released through sweating and can cause additional problems. Individuals who have complete spinal cord injuries do not sweat below the level of injury, therefore decreasing the efficiency of the skin to cool down the body. Excessive sweating, on the other hand, can cause social problems and body odor.

Recreational therapists are aware of the environment and activity as it relates to body temperature. Therapists problem solve to reduce the chances of heat stroke and closely monitor clients who are at a high risk for health issues related to heat. Depending on the intensity of the activity and the temperature of the day, the activity may be contraindicated for some.

Sweating can also cause problems because it creates a moist area. Skin breakdowns become more likely, transfers can be more difficult because of increased friction, and infection risk is increased because bacteria have a more hospitable area in which to grow. Precautions need to be taken to keep sensitive areas dry.

Recreational therapists document the specific actions taken to cool body temperature when appropriate to diagnosis. For example, "Therapist recommended that client carry a cool water bottle and washcloth in backpack to cool down body on hot days. Client demonstrated ability to independently plan for and use cooling agents when outdoors in the heat."

### Cross References

In *Recreational Therapy for Specific Diagnoses and Conditions, First Edition*, ICF code b830 Other Functions of the Skin is listed in two chapters: Pressure Ulcers and Sickle Cell Disease.

In *Recreational Therapy Basics, Techniques, and Interventions, First Edition*, there are no references for ICF code b830 Other Functions of the Skin.

### b840 Sensation Related to the Skin

Sensations related to the skin such as itching, burning sensation, and tingling.

Inclusions: impairments such as pins and needles sensation and crawling sensation

Exclusion: sensation of pain (b280)

Recreational therapists are not likely to score b840 Sensation Related to the Skin. However, recreational therapists know about such sensations and work with them in therapy sessions. Sensations of the skin such as pins and needles, crawling sensations, itching, burning, and tingling have different causes. The feeling of pins and needles is commonly felt when there is lack of blood flow to the area. Crawling sensations may be induced by drugs that cause hallucinations. Itching and burning can be caused by an irritant and tingling may be the result of nerve damage. The cause must first be identified to treat the problem. Specific diagnoses often have characteristic sensations.

In most cases, with the exception of nerve damage, odd sensations of the skin are short-lived and have simple cures. For example, the feeling of pins and needles can be halted by increasing blood flow to the area through repositioning and rubbing the affected area to promote blood flow. Itching and burning caused by an irritant can often be treated by using a topical medication to reduce the reaction and avoiding the irritant. Crawling sensations that are drug induced will commonly cease once the drug is no longer taken.

Sometimes adaptations need to be made for clients who are not able to monitor and act on their own. For example, a client may complain about pins and needles but lack the cognitive ability to understand that moving the affected area will help the situation. The recreational therapist should document the concern about restricted blood flow and be sure to add monitoring the client's position on a routine basis to the treatment plan. In cases where medications cause uncomfortable sensations that cannot be altered, the therapist may implement relaxation, mental imagery, or other techniques to help the client increase tolerance of sensations.

### Cross References

In *Recreational Therapy for Specific Diagnoses and Conditions, First Edition*, ICF code b840 Sensation Related to the Skin is listed in five chapters: Burns, Guillain-Barré Syndrome, Multiple Sclerosis, Pressure Ulcers, and Sickle Cell Disease.

In *Recreational Therapy Basics, Techniques, and Interventions, First Edition*, there are no references for ICF code b840 Sensation Related to the Skin.

### b849 Functions of the Skin, Other Specified and Unspecified

## Functions of the Hair and Nails (b850 - b869)

### b850 Functions of the Hair

Functions of the hair, such as protection, coloration, and appearance.

Inclusions: functions of growth of hair, pigmentation of hair, location of hair; impairments such as loss of hair or alopecia

Recreational therapists are not likely to score b850 Functions of the Hair. However, recreational therapists are aware of the functions of hair in activities and report on issues as they impact activity performance and participation. For example, clients who have hair loss may have lower self-esteem, confidence, and body image. Hair loss may require added head protection in sunny weather and in cold weather. Use of a wig may require the therapist to assist the client in problem solving for wig care in specific situations such as rain or physical activity.

Recreational therapists document the specific hair problem, the specific care that is required in activities, the client's ability to perform and problem solve for such care, and special precautions taken by the therapist to ensure protection and optimal conditions. For example, "Client instructed on importance of keeping head warm in cold weather. Client able to verbally repeat information independently and demonstrate ability to protect head in cold weather as observed during community integration training session." In addition to the issues discussed, therapists also document any noted hair changes and action taken, such as "When brushing hair prior to therapy session, excessive hair loss in brush was noted. Client reports that this is a new occurrence and is concerned. Nursing notified and informed client that hair loss is a side effect of XYZ medication."

### Cross References

In *Recreational Therapy for Specific Diagnoses and Conditions, First Edition*, there are no references for ICF code b850 Functions of the Hair.

In *Recreational Therapy Basics, Techniques, and Interventions, First Edition*, there are no references for ICF code b850 Functions of the Hair.

### b860 Functions of the Nails

Functions of the nails, such as protection, scratching, and appearance.

Inclusions: growth and pigmentation of nails, quality of nails

Recreational therapists are not likely to score b860 Functions of the Nails. However, recreational therapists are aware of functions of the nails in activities and report on issues as they impact activity performance and participation. For example, clients who have brittle nails may have changes in the structure of fingernails and toenails that lead to splitting. Other clients may have behaviors that impair the functions of the nails, such as biting the nails. Both may increase the risk of infection, so therapists are aware of thorough hand washing and protective measures, such as gloves, during activities. Irritating chemicals that could enter the skin should be avoided.

Nail funguses can cause concerns about appearance. They may also be somewhat contagious, so precautions may need to be taken. Systemic medicines used to treat nail fungus can have side effects that the therapist needs to be aware of.

Recreational therapists document the specific nail problem, the specific care that is required during activities, the client's ability to perform and problem solve for such care, and special precautions taken by the therapist to ensure protection and optimal conditions. In addition to the issues discussed, therapists also document any noted nail changes and action taken. For example, "Client's nails are now long enough to use for peeling an orange."

### Cross References

In *Recreational Therapy for Specific Diagnoses and Conditions, First Edition*, there are no references for ICF code b8560 Functions of the Nails.

In *Recreational Therapy Basics, Techniques, and Interventions, First Edition*, there are no references for ICF code b8560 Functions of the Nails.

### b869 Functions of the Hair and Nails, Other Specified and Unspecified

### b898 Functions of the Skin and Related Structures, Other Specified

### b899 Functions of the Skin and Related Structures, Unspecified

### References

Armstrong, D. G., Holtz-Neiderer, K., Wendel, C., Mohler, M. J., Kimbriel, H. R., & Lavery, L. (2007). Skin temperature monitoring reduces the risk for diabetic foot ulceration in high-risk patients. The *American Journal of Medicine, 120*(12), 1042-1046.

Gorecki, C., Brown, J. M., Nelson, E. A., Briggs, M., Schoonhoven, L., Dealey, C., Defloor, T., & Nixon, J. (2009). Impact of pressure ulcers on quality of life in older patients: A systematic review. *Journal of the American Geriatrics Society, 57*(7), 1175-1183.

Leite, V. B. E. & Faro, A. C. M. (2006). Identification of factors associated to pressure sores in paraplegic individuals and related to leisure activities. *ACTA FISIATR, 13*(1), 21-25.

Lemieux, J., Maunsell, E., & Provencher, L. (2008). Chemotherapy-induced alopecia and effects on quality of life among women with breast cancer: A literature review. *Psycho-Oncology, 17*(4), 317-332.

McCaffrey, C. N. (2006). Major stressors and their effects on the well-being of children with cancer. *Journal of Pediatric Nursing, 21*(1), 59-66.

# Body Structures

*Heather R. Porter*

Body Structures is a list of the anatomical parts of the body used to indicate the extent, nature, and location of an impairment. It is divided into eight chapters.

## Scoring

Recreational therapists usually will not score codes in this component. However, it is important for therapists to understand how to read the scoring of this component for interpretative purposes.

*Body structures* are anatomical parts of the body such as organs, limbs, and their components.

*Impairments* are problems in body functions or structures representing a significant deviation or loss.

To score a Body Structures impairment the therapist first identifies the appropriate code to score using the General Coding Guidelines shown below.

## General Coding Guidelines (WHO, 2001)

- Choose the appropriate codes that best reflect the body structure that is the purpose of the encounter.
- Only choose codes that are relevant to the context of the health condition. For example, if a person has impairments of the heart, but is being evaluated for neurological functioning, only neurological functioning should be coded.
- Do not make assumptions about a client's functioning based on a Body Structures impairment. Each function should be evaluated and scored separately. For example, a moderate structure impairment of the heart (s4100 Heart) does not mean there will be difficulty with b4550 General Physical Endurance.
- Only choose codes that reflect the specific predefined timeframe. Functions that relate to a timeframe outside of the predefined timeframe should not be coded.
- Use the most specific code whenever possible. For example, if a client has an impairment of the knee joint score the specific code of s75011 Knee Joint rather than the broad code of s7501 Structure of Lower Leg.

The code is written down in its entirety. This includes the letter and number (all Body Structures codes begin with the letter s). A decimal point is placed after the code. After the decimal point, the score for the first qualifier, second qualifier, and third qualifier are placed in this order. There are two recommended qualifiers and one suggested qualifier:

- Extent of Impairment (recommended)
- Nature of Impairment (recommended)
- Location of Impairment (suggested)

The scoring for the qualifiers is shown in Table 10.

## Table 10: Body Structures Qualifiers (WHO, 2001)

### Qualifier 1. Extent of Impairment

0: NO impairment, 0-4% (none, absent, negligible…)
1: MILD impairment, 5-24% (slight, low…)
2: MODERATE impairment, 25-49% (medium, fair…)
3: SEVERE impairment, 50-95% (high, extreme…)
4: COMPLETE impairment, 96-100% (total)
8: not specified
9: not applicable

### Qualifier 2. Nature of Impairment

0: no change in structure
1: total absence
2: partial absence
3: additional part
4: aberrant dimensions
5: discontinuity
6: deviating position
7: qualitative changes in structure, including accumulation of fluid
8: not specified
9: not applicable

### Qualifier 3. Location of Impairment

0: more than one region

1: right
2: left
3: both sides
4: front
5: back
6: proximal
7: distal
8: not specified

9: not applicable

*Example*: A client has a mild deviating position impairment of the right upper arm. The Body Structures code for upper arm is s7300 Structure of Upper Arm. The code appropriately written would look like this: s7300.161.

# Chapter 1 Structures of the Nervous System

In *Recreational Therapy for Specific Diagnoses and Conditions, First Edition*, ICF code s1 Structures of the Nervous System and its subcategories are listed in 13 chapters: Back Disorders and Back Pain, Borderline Personality Disorder, Cerebrovascular Accident, Epilepsy, Fibromyalgia and Juvenile Fibromyalgia, Guillain-Barré Syndrome, Hearing Loss, Multiple Sclerosis, Parkinson's Disease, Spina Bifida, Spinal Cord Injury, Substance-Related Disorders, and Traumatic Brain Injury.

In *Recreational Therapy Basics, Techniques, and Interventions, First Edition*, treatment for ICF code s1 Structures of the Nervous System and its subcategories are discussed in four chapters: Consequences of Inactivity, Parameters and Precautions, Psychoneuroimmunology, and Cognitive Retraining and Rehabilitation.

## s110 Structure of Brain

- *s1100 Structure of Cortical Lobes*
  - *s11000 Frontal Lobe*
  - *s11001 Temporal Lobe*
  - *s11002 Parietal Lobe*
  - *s11003 Occipital Lobe*
  - *s11008 Structure of Cortical Lobes, Other Specified*
  - *s11009 Structure of Cortical Lobes, Unspecified*
- *s1101 Structure of Midbrain*
- *s1102 Structure of Diencephalon*
- *s1103 Basal Ganglia and Related Structures*
- *s1104 Structure of Cerebellum*
- *s1105 Structure of Brain Stem*
  - *s11050 Medulla Oblongata*
  - *s11051 Pons*
  - *s11058 Structure of Brain Stem, Other Specified*
  - *s11059 Structure of Brain Stem, Unspecified*
- *s1106 Structure of Cranial Nerves*
- *s1108 Structure of Brain, Other Specified*
- *s1109 Structure of Brain, Unspecified*

In *Recreational Therapy for Specific Diagnoses and Conditions, First Edition*, ICF code s110 Structure of Brain is listed in eight chapters: Borderline Personality Disorder, Cerebrovascular Accident,

Epilepsy, Hearing Loss, Multiple Sclerosis, Parkinson's Disease, Substance-Related Disorders, and Traumatic Brain Injury.

In *Recreational Therapy Basics, Techniques, and Interventions, First Edition*, treatment for ICF code s110 Structure of Brain is discussed in two chapters: Parameters and Precautions and Cognitive Retraining and Rehabilitation.

## s120 Spinal Cord and Related Structures

- *s1200 Structure of Spinal Cord*
  - *s12000 Cervical Spinal Cord*
  - *s12001 Thoracic Spinal Cord*
  - *s12002 Lumbosacral Spinal Cord*
  - *s12003 Cauda Equina*
  - *s12008 Structure of Spinal Cord, Other Specified*
  - *s12009 Structure of Spinal Cored, Unspecified*
- *s1201 Spinal Nerves*
- *s1208 Spinal Cord and Related Structures, Other Specified*
- *s1209 Spinal Cord and Related Structure, Unspecified*

In *Recreational Therapy for Specific Diagnoses and Conditions, First Edition*, ICF code s120 Spinal Cord and Related Structures is listed in four chapters: Back Disorders and Back Pain, Guillain-Barré Syndrome, Multiple Sclerosis, and Spinal Cord Injury.

## s130 Structure of Meninges

## s140 Structure of Sympathetic Nervous System

## s150 Structure of Parasympathetic Nervous System

## s198 Structure of the Nervous System, Other Specified

## s199 Structure of the Nervous System, Unspecified

# Chapter 2 The Eye, Ear, and Related Structures

### s210 Structure of Eye Socket

### s220 Structure of Eyeball

- *s2200 Conjunctiva, Sclera, Choroid*
- *s2201 Cornea*
- *s2202 Iris*
- *s2203 Retina*
- *s2204 Lens of Eyeball*
- *s2205 Vitreous Body*
- *s2208 Structure of Eyeball, Other Specified*
- *s2209 Structure of Eyeball, Unspecified*

In *Recreational Therapy for Specific Diagnoses and Conditions, First Edition*, ICF code s220 Structure of Eyeball is listed in one chapter: Visual Impairments and Blindness.

### s230 Structures Around the Eye

- *s2300 Lachrymal Gland and Related Structures*
- *s2301 Eyelid*
- *s2302 Eyebrow*
- *s2303 External Ocular Muscles*
- *s2308 Structures Around Eye, Other Specified*
- *s2309 Structure Around Eye, Unspecified*

In *Recreational Therapy for Specific Diagnoses and Conditions, First Edition*, ICF code s230 Structures Around the Eye is listed in one chapter: Visual Impairments and Blindness.

### s240 Structure of External Ear

In *Recreational Therapy for Specific Diagnoses and Conditions, First Edition*, ICF code s240 Structure of External Ear is listed in one chapter: Hearing Loss.

### s250 Structure of Middle Ear

- *s2500 Tympanic Membrane*
- *s2501 Eustachian Canal*
- *s2502 Ossicles*
- *s2508 Structure of Middle Ear, Other Specified*
- *s2509 Structure of Middle Ear, Unspecified*

In *Recreational Therapy for Specific Diagnoses and Conditions, First Edition*, ICF code s250 Structure of Middle Ear is listed in one chapter: Hearing Loss.

### s260 Structure of Inner Ear

- *s2600 Cochlea*
- *s2601 Vestibular Labyrinth*
- *s2602 Semicircular Canals*
- *s2603 Internal Auditory Meatus*
- *s2608 Structure of Inner Ear, Other Specified*
- *s2609 Structure of Inner Ear, Unspecified*

In *Recreational Therapy for Specific Diagnoses and Conditions, First Edition*, ICF code s260 Structure of Inner Ear is listed in one chapter: Hearing Loss.

### s298 Eye, Ear, and Related Structures, Other Specified

### s299 Eye, Ear, and Related Structure, Unspecified

# Chapter 3 Structures Involved in Voice and Speech

## s310 Structure of Nose

- *s3100 External Nose*
- *s3101 Nasal Septum*
- *s3102 Nasal Fossae*
- *s3108 Structure of Nose, Other Specified*
- *s3109 Structure of Nose, Unspecified*

## s320 Structure of Mouth

- *s3200 Teeth*
- *s3201 Gums*
- *s3202 Structure of Palate*
  - *s32020 Hard Palate*
  - *s32021 Soft Palate*
- *s3203 Tongue*
- *s3204 Structure of Lips*
  - *s32040 Upper Lip*
  - *s32041 Lower Lip*
- *s3208 Structure of Mouth, Other Specified*
- *s3209 Structure of Mouth, Unspecified*

In *Recreational Therapy for Specific Diagnoses and Conditions, First Edition*, ICF code s320 Structure of Mouth is listed in two chapters: Diabetes Mellitus and Feeding and Eating Disorders.

## s330 Structure of Pharynx

- *s3300 Nasal Pharynx*
- *s3301 Oral Pharynx*
- *s3308 Structure of Pharynx, Other Specified*
- *s3309 Structure of Pharynx, Unspecified*

## s340 Structure of Larynx

- *s3400 Vocal Folds*
- *s3408 Structure of Larynx, Other Specified*
- *s3409 Structure of Larynx, Unspecified*

## s398 Structures Involved in Voice and Speech, Other Specified

## s399 Structures Involved in Voice and Speech, Unspecified

# Chapter 4 Structures of the Cardiovascular, Immunological, and Respiratory Systems

In *Recreational Therapy for Specific Diagnoses and Conditions, First Edition*, ICF code s4 Structures of the Cardiovascular, Immunological, and Respiratory Systems and its subcategories are listed in seven chapters: Amputation and Prosthesis, Chronic Obstructive Pulmonary Disease, Heart Disease, Obesity, Sickle Cell Disease, Spinal Cord Injury, and Substance-Related Disorders.

In *Recreational Therapy Basics, Techniques, and Interventions, First Edition*, treatment for ICF code s4 Structures of the Cardiovascular, Immunological, and Respiratory Systems and its subcategories are discussed in one chapter: Consequences of Inactivity.

## s410 Structure of Cardiovascular System

- *s4100 Heart*
  - o  *s41000 Atria*
  - o  *s41001 Ventricles*
  - o  *s41008 Structure of Heart, Other Specified*
  - o  *s41009 Structure of Heart, Unspecified*
- *s4101 Arteries*
- *s4102 Veins*
- *s4103 Capillaries*
- *s4108 Structures of Cardiovascular System, Other Specified*
- *s4109 Structures of Cardiovascular System, Unspecified*

In *Recreational Therapy for Specific Diagnoses and Conditions, First Edition*, ICF code s410 Structure of Cardiovascular System is listed in four chapters: Amputation and Prosthesis, Heart Disease, Obesity, and Sickle Cell Disease.

In *Recreational Therapy Basics, Techniques, and Interventions, First Edition*, treatment for ICF code s410 Structure of Cardiovascular System is discussed in one chapter: Consequences of Inactivity.

## s420 Structure of Immune System

- *s4200 Lymphatic Vessels*
- *s4201 Lymphatic Nodes*
- *s4202 Thymus*
- *s4203 Spleen*
- *s4204 Bone Marrow*
- *s4208 Structures of Immune System, Other Specified*
- *s4209 Structures of Immune System, Unspecified*

In *Recreational Therapy for Specific Diagnoses and Conditions, First Edition*, ICF code s420 Structure of Immune System is listed in one chapter: Amputation and Prosthesis.

## s430 Structure of Respiratory System

- *s4300 Trachea*
- *s4301 Lungs*
  - o  *s43010 Bronchial Tree*
  - o  *s43011 Alveoli*
  - o  *s43018 Structure of Lungs, Other Specified*
  - o  *s43019 Structure of Lungs, Unspecified*
- *s4302 Thoracic Cage*
- *s4303 Muscles of Respiration*
  - o  *s43030 Intercostal Muscles*
  - o  *s43031 Diaphragm*
  - o  *s43038 Muscles of Respiration, Other Specified*
  - o  *s43039 Muscles of Respiration, Unspecified*
- *s4308 Structure of Respiratory System, Other Specified*
- *s4309 Structure of Respiratory System, Unspecified*

In *Recreational Therapy for Specific Diagnoses and Conditions, First Edition*, ICF code s430 Structure of Respiratory System is listed in four chapters: Chronic Obstructive Pulmonary Disease, Obesity, Spinal Cord Injury, and Substance-Related Disorders.

In *Recreational Therapy Basics, Techniques, and Interventions, First Edition*, treatment for ICF code s430 Structure of Respiratory System is discussed in one chapter: Consequences of Inactivity.

**s498 Structures of the Cardiovascular, Immunological, and Respiratory Systems, Other Specified**

**s499 Structures of the Cardiovascular, Immunological, and Respiratory Systems, Unspecified**

# Chapter 5 Structures Related to the Digestive, Metabolic, and Endocrine Systems

In *Recreational Therapy for Specific Diagnoses and Conditions, First Edition*, ICF code s5 Structures Related to the Digestive, Metabolic, and Endocrine Systems and its subcategories are listed in two chapters: Feeding and Eating Disorders and Substance-Related Disorders.

## s510 Structure of Salivary Glands

## s520 Structure of Esophagus

## s530 Structure of Stomach

## s540 Structure of Intestine

- s5400 Small Intestine
- s5401 Large Intestine
- s5408 Structure of Intestine, Other Specified
- s5409 Structure of Intestine, Unspecified

## s550 Structure of Pancreas

## s560 Structure of Liver

In *Recreational Therapy for Specific Diagnoses and Conditions, First Edition*, ICF code s560

Structure of Liver is listed in one chapter: Substance-Related Disorders.

## s570 Structure of Gall Bladder and Ducts

## s580 Structure of Endocrine Glands

- s5800 Pituitary Gland
- s5801 Thyroid Gland
- s5802 Parathyroid Gland
- s5803 Adrenal Gland
- s5808 Structure of Endocrine Glands, Other Specified
- s5809 Structure of Endocrine Glands, Unspecified

## s598 Structures Related to the Digestive, Metabolic, and Endocrine Systems, Other Specified

## s599 Structures Related to the Digestive, Metabolic, and Endocrine Systems, Unspecified

# Chapter 6 Structures Related to the Genitourinary and Reproductive Systems

## s610 Structure of Urinary System

- s6100 Kidney
- s6101 Ureters
- s6102 Urinary Bladder
- s6103 Urethra
- s6108 Structure of Urinary System, Other Specified
- s6109 Structure of Urinary System, Unspecified

## s620 Structure of Pelvic Floor

## s630 Structure of Reproductive System

- s6300 Ovaries
- s6301 Structure of Uterus
  - s63010 Body of Uterus
  - s63011 Cervix
  - s63012 Fallopian Tubes
  - s63018 Structure of Uterus, Other Specified
  - s63019 Structure of Uterus, Unspecified
- s6302 Breast and Nipple
- s6303 Structure of Vagina and External Genitalia
  - s63030 Clitoris
  - s63031 Labia Majora
  - s63032 Labia Minora
  - s63033 Vaginal Canal
- s6304 Testes
- s6305 Structure of the Penis
  - s63050 Glans Penis
  - s63051 Shaft of Penis
  - s63058 Structure of Penis, Other Specified
  - s63059 Structure of Penis, Unspecified
- s6306 Prostate
- s6308 Structures of Reproductive Systems, Other Specified
- s6309 Structures of Reproductive Systems, Unspecified

## s698 Structures Related to the Genitourinary and Reproductive Systems, Other Specified

## s699 Structures Related to the Genitourinary and Reproductive Systems, Unspecified

# Chapter 7 Structures Related to Movement

In *Recreational Therapy for Specific Diagnoses and Conditions, First Edition*, ICF code s7 Structures Related to Movement and its subcategories are listed in 14 chapters: Back Disorders and Back Pain, Burns, Chronic Obstructive Pulmonary Disease, Feeding and Eating Disorders, Hearing Loss, Multiple Sclerosis, Obesity, Osteoarthritis, Osteoporosis, Rheumatoid Arthritis, Sickle Cell Disease, Spina Bifida, Spinal Cord Injury, and Total Joint Replacement.

In *Recreational Therapy Basics, Techniques, and Interventions, First Edition*, treatment for ICF code s7 Structures Related to Movement and its subcategories are discussed in four chapters: Activity and Task Analysis, Body Mechanics and Ergonomics, Consequences of Inactivity, and Parameters and Precautions.

## s710 Structure of Head and Neck Region

- *s7100 Bones of Cranium*
- *s7101 Bones of Face*
- *s7102 Bones of Neck Region*
- *s7103 Joints of Head and Neck Region*
- *s7104 Muscles of Head and Neck Region*
- *s7105 Ligaments and Fasciae of Head and Neck Region*
- *s7108 Structures of Head and Neck Region, Other Specified*
- *s7109 Structure of Head and Neck Region, Unspecified*

In *Recreational Therapy for Specific Diagnoses and Conditions, First Edition*, ICF code s710 Structure of Head and Neck Region is listed in three chapters: Hearing Loss, Rheumatoid Arthritis, and Spinal Cord Injury.

## s720 Structure of Shoulder Region

- *s7200 Bones of Shoulder Region*
- *s7201 Joints of Shoulder Region*
- *s7202 Muscles of Shoulder Region*
- *s7203 Ligaments and Fasciae of Shoulder Region*
- *s7208 Structure of Shoulder Region, Other Specified*
- *s7209 Structure of Shoulder Region, Unspecified*

In *Recreational Therapy for Specific Diagnoses and Conditions, First Edition*, ICF code s720 Structure of Shoulder Region is listed in one chapter: Rheumatoid Arthritis.

## s730 Structure of Upper Extremity

- *s7300 Structure of Upper Arm*
  - o *s73000 Bones of Upper Arm*
  - o *s73001 Elbow Joint*
  - o *s73002 Muscles of Upper Arm*
  - o *s73003 Ligaments and Fasciae of Upper Arm*
  - o *s73008 Structure of Upper Arm, Other Specified*
  - o *s73009 Structure of Upper Arm, Unspecified*
- *s7301 Structure of Forearm*
  - o *s73010 Bones of Forearm*
  - o *s73011 Wrist Joint*
  - o *s73012 Muscles of Forearm*
  - o *s73013 Ligaments and Fasciae of Forearm*
  - o *s73018 Structure of Forearm, Other Specified*
  - o *s73019 Structure of Forearm, Unspecified*
- *s7302 Structure of Hand*
  - o *s73020 Bones of Hand*
  - o *s73021 Joints of Hand and Fingers*
  - o *s73022 Muscles of Hand*
  - o *s73023 Ligaments and Fasciae of Hand*
  - o *s73028 Structure of Hand, Other Specified*
  - o *s73029 Structure of Hand, Unspecified*
- *s7308 Structure of Upper Extremity, Other Specified*
- *s7309 Structure of Upper Extremity, Unspecified*

In *Recreational Therapy for Specific Diagnoses and Conditions, First Edition*, ICF code s730 Structure of Upper Extremity is listed in two chapters: Osteoarthritis and Rheumatoid Arthritis.

In *Recreational Therapy Basics, Techniques, and Interventions, First Edition*, treatment for ICF code s730 Structure of Upper Extremity is discussed in one chapter: Activity and Task Analysis.

## s740 Structure of Pelvic Region

- *s7400 Bones of Pelvic Region*
- *s7401 Joints of Pelvic Region*
- *s7402 Muscles of Pelvic Region*
- *s7403 Ligaments and Fasciae of Pelvic Region*

- *s7408 Structure of Pelvic Region, Other Specified*
- *s7409 Structure of Pelvic Region, Unspecified*

In *Recreational Therapy Basics, Techniques, and Interventions, First Edition*, treatment for ICF code s740 Structure of Pelvic Region is discussed in one chapter: Parameters and Precautions.

## s750 Structure of Lower Extremity

- *s7500 Structure of Thigh*
  - o *s75000 Bones of Thigh*
  - o *s75001 Hip Joint*
  - o *s75002 Muscles of Thigh*
  - o *s75003 Ligaments and Fasciae of Thigh*
  - o *s75008 Structure of Thigh, Other Specified*
  - o *s75009 Structure of Thigh, Unspecified*
- *s7501 Structure of Lower Leg*
  - o *s75010 Bones of Lower Leg*
  - o *s75011 Knee Joint*
  - o *s75012 Muscles of Lower Leg*
  - o *s75013 Ligaments and Fasciae of Lower Leg*
  - o *s75018 Structure of Lower Leg, Other Specified*
  - o *s75019 Structure of Lower Leg, Unspecified*
- *s7502 Structure of Ankle and Foot*
  - o *s75020 Bones of Ankle and Foot*
  - o *s75021 Ankle Joint and Joints of Foot and Toes*
  - o *s75022 Muscles of Ankle and Foot*
  - o *s75023 Ligaments and Fascia of Ankle and Foot*
  - o *s75028 Structure of Ankle and Foot, Other Specified*
  - o *s75029 Structure of Ankle and Foot, Unspecified*
- *s7508 Structure of Lower Extremity, Other Specified*
- *s7509 Structure of Lower Extremity, Unspecified*

In *Recreational Therapy for Specific Diagnoses and Conditions, First Edition*, ICF code s750 Structure of Lower Extremity is listed in five chapters: Multiple Sclerosis, Osteoarthritis, Osteoporosis, Rheumatoid Arthritis, and Total Joint Replacement.

In *Recreational Therapy Basics, Techniques, and Interventions, First Edition*, treatment for ICF code s750 Structure of Lower Extremity is discussed in one chapter: Parameters and Precautions.

## s760 Structure of Trunk

- *s7600 Structure of Vertebral Column*
  - o *s76000 Cervical Vertebral Column*
  - o *s76001 Thoracic Vertebral Column*
  - o *s76002 Lumbar Vertebral Column*
  - o *s76003 Sacral Vertebral Column*
  - o *s76004 Coccyx*
  - o *s76008 Structure of Vertebral Column, Other Specified*
  - o *s76009 Structure of Vertebral Column, Unspecified*
- *s7601 Muscles of Trunk*
- *s7602 Ligaments and Fasciae of Trunk*
- *s7608 Structure of Trunk, Other Specified*
- *s7609 Structure of Trunk, Unspecified*

In *Recreational Therapy for Specific Diagnoses and Conditions, First Edition*, ICF code s760 Structure of Trunk is listed in five chapters: Back Disorders and Back Pain, Multiple Sclerosis, Osteoporosis, Sickle Cell Disease, and Spina Bifida.

In *Recreational Therapy Basics, Techniques, and Interventions, First Edition*, treatment for ICF code s760 Structure of Trunk is discussed in one chapter: Parameters and Precautions.

## s770 Additional Musculoskeletal Structures Related to Movement

- *s7700 Bones*
- *s7701 Joints*
- *s7702 Muscles*
- *s7703 Extra-articular Ligaments, Fasciae, Extramuscular Aponeuroses, Retinacula, Septa, Bursae, Unspecified*
- *s7708 Additional Musculoskeletal Structures Related to Movement, Other Specified*
- *s7709 Additional Musculoskeletal Structures Related to Movement, Unspecified*

In *Recreational Therapy for Specific Diagnoses and Conditions, First Edition*, ICF code s770 Additional Musculoskeletal Structures Related to Movement is listed in two chapters: Back Disorders and Back Pain and Osteoarthritis.

## s798 Structures Related to Movement, Other Specified

## s799 Structures Related to Movement, Unspecified

# Chapter 8 Skin and Related Structures

In *Recreational Therapy for Specific Diagnoses and Conditions, First Edition*, ICF code s8 Skin and Related Structures and its subcategories are listed in four chapters: Amputation and Prosthesis, Burns, Parkinson's Disease, and Pressure Ulcers.

## s810 Structure of Areas of Skin

- s8100 Skin of Head and Neck Region
- s8101 Skin of the Shoulder Region
- s8102 Skin of Upper Extremity
- s8103 Skin of Pelvic Region
- s8104 Skin of Lower Extremity
- s8105 Skin of Trunk and Back
- s8108 Structure of Areas of Skin, Other Specified
- s8109 Structure of Areas of Skin, Unspecified

In *Recreational Therapy for Specific Diagnoses and Conditions, First Edition*, ICF code s810 Structure of Areas of Skin is listed in three chapters: Burns, Parkinson's Disease, and Pressure Ulcers.

## s820 Structure of Skin Glands

- s8200 Sweat Glands
- s8201 Sebaceous Glands
- s8208 Structure of Skin Glands, Other Specified
- s8209 Structure of Skin Glands, Unspecified

## s830 Structure of Nails

- s8300 Finger Nails
- s8301 Toe Nails
- s8308 Structure of Nails, Other Specified
- s8309 Structure of Nails, Unspecified

## s840 Structure of Hair

## s898 Skin and Related Structures, Other Specified

## s899 Skin and Related Structures, Unspecified

# Activities and Participation

*Heather R. Porter*

Activities and Participation contain some of the most important codes for recreational therapy practice. Included in this section are the activities of learning, performing tasks, communication, mobility, self-care, interpersonal interactions, major life areas, and community and social life. Everything we *do* as humans is included here. It is divided into nine chapters.

## Relationship between Activities and Participation and Other ICF Sections

When problems are seen in a client's ability to do activities or participate in the community, the problems can usually be traced to an impaired body function or body structure deficit. Determining treatment requires understanding the underlying cause of the problem. What recreational therapists see in their practice is a deficit at the activities and participation level. What they need to do to treat the problem is to find the underlying problem in body function or body structure.

A body function is a skill or ability to carry out a defined task or action. In some cases the client will be able to consciously modify performance, while in other cases the client will be unable to do so. Some examples of the types of body functions listed by the World Health Organization include b1400 Sustaining Attention, b4101 Heart Rhythm, and b3302 Speed of Speech.

Some tasks cannot be performed because the body structure required to perform the task is no longer functioning. Some of the structures include s1200 Structure of Spinal Cord and s740 Structure of Pelvic Region.

To understand how the codes interact, let's consider a client who has a problem with balance while bowling. One body structure code to check is the s2601 Vestibular Labyrinth in the inner ear. The Body Functions code is b2351 Vestibular Function of Balance. If either of these codes shows a deficit, the client will probably have trouble with balance. Treatment in this case would most likely consist of finding adaptations that allow the client to continue bowling using codes in Environmental Factors e1 Products and Technology.

However, there are other possibilities. One of the most important is that the client may not be strong enough to handle the weight of a bowling ball. One of the b730 Muscle Power Functions may be the problem. (There are many other possibilities.)

The therapist's responsibility is to document more than the problem with bowling. The therapist and the rest of the treatment team should find the appropriate codes to document the observation at the body function and/or body structure level. In this example, documenting the weakness of the client will allow the therapist to carry out appropriate treatment with the goal of making the client strong enough to bowl.

All the parts of the ICF tie together to create a picture of the whole person. It is important to code appropriately in all sections of the codes to be sure the picture is accurate.

## Scoring

Recreational therapists score Activities and Participation (A&P) codes in many practice settings.

*Activity* is the execution of a task or action by a client.

*Activity limitations* are difficulties a client may have in executing activities.

*Capacity* is a client's ability to execute an activity in a standardized testing environment, such as the therapy gym or clinic.

*Participation* is involvement in a life situation.

*Participation restrictions* are problems a client may experience with involvement in life situations.

*Performance* is a client's ability to participate in a life situation. These include activities in the client's real-life environment, such as a client's neighborhood, church, grocery store, senior center, or home.

*Assistance* is the use of assistive devices or personal assistance. Personal assistance includes both hands-on assistance, such as providing moderate assistance for a transfer, and non-hands-on assistance, such as cueing and emotional support.

*Environmental factors (EF)* make up the physical, social, and attitudinal environment in which people live. Environmental factors (referred to as e-codes) are a separate component of the ICF discussed in the next section of the book. These e-codes will commonly be attached to A&P codes, as shown in some of the A&P examples.

To score an A&P difficulty the therapist first identifies the appropriate code to score using the General Coding Guidelines shown below.

The code is written down in its entirety. This includes the letter and number (all A&P codes begin with the letter d). A decimal point is placed after the code. After the decimal point there are four qualifiers and an additional fifth qualifier that is still in development.

## General Coding Guidelines (WHO, 2001)

- Choose the appropriate codes that best reflect the client's functioning as it relates to the purpose of the encounter.
- Only choose codes that are relevant to the context of the health condition. For example, if a person has difficulty with d6500 Making and Repairing Clothes, but is being evaluated for community mobility (d460 Moving Around in Different Locations) only mobility functioning should be coded.
- Do not make inferences about a client's functioning in other areas based on an A&P difficulty. Each function should be evaluated and then scored separately. For example, just because a person has a moderate difficulty with d450 Walking it does not mean that the client will have difficulty with d460 Moving Around in Different Locations.
- Only choose codes that reflect the specific predefined timeframe. Functions that relate to a timeframe outside of the predefined timeframe should not be coded.
- Use the most specific code whenever possible. For example, if a client has difficulty with manipulating small game pieces, score the specific code of d4402 Manipulating rather than the broader code of d440 Fine Hand Use.

## Table 11: Activities and Participation Qualifiers (WHO, 2001)

### All Qualifiers

0: NO difficulty, 0-4% (none, absent, negligible…)
1: MILD difficulty, 5-24% (slight, low…)
2: MODERATE difficulty, 25-49% (medium, fair…)
3: SEVERE difficulty, 50-95% (high, extreme…)
4: COMPLETE difficulty, 96-100% (total)
8: not specified
9: not applicable

The scoring for A&P is shown in Table 11. There are four qualifiers. The first and second qualifiers are required. The third and fourth qualifiers are optional.

- 1st Qualifier (required): Performance (with assistance)
- 2nd Qualifier (required): Capacity (without assistance)
- 3rd Qualifier (optional): Capacity (with assistance)
- 4th Qualifier (optional): Performance (without assistance)

Example: A six-year-old client named Sarah is admitted to an inpatient physical rehabilitation center. Her shyness in peer group play in the hospital playroom causes her severe difficulty with engagement in play. When the therapist (e355 Health Professionals) provides encouraging words and gently guides her into group play activities, her level of difficulty with engagement decreases to mild difficulty. The therapist conducts a home visit and asks her mother to invite two of Sarah's friends to the home. While at home, Sarah requires minimal verbal cues from her mother (e310 Immediate Family) to engage in play with her friends. With this prompting Sarah initiates and engages in play without any difficulty. The A&P code for play is d9200 Play. The code appropriately written using all four qualifiers and related e-codes would look like this: d9200.0 3 1 1 e355+2, e310+1. Scoring A&P qualifiers can be complex. The rest of the introduction will continue this example to show how the values for these qualifiers were assigned.

### First Qualifier (required)

The first qualifier (performance with assistance) indicates the client's level of difficulty participating in a life situation with all usual and realistic supports (facilitators) and constraints (barriers).

*Example*: The real-life setting is the client's home. The usual and realistic facilitator is the mother's prompting. Since Sarah plays with no problems when the mother's prompting is available, she scores a 0 for no difficulty. Although she requires some assistance from her mother, the mother's assistance is usual and realistic. When this assistance is provided, there is no residual difficulty. The score would be written out like this: d9200.0 _ _ _.

### Meaning of the Score

Level of difficulty with participation in a life situation with usual and realistic assistance. This score tells us how much help the client needs to do this activity in real life with the usual and realistic supports in place.

### Key points

*Exclude any assistance offered by the therapist*: Assistance provided by the therapist is not a usual and realistic facilitator in a client's life because the therapist will not be part of the client's life after discharge. Only facilitators and barriers that are in the client's usual real-life situation are considered. This does not mean that the therapist cannot offer assistance in a real-life setting if it is needed, but the therapist must exclude his/her assistance from the total picture to arrive at an appropriate score for the first qualifier. For example, if the therapist was providing the prompting for Sarah to engage in play instead of her mother, the first qualifier would be scored a 1 for mild difficulty because in a real-life setting (when the therapist is not there), Sarah would have mild difficulty engaging in play.

*Only score residual difficulty*: When assistance is provided, the therapist scores the amount of residual or unattended difficulty. This is the difficulty that is left over after counting in the usual assistance. So, if a client has moderate difficulty participating in a life situation and the client's spouse provides assistance to the client so that no difficulty remains, the client would be scored as having no difficulty. If a spouse provides a client with assistance but the client still struggles with the task by continuing to exhibit mild difficulty with the task despite the assistance, the client would be scored as having mild difficulty. This is a very different way of thinking for therapists. Basically, it challenges health professionals to say, "It

doesn't matter if the client needs minimal assistance to engage in play, her mom provides the prompting that she needs. There is no difficulty here." As health professionals we have been trained to see any deviation from independence as a problem. The ICF design reflects the true disability movement. If there are things in our environments that make up for our limitations, and we all have limitations of one kind or another, we should not be labeled as deficient.

*Score the average or the highest level of difficulty*: The first qualifier is supposed to represent the client's level of functioning in his/her real-life setting when an average number of barriers and facilitators are present. This level of functioning can be very difficult to obtain. Recreational therapists who work in rehabilitation settings may only have the opportunity to do integration training one or two times with a client before s/he is discharged, making it difficult to get a true gauge of the average number of barriers and facilitators present in a specific life situation. For example, all of the barriers or facilitators may not be present or the average may be misrepresented, leading the therapist to an invalid score. Another problem is that life situations are always changing. For example, in one moment a family can be very supportive and helpful and in another moment an argument can break out causing the family to withdraw from the client and refuse to offer assistance. Consequently, the score assigned should try to reflect the average based on the therapist's best clinical judgment. If the average level is difficult to obtain, the average does not accurately depict what happens most of the time, or the therapist has not had enough interaction with the client to calculate an average, the therapist may use the score that denotes the highest level of difficulty. In some cases, the therapist may assign a score that reflects the presence of the highest barriers and lowest facilitators, to denote the worst-case scenario. The goal is to assign an accurate score that will lead to the best results for the client.

*When to score this qualifier*: It is unlikely that a therapist working in inpatient rehabilitation or acute care will have enough information on admission to score this qualifier. Therapists usually do not use integration training until later in the client's stay when s/he is medically stable. While it is possible to use the available information and clinical judgment to estimate the client's anticipated level of difficulty with a specific life situation, it is usually better to leave the qualifier blank until a more accurate score can be given. Do not use the score 8 (not specified) or 9 (not applicable). A blank space indicates that the qualifier is not being used. If this is a readmission for the same diagnosis with no significant change in the client's condition, then the therapist will be able to score this qualifier fairly accurately using information from the client and other sources. When integration training is started or more real-life situations are encountered later in the client's stay, the therapist will be able to score this qualifier much more accurately.

### Second Qualifier (required)

The second qualifier (capacity without assistance) indicates the client's level of difficulty with an activity in a standardized testing environment without any assistance from a person or device.

*Example*: The standard environment is the hospital playroom where children play on their own. When assistance is not provided, Sarah has severe difficulty engaging in play. She chooses to withdraw from the activity area more than 50% of the time. This equates to severe difficulty, as shown in Table 11, and is scored as a 3. The score for d9200 Play, including the first two qualifiers, would be written out like this: d9200.0 3 _ _.

### Meaning of the Score

Level of difficulty with an activity in a standard environment without assistance from a person or device. This score tells us the client's baseline of functioning in a standardized testing environment when no assistance is being given. Baseline data is used to set treatment goals and objectives and measure progress.

### Key points

*Provide assistance if unsafe or unethical*: Clients are never asked to perform a task or action that has the potential to cause the client harm. If it is unethical or unsafe to withhold personal assistance or a device, the therapist uses professional judgment through informal and formal assessment tools to arrive at an anticipated level of difficulty that would be present if the assistance or device was not provided.

*Score the average or highest level of difficulty*: As with the first qualifier, a client's level of difficulty with an activity can vary due to many variables, such as mood, motivation, and time of day. Therapists

choose the average difficulty level from all of those observed for the activity. If the average level is difficult to obtain, the average does not accurately depict what happens most of the time, or the therapist has not had enough interaction with the client to calculate an average, the therapist may use the score that denotes the highest level of difficulty.

*How to assess baseline functioning*: Therapists assess this function by providing the client with a task or requesting an action in a standardized testing environment and assessing the client's response. Some examples: "Can you please read this to me?" "Do you remember my name?" "Can you raise your arm over your head?" It can be difficult to obtain a true baseline, even in a standardized testing environment. The culprits that affect the baseline are mostly related to the client and the environment. A client's level of functioning can vary from day to day, with the time of day, and because of who is around. Likewise, the therapy clinic may be quiet in the morning and noisy in the afternoon. Consequently, the score that the therapist assigns should try to best reflect the average.

### Third Qualifier (optional)

The third qualifier (capacity with assistance) indicates the client's level of difficulty with a task or action in a standardized testing environment with the assistance of a person or device.

*Example*: The standardized testing environment is the hospital playroom. When assistance is provided by the therapist, Sarah has mild difficulty engaging in play. With the therapist helping her get started in activities, she is able to continue playing more than 75% of the time, so she would score a 2 for moderate difficulty. The score for d9200 Play, including the first three qualifiers, would be written out like this: d9200.0 3 2 _.

### Meaning of the Score

Level of difficulty with an activity in a standardized testing environment with assistance from a person or device. This score tells us how much difficulty a client has with an activity in a standardized testing environment when help from a person or device is provided. This represents the client's optimal level of functioning in the standardized testing environment, in this example, the hospital.

## Key points

*Only score residual difficulty*: When assistance is provided, the therapist scores the amount of residual or unattended difficulty. This is the difficulty that is left over after counting in the assistance provided in the standardized testing environment. So, if a client has moderate difficulty participating in a task and the therapist provides assistance to the client so that no difficulty remains, the client would be scored as having no difficulty. If a therapist provides a client with assistance but the client continues to exhibit mild difficulty with the task despite the assistance, the client would be scored as having mild difficulty. This is a very different way of thinking for therapists. Therapists usually score the level of assistance that the client requires. Here the therapist scores only the level of difficulty that remains outside of the assistance provided. The reasoning is the same as the first qualifier. If there are things in our usual or clinical environments that make up for our limitations, we should not be labeled as deficient.

*Score the average or the highest level of difficulty*: Like the second qualifier, it can be difficult to get a true score due to the many variables that can affect a client's level of functioning within a standardized testing environment. Consequently, the score that the therapist assigns should try to best reflect the average. If the average level is difficult to obtain, the average does not accurately depict what happens most of the time, or the therapist has not had enough interaction with the client to calculate an average, the therapist may use the score that denotes the highest level of difficulty.

### Fourth Qualifier (optional but highly recommended)

The fourth qualifier (performance without assistance) indicates the client's level of difficulty participating in a life situation without assistance from another person or the use of a device with consideration of environmental factors (and personal factors, although not recorded in the ICF) that could influence the client's performance.

*Example*: The real-life setting is the client's home. The usual and realistic facilitator is the mother's prompting. If this assistance from the mother's prompting is taken away, Sarah would have mild difficulty engaging in play in her real-life environment. The mother has observed that Sarah will leave her friends about 10% of the time because

of frustration with not being able to do something, so she would have a score of 1 for mild difficulty. The score for d9200 Play, with all of the qualifiers, would be written out like this: d9200.0 3 1 1.

### Meaning of the Score

Level of difficulty that a client has participating in a life situation without assistance. This score tells us the worst-case scenario: If the client is participating in this specific activity in his/her real-life environment and s/he has no assistance from a person or a device, which is possible at any time, this is how much difficulty the client would have with the activity.

When compared to the first qualifier (performance), it highlights the effect of environmental factors on the client's level of difficulty in a life situation. The question is, what is it specifically that causes this difference? If we can identify the causes, then there is a chance that we can improve the situation by encouraging continuation of positive influences (facilitators) and eliminating or reducing negative influences (barriers). The facilitators and barriers are shown with Environmental Factors. Although there are several ways to list Environmental Factors, the most effective way is to attach them to A&P codes to highlight variables that are affecting a client's level of difficulty. See the Environmental Factors chapter for more information about this.

In the ICF, this qualifier is identified as being optional. Only the first two qualifiers are required. We strongly suggest that therapists complete the fourth qualifier whenever possible for the following reasons:

*Better reflection of true performance*: The first qualifier (performance with assistance) reflects the norm and the fourth qualifier (performance without assistance) reflects the worst-case scenario. As therapists, we understand that situations can change quickly and the client needs to be prepared to deal with challenges. There will be times when things go better than the norm and other times when things go worse. For planning purposes, it is important to know how much worse the situation can get.

*Performance without assistance is not clearly deduced*: When looking at just the first qualifier, it can be unclear in some cases how much difficulty the client would have participating in life situations if assistance was taken away, especially if Environmental Factor codes are not attached to the A&P

code. For example, the first qualifier may reflect that the client has no difficulty with d630 Preparing Meals in a life situation with usual and realistic supports and constraints. This is misleading to the reader because it doesn't disclose the reason she has no difficulty in preparing meals is because her sister (e310 Immediate Family) helps her with 75% of the work. Now, if an Environmental Factor code (e-code) was attached to the A&P code to reflect the help from the sister and it was rated a substantial facilitator (d630.0 _ _ _ e310+3), the reader could see that if the facilitator was taken away, the client would have severe difficulty with the task of d630 Preparing Meals. The first qualifier 0 would become a 3 without the sister's help. So, e-codes help. But even if e-codes are attached to A&P codes, the reader may still not be able to get a clear picture of the worst-case scenario if the assistance is not provided. Health professionals may not attach all of the appropriate e-codes. There may be so many e-codes that the reader can't figure out what the client's level of difficulty would be if the assistance was not provided. A client's participation in real-life situations is a strong focus of recreational therapy practice. By scoring the fourth qualifier we can provide more accurate levels of real-life functioning.

*Promotes attention to environmental factors*: When we can easily see the difference in functioning between the first and fourth qualifier, it highlights the importance of environmental factors that are causing the difference. Disparities get attention. The more disparities that are reflected between the first and fourth qualifier, the more attention it can bring to reviewers of the importance of encouraging and promoting facilitators and eliminating or reducing barriers that are outside of the immediate person. Changes in the environment can play a large role in making changes in health.

### Key points

*Exclude assistance from all sources*: When determining the score for this qualifier, the therapist uses clinical judgment (in most cases) to determine the level of difficulty that a client would have participating in a specific life situation without assistance from a person or device. This includes assistance not only from the therapist, but also from any other person who would help the client with participation in the specific life situation including other healthcare professionals, family, and friends.

*Provide assistance if unsafe or unethical*: Like the second qualifier, clients are never asked to participate in a life situation that has the potential to cause the client harm. In this case, the therapist would use professional judgment through informal and formal assessment tools to arrive at an anticipated level of difficulty if the assistance or device was not provided.

*Score the average or highest level of difficulty*: Like the previous qualifiers, identifying a true score is almost impossible because of the constant fluctuation of internal and external variables that can affect a client's level of functioning. Consequently, the score that the therapist assigns should reflect the average. Like the first qualifier, it can be difficult for recreational therapists who work in a rehabilitation setting to identify an accurate score for this qualifier due to the often-limited number of integration training sessions with clients. If the average level is difficult to obtain, the average does not accurately depict what happens most of the time, or the therapist has not had enough interaction with the client to calculate an average, the therapist may use the score that reflects the presence of the highest barriers and lowest facilitators, to denote the worst-case scenario.

### Fifth Qualifier

The fifth qualifier is currently not shown or scored. It is unknown and is still in development. It is possible that it might be used to reflect the client's level of involvement in the activity or subjective satisfaction.

### Blended Scores

A&P codes are all blended activities. What this means is that they are comprised of multiple skill sets. For example, d4554 Swimming is defined as "propelling the whole body through water by means of limb and body movements without taking support from the ground underneath." This requires many skills including; mobility of joints (b710 Mobility of Joint Functions), upper body and lower body strength (b730 Muscle Power Functions), endurance (b740 Muscle Endurance Functions), and control and coordination of voluntary movements (b7601 Control of Complex Voluntary Movements, b7602 Coordination of Voluntary Movements).

It is important not to get caught up in just the Body Functions skills, but to look also at the A&P questions, how well does the client swim? Regardless of how it is done, as long as it's swimming of some kind, the therapist scores the amount of difficulty the client has with swimming from one point to another. We suggest scoring the level of difficulty for the part of the task the client needs the most help with. It really doesn't matter that the client can do the backstroke with no difficulty. If s/he has moderate difficulty with the crawl stroke, the activity of swimming is scored as moderate difficulty.

A&P codes that include a variety of activities can also pose a problem. For example, d9201 Sports is defined as "engaging in competitive and informal or formally organized games or athletic events, performed alone or in a group, such as bowling, gymnastics, or soccer." If a client participates in three different sports and has different average levels of difficulty for each sport, there can be a problem in scoring. Let's say the client had mild difficulty engaging in bowling, moderate difficulty with baseball, and severe difficulty with tennis. In this case, the therapist would need to choose the maximum level of difficulty the client has with sports (severe difficulty with tennis in this example).The appropriate way to blend scores is not settled yet, so therapists will need to score codes as they feel is appropriate and stay aware of the latest thinking in the field.

### Addition of a Participation Level Score

When scoring codes in d9 Community, Social, and Civic Life, we suggested that recreational therapists consider documenting the extent of participation. For example, writing in an additional Dehn (1995) code to the right of the scored ICF code. The Dehn code is not part of the ICF. It is an additional code that could help clarify a client's level of participation. If there were no problems with participation in d9205 Socializing, but the client was a spectator rather than a participant, the scoring would look like d9205.0 0 0 0 Dehn level +1.

Dehn levels are discussed in the *Leisure Step Up* (Dehn, 1995) and in the Community Participation chapter of *Recreational Therapy Basics, Techniques, and Interventions.*

### References

Dehn, D. (1995). *Leisure Step Up.* Ravensdale, WA: Idyll Arbor.

# Chapter 1 Learning and Applying Knowledge

This chapter is about learning, applying the knowledge that is learned, thinking, solving problems, and making decisions.

### Sample Scoring for Learning and Applying Knowledge

- A three-year-old child in a medical day program is learning to copy actions with single objects, such as banging a block on the floor to make a noise (d130 Copying). When the therapist does something with the block and places it in the child's hand, 70% of the time the child just holds it and does nothing with it. The other 30% of the time, he interacts with the block as the therapist did. With maximum multi-modal cueing and hand-over-hand assistance, the child's ability to copy the therapist improves to 60%. The correct scoring of d130 Copying would look like this: d130._ 3 2 _.
- An adult client with paraplegia in a physical rehab facility has difficulty solving complex problems related to community participation (d1751 Solving Complex Problems). When he desires to engage in a community task, such as going to the movies with his two young children, he has to problem solve for various issues prior to going out including accessibility, controlling children, and mobility skills. Typically, the client struggles with problem solving for about 20% of the tasks because it is a new experience for him. He never had to problem solve for such things prior to his injury. The correct scoring of d1751 Solving Complex Problems would look like this: d1715._ 1 _ _.
- A 12-year-old boy in an inpatient psychiatric facility struggles with fitting in with his peer group. Many of his peers play soccer and he has never played. He refuses to join the local team because he thinks kids will make fun of him because he doesn't know how to play. The recreational therapist teaches him the basic rules of the game, along with some basic soccer moves (d1551 Acquiring Complex Skills). Through this instruction, he was able to learn about 60% of the rules and moves and now looks forward to joining the local team in the fall. The correct scoring for d1551 Acquiring Complex Skills would look like this: d1551._ 2 _ _ (soccer).

This section is the cousin to Body Functions b1 Mental Functions. The Body Functions chapter reflects brain functions and the Activities and Participation chapter reflects brain activities. It is very difficult for the clinician to differentiate between the two because recreational therapists use activities to determine the functioning of the brain. For example, a therapist presents the client with a problem-solving activity to assess the brain function of problem solving. Examples of codes that are closely related include:

- b1646 Problem-Solving versus d175 Solving Problems.
- b1400 Sustaining Attention versus d160 Focusing Attention.
- b1720 Simple Calculation versus d150 Learning to Calculate.

Consequently, much of the description on how to assess, treat, and document for cognitive and mental tasks is in Body Functions b1 Mental Functions.

### Assessment of Learning and Applying Knowledge

Recreational therapists utilize various methods to assess learning and applying knowledge including but not limited to interview, observation, functional testing, and standardized assessments. The skills in this section are vast. Consequently the assessment methods chosen will vary greatly. For example, assessment methods chosen to evaluate d115 Listening will be quite different from those chosen to evaluate d1751 Solving Complex Problems.

### Treatment of Learning and Applying Knowledge

Given that this section is comprised of a vast array of skills and tasks, it is difficult to suggest a general treatment strategy. Treatment will vary depending on the skills and the underlying components that are causing the difficulty.

### Evidence Review

Reviews of several studies are provided to highlight evidence-based practice related to learning and applying knowledge. This is only a sample of the evidence. A thorough review of the literature is needed to identify evidence-based practice interventions that reflect the needs and characteristics of individual clients.

Clare and Jones (2008) conducted a literature review of errorless learning. Errorless learning is the elimination of errors during the learning process through various means including: (1) breaking down the targeted task into small, discrete steps or units, (2) providing sufficient models before the client is asked to perform the target task, (3) encouraging the client to avoid guessing, (4) immediately correcting errors, and (5) carefully fading prompts. The review found that errorless learning was the most helpful for people with severe memory impairments following traumatic brain injury.

Kessels and Olde-Hensken (2009) conducted a study of 60 people (20 with severe dementia, 20 with mild to moderate dementia, and 20 without dementia). Participants were taught a new procedural task using errorless learning and trial-and-error learning. Errorless learning yielded significantly better learning outcomes for individual with mild to moderate dementia compared to trial-and-error learning.

Frank et al. (2009) conducted a study of 14 three month olds, 14 six month olds, and 12 nine month olds. Findings indicated that infants from three to nine months gradually increased their attention to faces. Younger infants were primarily attentive (showed fixation) to low-level perceptual salience which included the attractiveness of basic perceptual features such as color, luminance, and motion. Since attention to faces gradually increases with age, the authors conclude that "in early infancy, a weak bias for faces may suffice to spur learning about conspecifics across a variety of real world contexts" (p. 168).

Kester et al. (2006) conducted a study of 15 adolescents with schizophrenia evaluating decision-making abilities using the *Iowa Gambling Task*. Findings indicated that the adolescents "allocated significantly more attention to monetary gains than losses encountered during the task, suggesting a hypersensitivity to rewards and relative insensitivity to future consequences" (p. 113). The authors suggest that this may make adolescents with schizophrenia more vulnerable to substance abuse.

Malouff, Thorsteinsson, and Schutte (2007) conducted a meta-analysis of 31 studies examining the efficacy of problem solving therapy. Problem solving therapy includes applying a problem solving orientation to life and using rational problem solving skills. Problem solving orientation to life includes appraising problems as challenges, thinking that problems can be solved, and realizing that effective problem solving tends to require time and systematic effort. Rational problem solving includes attempting to identify the problem when it occurs, defining a problem, attempting to understand the problem, setting goals related to the problem, generating alternative solutions, evaluating and choosing the best alternatives, implementing the chosen alternatives, evaluating the efficacy of the effort at problem solving, and then returning to any of the steps, as needed, to try again. Steps are typically discussed as well as written down and guided practice is provided. Findings indicated that problem solving therapy "tends to be effective in treating mental or physical health problems" (p. 53).

Kasari, Freeman, and Paparella (2006) conducted a study of 58 children with autism aged three to four. Children were randomized into one of three groups: joint attention intervention, symbolic play intervention, and control group. The intervention in the joint attention and symbolic play groups were conducted 30 minutes daily for five to six weeks. Both groups consisted of five minutes of table activity and about 20 minutes of milieu teaching on the floor to enhance generalization and flexible learning. The joint attention group focused on teaching joint attention skills: imitation of the child and engineered play routines. The play intervention group focused on improving symbolic play using object combinations that were increasingly more symbolic. Both groups improved significantly over the control group. The joint attention group showed increased responsiveness to joint attention and more child-initiated joint attention in mother-child interactions. The symbolic play group showed more diverse symbolic play in mother-child interactions, as well as higher play levels. A manual was developed for this study. It may be requested through the first author.

Van Tilborg, Kessles, and Hulstijn conducted a study of 10 patients with mild dementia. Participants were taught how to use a microwave oven and a coffee machine within five 15-minute sessions.

Participants were taught one of the skills using implicit learning methods (modeling) and the other using explicit learning methods (providing verbal cues). Both methods were found to be effective in helping the participants acquire new daily life skills.

Lawson and Dunn (2008) conducted a study of 53 typically developing children ages three years two months to five years six months. The researchers completed a sensory profile on each child and observed the children in play to examine the relationship between sensory processing and play preferences. Results indicated that children who had a tendency to avoid stimulation had less variation in body positions during play. They were content to stay in one position and continue playing. "This may be an effort to control the amount of stimulation they receive from the toy they are playing with and their surroundings" (p. 7). Consequently, the child might only move if directed by the teacher or if the play area became over-stimulating. Recreational therapists who work with children who avoid stimulation might consider several adaptations. The therapists might introduce new activities while maintaining a comfortable level of stimulation. They might bring new play activities to the child or bring children to the child who avoids stimulation rather than ask the child to join others in play. Children who were more sensory avoidant preferred pretend toys and miniature vehicles. They were content to engage in solitary fantasy play. Sensation-seeking children preferred creative arts toys and building materials with no specific toy preference. They were interested in novel stimuli and more likely to engage in social group play. "As we begin to understand what young children prefer and why, we should use this information to offer children toys that will motivate them to play longer and engage in higher levels of play" (p. 9).

### Cross References

In *Recreational Therapy for Specific Diagnoses and Conditions, First Edition*, ICF code d1 Learning and Applying Knowledge and its subcategories are listed in 26 chapters: Amputation and Prosthesis, Attention-Deficit/Hyperactivity Disorder, Autism Spectrum Disorder, Burns, Cancer, Cerebral Palsy, Cerebrovascular Accident, Chronic Obstructive Pulmonary Disease, Diabetes Mellitus, Epilepsy, Generalized Anxiety Disorder, Hearing Loss, Intellectual Disability, Major Depressive Disorder,

Multiple Sclerosis, Neurocognitive Disorders, Oppositional Defiant Disorder and Conduct Disorder, Parkinson's Disease, Post-Traumatic Stress Disorder, Schizophrenia Spectrum and Other Psychotic Disorders, Sickle Cell Disease, Spina Bifida, Spinal Cord Injury, Substance-Related Disorders, Traumatic Brain Injury, and Visual Impairments and Blindness.

In *Recreational Therapy Basics, Techniques, and Interventions, First Edition*, treatment for ICF code d1 Learning and Applying Knowledge and its subcategories are discussed in 24 chapters: Activity and Task Analysis, Education and Counseling, Parameters and Precautions, Stress, Adaptive Sports, Adventure Therapy, Aquatic Therapy, Behavior Strategies and Interventions, Bibliotherapy, Cognitive Behavioral Counseling, Cognitive Retraining and Rehabilitation, Community Problem Solving, Disability Rights: Education and Advocacy, Errorless Learning, Group Psychotherapy Techniques, Leisure Education and Counseling, Mind-Body Interventions, Montessori Method, Physical Activity, Reality Orientation, Sensory Interventions, Social Skills Training, Therapeutic Thematic Arts Programming, and Wheelchair Mobility.

### Purposeful Sensory Experiences (d110 - d129)

Purposeful Sensory Experiences comprises the activities of watching, listening, and other purposeful sensing. A description will follow each code directing the therapist to the appropriate codes that impact a person's ability to perform the activity. In general a person needs to be conscious and have skills on some level of mental attention. Refer to b110 Consciousness Functions and b140 Attention Functions for information on how to assess, treat, document, and adapt for these precursor skills of d110 - d129 Purposeful Sensory Experiences

### d110 Watching

Using the sense of seeing intentionally to experience visual stimuli, such as watching a sporting event or children playing.

The purposeful use of sensory experiences does not mean that the client interprets the sensory experiences correctly. For example, a client who has dementia may actively use his sense of seeing to watch television, but he may not be able to correctly interpret what he is seeing due to cognitive impairments. He is not successfully watching.

To be able to use watching to intentionally experience visual stimuli a client needs to possess the skills mentioned at the beginning of the code set (b110 Consciousness Functions and b140 Attention Functions) and have vision (b210 - b229 Seeing and Related Functions). Refer to those code sets for information on how to assess, treat, document, and adapt for consciousness and seeing functions that are needed for watching.

Recreational therapists document the extent of difficulty a client has with watching. For example, client has moderate difficulty watching films at home without assistance (d110._ _ _ 2).

### Cross References

In *Recreational Therapy for Specific Diagnoses and Conditions, First Edition*, ICF code d110 Watching is listed in one chapter: Neurocognitive Disorders.

In *Recreational Therapy Basics, Techniques, and Interventions, First Edition*, treatment for ICF code d110 Watching is discussed in three chapters: Activity and Task Analysis, Sensory Interventions, and Social Skills Training.

### d115 Listening

Using the sense of hearing intentionally to experience auditory stimuli, such as listening to a radio, music, or a lecture.

The purposeful use of sensory experiences does not mean that the client interprets the sensory experiences correctly. For example, a client who has dementia may actively use his sense of listening to listen to a radio program, but he may not be able to correctly interpret what he is hearing due to cognitive impairments. He is not successfully listening.

To be able to use listening to intentionally experience auditory stimuli, the client needs to possess the skills mentioned at the beginning of the code set (b110 Consciousness Functions and b140 Attention Functions) and have the sense of hearing (b230 Hearing Functions). Refer to those codes for information on how to assess, treat, document, and adapt for consciousness and hearing functions that are needed for listening.

Recreational therapists document the extent of difficulty a client has with listening. For example,

client has mild difficulty listening to others when playing a board game in the clinic without assistance from others (d115._ 1 _ _).

### Cross References

In *Recreational Therapy for Specific Diagnoses and Conditions, First Edition*, ICF code d115 Listening is listed in one chapter: Neurocognitive Disorders.

In *Recreational Therapy Basics, Techniques, and Interventions, First Edition*, treatment for ICF code d115 Listening is discussed in three chapters: Activity and Task Analysis, Sensory Interventions, and Social Skills Training.

### d120 Other Purposeful Sensing

Using the body's other basic senses intentionally to experience stimuli, such as touching and feeling textures, tasting sweets, or smelling flowers.

The purposeful use of sensory experiences does not mean that the client interprets the sensory experiences correctly. For example, a client who has dementia may actively use a basic sense, but he may not be able to correctly interpret what he is experiencing due to cognitive impairments. He is not successful at purposeful sensing.

To be able to use other purposeful sensing to experience stimuli, such as touching and feeling textures, tasting sweets, or smelling flowers, a client needs to have the skills mentioned at the beginning of the code set (b110 Consciousness Functions and b140 Attention Functions) and have the sense of touch, taste, and smell (b265 Touch Function, b250 Taste Function, and b255 Smell Function). Refer to those codes for information on how to assess, treat, document, and adapt for consciousness and touch, taste, and smell functions that are needed for other purposeful sensing.

Recreational therapists document the extent of difficulty a client has with other purposeful sensing. For example, client has moderate difficulties with touching and feeling textures in the community to compensate for vision loss despite receiving verbal cues from others (d120.2 _ _ _).

### Cross References

In *Recreational Therapy for Specific Diagnoses and Conditions, First Edition*, ICF code d120 Other Purposeful Sensing is listed in one chapter: Amputation and Prosthesis.

In *Recreational Therapy Basics, Techniques, and Interventions, First Edition*, treatment for ICF code d120 Other Purposeful Sensing is discussed in two chapters: Sensory Interventions and Social Skills Training.

### d129 Purposeful Sensory Experiences, Other Specified and Unspecified

### Basic Learning (d130 - d159)

Basic learning comprises the activities of copying, rehearsing, learning to read, learning to write, learning to calculate, and acquiring skills. A description will follow each code directing the therapist to the appropriate b1 Mental Functions codes that impact a person's ability to perform the activity. In general a person needs to be conscious, and have skills on some level of mental attention, memory, and perception to perform the activities in this section. Refer to b110 Consciousness Functions, b140 Attention Functions, b144 Memory Functions, and b156 Perceptual Functions for information on how to assess, treat, document, and adapt for these precursor skills of d130 - d159 Basic Learning.

### d130 Copying

Imitating or mimicking as a basic component of learning, such as copying a gesture, a sound, or the letters of an alphabet.

To be able to mimic a basic component of learning, such as copying a gesture, sound, or letter of the alphabet, a variety of mental and physical skills are needed, including those mentioned at the beginning of this code set. The specific skills will vary depending on the desired activity. For example, mimicking a sound requires different skills than copying a gesture. The therapist will need to determine the components of the specific activity through task analysis. Once the components are identified, specific problem areas can be identified and then referred to in this book for information on how to assess, treat, document, and adapt for the specific skill. For example, if the client is having problems with joint mobility impacting her ability to mimic a hand gesture, then the therapist would refer to b710 Mobility of Joint Functions for information on how to assess, treat, document, and adapt for the problem.

Recreational therapists document the extent of difficulty a client has with copying. For example, cli-

ent has moderate difficulty copying facial expressions in the therapy room when prompted to do so by the therapist (d130._ _ 2 _).

### Cross References

In *Recreational Therapy for Specific Diagnoses and Conditions, First Edition*, ICF code d130 Copying is listed in four chapters: Attention-Deficit/Hyperactivity Disorder, Epilepsy, Schizophrenia Spectrum and Other Psychotic Disorders, and Traumatic Brain Injury.

In *Recreational Therapy Basics, Techniques, and Interventions, First Edition*, treatment for ICF code d130 Copying is discussed in three chapters: Activity and Task Analysis, Sensory Interventions, and Social Skills Training.

### d135 Rehearsing

Repeating a sequence of events or symbols as a basic component of learning, such as counting by tens or practicing the recitation of a poem.

To be able to repeat a sequence of events or symbols, such as counting by tens or practicing the recitation of a poem, the client requires a variety of mental and/or physical skills, including those mentioned at the beginning of this code set. The specific skills will vary depending on the desired activity. For example, repeating a dance sequence requires different skills than reciting a poem. The therapist will need to determine the components of the specific activity through task analysis. Once the components are identified, specific problem areas can be identified and then referred to in this book for information on how to assess, treat, document, and adapt for the specific skill. For example, if the client is having problems with memory impacting his ability to recite a poem, then the therapist would refer to b144 Memory Functions for information on how to assess, treat, document, and adapt for the problem.

Recreational therapists document the extent of difficulty a client has with rehearsing. For example, client has severe difficulty repeating the sequence for accessing Facebook at home without assistance (d135._ _ _ 3).

### Cross References

In *Recreational Therapy for Specific Diagnoses and Conditions, First Edition*, ICF code d135 Rehearsing is listed in four chapters: Attention-Deficit/Hyperactivity            Disorder,            Epilepsy,

Schizophrenia Spectrum and Other Psychotic Disorders, and Traumatic Brain Injury.

In *Recreational Therapy Basics, Techniques, and Interventions, First Edition*, treatment for ICF code d135 Rehearsing is discussed in four chapters: Activity and Task Analysis, Aquatic Therapy, Reality Orientation, and Social Skills Training.

### d140 Learning to Read

Developing the competence to read written material (including Braille) with fluency and accuracy, such as recognizing characters and alphabets, sounding out words with correct pronunciation, and understanding words and phrases.

To learn to read written material (including Braille) with fluency and accuracy, a variety of mental and/or physical skills are needed, including those mentioned at the beginning of this code set. The specific skills will vary depending on the desired activity. For example, sounding out letters requires different skills than recognizing Braille words. The following additional basic precursor skills should also be considered:

- *For sounding out letters and words*: b310 Voice Functions, b320 Articulation Functions, b330 Fluency and Rhythm of Speech Functions, b340 Alternative Vocalization Functions, and b230 Hearing Functions.
- *For reading written words*: b167 Mental Functions of Language, b210 Seeing Functions.
- *For reading Braille words*: b1564 Tactile Perception.

The therapist will need to determine the components of the specific activity through task analysis. Once the components are identified, specific problem areas can be identified and then referred to in this book for information on how to assess, treat, document, and adapt for the specific skill. For example, if the client is having problems with attention that are impacting her ability to read written words, then the therapist would refer to b140 Attention Functions for information on how to assess, treat, document, and adapt for the problem.

Recreational therapists document the extent of difficulty a client has with learning to read. For example, client has moderate difficulty learning to read activity directions in the clinic when assistance is not provided (d140._ 2 _ _).

### Cross References

In *Recreational Therapy for Specific Diagnoses and Conditions, First Edition*, ICF code d140 Learning to Read is listed in four chapters: Attention-Deficit/Hyperactivity Disorder, Epilepsy, Schizophrenia Spectrum and Other Psychotic Disorders, and Traumatic Brain Injury.

In *Recreational Therapy Basics, Techniques, and Interventions, First Edition*, there are no references for ICF code d140 Learning to Read.

### d145 Learning to Write

Developing the competence to produce symbols that represent sounds, words, or phrases in order to convey meaning (including Braille writing), such as spelling effectively and using correct grammar.

To learn to produce symbols that represent sounds, words, or phrases to convey meaning, a variety of mental and/or physical skills are needed, including those mentioned at the beginning of this code set. The specific skills will vary depending on the desired activity. For example, painting Chinese symbols requires different skills than writing a letter. The following additional basic precursor skills should also be considered:

- *Writing with sight*: b167 Mental Functions of Language, b210 Seeing Functions, d440 Fine Hand Use.
- *Writing without sight*: All of above except b210 Seeing Functions. Additionally, b1564 Tactile Perception.

The therapist will need to determine the components of the specific activity through task analysis. Once the components are identified, specific problem areas can be identified and then referred to in this book for information on how to assess, treat, document, and adapt for the specific skill. For example, if the client is having a problem with grasping a pen and it is impacting his ability to write, then the therapist would refer to d4401 Grasping for information on how to assess, treat, document, and adapt for the problem.

Recreational therapists document the extent of difficulty a client has with learning to write. For example, client has moderate difficulty learning to write in school when assistance is not provided (d145._ _ _ 2).

*Cross References*

In *Recreational Therapy for Specific Diagnoses and Conditions, First Edition*, there are no references for ICF code d145 Learning to Write.

In *Recreational Therapy Basics, Techniques, and Interventions, First Edition*, there are no references for ICF code d145 Learning to Write.

### d150 Learning to Calculate

Developing the competence to manipulate numbers and perform simple and complex mathematical operations, such as using mathematical signs for addition and subtraction and applying the correct mathematical operation to a problem.

To learn to manipulate numbers and perform simple and complex mathematical operations, a client needs a variety of mental and/or physical skills, including those mentioned at the beginning of this code set. The specific skills will vary depending on the desired activity. For example, adding two single digit numbers requires different skills than balancing a checkbook. The following additional basic precursor skills should also be considered: b172 Calculation Functions and b210 Seeing Functions, as well as d440 Fine Hand Use and b710 Mobility of Joint Functions for operation and manipulation of a pencil, calculator, etc. The therapist will need to determine the components of the specific activity through task analysis. Once the components are identified, specific problem areas can be identified and then referred to in this book for information on how to assess, treat, document, and adapt for the specific skill. For example, if the client is having problems with the mental skill of addition and it is impacting her ability to learn how to calculate, then the therapist would refer to b1720 Simple Calculation for information on how to assess, treat, document, and adapt for the problem.

Recreational therapists document the extent of difficulty a client has with learning to calculate. For example, client has mild difficulty learning to calculate items at the store despite assistance from the therapist (d150.1 _ _ _).

*Cross References*

In *Recreational Therapy for Specific Diagnoses and Conditions, First Edition*, there are no references for ICF code d150 Learning to Calculate.

In *Recreational Therapy Basics, Techniques, and Interventions, First Edition*, there are no references for ICF code d150 Learning to Calculate.

### d155 Acquiring Skills

Developing basic and complex competencies in integrated sets of actions or tasks so as to initiate and follow through with the acquisition of a skill, such as manipulating tools, or playing games like chess.

Inclusions: acquiring basic and complex skills

- *d1550 Acquiring Basic Skills*
  Learning elementary, purposeful actions, such as learning to manipulate eating utensils, a pencil, or a simple tool.

- *d1551 Acquiring Complex Skills*
  Learning integrated sets of actions so as to follow rules, and to sequence and coordinate one's movements, such as learning to play games like football or to use a building tool.

- *d1558 Acquiring Skills, Other Specified*
- *d1559 Acquiring Skills, Unspecified*
  There are two kinds of skills that are especially important for recreational therapists, leisure activity skills and skills related to advanced activities of daily living. Leisure activity skills are skills that allow an individual to "engage in any form of play, recreation, or leisure activity, such as informal or organized play and sports, programs of physical fitness, relaxation, amusement or diversion; going to art galleries, museums, cinemas, or theatres; engaging in crafts or hobbies; reading for enjoyment; playing musical instruments; sight seeing, tourism, and traveling for pleasure" (d920 Recreation and Leisure). Advanced activities of daily living include shopping, banking, related travel, and other complex activities required for daily life.

This code covers the ability of clients to learn new activity skills such as using the steps required for learning a new game, hobby, or sport. It is not the process of restoring lost skills and advancing developmental skills, such as improving memory skills or following directions. Skills development assumes that the client does not possess skills and the therapist is teaching the client how to learn those underlying skills.

Although recreational therapy uses the term leisure skills development, the ICF does not recognize this term. Because the ICF is client-centered rather than therapy-centered, it does not look at teaching; it looks at learning. Therefore, therapists determine a client's ability to acquire basic skills (d1550 Acquiring Basic Skills) and acquire complex skills (d1551 Acquiring Complex Skills) according to the extent of difficulty.

When the therapist is teaching the client how to learn skills, it is documented by using these two codes. The specific activity can be noted to the right of the scoring area. Many activity skills that are taught to a client can be scored under these two codes, although there are also many places in Activities and Participation that refer to specific leisure activity skills, such as d6505 Taking Care of Plants, Indoors and Outdoors or d6500 Making and Repairing Clothes. Therapists should be careful not to use the d920 Recreation and Leisure code set (in d9 Community, Social, and Civic Life) for leisure skills development because the d920 Recreation and Leisure code set reflects *participation* in a specific activity rather than *acquiring* activity skills needed to participate in that activity.

Recreational therapists document the extent of difficulty a client has with acquiring skills. For example, client has mild difficulty acquiring the complex skills of shooting a bow and arrow using a sip and puff in the clinic despite assistance from therapist (d1551._ _ 1 _).

### Cross References

In *Recreational Therapy for Specific Diagnoses and Conditions, First Edition*, ICF code d155 Acquiring Skills is listed in 10 chapters: Attention-Deficit/Hyperactivity Disorder, Autism Spectrum Disorder, Burns, Cerebrovascular Accident, Diabetes Mellitus, Epilepsy, Hearing Loss, Oppositional Defiant Disorder and Conduct Disorder, Schizophrenia Spectrum and Other Psychotic Disorders, and Traumatic Brain Injury.

In *Recreational Therapy Basics, Techniques, and Interventions, First Edition*, treatment for ICF code d155 Acquiring Skills is discussed in six chapters: Adaptive Sports, Aquatic Therapy, Cognitive Behavioral Counseling, Errorless Learning, Leisure Education and Counseling, and Social Skills Training.

### d159 Basic Learning Skills, Other Specified and Unspecified

## Applying Knowledge (d160 - d179)

Applying Knowledge comprises the activities of focusing attention, thinking, reading, writing, calculating, solving problems, and making decisions. Note that there is a difference in this section of *applying knowledge* compared to the previous section of *acquiring skills*. For example, in the previous section d140 Learning to Read addressed *learning* the skill whereas in this section d166 Reading addresses the *application* of the skill to read for the purpose of obtaining general knowledge or specific information. A description follows each code directing the therapist to other appropriate codes that impact a person's ability to perform the activity. In general a person needs to be conscious and have some level of mental attention to perform the activities in this section. Refer to b110 Consciousness Functions, b140 Attention Functions, and b160 Thought Functions for information on how to assess, treat, document, and adapt for these precursor skills of d160 - d179 Applying Knowledge.

### d160 Focusing Attention

Intentionally focusing on specific stimuli, such as by filtering out distracting noises.

To focus on specific stimuli and filter out distractions, a variety of mental skills are needed, including those mentioned at the beginning of this code set. More specifically one or more of the subcomponents of b140 Attention Functions (b1400 Sustaining Attention, b1401 Shifting Attention, b1402 Dividing Attention, b1403 Sharing Attention) are needed depending on the specific task that requires focused attention. The therapist will need to determine the components of the specific activity through task analysis. Once the components are identified, specific problem areas can be identified and then referred to in this book for information on how to assess, treat, document, and adapt for the specific skill. For example, if the client's problem with focusing attention in a group activity is impacting his ability to complete the task at hand, the therapist may refer to b1401 Shifting Attention for information on how to assess, treat, document, and adapt for the problem.

Recreational therapists document the extent of difficulty a client has with focusing attention. For example, client has moderate difficulty with focusing attention when building model cars at his friend's house when assistance is not provided (d160._ _ _ 2).

### Cross References

In *Recreational Therapy for Specific Diagnoses and Conditions, First Edition*, ICF code d160 Focusing Attention is listed in six chapters: Cerebrovascular Accident, Epilepsy, Generalized Anxiety Disorder, Intellectual Disability, Neurocognitive Disorders, and Traumatic Brain Injury.

In *Recreational Therapy Basics, Techniques, and Interventions, First Edition*, treatment for ICF code d160 Focusing Attention is discussed in four chapters: Stress, Adaptive Sports, Aquatic Therapy, and Social Skills Training.

### d163 Thinking

Formulating and manipulating ideas, concepts, and images, whether goal-oriented or not, either alone or with others, such as creating fiction, proving a theorem, playing with ideas, brainstorming, meditating, pondering, speculating, or reflecting.

Exclusions: Solving Problems (d175), Making Decisions (d177)

To formulate and manipulate ideas, concepts, and images a variety of mental skills are needed including those mentioned at the beginning of this code set. Additional skills that may be needed, depending on the complexity of the task, include subcomponents of b144 Memory Functions, b160 Thought Functions, b164 Higher-Level Cognitive Functions (b1640 Abstraction, b1641 Organization and Planning, b1642 Time Management, b1643 Cognitive Flexibility, b1644 Insight, b1645 Judgment, b1646 Problem-Solving). The therapist will need to determine the components of the specific activity through task analysis. Once the components are identified, specific problem areas can be identified and then referred to in this book for information on how to assess, treat, document, and adapt for the specific skill. For example, if client is having problems with abstraction that are impacting his ability to complete the thinking task at hand, the therapist may refer to b1640 Abstraction for information on how to assess, treat, document, and adapt for the problem.

Recreational therapists document the extent of difficulty a client has with thinking. For example, client has mild difficulty formulating ideas for writing a story during down time at the hospital when assistance is not provided (d163._ 1 _ _).

### Cross References

In *Recreational Therapy for Specific Diagnoses and Conditions, First Edition*, ICF code d163 Thinking is listed in seven chapters: Cerebrovascular Accident, Epilepsy, Generalized Anxiety Disorder, Major Depressive Disorder, Neurocognitive Disorders, Substance-Related Disorders, and Traumatic Brain Injury.

In *Recreational Therapy Basics, Techniques, and Interventions, First Edition*, treatment for ICF code d163 Thinking is discussed in four chapters: Activity and Task Analysis, Parameters and Precautions, Social Skills Training, and Therapeutic Thematic Arts Programming.

### d166 Reading

Performing activities involved in the comprehension and interpretation of written language (e.g., books, instructions, or newspapers in text or Braille), for the purpose of obtaining general knowledge or specific information.

Exclusions: Learning to Read (d140)

To perform reading activities involved in the comprehension and interpretation of written language, the client needs a variety of mental skills, including those mentioned at the beginning of this code set. More specifically, subcomponents of b144 Memory Functions, b167 Mental Functions of Language, and those skills needed for code d140 Learning to Read. For reading written words: b210 Seeing Functions. For reading Braille words: b1564 Tactile Perception. The therapist will need to determine the components of the specific activity through task analysis. Once the components are identified, specific problem areas can be identified and then referred to in this book for information on how to assess, treat, document, and adapt for the specific skill. For example, if the client is having a problem with feeling the raised Braille symbols and it is impacting her ability to comprehend and interpret the text, the therapist may refer to b1564 Tactile Perception for information on how to assess, treat, document, and adapt for the problem.

Recreational therapists document the extent of difficulty a client has with reading. For example, client has moderate difficulty reading activity instructions in the therapy room when assistance is not provided (d166._ 2 _ _).

### *Cross References*

In *Recreational Therapy for Specific Diagnoses and Conditions, First Edition*, ICF code d166 Reading is listed in five chapters: Cerebrovascular Accident, Epilepsy, Neurocognitive Disorders, Traumatic Brain Injury, and Visual Impairments and Blindness.

In *Recreational Therapy Basics, Techniques, and Interventions, First Edition*, treatment for ICF code d166 Reading is discussed in three chapters: Activity and Task Analysis, Disability Rights: Education and Advocacy, and Social Skills Training.

### *d170 Writing*

Using or producing symbols or language to convey information, such as producing a written record of events or ideas or drafting a letter.

Exclusions: learning to write (d145)

To perform writing activities involved in using or producing symbols or language to convey information, the client needs a variety of mental and physical skills, including those mentioned at the beginning of this code set. More specifically, the skills that are needed for the code d145 Learning to Write include b167 Mental Functions of Language. For writing with sight: b210 Seeing Functions and d440 Fine Hand Use. For writing without sight: b1564 Tactile Perception and d440 Fine Hand Use. Depending on the complexity of the writing activity, subcomponents of b164 Higher-Level Cognitive Functions may also be needed. The therapist will need to determine the components of the specific activity through task analysis. Once the components are identified, specific problem areas can be identified and then referred to in this book for information on how to assess, treat, document, and adapt for the specific skill. For example, if the client is having problems with organizing skills that are impacting his ability to organize a letter, the therapist may refer to b1641 Organization and Planning for information on how to assess, treat, document, and adapt for the problem.

Recreational therapists document the extent of difficulty a client has with writing. For example, at home, client has severe difficulty writing a letter to her friend when assistance is not provided (d170._ _ _ 3).

### *Cross References*

In *Recreational Therapy for Specific Diagnoses and Conditions, First Edition*, ICF code d170 Writing is listed in five chapters: Cerebrovascular Accident, Epilepsy, Multiple Sclerosis, Neurocognitive Disorders, and Traumatic Brain Injury.

In *Recreational Therapy Basics, Techniques, and Interventions, First Edition*, treatment for ICF code d170 Writing is discussed in three chapters: Activity and Task Analysis, Bibliotherapy, and Social Skills Training.

### *d172 Calculating*

Performing computations by applying mathematical principles to solve problems that are described in words and producing or displaying the results, such as computing the sum of three numbers or finding the result of dividing one number by another.

Exclusions: Learning to Calculate (d150)

To perform computations by applying mathematical principles to solve problems, the client needs a variety of mental and physical skills, including those mentioned at the beginning of this code set. Specific required skills include the ones that are needed for code d150 Learning to Calculate, b172 Calculation Functions, b210 Seeing Functions, d440 Fine Hand Use, and b710 Mobility of Joint Functions. Depending on the complexity of the calculating activity, subcomponents of b164 Higher-Level Cognitive Functions may also be needed. The therapist will need to determine the components of the specific activity through task analysis. Once the components are identified, specific problem areas can be identified and then referred to in this book for information on how to assess, treat, document, and adapt for the specific skill. For example, if the client is having difficulty with problem solving that is impacting her ability to perform computations, the therapist may refer to b1646 Problem-Solving for information on how to assess, treat, document, and adapt for the problem.

Recreational therapists document the extent of difficulty a client has with calculating. For example, client has moderate difficulty with simple addition at the store when assistance is not provided (d172._ _ _ 2).

### Cross References

In *Recreational Therapy for Specific Diagnoses and Conditions, First Edition*, ICF code d172 Calculating is listed in four chapters: Cerebrovascular Accident, Epilepsy, Neurocognitive Disorders, and Traumatic Brain Injury.

In *Recreational Therapy Basics, Techniques, and Interventions, First Edition*, treatment for ICF code d172 Calculation Functions is discussed in one chapter: Social Skills Training.

### d175 Solving Problems

Finding solutions to questions or situations by identifying and analyzing issues, developing options and solutions, evaluating potential effects of solutions, and executing a chosen solution, such as in resolving a dispute between two people.

Inclusions: solving simple and complex problems

Exclusions: thinking (d163), making decisions (d177)

- *d1750 Solving Simple Problems*
  Finding solutions to a simple problem involving a single issue or question, by identifying and analyzing the issue, developing solutions, evaluating the potential effects of the solutions, and executing a chosen solution.

- *d1751 Solving Complex Problems*
  Finding solutions to a complex problem involving multiple and interrelated issues, or several related problems, by identifying and analyzing the issue, developing solutions, evaluating the potential effects of the solutions, and executing a chosen solution.

- *d1758 Solving Problems, Other Specified*
- *d1759 Solving Problems, Unspecified*
  Finding solutions to questions or situation by identifying and analyzing issues, developing options and solutions, evaluating potential effects of solutions, and executing a chosen solution requires a variety of mental and possibly physical skills, including those mentioned at the beginning of this code set. More specifically, b164 Higher-Level Cognitive Functions along with b160 Thought Functions and b144 Memory Functions may be required. The therapist will need to determine the

components of the specific activity through task analysis. Once the components are identified, specific problem areas can be identified and then referred to in this book for information on how to assess, treat, document, and adapt for the specific skill. For example, if the client's difficulty with short-term memory is impacting her ability to solve problems, the therapist may refer to b1440 Short-Term Memory for information on how to assess, treat, document, and adapt for the problem.

Recreational therapists document the extent of difficulty a client has with solving problems. For example, client has moderate difficulty solving complex problems in the clinic related to social situations despite assistance from therapist (d1751._ _ 2 _).

### Cross References

In *Recreational Therapy for Specific Diagnoses and Conditions, First Edition*, ICF code d175 Solving Problems is listed in 13 chapters: Cerebrovascular Accident, Epilepsy, Generalized Anxiety Disorder, Intellectual Disability, Major Depressive Disorder, Multiple Sclerosis, Neurocognitive Disorders, Post-Traumatic Stress Disorder, Schizophrenia Spectrum and Other Psychotic Disorders, Spina Bifida, Spinal Cord Injury, Traumatic Brain Injury, and Visual Impairments and Blindness.

In *Recreational Therapy Basics, Techniques, and Interventions, First Edition*, treatment for ICF code d175 Solving Problems is discussed in five chapters: Adaptive Sports, Adventure Therapy, Community Problem Solving, Group Psychotherapy Techniques, and Wheelchair Mobility.

### d177 Making Decisions

Making a choice among options, implementing the choice, and evaluating the effects of the choice, such as selecting and purchasing a specific item, or deciding to undertake and undertaking one task from among several tasks that need to be done.

Exclusions: thinking (d163), solving problems (d175)

To make a choice among options, implement the choice, and evaluate the effects of the choice, the client needs a variety of mental and possibly physical skills, including those mentioned at the beginning of this code set. More specifically b164 Higher-Level Cognitive Functions along with b160 Thought Functions and b144 Memory Functions may be required. Physical skills, such as d170 Writing may be required for tasks like writing options on paper to help make decisions. The therapist will need to determine the components of the specific activity through task analysis. Once the components are identified, specific problem areas can be identified and then referred to in this book for information on how to assess, treat, document, and adapt for the specific skill. For example, if the client has difficulty being optimistic (perhaps feeling that it doesn't matter what choice she makes because it will always result in a negative outcome), the therapist may refer to b1265 Optimism for information on how to assess, treat, document, and adapt for the problem.

Recreational therapists document the extent of difficulty a client has with making decisions. For example, client has mild difficulty making activity-related decisions in the clinic when assistance is not provided (d177._ 1 _ _).

*Cross References*

In *Recreational Therapy for Specific Diagnoses and Conditions*, ICF-CY code d250 Managing One's Own Behavior, which is not in the current version of the ICF, is listed in 15 chapters: Borderline Personality Disorder, Cerebral Palsy, Epilepsy, Feeding and Eating Disorders, Gambling Disorder, Generalized Anxiety Disorder, Intellectual Disability, Obesity, Oppositional Defiant Disorder and Conduct Disorder, Post-Traumatic Stress Disorder, Schizophrenia Spectrum and Other Psychotic Disorders, Sickle Cell Disease, Spina Bifida, Substance-Related Disorders, and Traumatic Brain Injury. ICF code d177 Making Decisions is probably the best place to look for a replacement.

In *Recreational Therapy for Specific Diagnoses and Conditions, First Edition*, ICF code d177 Making Decisions is listed in eight chapters: Attention-Deficit/Hyperactivity Disorder, Cerebrovascular Accident, Chronic Obstructive Pulmonary Disease, Epilepsy, Intellectual Disability, Major Depressive Disorder, Neurocognitive Disorders, and Traumatic Brain Injury.

In *Recreational Therapy Basics, Techniques, and Interventions, First Edition*, treatment for ICF code d177 Making Decisions is discussed in four chapters:

Activity and Task Analysis, Education and Counseling, Mind-Body Interventions, and Wheelchair Mobility.

### d179 Applying Knowledge, Other Specified and Unspecified

### d198 Learning and Applying Knowledge, Other Specified

In *Recreational Therapy Basics, Techniques, and Interventions, First Edition*, treatment for ICF code d198 Learning and Applying Knowledge, Other Specified is discussed in one chapter: Education and Counseling.

### d199 Learning and Applying Knowledge, Unspecified

*References*

Clare, L. & Jones, R. S. P. (2008). Errorless learning in the rehabilitation of memory impairment: A critical review. *Neuropsychology Review, 18*(1), 1-23.

Frank, M. C., & Vul, E., & Johnson, S. P. (2009). Development of infants' attention to faces during the first year. *Cognition, 110*(2), 160-170.

Kasari, C., Freeman, S., & Paparella, T. (2006). Joint attention and symbolic play in young children with autism: A randomized controlled intervention study. *Journal of Child Psychology and Psychiatry, 47*(6), 611-620.

Kessels, R. P. C. & Olde-Hensken, L. M. G. (2009). Effects of errorless skill learning in people with mild-to-moderate or severe dementia: A randomized controlled pilot study. *NeuroRehabilitation, 25*(4), 307-312.

Kester, H. M., Sevy, S., Yechiam, E., Burdick, K. E., Cervellione, K. L., & Kumra, S. (2006). Decision-making impairments in adolescents with early-onset schizophrenia. *Schizophrenia Research, 85*(1-3), 113-123.

Lawson, L. M. & Dunn, W. (2008). Children's sensory processing patterns and play preferences. *Annual in Therapeutic Recreation, XVI*, 1-14.

Malouff, J. M., Thorsteinsson, E. B., & Schutte, N. (2007). The efficacy of problem solving therapy in reducing mental and physical health problems: A meta-analysis. *Clinical Psychology Review, 27*(1), 46-57.

Van Tilborg, I. A., Kessles, R. P. C., & Hulstijn, W. (2011). How should we teach everyday skills in dementia? A controlled study comparing implicit and explicit training methods. *Clinical Rehabilitation, 25*(7), 638-648.

# Chapter 2 General Tasks and Demands

This chapter is about general aspects of carrying out single or multiple tasks, organizing routines, and handling stress. These items can be used in conjunction with more specific tasks or actions to identify the underlying features of the execution of tasks under different circumstances.

***Sample Scoring of General Tasks and Demands***

- In a clinic setting, a child requires 25% assistance (moderate difficulty = 2) to build a simple five-block tower (d2100 Undertaking a Simple Task). When assistance is provided by the recreational therapist, the child is able to complete the task without any difficulty (no difficulty = 0). The correct scoring of d2100 Undertaking a Simple Task would look like this: d2100._ 2 0 _.
- In a community setting, a client who sustained a traumatic brain injury utilizes a calendar app on his iPad to help him manage his time (d2303 Managing One's Own Activity Level). With this technology he is able to manage his time independently (no difficulty = 0). On days when he does not have his iPad, he requires approximately 75% assistance to manage his time for the day (severe difficulty = 3). The correct scoring for d2303 Managing One's Own Activity Level would look like this: d2303.0 _ _ 3.

This chapter is about *tasks*. A task is the direct effort of one person or a group to complete a goal. A task generally occurs in a sequential order and has a beginning point and a target outcome. This chapter is also about *demands*. A demand is either an internal or an external motivation to take action to fulfill a need. The majority of work done with a client can be boiled down to helping clients master tasks to fulfill demands.

The World Health Organization recognizes the ability to complete many different tasks as the basis for taking care of oneself and fitting into one's community. Because of the importance of being able to undertake and complete all types of tasks, the World Health Organization made tasks its own, major chapter in its system of categorization. Therapists are expected to assess the client's ability to perform these functions and provide interventions when appropriate. To be able to do this, it helps to understand what types of skills are included in each of the subcategories of d2 General Tasks and Demands.

The category of d2 General Tasks and Demands is divided into four subcategories: (1) undertaking a single task, (2) undertaking multiple tasks, (3) carrying out daily routine, and (4) handling stress and other psychological demands. The rest of this chapter will explain each of these subcategories and provide suggestions and guidelines for recreational therapy interventions. As discussed in the introduction to Activities and Participation, d2 General Tasks and Demands requires the therapist to understand the other parts of the ICF because the tasks rely on physical, mental, social, or psychological body functions; body structures; and environmental factors.

Notice that d2 General Tasks and Demands categories include d230 Carrying Out Daily Routine and d240 Handling Stress and Other Psychological Demands. At first it might seem like these two categories don't belong in this section. The reason that they are included is because the ability to carry out a daily routine is a general life task and handling stress and other psychological demands is part of our everyday lives.

When problems are seen in a client's ability to perform a task, it is usually a result of an impaired body function, a body structure deficit, or an inappropriate environment. The one most amenable to treatment is a problem with a body function.

In some cases the client will be able to consciously modify body function performance while in other cases the client will be unable to do so. Some examples of the types of body functions listed by the World Health Organization include b1400 Sustaining Attention and b3302 Speed of Speech. The therapist's job is to compare the client's performance against the task analysis of the activity. The client's ability or inability to perform each of the functions that are part of the task in the correct sequence helps the therapist identify where functional breakdown occurs.

To address isolated skills, the therapist has to understand the body functions required to carry out the skill. For example, a therapist must understand the basic anatomy of the brain and how it works. This understanding helps the therapist appreciate the theory of neuroplasticity, as it relates to adaptability, flexibility, and malleability of brain cells, and cognitive retraining, which help enhance cognitive functioning. If the therapist doesn't understand the workings of the brain, then s/he will not be able to grasp the value of interventions.

As an example, let's look at a recreational therapist on a healthcare team working with a client who has difficulty undertaking a single task of repotting a plant. By watching the client try to pot the plant, the therapist finds that the client has difficulty because she has tremors in both of her hands. This would be noted as a problem with b765 Involuntary Movement Functions. The therapist also notes that the client is neglecting the tools and supplies on the left side of the table because of a problem with left neglect documented as b2101 Visual Field Functions. After the recreational therapist reports these problems to the team, the occupational therapist searches her database for tasks that require visual field functions and together both therapists work on a unified approach to address this impairment. The physical therapist and physician work on a combined treatment and medication protocol to reduce problems with involuntary movement. The recreational therapist will be able to report on the success of the interventions by continued observation of the client in activities.

### Assessment of General Tasks and Demands

Recreational therapists utilize various methods to assess tasks, demands, daily routine, stress and psychological demands, and behavior, including but not limited to interview, observation, functional testing, and standardized assessments. The skills in this section are vast. Consequently the assessment methods chosen will vary greatly. For example, assessment methods chosen to evaluate "undertaking a single task" will be quite different from those chosen to evaluate "managing one's behavior."

### Treatment of General Tasks and Demands

The first three subcategories under d2 General Tasks and Demands relate to the ability to *act*. The fourth subcategory relates to the client's ability to regulate his/her emotional *reaction* to demands. The therapist will use a variety of techniques when addressing client impairments related to d2 General Tasks and Demands.

### Evidence Review

Reviews of several studies are provided below to highlight evidence-based practice related to d2 General Tasks and Demands. This is only a sample of the evidence. A thorough review of the literature is needed to identify evidence-based practice interventions that are reflective of the needs and characteristics of the individual client.

Richardson, Ong, and Sim (2008) conducted a qualitative study on eight adults living with chronic widespread pain (CWP). Findings indicated that people with CWP took longer to carry out everyday tasks, had disrupted daily routines, and required changes to how they managed their time. Some made successful adaptations, but others experienced feelings of lack of control. "Regaining control over time is an important element in coping with chronic pain, and helping patients to regain such control has potential as a target for health professionals involved in pain management" (p. NA).

Scott-Sheldon et al., (2008) conducted a meta-analysis of the literature relate to HIV+ adults and stress management (35 randomized controlled trials, 46 different stress management interventions, 3,077 participants). Findings indicate that stress management interventions for adults who are HIV+ significantly improve mental health and quality of life, but did not result in any immunological or hormonal benefits.

Bernheimer and Weisner (2007) conducted a 15-year longitudinal study of the daily lives of 102 families that had children with disabilities. A major theme was the need to make changes to their daily routine of activities based on needed accommodations, how the child impacted the parents' daily routine, the parents' goals and values, and attempts to maintain sustainability of daily routines. The authors noted that "no intervention, no matter how well designed or implemented, will have an impact if it cannot find a slot in the daily routines of an organization, family, or individual. The information and practices that make up the intervention must fit into the existing beliefs and practices already in place. The accommodations that parents make in their daily routines show that family routines and practices can and do change — that interventions can indeed find their places. The practitioner participates in this 'conversation' between the social structural constraints and opportunities of families and communities, the beliefs and values of parents, and the valuable contributions of the intervention." (p. 199).

Wilson (2006) conducted a study of 780 kindergarten and first grade children from seven rural low- to middle-class Pacific Northwest schools to evaluate behavior strategies the children used to gain entry to ongoing play. Strategies included wait and watch, eye contact, smile or laugh, approach, join in, imitate, agree, share, give information, request info, direct request, make "me" statement, make a feeling statement, disagree, demand, take toy, and be aggressive. Wilson found that aggressive/rejected children initially refrained from using aggressive entry strategies, but showed a steady increase in the use of such strategies after experiencing rejection. The author notes that the "inability to regulate negative affect may be an important mechanism in the peer relationship and conduct problems of these children. Frustration and other negative affect generated by social failure may result in a disorganization of previous levels of functioning, causing aggressive/rejected children to resort to entry behaviors that are well learned but inappropriate, such as aggression" (p. 474). Shyness and fear contributed to low-risk entry strategies, such as watching.

Guo and Lee (2010) conducted a qualitative study of 14 adult women with rheumatoid arthritis to explore the role of leisure in coping with stress. Findings indicated that participants utilized leisure to release stress. They used leisure to escape stress, to express negative emotions brought on by stress, to relax from stress, to enhance their moods, and as a means to be with friends and others to release stress. "This study provides evidence that leisure serves as a useful and unique agent and contributes to the rehabilitation process of people with RA" (p. 100).

Russoniello et al. (2008) conducted a study of 150 fourth grade students in North Carolina whose school was destroyed by flooding from Hurricane Floyd to assess the effectiveness of recreational therapy group interventions on symptoms of PTSD. Students received a five weekly recreational therapy interventions consisting of 60 minutes aimed at addressing emotional trauma, acting out behaviors,

and poor concentration on academic tasks. Sessions were conducted by trained recreational therapy students. Each session consisted of three 20-minute sessions. The first 20 minutes consisted of developmentally appropriate gross motor physical activity to promote concentration and on-task behavior in the classroom. The second 20-minutes contained didactic content designed to help the children become aware of PTSD symptoms and teach self-regulatory methods. Techniques included deep breathing; meditation; reversing negative and increasing positive thought processes; identifying, labeling, and appropriately processing emotions; and methods to improve how the students viewed themselves. Topics discussed included stress, identifying symptoms of stress, controlling emotions, diaphragmatic breathing, and positive thinking. During the remaining 20 minutes the children again engaged in gross motor physical activity aimed at applying the information learned and reinforcing the use of activity to reduce stress and promote healthy involvement with others. PTSD symptoms were significantly reduced from pre to post testing. There was an increased use of positive and decreased use of negative coping strategies.

***Cross References***

In *Recreational Therapy for Specific Diagnoses and Conditions, First Edition*, ICF code d2 General Tasks and Demands and its subcategories are listed in 38 chapters: Amputation and Prosthesis, Attention-Deficit/Hyperactivity Disorder, Autism Spectrum Disorder, Back Disorders and Back Pain, Borderline Personality Disorder, Burns, Cancer, Cerebral Palsy, Cerebrovascular Accident, Chronic Obstructive Pulmonary Disease, Diabetes Mellitus, Epilepsy, Feeding and Eating Disorders, Fibromyalgia and Juvenile Fibromyalgia, Gambling Disorder, Generalized Anxiety Disorder, Guillain-Barré Syndrome, Hearing Loss, Heart Disease, Intellectual Disability, Major Depressive Disorder, Multiple Sclerosis, Neurocognitive Disorders, Obesity, Oppositional Defiant Disorder and Conduct Disorder, Osteoarthritis, Osteoporosis, Parkinson's Disease, Post-Traumatic Stress Disorder, Rheumatoid Arthritis, Schizophrenia Spectrum and Other Psychotic Disorders, Sickle Cell Disease, Spina Bifida, Spinal Cord Injury, Substance-Related Disorders, Total Joint Replacement, Traumatic Brain Injury, and Visual Impairments and Blindness.

In *Recreational Therapy Basics, Techniques, and Interventions, First Edition*, treatment for ICF code d2 General Tasks and Demands and its subcategories are discussed in 36 chapters: Activity and Task Analysis, Adjustment and Response to Disability, Education and Counseling, Parameters and Precautions, Participation, Stress, Activity Pattern Development, Adaptive Sports, Adventure Therapy, Anger Management, Animal Assisted Therapy, Aquatic Therapy, Assertiveness Training, Balance Training, Behavior Strategies and Interventions, Bibliotherapy, Cognitive Behavioral Counseling, Cognitive Retraining and Rehabilitation, Community Problem Solving, Energy Conservation Techniques, Errorless Learning, Group Psychotherapy Techniques, Leisure-Based Stress Coping, Leisure Education and Counseling, Life Review, Medical Play and Preparation, Mind-Body Interventions, Montessori Method, Neuro-Developmental Treatment, Physical Activity, Reality Orientation, Sensory Interventions, Social Skills Training, Stress Management and Coping, Therapeutic Thematic Arts Programming, and Values Clarification.

### d210 Undertaking a Single Task

Carrying out simple or complex and coordinated actions related to the mental and physical components of a single task, such as initiating a task, organizing time, space, and materials for a task, pacing task performance, and carrying out, completing, and sustaining a task.

Inclusions: undertaking a simple or complex task; undertaking a single task independently or in a group

Exclusions: acquiring skills (d155); solving problems (d175); making decisions (d177); undertaking multiple tasks (d220)

- *d2100 Undertaking a Simple Task*
  Preparing, initiating, and arranging the time and space required for a simple task; executing a simple task with a single major component, such as reading a book, writing a letter, or making one's bed.

- *d2101 Undertaking a Complex Task*
  Preparing, initiating, and arranging the time and space for a single complex task; executing a complex task with more than one component, which may be carried out in sequence or simulta-

neously, such as arranging the furniture in one's home or completing an assignment for school.

- *d2102 Undertaking a Single Task Independently*
  Preparing, initiating, and arranging the time and space for a simple or complex task; managing and executing a task on one's own and without the assistance of others.

- *d2103 Undertaking a Single Task in a Group*
  Preparing, initiating, and arranging the time and space for a single task, simple or complex; managing and executing a task with people who are involved in some or all steps of the task.

- *d2108 Undertaking Single Tasks, Other Specified*
- *d2109 Undertaking Single Tasks, Unspecified*
  A single task can be either a very simple action such as turning on a light or a very complex task such as determining the area of a pentagram. A single task usually involves both mental and physical components. For example, when a client walks into a dark room s/he realizes that the light needs to be turned on so that s/he can see and reaches out for the wall switch to turn on the light. The actions required for a single task would include initiating the action; organizing the time needed, the space needed, and materials required for completing the action; maintaining a reasonable pace of activity; and sustaining the mental and physical actions needed to carry out and complete the activity.

The skill of undertaking a single task requires the use of many skills. This is why it is referred to as an *application* skill. All Activities and Participation categories are application skills. Undertaking a single task is the application of isolated skills related to body functions, such as voluntary movement and visual field functions. Therapists evaluate a client's ability to perform application skills, but to address the problem, the isolated skills that make up the task must be evaluated, problems clearly identified, and methods to improve the client's performance developed. To identify the specific isolated skills of a task, the therapist conducts a task analysis. Once specific deficits are identified, the therapist designs a treatment plan to restore, develop, or adapt for the problem. Consult the ICF codes in this book for information on a specific dysfunction.

Many clients need to have interventions directed at the level of undertaking a simple task. For example, clients with brain injuries, chronic mental illness, and developmental disabilities will often be working on this level. At this level the recreational therapist is likely to be teaching the client skills related to specific activities such as playing bingo, swimming, making a clay pot, ordering from a restaurant menu, making a phone call, playing cards, and yoga. Problems with d155 Acquiring Skills will probably also need to be addressed.

As clients increase their skill levels they will be better equipped to give their attention to more than one task at a time. If a client has been able to overlearn an activity skill, it will be easier for him/her to integrate more than one activity at a time. The therapist will help a client succeed if s/he does not push the client too fast into working on multiple tasks.

Recreational therapists document the extent of difficulty a client has with undertaking a single task. For example, client has mild difficulty undertaking the simple task of feeding the family dog at home when assistance is not provided (d2100._ _ _ 1).

### Cross References

In *Recreational Therapy for Specific Diagnoses and Conditions, First Edition*, ICF code d210 Undertaking a Single Task is listed in six chapters: Autism Spectrum Disorder, Intellectual Disability, Neurocognitive Disorders, Schizophrenia Spectrum and Other Psychotic Disorders, Spina Bifida, and Traumatic Brain Injury.

In *Recreational Therapy Basics, Techniques, and Interventions, First Edition*, treatment for ICF code d210 Undertaking a Single Task is discussed in eight chapters: Activity and Task Analysis, Stress, Adaptive Sports, Adventure Therapy, Aquatic Therapy, Errorless Learning, Mind-Body Interventions, and Social Skills Training.

### d220 Undertaking Multiple Tasks

Carrying out simple or complex and coordinated actions as components of multiple, integrated, and complex tasks in sequence or simultaneously.

Inclusions: undertaking multiple tasks; completing multiple tasks; undertaking multiple tasks independently and in a group

Exclusions: acquiring skills (d155); solving problems (d175); making decisions (d177); undertaking a single task (d210)

- *d2200 Carrying Out Multiple Tasks*
  Preparing, initiating, and arranging the time and space needed for several tasks, and managing and executing several tasks, together or sequentially.

- *d2201 Completing Multiple Tasks*
  Completing several tasks, together or sequentially.

- *d2202 Undertaking Multiple Tasks Independently*
  Preparing, initiating, and arranging the time and space for multiple tasks, and managing and executing several tasks together or sequentially, on one's own and without the assistance of others.

- *d2203 Undertaking Multiple Tasks in a Group*
  Preparing, initiating, and arranging the time and space for multiple tasks, and managing and executing several tasks together or sequentially with others who are involved in some or all steps of the multiple tasks.

- *d2208 Undertaking Multiple Tasks, Other Specified*

- *d2209 Undertaking Multiple Tasks, Unspecified*

In a clinical setting (either inpatient or outpatient) the types of challenges that a therapist presents to clients tend to be single task challenge. This is because it is easier to evaluate a client's actual skill level when the therapist has to look at one skill at a time. However, life in the community is seldom that simple and planned. The ability to juggle many different demands at the same time requires a complex set of skills that are hard to define and harder to measure. Often, when a client fails to complete multiple tasks, it is hard for the therapist to determine if the client failed because s/he was not able to perform a specific skill in one of the many tasks being evaluated or if s/he was not able to integrate the "higher level" skill of planning and coordinating multiple tasks.

As an example, the therapist sets up a situation in which a group of clients are in the kitchen making a complete meal. One group of clients is responsible for preparing the chef salad, another group is responsible for making cornbread, and a third group is responsible for making chocolate chip cookies. One of the clients making the cookies, Barbara, is given the task of listening to Steve (another client) read the recipe out loud, measuring out the ingredients, and mixing the cookie dough. When the dinner is all done and the cookies baked, everyone takes one bite and spits the cookie out. It appears that Barbara put in two *tablespoons* of salt instead of one-eighth *teaspoon* of salt. Did Barbara fail to measure the salt correctly because she could not handle a set of tasks read to her step-by-step (d2103 Undertaking a Single Task in a Group) or did she get distracted because of others working on different tasks (d2203 Undertaking Multiple Tasks in a Group)? In the first case the impairment may be related to listening, reading, or a lack of basic kitchen skills. In the second case the impairment may be related to an inability to execute a sequential attention span (being able to pay attention to one task, move on to the next task, ignoring things she didn't need to pay attention to, and so forth), an inability to prioritize actions, or a lack of ability to observe someone else using a tablespoon to measure salt for the cornbread while she needed to use a quarter teaspoon to measure salt for the cookies.

Because many of the tasks related to recreation and leisure involve multiple tasks, the recreational therapist needs to become very skilled in observing clients engaged in multiple tasks and identifying the area(s) of impairment. It is important to distinguish an impairment because of a lack of skill related to a simple task from a lack of skill related to juggling multiple tasks. This is especially true for the therapist working with clients in a community setting.

The ICF makes a distinction between carrying out multiple tasks and completing multiple tasks. A client can be good at preparing, initiating, arranging time and space, and managing and executing several tasks, but that does not necessarily equate to being able to complete the tasks. For example, a client may be able to manage and carry out the tasks needed to organize a family vacation, including making phone calls for camping sites, evaluating the calendar and individual family members' schedules, and looking at a map. But that does not mean that the vacation gets fully planned and carried out. The ability to complete several tasks together or sequentially often requires greater integration of cognitive and personality traits, such as persistence, confidence, and problem solving.

The observation of failure in carrying out, undertaking, or completing multiple tasks will require the therapist to conduct a task analysis to further determine the specific dysfunction hindering capacity or performance. Once the specific dysfunction is identified, the therapist identifies and implements a treatment plan to optimize functioning.

This is the level where many recreational therapists address a client's ability to engage in leisure activities, including the steps needed to get to the movie theater, take a trip downtown to go shopping, or go to a baseball game. The *Community Integration Program* (Armstrong & Lauzen, 1994) is a set of twenty-two assessment and treatment protocol modules used by recreational therapists to address skills at the multiple task level. This is also an appropriate level to work on the concept of leisure balance: that the combined set of leisure activities the client engages in on a regular basis is balanced between physical, cognitive, social, and emotional development opportunities.

Just as the progression from undertaking a simple task to undertaking multiple tasks represents the skills to take an action and execute it in a progressively more complex and stimulating situation, the move from undertaking multiple tasks to carrying out a daily routine represents another significant jump in ability.

Recreational therapists document the extent of difficulty a client has with undertaking multiple tasks. For example, client has moderate difficulty undertaking multiple tasks independently when preparing a meal for her friends at home (d2202._ _ _ 2).

### Cross References

In *Recreational Therapy for Specific Diagnoses and Conditions, First Edition*, ICF code d220 Undertaking Multiple Tasks is listed in five chapters: Autism Spectrum Disorder, Intellectual Disability, Neurocognitive Disorders, Schizophrenia Spectrum and Other Psychotic Disorders, and Spina Bifida.

In *Recreational Therapy Basics, Techniques, and Interventions, First Edition*, treatment for ICF code d220 Undertaking Multiple Tasks is discussed in five chapters: Activity and Task Analysis, Stress, Aquatic Therapy, Mind-Body Interventions, and Social Skills Training.

### d230 Carrying Out Daily Routine

Carrying out simple or complex and coordinated actions in order to plan, manage, and complete the requirements of day-to-day procedures or duties, such as budgeting time and making plans for separate activities throughout the day.

Inclusions: managing and completing the daily routine; managing one's own activity level

Exclusion: undertaking multiple tasks (d220)

- *d2301 Managing Daily Routine*
  Carrying out simple or complex and coordinated actions in order to plan and manage the requirements of day-to-day procedures or duties.

- *d2302 Completing the Daily Routine*
  Carrying out simple or complex and coordinated actions in order to complete the requirements of day-to-day procedures or duties.

- *d2303 Managing One's Own Activity Level*
  Carrying out actions and behaviors to arrange the requirements in energy and time day-to-day procedures or duties.

- *d2308 Carrying Out Daily Routine, Other Specified*
- *d2309 Carrying Out Daily Routine, Unspecified*

Once a client has managed to undertake and complete a single task and multiple tasks, the next step up in complexity is being able to carry out a daily routine. This includes the client's ability to follow routines, manage a daily routine, and subsequently complete a daily routine. As part of the daily routine, this code grouping also covers the client's ability to manage his/her energy and respond to changes in the daily routine, as well as manage time and adapt to time demands.

While undertaking a simple task generally relates to having the skills necessary to carry out a specific activity, such as walking to the store, and undertaking multiple tasks generally relates to having the ability to sequentially pay attention to and carry out numerous activities at one time, such as talking to a friend who is walking with you to the store or creating a shopping list as you walk, carrying out a daily routine generally relates to how well you are able to get done what needs to get done. This includes making sure that you go to the store in time to fix dinner, arranging with your friend to walk with you, and ensuring that you have a means to pay for the food.

Just as with d220 Undertaking Multiple Tasks, the ICF makes a distinction between managing (d2301 Managing Daily Routine) and completing (d2302 Completing the Daily Routine). Managing daily routine refers to the client's ability to carry out

actions in order to plan and manage his/her daily responsibilities and duties. This might include making a to-do list, looking at all of the tasks of the day and arranging them in an optimal manner, considering transportation schedules that affect abilities to carry out tasks, considering the impact of tasks on other tasks that need to be done, and actually carrying out multiple tasks. This is different from completing a daily routine, which reflects the client's ability to follow through and accomplish all of the daily routine.

Within the daily routine, there are also additional challenges, such as managing activity level. We only have so much energy and time to do what we want or need to do. It is not about managing the routine or completing the routine, but the client's ability to arrange actions and behaviors to allow for time and energy constraints. For example, a client with multiple sclerosis may be able to plan and manage a daily routine and even complete it, but at the end of the day she is so fatigued that she is having multiple falls. Clients who have disorders that impact their energy level, such as multiple sclerosis, chronic fatigue syndrome, fibromyalgia, and bipolar disorder, have to pay particular attention to the impact of their activity level on health. Clients with disorders that impact their ability to remember all that needs to be done, such as clients with early Alzheimer's disease, autism, or stroke, will be working on adaptations to keep track of all the tasks.

Engaging in a daily routine also requires flexibility. For example, the client may need to manage changes in the daily routine, manage time if a task takes longer than expected, and adapt to other time demands, such as eating breakfast on the run to be at work on time.

Therapists are aware of the secondary problems caused by poor management and execution of a daily routine and activity level, such as increased stress and inappropriate demands on the physical, mental, social, and emotional functions. Therapists are also careful to fully evaluate the dysfunction to find underlying causes in the daily routine and activity level that can be remediated. Specific treatment interventions will vary depending on the individual needs of the client.

Recreational therapists document the extent of difficulty a client has with carrying out a daily routine. For example, client has severe difficulty managing one's activity level to prevent adverse when alone at home (d2303._ _ _ 3).

### Cross References

In *Recreational Therapy for Specific Diagnoses and Conditions, First Edition*, ICF code d230 Carrying Out Daily Routine is listed in 22 chapters: Amputation and Prosthesis, Autism Spectrum Disorder, Back Disorders and Back Pain, Borderline Personality Disorder, Cancer, Cerebrovascular Accident, Epilepsy, Generalized Anxiety Disorder, Hearing Loss, Heart Disease, Intellectual Disability, Major Depressive Disorder, Multiple Sclerosis, Neurocognitive Disorders, Parkinson's Disease, Post-Traumatic Stress Disorder, Rheumatoid Arthritis, Spina Bifida, Spinal Cord Injury, Total Joint Replacement, Traumatic Brain Injury, and Visual Impairments and Blindness.

In *Recreational Therapy Basics, Techniques, and Interventions, First Edition*, treatment for ICF code d230 Carrying Out Daily Routine is discussed in 12 chapters: Stress, Activity Pattern Development, Balance Training, Community Problem Solving, Energy Conservation Techniques, Leisure Education and Counseling, Mind-Body Interventions, Neuro-Developmental Treatment, Reality Orientation, Sensory Interventions, Social Skills Training, and Values Clarification.

### d240 Handling Stress and Other Psychological Demands

Carrying out simple or complex and coordinated actions to manage and control the psychological demands required to carry out tasks demanding significant responsibilities and involving stress, distraction, or crises, such as driving a vehicle during heavy traffic or taking care of many children.

Inclusions: handling responsibilities; handling stress and crisis

- *d2400 Handling Responsibilities*
  Carrying out simple or complex and coordinated actions to manage the duties of task performance and to assess the requirements of these duties.

- *d2401 Handling Stress*
  Carrying out simple or complex and coordinated actions to cope with pressure, emergencies, or stress associated with task performance.

- *d2402 Handling Crisis*
  Carrying out simple or complex and coordinated actions to cope with decisive turning points in a situation or times of acute danger or difficulty.

- *d2408 Handling Stress and Other Psychological Demands, Other Specified*
- *d2409 Handling Stress and Other Psychological Demands, Unspecified*

This section looks at how the client handles the psychological demands required to carry out tasks. While carrying out a daily routine revolves around the self-management of time, resources, and duties, the ability to handle stress and other psychological demands is the ability to self-regulate responses to situations that tax the client's capabilities.

This code group defines the distinctions between, and increasing levels of difficulty of, handling responsibilities, stress, and crisis. Handling responsibilities is about doing the things for which one is accountable, such as feeding the dog, watching the kids play in the pool to make sure they are safe, or preparing meals for the family. Handling stress, such as functioning in a chaotic environment or meeting pressing deadlines, is more difficult. Handling crisis adds the element of potential harm from the situation, such as a health problem in the community or being in an unsafe environment.

Stress is a huge topic and a central feature of many of the treatments provided by recreational therapists. The companion book, *Recreational Therapy Basics, Techniques, and Interventions*, provides a chapter with background information about Stress and another chapter on techniques for Stress Management and Coping.

Recreational therapists document the extent of difficulty a client has with handling stress and other psychological demands. For example, client has moderate difficulty handling stress when playing sports in the community despite assistance from others (d2401._ _ _ 2).

### Cross References

In *Recreational Therapy for Specific Diagnoses and Conditions, First Edition*, ICF code d240 Handling Stress and Other Psychological Demands is listed in 36 chapters: Amputation and Prosthesis, Attention-Deficit/Hyperactivity Disorder, Autism Spectrum Disorder, Back Disorders and Back Pain, Borderline Personality Disorder, Burns, Cancer,

Cerebral Palsy, Cerebrovascular Accident, Chronic Obstructive Pulmonary Disease, Diabetes Mellitus, Epilepsy, Feeding and Eating Disorders, Fibromyalgia and Juvenile Fibromyalgia, Gambling Disorder, Generalized Anxiety Disorder, Guillain-Barré Syndrome, Hearing Loss, Heart Disease, Intellectual Disability, Major Depressive Disorder, Multiple Sclerosis, Neurocognitive Disorders, Obesity, Oppositional Defiant Disorder and Conduct Disorder, Osteoarthritis, Parkinson's Disease, Post-Traumatic Stress Disorder, Rheumatoid Arthritis, Schizophrenia Spectrum and Other Psychotic Disorders, Sickle Cell Disease, Spina Bifida, Spinal Cord Injury, Substance-Related Disorders, Traumatic Brain Injury, and Visual Impairments and Blindness.

In *Recreational Therapy Basics, Techniques, and Interventions, First Edition*, treatment for ICF code d240 Handling Stress and Other Psychological Demands is discussed in 23 chapters: Activity and Task Analysis, Adjustment and Response to Disability, Education and Counseling, Parameters and Precautions, Participation, Stress, Activity Pattern Development, Anger Management, Animal Assisted Therapy, Assertiveness Training, Bibliotherapy, Cognitive Behavioral Counseling, Group Psychotherapy Techniques, Leisure-Based Stress Coping, Leisure Education and Counseling, Life Review, Medical Play and Preparation, Montessori Method, Physical Activity, Reality Orientation, Social Skills Training, Stress Management and Coping, and Values Clarification.

### d298 General Tasks and Demands, Other Specified

### d299 General Tasks and Demands, Unspecified

### References
Armstrong, M. & Lauzen, S. (1994). *Community Integration Program.* Ravensdale, WA: Idyll Arbor.

Bernheimer, L. P. & Weisner, T. S. (2007). "Let me just tell you what I do all day...": The family story at the center of intervention research and practice. *Infants and Young Children, 20*(3), 192-201.

Guo, L. & Lee, Y. (2010). Examining the role of leisure in the process of coping with stress in adult women with rheumatoid arthritis. *Annual in Therapeutic Recreation, 18*, 100-113.

Richardson, J. C., Ong, B. N., & Sim, J. (2008). Experiencing and controlling time in everyday life with chronic widespread pain: A qualitative study, *BMC Musculoskeletal Disorders, 9*(3).

Russoniello, C. V., O'Brien, K., McGhee, S. A., & Skalko, T. K. (2008). Reducing symptoms of posttraumatic stress in children after a natural disaster: A recreational therapy intervention. *Annual in Therapeutic Recreation, XVI*, 15-28.

Sheldon, L. J., Kalichman, S. C., Carey, M. P., & Fielder, R. L. (2008). Stress management interventions for HIV+ adults: A meta-analysis of randomized controlled trials, 1989 to 2006. *Health Psychology, 27*(2), 129-139.

Wilson, B. J. (2006). The entry behavior of aggressive/rejected children: The contributions of status and temperament. *Social Development, 15*(3), 463-479.

# Chapter 3 Communication

This chapter is about general and specific features of communicating by language, signs, and symbols, including receiving and producing messages, carrying on conversations, and using communication devices and techniques.

### *Sample Scoring of Communication Codes*

- A client sustained a traumatic brain injury. In the clinic, when presented with simple verbal commands, such as raising his arm, the client responds with the correct action 60% of the time (severe difficulty = 3) despite his ability to perform such movements. Through clinical observation and additional testing the therapist determines that the problem is in d310 Communicating with — Receiving — Spoken Messages. With hand-over-hand assistance and demonstrative cues added to verbal commands, the client performs the actions 100% of the time (no difficulty = 0). The complete scoring for code d310 Communicating with — Receiving — Spoken Messages would look like this: d310._ 3 0 _.
- A client has schizophrenia. Secondary to delusions and hallucinations, the client has difficulty maintaining a conversation with another person in the clinic and in the community (d3550 Discussion with One Person). In the clinic, he has difficulty maintaining a conversation with a peer about 30% of the time (moderate difficulty = 2). With re-direction and cueing from the therapist, his difficulty reduces to about 20% of the time (mild difficulty = 1). In the community, his delusions and hallucinations are more frequent and intense resulting in 75% failure in maintaining a conversation with a peer (severe difficulty = 3). With re-direction and cueing from the therapist in the community, his difficulty is about 60% (severe difficulty = 3). The complete scoring for code d3550 Discussion with One Person would look like this: d3550.3 2 1 3.

Communication is the process of conveying information. The sender conveys verbal and non-verbal messages to the receiver. Ideally, the sender verifies that the receiver understood the message by observing the receiver's feedback, and sends new messages as needed until the receiver fully understands the message. Despite the best intentions from both the sender and the receiver, communication can be easily misunderstood due to many variables that affect this complex process — words and phrases can have various meanings; the sender or receiver may have social or communication impairments; communication equipment might fail; the environment might not be conducive to effective communication; interest in the message may vary thus impacting attention; information might be too complex; linguistic ability, dialect, and accent can cause confusion; and the emotional state of the people involved can get in the way.

Communication difficulties are not an isolated problem. Communication difficulties can impact engagement in life activities and ultimately affect quality of life. For example, a study by Davidson et al. (2008) compared older adults with aphasia to older adults who did not have aphasia. All of them lived independently in the community. Findings indicated that older adults with aphasia, when compared to their peers without aphasia, initiated conversation less, had fewer friends, had smaller social networks, visited a lesser variety of community places, had increased occurrences of communication breakdown, played more of a passive and listening role in group interactions and conversations, watched more television, had less involvement in sports and hobbies, and had fewer occurrences of initiating plans with friends. The authors noted that programs are needed to address social participation and quality of life for older adults in the community. The programs need to address these issues in acute and rehabilitative care and provide continued services post discharge. This is one example that highlights how an underlying communication problem impacts not only communication skills, but also leisure engagement, social skills, and quality of life.

Communication is also an integral component of the therapy process. When thinking about the skills a recreational therapist teaches a client, it is hard to think of any that don't require some form of communication. Physicians can treat illness without communicating with their clients, although treatment may not be optimal. Recreational therapists, on the other hand, are almost always working on activities that require explanation (receptive communication) or the client's interaction with others (expressive communication). Even the simple act of finding out what a client likes to do requires both of these kinds of communication.

### Assessment of Communication

In the absence of specific known Body Function issues and Environmental and Personal Factor barriers, assessing deficits and issues related to communication can be a complicated task. The therapist will note first that something is going wrong in the interaction. Perhaps questions are answered inappropriately, instructions may be consistently misunderstood, or psychological issues may get in the way of conversation and discussion. Most of these problems will be the result of deficits in Body Functions (most notably b1 Mental Functions and b3 Voice and Speech Functions), and/or Environmental and Personal Factors such as culture or communication devices. If a client exhibits a communication impairment in d3 Communication, further assess the client to determine the underlying Body Functions and/or Environmental and Personal Factors contributing to the impairment. Once the underlying and contributing impairments or issues have been identified, appropriate interventions can be planned and implemented.

The consequences of communication problems will be seen in many other areas of Activities and Participation. Some of the possible areas are given in this chapter, but be sure to look for other possibilities when working with a client.

### Treatment of Communication

Recreational therapists consult the client's speech therapist to identify recovery and compensatory treatment interventions that can be carried over into recreational therapy sessions. Recovery-based interventions may include the use of specific communication strategies, such as tapping one's finger on the table for each syllable when talking to help the client decrease his rate of speech, over pronunciation of each syllable to increase speech clarity, practicing specific words, syllables, or letter blends that relate to recreation and social speech, or "hollering" during conversation to increase speech volume. Compensatory strategies include the use of communication boards, augmentative communication devices, text to speech, use of gestures/body lan-

guage, writing, texting, signing, and other methods to communication that align with the client's strengths.

Recreational therapists are also aware of the variables in recreation and community activities that can impact communication skills. For example, when feeling stress, anxiety, or pressure to perform, speech production can be more difficult. For example, it can be difficult to find the right word or to slow down the rate of speech. These difficulties result in other problems, such as a withdrawal from recreation and community activities, which ultimately impacts health and quality of life. Within a social context, there are also other variables that effect communication skills, including peer expectations such as a "quick come back" to a remark or appropriate use slang. The social situation itself can also induce particular feelings and concerns that can hinder communication skills when a client feels too self-conscious to talk. Recreational therapists help clients problem solve for these variables and address underlying issues (e.g., self-confidence, assertiveness) with the goal of improving social communication skills.

### Evidence Review

Several studies are provided below to highlight evidence-based practice related to communication. This is only a sample of the evidence. A thorough review of the literature is needed to identify evidence-based practice interventions that reflect the needs and characteristics of an individual client.

Dahlberg et al. (2007) implemented a 12-session interdisciplinary social skills training program (12 weeks, 1.5 hours per week, eight participants at a time in the group). The treatment was based on *Social Skills and Traumatic Brain Injury: A Workbook for Group Treatment* by Hawley and Newman (2006). The 52 adults who participated in the study were one year post TBI, discharged from a TBI rehab program, Rancho Los Amigos VI or higher, and had sufficient recall skills. They also had an impairment in social communication skills. Follow-up was conducted at three, six, and nine months after program participation. Post participation, participants had improved social communication skills that were maintained at follow-up and overall life satisfaction improved. The sessions were

- Session 1: Group overview, learning the skills of a group communicator.

- Session 2: Self-assessment and goal setting.
- Session 3: Presenting yourself successfully and starting conversations.
- Session 4: Developing conversation strategies and using feedback.
- Session 5: Being assertive and solving problems.
- Session 6: Practice in the community.
- Session 7: Developing social confidence through positive self-talk.
- Session 8: Setting and respecting social boundaries.
- Session 9: Video taping and problem solving.
- Session 10: Video review and feedback.
- Session 11: Conflict resolution.
- Session 12: Closure and celebration.

DeRosier et al. (2011) implemented a 15-session social skills group to improve social skills and social relationships. The sessions lasted 15 weeks with one hour per week. The group was led by two professionals with experience in facilitating social skills development in children with high-level autism spectrum disorders (ASD). Twenty-seven eight-to-twelve-year-old children in the experimental group, along with their parents, received the intervention, while 28 matched children served as the control group. Sessions included didactic instruction combined with active practice, such as role playing, modeling, and hands-on activities. A manual was strictly followed. Concepts were reviewed and practiced in the sessions, as well as through community-based activities completed with the family. Children in the experimental group exhibited significantly greater mastery of social skills compared to children in the control group, particularly in the areas of social awareness, social communication, social motivation, and social mannerisms. Parents in the experimental group also reported greater self-efficacy for helping their children successfully navigate social situations compared to parents in the control group.

Kurtz and Mueser (2008) conducted a meta-analysis of randomized, controlled trials on social skills training (SST) for schizophrenia (22 studies, 1,521 clients). They found SST to be effective in improving social skills, daily living skills, community functioning, and reducing negative symptoms. SST was found to have a small effect on symptoms and relapse. Overall, the results support the efficacy of SST for improving psychosocial functioning in schizophrenia. Techniques that were found to be helpful in SST included role playing, practicing behaviors, social reinforcement, and willingness of the individual to use existing skills. Interestingly, role-play tests are strongly related to overall psychosocial functioning in schizophrenia.

Goldstein and Schwade (2008) conducted a study of sixty 9.5-month-old children without disability. Mothers were asked to provide models of vocal production timed to be either contingent or non-contingent on their infant's babbling. Infants that received contingent feedback quickly restructured their babbling to incorporate phonological patterns from their mother's speech, whereas the infants that received non-contingent feedback did not. Consequently, infants learned new vocal forms by discovering phonological patterns in their mother's contingent speech and then generalizing from these patterns. The authors noted that "in our view, infants' pre-linguistic vocalizations, and caregivers' reactions to those immature sounds, create opportunities for social learning that affords infants knowledge of phonology. Socially guided learning is thus an important mechanism in early vocal development, laying the foundation for advances in communication and language" (p. 522).

Crawford, Gray, and Woolhiser (2012) conducted a longitudinal study of 11 individuals aged 12-15 diagnosed with high-level autism and/or Asperger's. The children participated in a public school social skills training program conducted by recreational therapists. Students received weekly individual social skills development sessions that focused on social deficits and skill acquisition. Following the session, leisure education homework and practice sessions were assigned to the students and their parents and teachers through regularly scheduled meetings, phone conversations, and a social skills notebook. Homework assignments were frequently associated with bi-monthly social clubs. The participants would be asked, for example, to introduce themselves to someone new or practice scripted social invitations. A notebook was continuously updated with social experiences to act as a prompt for conversations. Field trips were provided with a trio of students to work on targeted behaviors in a real-life environment and receive feedback. Teachers additionally monitored quality and frequency of social interactions with peers. The focus of individual sessions changed based on the collective record of social performance. The program ran year round to minimize atrophy of skills. For example, during the summer, individual sessions occurred in the student's home or public library and bi-monthly field trips continued. Two case studies are reviewed in depth to highlight the positive outcomes of the program. A subsequent manuscript will be written to highlight data outcomes.

***Cross References***

In *Recreational Therapy for Specific Diagnoses and Conditions, First Edition*, ICF code d3 Communication and its subcategories are listed in 14 chapters: Autism Spectrum Disorder, Borderline Personality Disorder, Cerebral Palsy, Cerebrovascular Accident, Hearing Loss, Intellectual Disability, Major Depressive Disorder, Multiple Sclerosis, Neurocognitive Disorders, Oppositional Defiant Disorder and Conduct Disorder, Schizophrenia Spectrum and Other Psychotic Disorders, Sickle Cell Disease, Traumatic Brain Injury, and Visual Impairments and Blindness.

In *Recreational Therapy Basics, Techniques, and Interventions, First Edition*, treatment for ICF code d3 Communication and its subcategories are discussed in 12 chapters: Activity and Task Analysis, Adventure Therapy, Anger Management, Animal Assisted Therapy, Aquatic Therapy, Assertiveness Training, Bibliotherapy, Cognitive Behavioral Counseling, Cognitive Retraining and Rehabilitation, Montessori Method, Social Skills Training, and Therapeutic Thematic Arts Programming.

## Communicating — Receiving (d310 - d329)

### d310 Communicating with — Receiving — Spoken Messages

Comprehending literal and implied meanings of messages in spoken language, such as understanding that a statement asserts a fact or is an idiomatic expression.

Communicating with — Receiving — Spoken Messages is commonly scored by recreational therapists in the context of functional activities, such as play, recreation, leisure, and community activities. Comprehending literal and implied meanings of messages in spoken language requires the integration

of many skills including b230 Hearing Functions, b1670 Reception of Language, b140 Attention Functions, and b1560 Auditory Perception. Deficits could affect functioning in other activities, such as d6200 Shopping, d660 Assisting Others, all the skills listed in d7 Interpersonal Interactions and Relationships, and all the skills in d9 Community, Social, and Civic Life.

If deficits are noted in this area, conduct a task analysis to determine the specific problem areas and then refer to the related codes in this book for further guidance on how to assess, treat, document, and adapt for the dysfunctions found.

Recreational therapists document the extent of difficulty a client has. For example, a client has mild difficulty comprehending simple statements during therapy sessions when assistance is not provided (d310._ 1 _ _).

***Cross References***

In *Recreational Therapy for Specific Diagnoses and Conditions, First Edition*, ICF code d310 Communicating with — Receiving — Spoken Messages is listed in two chapters: Hearing Loss and Schizophrenia Spectrum and Other Psychotic Disorders.

In *Recreational Therapy Basics, Techniques, and Interventions, First Edition*, treatment for ICF code d310 Communication with — Receiving — Spoken Messages is discussed in two chapters: Activity and Task Analysis and Social Skills Training.

### d315 Communicating with — Receiving — Nonverbal Messages

Comprehending the literal and implied meanings of messages conveyed by gestures, symbols, and drawings, such as realizing that a child is tired when she rubs her eyes or that a warning bell means that there is a fire.

Inclusions: communicating with — receiving — body gestures, general signs and symbols, drawings, and photographs

- *d3150 Communicating with — Receiving — Body Gestures*
  Comprehending the meaning conveyed by facial expressions, hand movements or signs, body postures, and other forms of body language.

- *d3151 Communicating with — Receiving — General Signs and Symbols*
  Comprehending the meaning represented by public signs and symbols, such as traffic signs, warning symbols, musical or scientific notations, and icons.

- *d3152 Communicating with — Receiving — Drawings and Photographs*
  Comprehending the meaning represented by drawings (e.g., line drawings, graphic designs, paintings, three-dimensional representations), graphs, charts, and photographs such as understanding that an upward line on a height chart indicates that a child is growing.

- *d3158 Communicating with — Receiving — Nonverbal Messages, Other Specified*

- *d3159 Communicating with — Receiving — Nonverbal Messages, Unspecified*

Communication with — Receiving — Nonverbal Messages is commonly scored by recreational therapists in the context of functional activities such as play, recreation, leisure, and community activities. Comprehending the literal and implied meanings of messages conveyed by gestures, symbols, and drawings requires the integration of many skills including b1672 Integrative Language Functions, b210 Seeing Functions, b140 Attention Functions, b1561 Visual Perception, b1640 Abstraction, and, perhaps, b16702 Reception of Sign Language. Deficits could affect functioning in other activities, such as d350 Conversation, d860 Basic Economic Transactions, d9201 Sports, and d475 Driving.

If deficits are noted in this area, conduct a task analysis to determine the specific problem areas and then refer to the related codes in this book for further guidance on how to assess, treat, document, and adapt for the dysfunction found. Document the treatment using both this code and the code for the specific problem area being treated.

Recreational therapists document the extent of difficulty a client has. For example, a client has moderate difficulty comprehending body language of peers in a community setting when assistance is not provided (d3150._ _ _ 2).

### Cross References

In *Recreational Therapy for Specific Diagnoses and Conditions, First Edition*, ICF code d315 Communicating with — Receiving — Nonverbal Messages is listed in three chapters: Autism Spectrum Disorder, Schizophrenia Spectrum and Other Psychotic Disorders, and Visual Impairments and Blindness.

In *Recreational Therapy Basics, Techniques, and Interventions, First Edition*, treatment for ICF code d315 Communicating with — Receiving — Nonverbal Messages is discussed in one chapter: Social Skills Training.

### d320 Communicating with — Receiving — Formal Sign Language Messages

Receiving and comprehending messages in formal sign language with literal and implied meaning.

Communicating with — Receiving — Formal Sign Language Messages is commonly scored by recreational therapists in the context of functional activities, such as play, recreation, leisure, and community activities. Receiving and comprehending messages in formal sign language with literal and implied meaning requires the integration of many skills including b140 Attention Functions, b144 Memory Functions, and b16702 Reception of Sign Language. Deficits could affect functioning in other activities such as d350 Conversation, d140 Learning to Read, d810 - d839 Education, and d920 Recreation and Leisure.

If deficits are noted in this area, conduct a task analysis to determine the specific problem areas and then refer to the related codes in this book for further guidance on how to assess, treat, document, and adapt for the dysfunction found. Document the treatment using both this code and the code for the specific problem area being treated.

Recreational therapists document the extent of difficulty a client has. For example, a client has mild difficulty comprehending simple sign language in the clinic when assistance is not provided (d320._ 1 _ _).

### Cross References

In *Recreational Therapy for Specific Diagnoses and Conditions, First Edition*, there are no references for ICF code d320 Communicating with — Receiving — Formal Sign Language Messages.

In *Recreational Therapy Basics, Techniques, and Interventions, First Edition*, there are no references for ICF code d320 Communicating with — Receiving — Formal Sign Language Messages.

### d325 Communicating with — Receiving — Written Messages

Comprehending the literal and implied meanings of messages that are conveyed through written language (including Braille), such as following political events in the daily newspaper or understanding the intent of religious scripture.

Communicating with — Receiving — Written Messages is commonly scored by recreational therapists in the context of functional activities such as recreation, leisure, and community activities. Comprehending the literal and implied meanings of messages that are conveyed through written language (including Braille) requires the integration of many skills such as b140 Attention Functions, b144 Memory Functions, b16701 Reception of Written Language, and b210 Seeing Functions (b1564 Tactile Perception for Braille). Deficits could affect functioning in other activities including d166 Reading, d6200 Shopping, and, if reading skills are needed to understand craft directions, d9203 Crafts.

If deficits are noted in this area, conduct a task analysis to determine the specific problem areas and then refer to the related codes in this book for further information on how to assess, treat, document, and adapt for the dysfunction found. Document the treatment using both this code and the code for the specific problem area being treated.

Recreational therapists document the extent of difficulty a client has. For example, client has severe difficulty comprehending short written stories in the clinic when assistance is not provided (d325._3 _ _).

### Cross References

In *Recreational Therapy for Specific Diagnoses and Conditions, First Edition*, ICF code d325 Communicating with — Receiving — Written Messages is listed in one chapter: Schizophrenia Spectrum and Other Psychotic Disorders.

In *Recreational Therapy Basics, Techniques, and Interventions, First Edition*, treatment for ICF code d325 Communicating with — Receiving — Written Messages is discussed in two chapters: Activity and Task Analysis and Social Skills Training.

### d329 Communicating — Receiving, Other Specified or Unspecified

## Communicating — Producing (d330 - d349)

### d330 Speaking

Producing words, phrases, and longer passages in spoken messages with literal and implied meaning, such as expressing a fact or telling a story in oral language.

Speaking is commonly scored by recreational therapists in the context of functional activities such as play, recreation, leisure, and community activities. Producing words, phrases, and longer passages in spoken messages with literal and implied meaning, requires the integration of many skills including b160 Thought Functions, b1641 Organization and Planning, and b16710 Expression of Spoken Language. Deficits in d330 Speaking could affect functioning in many other activities, including d355 Discussion, d620 Acquisition of Goods and Services, d7200 Forming Relationships, d845 Acquiring, Keeping, and Terminating a Job, d9205 Socializing, and d910 Community Life.

If deficits are noted in this area, conduct a task analysis to determine the specific problem areas and then refer to the related codes in this book for further guidance on how to assess, treat, document, and adapt for the dysfunction found. Document the treatment using both this code and the code for the specific problem area being treated.

Recreational therapists document the extent of difficulty a client has with speaking. For example, client has mild difficulty producing words when under stress in a community setting when assistance is not provided (d330._ _ _ 1).

### Cross References

In *Recreational Therapy for Specific Diagnoses and Conditions, First Edition*, ICF code d330 Speaking is listed in two chapters: Hearing Loss and Schizophrenia Spectrum and Other Psychotic Disorders.

In *Recreational Therapy Basics, Techniques, and Interventions, First Edition*, treatment for ICF code d330 Speaking is discussed in three chapters: Activity and Task Analysis, Montessori Method, and Social Skills Training.

### d335 Producing Nonverbal Messages

Using gestures, symbols, and drawings to convey messages, such as shaking one's head to indicate disagreement or drawing a picture or diagram to convey a fact or complex idea.

Inclusions: producing body gestures, signs, symbols, drawings, and photographs

- *d3350 Producing Body Language*
  Conveying messages by movements of the body, such as facial gestures (e.g., smiling, frowning, wincing), arm and hand movements, and postures (e.g., embracing to indicate affection).

- *d3351 Producing Signs and Symbols*
  Conveying meaning by using signs and symbols (e.g., icons, Bliss board, scientific symbols) and symbolic notations systems, such as using musical notation to convey a melody.

- *d3352 Producing Drawings and Photographs*
  Conveying meaning by drawing, painting, sketching, and making diagrams, pictures, or photographs, such as drawing a map to give someone directions to a location.

- *d3358 Producing Nonverbal Messages, Other Specified*

- *d3359 Producing Nonverbal Messages, Unspecified*

Producing Nonverbal Messages is commonly scored by recreational therapists in the context of functional activities such as play, recreation, leisure, and community activities. Using gestures, symbols, and drawings to convey messages requires the integration of many skills including b160 Thought Functions, b1641 Organization and Planning, skills listed in b7 Neuromusculoskeletal and Movement-Related Functions to make physical gestures, and b1672 Integrative Language Functions. Deficits could affect functioning in other activities such as d175 Solving Problems, d172 Calculating, d9201 Sports, d9203 Crafts, and d7200 Forming Relationships.

If deficits are noted in this area, conduct a task analysis to determine the specific problem areas and then refer to the related codes in this book for further guidance on how to assess, treat, document, and adapt for the dysfunction found. Document the treatment using both this code and the code for the specific problem area being treated.

Recreational therapists document the extent of difficulty a client has with producing nonverbal messages. For example, a client is unable to produce words and therefore commonly draws pictures and utilizes gestures to convey thoughts and needs. He has mild difficulty communicating in the clinic when assistance is not provided (d335._ 1 _ _).

### Cross References

In *Recreational Therapy for Specific Diagnoses and Conditions, First Edition*, ICF code d335 Producing Nonverbal Messages is listed in three chapters: Autism Spectrum Disorder, Schizophrenia Spectrum and Other Psychotic Disorders, and Visual Impairments and Blindness.

In *Recreational Therapy Basics, Techniques, and Interventions, First Edition*, treatment for ICF code d335 Producing Nonverbal Messages is discussed in three chapters: Activity and Task Analysis, Aquatic Therapy, and Social Skills Training.

### d340 Producing Messages in Formal Sign Language

Conveying, with formal sign language, literal and implied meaning.

Producing Messages in Formal Sign Language is commonly scored by recreational therapists in the context of functional activities such as play, recreation, leisure, and community activities. Conveying literal and implied meaning using formal sign language requires the integration of many skills including b710 Mobility of Joint Functions, b7202 Mobility of Carpal Bones, b735 Muscle Tone Functions, b765 Involuntary Movement Functions, b160 Thought Functions, b16712 Expression of Sign Language, and b1672 Integrative Language Functions. Deficits could affect functioning in other activities such as d7200 Forming Relationships, d910 Community Life, d9200 Play, d810 - d839 Education, and d840 - d859 Work and Employment.

If deficits are noted in this area, the recreational therapist conducts a task analysis to determine the specific problem areas and then refers to the related codes in this book for further guidance on how to assess, treat, document, and adapt for the dysfunction found. Document the treatment using both this code and the code for the specific problem area being treated.

Recreational therapists document the extent of difficulty a client has with producing messages in formal sign language. For example, client has mild difficulty producing messages using formal sign language with friends in the community when assistance is not provided (d340._ _ _ 1).

### Cross References

In *Recreational Therapy for Specific Diagnoses and Conditions, First Edition*, there are no references for ICF code d340 Producing Messages in Formal Sign Language.

In *Recreational Therapy Basics, Techniques, and Interventions, First Edition*, there are no references for ICF code d340 Producing Messages in Formal Sign Language.

### d345 Writing Messages

Producing the literal and implied meanings of messages that are conveyed through written language, such as writing a letter to a friend.

Writing Messages is commonly scored by recreational therapists in the context of functional activities such as play, recreation, leisure, and community activities. Producing the literal and implied meanings of messages that are conveyed through written language requires the integration of the skills listed in b7 Neuromusculoskeletal and Movement-Related Functions related to using the hand for writing such as b710 Mobility of Joint Functions and b735 Muscle Tone Functions. Other required skills include d440 Fine Hand Use for picking up, grasping, manipulating, and releasing a writing utensil; d170 Writing; and b16711 Expression of Written Language. Deficits could affect functioning in other activities such as d810 - d839 Education, d840 - d859 Work and Employment, and d660 Assisting Others.

If deficits are noted in this area, conduct a task analysis to determine the specific problem areas and then refer to the related codes in this book for further guidance on how to assess, treat, document, and adapt for the dysfunction found. Document the treatment using both this code and the code for the specific problem area being treated.

Recreational therapists document the extent of difficulty a client has with writing messages. For example, client has mild difficulty writing personalized notes to family and friends when assistance is not provided at home (d345._ _ _ 1).

### Cross References

In *Recreational Therapy for Specific Diagnoses and Conditions, First Edition*, ICF code d345 Writing Messages is listed in one chapter: Schizophrenia Spectrum and Other Psychotic Disorders.

In *Recreational Therapy Basics, Techniques, and Interventions, First Edition*, treatment for ICF code d345 Writing Messages is discussed in two chapters: Activity and Task Analysis and Social Skills Training.

## d349 Communication — Producing, Other Specified and Unspecified

## Conversation and Use of Communication Devices and Techniques (d350 - d369)

### d350 Conversation

Starting, sustaining, and ending an interchange of thoughts and ideas, carried out by means of spoken, written, sign, or other forms of language, with one or more people one knows or who are strangers, in formal or casual settings.

Inclusions: Starting, sustaining, and ending a conversation; conversing with one or many people

- *d3500 Starting a Conversation*
  Beginning a dialogue or interchange, such as by introducing oneself, expressing customary greetings, and introducing a topic or asking questions.

- *d3501 Sustaining a Conversation*
  Continuing and shaping a dialogue or interchange by adding ideas, introducing a new topic or retrieving a topic that has been previously mentioned, as well as by taking turns in speaking or signing.

- *d3502 Ending a Conversation*
  Finishing a dialogue or interchange with customary termination statements or expressions and by bringing closure to the topic under discussion.

- *d3503 Conversing with One Person*
  Initiating, maintaining, shaping, and terminating a dialogue or interchange with one person, such as in discussing the weather with a friend.

- *d3504 Conversing with Many People*
  Initiating, maintaining, shaping, and terminating a dialogue or interchange with more than one individual, such as in starting and participating in a group interchange.

- *d3508 Conversation, Other Specified*
- *d3509 Conversation, Unspecified*

Conversation is commonly scored by recreational therapists in the context of functional activities such as play, recreation, leisure, and community activities. This code requires the integration of many skills including b110 Consciousness Functions, b122 Global Psychosocial Functions, b1260 Extraversion, b1304 Impulse Control, b140 Attention Functions, b144 Memory Functions, b1560 Auditory Perception, b1561 Visual Perception, b1603 Control of Thought, and many more. Deficits could affect functioning in other activities including d910 Community Life, d810 - d839 Education, d840 - d859 Work and Employment, d660 Assisting Others, d9205 Socializing, d9201 Sports, d9300 Organized Religion, d7200 Forming Relationships, and d770 Intimate Relationships.

If deficits are noted in this area, conduct a task analysis to determine the specific problem areas and then refer to the related codes in this book for further guidance on how to assess, treat, document, and adapt for the dysfunction found. Document the treatment using both this code and the code for the specific problem area being treated.

Recreational therapists document the extent of difficulty a client has with conversation. For example, client has moderate difficulty sustaining a conversation with the therapist during therapy sessions despite prompting from therapist (d3501._ _ 2 _).

### Cross References

In *Recreational Therapy for Specific Diagnoses and Conditions, First Edition*, ICF code d350 Conversation is listed in six chapters: Autism Spectrum Disorder, Borderline Personality Disorder, Hearing Loss, Major Depressive Disorder, Schizophrenia Spectrum and Other Psychotic Disorders, and Traumatic Brain Injury.

In *Recreational Therapy Basics, Techniques, and Interventions, First Edition*, treatment for ICF code d350 Conversation is discussed in three chapters: Activity and Task Analysis, Community Participa-

tion: Integration, Transitioning, and Inclusion, and Social Skills Training.

### *d355 Discussion*

Starting, sustaining, and ending an examination of a matter, with arguments for or against, or debate carried out by means of spoken, written, sign, or other forms of language, with one or more people one knows or who are strangers, in formal or casual settings.

Inclusions: discussion with one person or many people

- *d3550 Discussion with One Person*
  Initiating, maintaining, shaping, or terminating an argument or debate with one person.

- *d3551 Discussion with Many People*
  Initiating, maintaining, shaping, or terminating an argument or debate with more than one individual.

- *d3558 Discussion, Other Specified*
- *d3559 Discussion, Unspecified*

Discussion is commonly scored by recreational therapists in the context of functional activities such as play, recreation, leisure, and community activities. Discussion requires the integration of many skills including b110 Consciousness Functions, b122 Global Psychosocial Functions, b1260 Extraversion, b1304 Impulse Control, b140 Attention Functions, b144 Memory Functions, b1560 Auditory Perception, b1561 Visual Perception, b1603 Control of Thought, and many more. Deficits could affect functioning in other activities such as d910 Community Life, d810 - d839 Education, d840 - d859 Work and Employment, d9201 Sports, d9300 Organized Religion, d7200 Forming Relationships, and d770 Intimate Relationships.

If deficits are noted in this area, conduct a task analysis to determine the specific problem areas and then refer to the related codes in this book for further guidance on how to assess, treat, document, and adapt for the dysfunction found. Document the treatment using both this code and the code for the specific problem area being treated.

Recreational therapists document the extent of difficulty a client has with discussion. For example, client has mild difficulty initiating a discussion with one person when attending activities at the local senior center when assistance is not provided (d3550._ _ _ 1).

### Cross References

In *Recreational Therapy for Specific Diagnoses and Conditions, First Edition*, ICF code d355 Discussion is listed in three chapters: Borderline Personality Disorder, Oppositional Defiant Disorder and Conduct Disorder, and Traumatic Brain Injury.

In *Recreational Therapy Basics, Techniques, and Interventions, First Edition*, treatment for ICF code d355 Discussion is discussed in one chapter: Social Skills Training.

## d360 Using Communication Devices and Techniques

Using devices, techniques, and other means for the purposes of communicating, such as calling a friend on the telephone.

Inclusions: using telecommunication devices, using writing machines and communication techniques

- *d3600 Using Telecommunication Devices*
  Using telephones and other machines, such as facsimile or telex machines, as a means of communication.

- *d3601 Using Writing Machines*
  Using machines for writing, such as typewriters, computers, and Braille writers, as a means of communication.

- *d3602 Using Communication Techniques*
  Performing actions and tasks involved in techniques for communicating, such as reading lips.

- *d3608 Using Communication Devices and Techniques, Other Specified*
- *d3609 Using Communication Devices and Techniques, Unspecified*

Using Communication Devices and Techniques is commonly scored by recreational therapists in the context of functional activities such as play, recreation, leisure, and community activities. Using devices, techniques, and other means for the purposes of communicating requires the integration of many skills including b140 Attention Functions, b144 Memory Functions, b1564 Tactile Perception, b210 Seeing Functions, b230 Hearing Functions, b2702 Sensitivity to Pressure, and b3 Voice and Speech Functions. ICF codes in b7 Neuromusculoskeletal

and Movement-Related Functions also plays a role when these functions are needed to operate the specific communication device. Look especially at b710 Mobility of Joint Functions, b730 Muscle Power Functions, b735 Muscle Tone Functions, b760 Control of Voluntary Movement Functions, and b765 Involuntary Movement Functions. Deficits could affect functioning in other activities such as d350 Conversation, d355 Discussion, d155 Acquiring Skills, d175 Solving Problems, d2402 Handling Crisis, d7200 Forming Relationships, d910 Community Life, d810 - d839 Education, and d840 - d859 Work and Employment.

If deficits are noted in this area, conduct a task analysis to determine the specific problem areas and then refer to the related codes in this book for further information on how to assess, treat, document, and adapt for the dysfunction found. Document the treatment using both this code and the code for the specific problem area being treated.

Recreational therapists document the extent of difficulty a client has with using communication devices and techniques. For example, client has moderate difficulty communicating with friends on the computer through Facebook in the clinic when assistance is not provided (d3601._ 1 _ _).

### Cross References

In *Recreational Therapy for Specific Diagnoses and Conditions, First Edition*, ICF code d360 Using Communication Devices and Techniques is listed in four chapters: Hearing Loss, Intellectual Disability, Multiple Sclerosis, and Traumatic Brain Injury.

In *Recreational Therapy Basics, Techniques, and Interventions, First Edition*, treatment for ICF code d360 Using Communication Devices and Techniques is discussed in two chapters: Activity and Task Analysis and Social Skills Training.

## d369 Conversation and Use of Communication Devices and Techniques, Other Specified and Unspecified

## d398 Communication, Other Specified

## d399 Communication, Unspecified

### References

Crawford, M. E., Gray, C., & Woolhiser, J. (2012). Design and delivery of a public school social skills training program for youth with autism spectrum disorders: A five year retrospective of the school/community/home (SCH) model of social skills development. *Annual in Therapeutic Recreation, 20,* 17-35.

Damon, W., Lerner, R. M., Kuhn, D., & Siegler, R. (2006). *Handbook of child psychology*, 6th edition. New York: John Wiley & Sons.

Dahlberg, C. A., Cusick, C. P., Hawley, L. A., Newman, J. K., Morey, C. E., Harrison-Felix, C. L., & Whiteneck, G. G. (2007). Treatment efficacy of social communication skills training after traumatic brain injury: A randomized treatment and deferred treatment controlled trial. *Arch Phys Med Rehabil, 88,* 1561-1573.

Davidson, B., Howe, T., Worrall, L., Hickson, L., & Togher, L. (2008). Social participation for older people with aphasia: The impact of communication disability on friendships. *Topics in Stroke Rehabilitation, 15*(4), 325-340.

DeRosier, M. E., Swick, D. C., Ornstein Davis, L., Sturtz McMillen, J., & Matthews, R. (2011). The efficacy of a social skills group intervention for improving social behaviors in children with high functioning autism spectrum disorders. *J Autism Dev Disord, 41,* 1033-1043.

Kurtz, M. M. & Mueser, K. T. (2008). A meta-analysis of controlled research on social skills training for schizophrenia. *Journal of Consulting and Clinical Psychology, 76*(3), 491-504.

Goldstein, M. H. & Schwade, J. A. (2008). Social feedback to infant's babbling facilitates rapid phonological learning. *Psychological Science, 19*(5), 515-523.

Hawley, L. & Newman, J. (2006). *Social skills and traumatic brain injury: A workbook for group treatment.* Denver: author.

Machado, J. M. & Machado, C. (2012). *Early childhood experiences in language arts: Early literacy.* Cengage Learning.

Mayo Clinic. (2012). Language development: Speech milestones for babies. Accessed via website http://www.mayoclinic.com/health/infant-development/AN01026.

NICHCY. (2010). Developmental milestones. Accessed via website http://nichcy.org/disability/milestones.

Shulman, B. B. & Capone, N. C. (2010). *Language development: Foundations, processes, and clinical implications.* Burlington, MA: Jones & Bartlett Publishers.

# Chapter 4 Mobility

This chapter is about moving by changing body position or location or by transferring from one place to another, by carrying, moving, or manipulating objects, by walking, running, or climbing, and by using various forms of transportation.

### *Sample Scoring of Mobility*

- In the clinic, the recreational therapist practices car transfers with a client — wheelchair to car and vice versa (d4200 Transferring Oneself While Sitting). The ability to transfer unassisted would not be safe, therefore it is not performed. With assistance, the client requires 40% assistance from the therapist (moderate difficulty = 2). During community integration training, the client required 75% assistance from the therapist (severe difficulty = 3). The correct scoring of d4200 Transferring Oneself While Sitting would look like this: d4200.3 _ 2 _.
- In the community setting, a client is being evaluated for using public transportation (d4702 Using Public Motorized Transportation). He is able to perform 70% of the required skills and tasks (moderate difficulty = 2). With assistance from the therapist, he is able to perform all of the necessary skills and tasks (no difficulty = 0). The correct scoring of d4702 Using Public Motorized Transportation would look like this: d4702.0 _ _ 2.

Prior to 2001 the term mobility generally referred to the ability to move from one place to another. For example, the 2000 *Dorland's Illustrated Medical Dictionary* defined mobility as "capability of movement, or being moved" (p. 1122). Most aspects of mobility were assigned to the physical therapist, who worked with walking, mobility, and related adaptive equipment, such as wheelchairs, walkers, canes, and splints, to help the client move from one place to another.

The scope of the term mobility has been greatly expanded by the World Health Organization. Mobility now encompasses walking and moving, using transportation options, and participating in many different types of activities, such as catching and running.

The scope of practice for the recreational therapist includes many elements of mobility training and enhancement. While it is common for a physical therapist to determine the type of walking and moving appropriate for a client after a disabling condition, it is often the recreational therapist who helps the client problem solve barriers to mobility, especially related to moving around the community and using adaptive mobility equipment for sports and recreational activities. The recreational therapist uses his/her specialized knowledge to help the client integrate the equipment and techniques into everyday life, as well as identify additional equipment and training that are needed to enhance community and leisure participation. To illustrate that the definition

of mobility has clearly moved into the scope of practice of the recreational therapist look at d465 Moving Around Using Equipment.

Individuals who have compromised mobility are not only at risk for decreased participation, but also poorer health condition. This highlights the importance of addressing mobility challenges. For example, physical performance limitations and participation restrictions are associated with increased healthcare costs (Chan et al., 2002; Guralnik et al., 2002; Foote & Hogan, 2001).

In addition to cost, reduced mobility negatively affects life participation. For example, in a study of 62 individuals with Parkinson's disease, mobility related quality of life affected participation (Duncan & Earhart, 2011). In regards to fine motor skills, a study of 103 individuals with cerebral palsy found that poorer upper extremity motor skills, including fine motor skills, were predictors for restriction in daily activities and participation (Van Meeteren et al., 2008).

Mobility, in the ICF, also relates to transportation, which raises concerns for people's health and participation. For example, Balfour and Kaplan (2002) found that people who lost access to public transportation (one of several neighborhood barriers to community engagement) were more likely to experience the onset of severe, self-reported functional limitations over the course of one year. In another study of older adults with knee pain, better availability of transportation was associated with increased community mobility.

### Assessment of Mobility

Specific techniques for assessing mobility are reviewed in each of the codes. Mobility, transportation skills, and use of transportation are commonly assessed through functional testing, observation, interview, and standardized tools, such as the *Fifty-Foot Walk Test* or the *Bus Utilization Skills Assessment*.

### Treatment of Mobility

Treatment of mobility has many parts. Some information is provided in this book, but more detailed descriptions of mobility training are available in the companion book, *Recreational Therapy Basics, Techniques, and Interventions.* Topics to investigate include Body Mechanics and Ergonomics, Balance Training, Constraint-Induced Movement Therapy, Motor Learning and Training Strategies, Neuro-Developmental Treatment, Transfers, Walking and Gait Training, and Wheelchair Mobility.

### Evidence Review

Reviews of several studies are provided to highlight evidence-based practice related to mobility. This is only a sample of the evidence. A thorough review of the literature is needed to identify evidence-based practice interventions that reflect the needs and characteristics of the individual client.

Maynard et al., (2010) conducted a retrospective review of 41 patients ages eight to 21 with pain-associated disability. Patients received an interdisciplinary inpatient rehabilitation program including physical therapy, occupational therapy, recreational therapy, medicine, nursing, pediatric psychology, neuropsychology, psychiatry, social work, and education. The program included a comprehensive mental health assessment, cognitive-behavioral pain management and coping skills training, differential reinforcement and shaping, systematic desensitization, additional therapeutic interventions, such as medication and complementary therapy, parent training, generalization, and discharge planning. Significant improvements were observed in school status, sleep, functional ability, and physical mobility at admission, discharge, and three-month follow-up.

Rand et al., (2010) conducted a study in which eleven participants post stroke (mean age 67) participated in a six-month exercise and recreation program consisting of two hours a week of physical exercise covering stretching, balance, and task-specific exercises based on the Fitness and Mobility Exercise program and one hour a week of recreation with social and physical activities, introduction to community-based exercise groups to expand knowledge about community resources, and a focus on learning new skills. Participants significantly improved in dual task, such as talking while walking, response inhibition, memory, knee strength, and walking speed.

Bedini (2008) conducted a study of 11 older adults with mild cognitive and physical limitations who were residing in an assisted living facility. They participated in a 10-week instructional program that taught the participants how to do magic tricks. The sessions demonstrated the trick, explained how the trick worked step by step, and instructed and guided participants to conduct the trick. The participants met twice a week for 20-45 minutes in small groups consisting of two to seven participants. The magic tricks were chosen to challenge memory, adding, sequencing, fine motor skills, spatial awareness, communication, and interpersonal interaction. Following the program, participants had decreased depression and negativity, increased motor skills, increased self-confidence and self-esteem, and increased socialization. Memory and cognitive stimulation showed relatively no change.

Snethen et al. (2011) reviewed the *Independence through Community Access and Navigation* (I-CAN) intervention designed to "support participation in community-based activities by providing access and skill acquisition in a community environment" (p. 35). The program consists of the development of a community resource manual, an assessment of leisure interests that are in the client's living situation or environment, interviewing techniques to ascertain the motivation for participation, risk assessment for physical activity, identification of positive and negative perceived consequences to participation, and beliefs about ability to succeed and barriers to participation. Goals are then set and an action plan is developed. The number and length of recreational therapy sessions will vary depending upon goals and client functioning. Outcomes of the program include "development of social skills, increased social interaction, increased community awareness, increased ability to navigate with maps and public transportation to access community services, increased planning and scheduling skills, increased well being, development of identity through activity participation, increased quality of life, larger social networks, and increased self-esteem through successful life experiences" (p. 37).

### Cross References

In *Recreational Therapy for Specific Diagnoses and Conditions, First Edition*, ICF code d4 Mobility and its subcategories are listed in 30 chapters: Amputation and Prosthesis, Autism Spectrum Disorder, Back Disorders and Back Pain, Burns, Cancer, Cerebral Palsy, Cerebrovascular Accident, Chronic Obstructive Pulmonary Disease, Diabetes Mellitus, Epilepsy, Fibromyalgia and Juvenile Fibromyalgia, Guillain-Barré Syndrome, Hearing Loss, Heart Disease, Intellectual Disability, Multiple Sclerosis, Neurocognitive Disorders, Obesity, Osteoarthritis, Osteoporosis, Parkinson's Disease, Pressure Ulcers, Rheumatoid Arthritis, Schizophrenia Spectrum and Other Psychotic Disorders, Sickle Cell Disease, Spina Bifida, Spinal Cord Injury, Total Joint Replacement, Traumatic Brain Injury, and Visual Impairments and Blindness.

In *Recreational Therapy Basics, Techniques, and Interventions, First Edition*, treatment for ICF code d4 Mobility and its subcategories are discussed in 20 chapters: Activity and Task Analysis, Body Mechanics and Ergonomics, Consequences of Inactivity, Stress, Activity Pattern Development, Adaptive Sports, Adventure Therapy, Animal Assisted Therapy, Aquatic Therapy, Balance Training, Community Problem Solving, Constraint-Induced Movement Therapy, Energy Conservation Techniques, Montessori Method, Motor Learning and Training Strategies, Neuro-Developmental Treatment, Physical Activity, Transfers, Walking and Gait Training, and Wheelchair Mobility.

## Changing and Maintaining Body Position (d410 - d429)

### d410 Changing Basic Body Position

Getting into and out of a body position and moving from one location to another, such as getting up out of a chair to lie down on a bed, and getting into and out of positions of kneeling and squatting.

Inclusion: Changing body position from lying down, from squatting or kneeling, from sitting or standing, bending and shifting the body's center of gravity

Exclusions: transferring oneself (d420)

- *d4100 Lying Down*
  Getting into and out of a lying down position or changing body position from horizontal to any other position, such as standing up or sitting down.

  Inclusion: getting into a prostrate position

- *d4101 Squatting*
  Getting into and out of the seated or crouched posture on one's haunches with knees closely drawn up or sitting on one's heels, such as may be necessary in toilets that are at floor level, or changing body position from squatting to any other position, such as standing up.

- *d4102 Kneeling*
  Getting into and out of a position where the body is supported by the knees with legs bent, such as during prayers, or changing body position from kneeling to any other position, such as standing up.

- *d4103 Sitting*
  Getting into and out of a seated position and changing body position from sitting down to any other position, such as standing up or lying down.

  Inclusions: Getting into a sitting position with bent legs or cross-legged; getting into a sitting position with feet supported or unsupported

- *d4104 Standing*
  Getting into and out of a standing position or changing body position from standing to any other position, such as lying down or sitting down.

- *d4105 Bending*
  Tilting the back downwards or to the side, at the torso, such as in bowing or reaching down for an object.

- *d4106 Shifting the Body's Center of Gravity*
  Adjusting or moving the weight of the body from one position to another while sitting, standing, or lying, such as moving from one foot to another while standing.

Exclusions: transferring oneself (d420), walking (d450)

- *d4108 Changing Basic Body Position, Other Specified*
- *d4109 Changing Basic Body Position, Unspecified*

For clients to be able to change or maintain body positions they need to work on the underlying functional skills associated with body position. There are four underlying principles associated with changing or maintaining body position. These are functions of the joints and bones, muscle functions, movement functions, and proprioceptive functions. There are many reasons that clients may have problems with changing and maintaining body positions. The impairments may originate from a loss of muscle (being out of shape, muscle degeneration, or deconditioning), loss of muscle control (through neurological or brain damage), loss of tissue mobility, loss of the sensory feedback, or impairment in processes that allow balance. Because the causes of impairment vary, so will the approaches taken by the recreational therapist.

The primary body tissues that allow individuals to change or maintain position are soft-tissue (muscle, connective tissue, and skin) and boney tissue (bones and the associated joint structure). Conditions that cause a reduction in tissue mobility include "(1) prolonged immobilization, (2) restricted mobility, (3) connective tissue or neuromuscular diseases, (4) tissue pathology due to trauma, and (5) congenital and acquired boney deformities" (Kisner & Colby, 1990, p. 109).

Refer to b7 Neuromusculoskeletal and Movement-Related Functions for information on how to assess, treat, document, and adapt for joint, bone, muscle, and movement functions.

Refer to Body Functions b2 Sensory Functions and Pain (specifically code b260 Proprioceptive Function) for information on how to assess, treat, document, and adapt for proprioceptive dysfunction.

Recreational therapists consult with the physical and occupational therapist for recommended techniques for changing body positions, for example the best techniques to move from sitting to supine. Techniques are based on client's abilities, limitations, precautions, and parameters including weight-bearing restrictions.

Techniques used by physical therapists and occupational therapists may need to be adapted to meet the needs of the client in different settings. For example, kneeling techniques for outdoor gardening may vary from how they are done indoors due to the lack of a sturdy support in the garden. Recreational therapists assist the client in problem solving for change of position and address the development of change of position skills in real-life environments. Below are common approaches to changing position.

- *Sit to stand*: Scoot to the edge of the seat, tuck the feet slightly behind the knees, place the hands on armrests, lean forward (nose over toes), push up using the leg muscles with the arms pushing up from the armrest for added support, fully stand to upright position.
- *Stand to sit*: Back up to the chair so that the back of the legs are touching the chair, reach back for the armrests while leaning slightly forward, slowly lower bottom onto the chair using the leg muscles and arms on the armrest for added support, readjust into a comfortable sitting position.
- *Lying to sitting*: While on a bed, roll onto the side facing the edge of the bed, flex the elbow and wrist of the arm on the bottom. While pushing up with the arm to a sitting position, swing the legs off the side of the bed. The final position is sitting on the edge of the bed with the legs dangling off the side.
- *Sitting to lying*: Sit down on the bed two thirds of the way up from the bottom, rotate the trunk and place the palms of both hands on the bed, swing the legs onto the bed one at a time, stretch out the legs and gently lower self onto the bed using the arms for support.
- *Stand to kneel*: Upper body support is helpful. Place the left hand on a sturdy support and step back one step with the left foot, place the right hand on the right knee, flex both knees until the left knee rests on ground and the right knee is at a 90° angle, slide the right foot backwards and gently lower the right knee onto the ground. If the right leg is weaker, it might be better to reverse the legs.
- *Kneel to stand*: Place the left hand on a sturdy support, slide the right foot forward to raise the right knee to a 90° angle, place the right hand on the right knee, push up into a standing position using the left hand on sturdy support and the

right hand on the right knee. If the right leg is weaker, it might be better to reverse the legs.

If difficulty is noted in the person's ability to change a body position, the specific problem is identified through task analysis and/or direct observation. Once the dysfunction is isolated, the therapist consults the specific function in this book to learn how to assess, document, treat, and adapt for the problem. Document the treatment using both this code and the code for the specific problem area being treated. For more specific treatment information the recreational therapist can also refer the companion book, *Recreational Therapy Basics, Techniques, and Interventions* for the chapters on Body Mechanics and Ergonomics, Balance Training, and Motor Learning and Training Strategies.

Recreational therapists document the extent of difficulty a client has with changing body position. For example, when assistance is not provided, client has mild difficulty getting into a seated yoga position at the community yoga class (d4103._ _ _ 1).

### Cross References

In *Recreational Therapy for Specific Diagnoses and Conditions, First Edition*, ICF code d410 Changing Basic Body Position is listed in eight chapters: Amputation and Prosthesis, Back Disorders and Back Pain, Chronic Obstructive Pulmonary Disease, Guillain-Barré Syndrome, Intellectual Disability, Parkinson's Disease, Pressure Ulcers, and Rheumatoid Arthritis.

In *Recreational Therapy Basics, Techniques, and Interventions, First Edition*, treatment for ICF code d410 Changing Basic Body Position is discussed in six chapters: Activity and Task Analysis, Body Mechanics and Ergonomics, Activity Pattern Development, Aquatic Therapy, Transfers, and Wheelchair Mobility.

### d415 Maintaining a Body Position

Staying in the same body position as required, such as remaining seated or remaining standing for work or school.

Inclusions: maintaining a lying, squatting, kneeling, sitting, and standing position

- *d4150 Maintaining a Lying Position*
  Staying in a lying position from some time as required, such as remaining in a prone position in bed.

  Inclusions: staying in a prone (face down or prostrate), supine (face upwards), or side-lying position

- *d4151 Maintaining a Squatting Position*
  Staying in a squatting position for some time as required, such as when sitting on the floor without a seat.

- *d4152 Maintaining a Kneeling Position*
  Staying in a kneeling position where the body is supported by the knees with legs bent for some time as required, such as during prayers in church.

- *d4153 Maintaining a Sitting Position*
  Staying in a seated position, on a seat or the floor, for some time as required, such as when sitting at a desk or table.

  Inclusions: staying in a sitting position with straight legs or cross-legged, with feet supported or unsupported

- *d4154 Maintaining a Standing Position*
  Staying in a standing position for some time as required, such as when standing in a queue.

  Inclusions: staying in a standing position on a slope, on slippery or hard surfaces

- *d4158 Maintaining a Body Position, Other Specified*
- *d4159 Maintaining a Body Position, Unspecified*
  Maintaining a body position requires the skills reviewed in the previous code set, d410 Changing Basic Body Position, although a greater degree of strength and control is needed to maintain the position in some instances. For example, maintaining a squatting position requires more strength and control than maintaining a lying position.

  The skill of maintaining a position means that there is no movement for a prolonged period of time, such as sitting still at a desk or standing during church. It does not encompass movement, such as shooting basketballs while standing. Therefore, therapists should be careful not to use this code for dynamic positions where there is movement within a position. Dynamic positions are not described separately in the ICF. Rather they are included in the various activities listed in the ICF. For example, throwing, catching, and reaching are in d445 Hand and Arm Use, jumping is in d455 Moving Around, and kicking is in d435 Moving Objects with Lower Extremities. These codes, although they indicate movement within a body position, do not require a specific body position for the function. They do not say, for example, that a person has to be standing in order to show full function with kicking. Kicking can be from any position including sitting or lying down.

Maintaining a position is often documented by the length of time that a person can hold the position and the level and/or type of assistance that is needed to maintain the position. For example, "Client able to maintain a standing position for eight minutes prior to fatigue. Client requires bilateral upper extremity support of table to maintain a standing position." "Client able to maintain an unsupported sitting position in the clinic for six minutes with 50% physical assistance from therapist (d4153.＿ ＿ 3 ＿)."

If difficulty is noted in the person's ability to maintain a body position, the specific problem is identified through task analysis and/or direct observation. Once the dysfunction is isolated, the therapist consults the specific function in this book to learn how to assess, document, treat, and adapt for the problem. Document the treatment using both this code and the code for the specific problem area being treated. Recreational therapists can also refer to the companion book, *Recreational Therapy Basics, Techniques, and Interventions* for specific treatment information in the chapters on Body Mechanics and Ergonomics, Balance Training, and Motor Learning and Training Strategies.

### Cross References

In *Recreational Therapy for Specific Diagnoses and Conditions, First Edition*, ICF code d415 Maintaining a Body Position is listed in 13 chapters: Amputation and Prosthesis, Cerebrovascular Accident, Chronic Obstructive Pulmonary Disease, Guillain-Barré Syndrome, Intellectual Disability, Multiple Sclerosis, Neurocognitive Disorders, Osteoarthritis, Osteoporosis, Parkinson's Disease, Rheumatoid Arthritis, Spina Bifida, and Traumatic Brain Injury.

In *Recreational Therapy Basics, Techniques, and Interventions, First Edition*, treatment for ICF code d415 Maintaining a Body Position is discussed in three chapters: Body Mechanics and Ergonomics, Aquatic Therapy, and Neuro-Developmental Treatment.

### d420 Transferring Oneself

Moving from one surface to another, such as sliding along a bench or moving from a bed to a chair, without changing body positions.

Inclusions: transferring oneself while sitting or lying

Exclusions: changing basic body position (d410)

- *d4200 Transferring Oneself While Sitting*
  Moving from a sitting position on a seat to another seat on the same or a different level, such as moving from a chair to a bed.

  Inclusions: moving from a chair to another seat, such as a toilet seat; moving from a wheelchair to a car seat

  Exclusions: changing basic body position (d410)

- *d4201 Transferring Oneself While Lying*
  Moving from one lying position to another on the same or a different level, such as moving from one bed to another.

  Exclusions: changing basic body position (d410)

- *d4208 Transferring Oneself, Other Specified*
- *d4209 Transferring Oneself, Unspecified*
  The ability to transfer to or from various surfaces is a basic skill required for many leisure activities. Scooting into a booth at a restaurant, moving from one seat to another in a canoe, or moving over on the couch so that a friend may join you to watch a movie are all activities that involve transferring. Clients who use wheeled mobility devices or who are in a bed in a healthcare setting have an even greater need to transfer to engage in leisure activities. Many activities require specialized seating, including snow mobiles, bicycles, cars, and horseback riding or take place using equipment that does not accommodate the size and structure of a wheelchair, but will allow a standard chair, including many picnic table designs and some restaurant seating. The recreational therapist working either in a clinical setting or in the community will need to know how to implement transfers and how to train clients to use transfers.

It is often the physical therapist or the occupational therapist that provides basic transfer training for clients. To help the client participate in activities, the recreational therapist needs to know how to safely implement or modify transfers for two reasons:

The first is that the recreational therapist will be expected to help the client transfer during activities. For example, a client using a wheelchair comes to the pool for aquatic therapy. The client's orders from his physician specify that the client needs to have moderate assistance to safely transfer from his wheelchair and the client needs to transfer to a bench to change his clothes. The recreational therapist needs to know how to implement the moderate assistance needed by the client so the client may change into swimming trunks.

The second is that some leisure activities will require modifications or special problem solving so that clients can engage in the activity. For example, a client using a wheelchair has decided to try out the hand-peddled bicycle that the recreational therapist has in the gym. Transferring to a bicycle seat is different from transferring to a chair so the client may need instruction to transfer safely and efficiently. The companion book, *Recreational Therapy Basics, Techniques, and Interventions,* includes a chapter entitled Transfers that has more information about how to assess, treat, adapt, and document transfers.

Recreational therapists document the extent of difficulty a client has with transfers. For example, when assistance is not provided, the client has moderate difficulty transferring from the wheelchair to the bench-swing at the playground (d4200._ _ _ 2).

### Cross References

In *Recreational Therapy for Specific Diagnoses and Conditions, First Edition,* ICF code d420 Transferring Oneself is listed in four chapters: Chronic Obstructive Pulmonary Disease, Guillain-Barré Syndrome, Multiple Sclerosis, and Spina Bifida.

In *Recreational Therapy Basics, Techniques, and Interventions, First Edition,* treatment for ICF code d420 Transferring Oneself is discussed in seven chapters: Activity and Task Analysis, Body Mechanics and Ergonomics, Aquatic Therapy, Community Problem Solving, Neuro-Developmental Treatment, Transfers, and Wheelchair Mobility.

### d429 Changing and Maintaining Body Position, Other Specified or Unspecified

## Carrying, Moving, and Handling Objects (d430 - d449)

### d430 Lifting and Carrying Objects

Raising up an object or taking something from one place to another, such as when lifting a cup or carrying a child from one room to another.

Inclusions: lifting, carrying in the hands or arms, or on shoulders, hip, back, or head; putting down

- *d4300 Lifting*
  Raising up an object in order to move it from a lower to a higher level, such as when lifting a glass from the table.

- *d4301 Carrying in the Hands*
  Taking or transporting an object from one place to another using the hands, such as when carrying a drinking glass or a suitcase.

- *d4302 Carrying in the Arms*
  Taking or transporting an object from one place to another using the arms and hands, such as when carrying a child.

- *d4303 Carrying on Shoulders, Hip, and Back*
  Taking or transporting an object from one place to another using the shoulders, hip, or back, or some combination of these, such as when carrying a large parcel.

- *d4304 Carrying on the Head*
  Taking or transporting an object from one place to another using the head, such when as carrying a container of water on the head.

- *d4305 Putting Down Objects*
  Using hands, arms, or other parts of the body to place an object down on a surface or place, such as when lowering a container of water to the ground.

- *d4308 Lifting and Carrying, Other Specified*
- *d4309 Lifting and Carrying, Unspecified*
  Lifting and carrying objects is such a basic skill that dysfunction could greatly inhibit a person's ability to participate in life activities. Our arms are used routinely throughout the day to lift and carry objects to meet our needs for work, play, recreation, and self-care. Impairments that can affect someone's

ability to lift, carry, and put down objects include upper extremity amputations, congenital arm deformities, severe rheumatoid arthritis, severe burns on the upper extremities, paralysis, weakness, involuntary motor impairments or tremors, muscle contractures, lifting restrictions from some other condition, cognitive problems, and devices that hinder a person's ability to transport items in the hands, such as holding onto a walker with two hands does not allow the person to carry something in the hands while walking.

Therapists document the specific dysfunction, the level of dysfunction that it causes with the activity, the level of assistance that is needed, and adaptations recommended. For example, "Client has a lifting restriction of five pounds that restricts the client from carrying his cello. Until lifting restrictions are removed, client is 100% dependent on his sister to transport the cello to weekly practice (b4303.0 _ _ 4)."

Proper body mechanics are to be used for lifting, carrying, and putting down objects to prevent injury.

If problems are anticipated, the therapist identifies the specific limitations and consults other healthcare professionals as needed to problem solve for alternative techniques. Some adaptations for lifting and putting down objects include scooping using the forearms and using adaptive devices such as a "reacher." Adaptations for carrying objects include the use of backpacks on the back or on the back of a wheelchair; baskets on a bike, walker or under a wheelchair; waist packs; pocketbooks; pockets; baby sling carriers; and bags, such as lightweight bags to hang on side of a walker.

Refer to Body Mechanics and Ergonomics in the companion book, *Recreational Therapy Basics, Techniques, and Interventions*, for specific treatment information.

### Cross References

In *Recreational Therapy for Specific Diagnoses and Conditions, First Edition*, ICF code d430 Lifting and Carrying Objects is listed in three chapters: Amputation and Prosthesis, Multiple Sclerosis, and Rheumatoid Arthritis.

In *Recreational Therapy Basics, Techniques, and Interventions, First Edition*, treatment for ICF code d430 Lifting and Carrying Objects is discussed in one chapter: Body Mechanics and Ergonomics.

### d435 Moving Objects with Lower Extremities

Performing, coordinated actions aimed at moving an object by using the legs and feet, such as kicking a ball or pushing pedals on a bicycle.

Inclusions: pushing with lower extremities; kicking

- *d4350 Pushing with Lower Extremities*
  Using the legs and feet to exert a force on an object to move it away, such as pushing a chair away with a foot.

- *d4351 Kicking*
  Using the legs and feet to propel something away, such as kicking a ball.

- *d4358 Moving Objects with Lower Extremities, Other Specified*
- *d4359 Moving Objects with Lower Extremities, Unspecified*

Moving objects with the lower extremities is common in sports and recreational activities, such as soccer and kickball. Impairments that can affect someone's ability to move objects with the lower extremities include lower extremity amputations; congenital leg deformities; severe rheumatoid arthritis or osteoarthritis in the hips, knees, and ankles; involuntary motor impairments, including tremors and clonus; leg joint restrictions such as limitations in knee flexion after knee replacement surgery; cognitive problems; paralysis; extreme weakness; muscle contractures; and devices that hinder a person's ability to move objects with the lower extremities, such as a knee-ankle-foot cast.

Therapists document the specific dysfunction, the level of dysfunction that it causes with the activity, the level of assistance that is needed, and adaptations recommended. For example, "Client's knee flexion is limited to 45°, which restricts the client from kicking the soccer ball with her daughter. She is independent in stopping the rolled soccer ball with lower extremities but is dependent in kicking it back to her daughter (d4351._ _ _ 4). Until knee flexion improves, client will play the part of goalie when practicing soccer with her daughter in the backyard."

If problems are anticipated, the therapist identifies the specific limitations and consults with other healthcare professionals as needed to problem solve for alternative techniques, such as designing a push stick so the client can send a soccer ball back to her daughter when practicing in the back yard. Some adaptations for moving objects with the lower extremities include the use of devices or modification of the activity, as in the example above.

Refer to chapters on Balance Training, Constraint Induced Movement Therapy, and Motor Learning and Training Strategies in the companion book, *Recreational Therapy Basics, Techniques, and Interventions*, for specific treatment information.

### Cross References

In *Recreational Therapy for Specific Diagnoses and Conditions, First Edition*, there are no references for ICF code d435 Moving Objects with Lower Extremities.

In *Recreational Therapy Basics, Techniques, and Interventions, First Edition*, treatment for ICF code d435 Moving Objects with Lower Extremities is discussed in one chapter: Body Mechanics and Ergonomics.

### d440 Fine Hand Use

Performing the coordinated actions of handling objects, picking up, manipulating, and releasing them using one's hand, fingers, and thumb, such as required to lift coins off a table or turn a dial or knob.

Inclusions: picking up, grasping, manipulating, and releasing

Exclusions: lifting and carrying objects (d430)

- *d4400 Picking Up*
  Lifting or taking up a small object with hands and fingers, such as when picking up a pencil.

- *d4401 Grasping*
  Using one or both hands to seize and hold something, such as when grasping a tool or a doorknob.

- *d4402 Manipulating*
  Using fingers and hands to exert control over, direct or guide something, such as when handling coins or other small objects.

- *d4403 Releasing*
  Using fingers and hands to let go or set free something so that it falls or changes position, such as when dropping an item of clothing.

- *d4408 Fine Hand Use, Other Specified*
- *d4409 Fine Hand Use, Unspecified*

Fine hand use can be affected by a variety of conditions including rheumatoid arthritis, Parkinson's disease, multiple sclerosis, stroke, brain injury, peripheral neuropathy, upper extremity amputations, upper extremity congenital deformities, severe burns on the upper extremities, carpal tunnel syndrome, trigger finger, and muscle contractures.

Fine hand use, previously called fine motor skills, fine coordination, and/or dexterity, is a primary component of many activities. To help clients improve fine hand use the therapist should have a basic understanding of hand grasps (Table 12) and of ways to improve client performance through modification of the environment.

Prior to addressing fine hand use functions, the therapist identifies any specific precautions or parameters, such as joint protection of the hands, and conducts an assessment of fine hand skills. Assessments that look at fine hand use include:

- *General Recreation Screening Tool* (GRST) for developmental disability and pediatric settings.
- *Comprehensive Evaluation in Recreational Therapy — Physical Disabilities* (CERT Phys/Dys) for people five years or older to measure function.
- *Recreation Early Development Screening Tool* (REDS) for individuals with severe developmental disabilities who are adaptively under one year of age.
- *Therapeutic Recreation Activity Assessment* (TRAA) for people age four and older who have some obvious loss including clients with brain trauma, developmental disabilities, psychiatric disorders, and/or clients who are receiving some manner of supportive care such as residents in nursing homes, group homes, or assisted living.
- *Jebsen-Taylor Hand Function Test* to measure hand function with seven subtests covering the hand functions required for daily activities.

**Table 12: Developmental Levels of Hand Grasps**

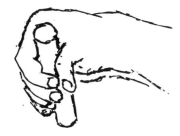

**Palmar Grasp:** Adducted Thumb. Generally developed by age five months.

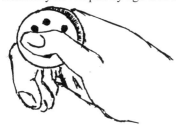

**Scissor Grasp:** Object held between side of finger and thumb. Generally developed by age eight months.

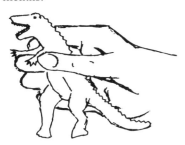

**Radial-Digital Grasp:** Object held between the thumb and fingers so that it is not touching the palm. Generally developed by age eight months.

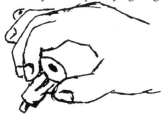

**3-Jaw Chuck Grasp:** Holding an object using the thumb and two fingers. Generally developed by age 10 months.

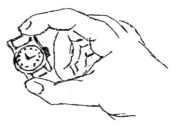

**Pincer Grasp:** The use of the index finger and the thumb to pick up and hold an object. Usually developed by age 10 months.

From burlingame, j. and Blaschko, T. (2010). *Assessment Tools for Recreational Therapy and Related Fields, Fourth Edition.* Ravensdale, WA: Idyll Arbor. Used with permission.

Fine hand use can also be assessed by asking the client to:

- Touch each finger to the thumb (finger thumb opposition).
- Make a fist and stretch out fingers (flexion and extension of fingers).
- Make a circle with the wrist (wrist rotation).
- Pinch the therapist's thumb or skin between thumb and index finger (pinch).
- Stretch out fingers straight to observe any finger deformities or contractures.
- Fan fingers open and closed (abduction and adduction of fingers).
- Bend palms and fingers up and down (wrist flexion and extension).
- With hand in a gentle fist, stretch out one finger and then put it back into the fist (do this with each finger and thumb to evaluate digit isolation).
- Pick up items. Place different size items in front of the client and observe the client's grasp (Table 12). Use items that are common in the client's typical life activities when possible. Items might include a penny, a card, a pen, a paint bottle, a game board box, etc. Observe the type of grasp the client uses to pick up each item. Ask the client to pick up a specific item using a specific grasp if the typical grasp is not used. For example, picking up a penny usually uses a pincer grasp. If the person slides the penny to the edge of the table and uses a scissor grasp, ask the person to try to pick it up with a pincer grip.

Therapists document the specific fine hand dysfunctions and the specific problem they cause with fine hand use, the level of assistance required, or the percentage or ratio of performance. For example: Client's intension tremors impact ability to manipulate objects smaller than two-inch diameter. Client has a severe difficulty picking up coins in the clinic using a pincer grasp with no assistance (d4400._3__). Client can pick up 16 out of 20 coins, one at a time, using a right pincer grasp with assistance of rubber finger grips.

Modalities used to improve fine hand use depend upon the underlying problems. Refer to the specific diagnosis for more information. In general:

- Conditions due to brain impairment such as stroke or brain injury: focus on the use of graduated fine hand activities and repetition to develop neural connections to promote fine hand use.

- Conditions due to joint impairments such as rheumatoid arthritis: focus on activity adaptation to protect joints. See b710 Mobility of Joint Functions for information on joint protection; also encourage routine gentle range of motion of the hands.

- Conditions resulting in peripheral neuropathy: focus on teaching the client how to compensate for difficulty with fine hand use by greater reliance on his/her vision and adapting objects so they are easier to handle.

- Conditions due to chronic neurological conditions such as multiple sclerosis and Parkinson's disease: focus on routine range of motion exercises for the fingers and hands along with activity adaptations to make it easier to handle objects.

- Conditions due to congenital deformities and overuse injury such as carpal tunnel syndrome or trigger finger: focus on adaptation of activities to make it easier to handle objects.

- Conditions that result in muscle contractures such as secondary complication of upper extremity paresis that is not routinely ranged or used in functional activities: focuses on release of contractures (if possible) through gentle passive range of motion and heat.

Common adaptations may include increasing the size of the object, using a universal cuff, and using stabilizing materials. Also consider substituting for the activity, for example switching from embroidery to plastic canvas work because it requires less fine hand skills.

Refer to Body Mechanics and Ergonomics in the companion book, *Recreational Therapy Basics, Techniques, and Interventions*, for more specific treatment information.

### Cross References

In *Recreational Therapy for Specific Diagnoses and Conditions, First Edition*, ICF code d440 Fine Hand Use is listed in 10 chapters: Amputation and Prosthesis, Cerebral Palsy, Cerebrovascular Accident, Guillain-Barré Syndrome, Intellectual Disability, Multiple Sclerosis, Osteoarthritis, Rheumatoid Arthritis, Schizophrenia Spectrum and Other Psychotic Disorders, and Spina Bifida.

In *Recreational Therapy Basics, Techniques, and Interventions, First Edition*, treatment for ICF code d440 Fine Hand Use is discussed in four chapters: Activity and Task Analysis, Body Mechanics and Ergonomics, Constraint-Induced Movement Therapy, and Montessori Method.

### d445 Hand and Arm Use

Performing the coordinated actions required to move objects or to manipulate them by using hands and arms, such as when turning door handles or throwing or catching an object.

Inclusions: pulling or pushing objects; reaching; turning, or twisting the hands or arms; throwing; catching

Exclusions: fine hand use (d440)

- *d4450 Pulling*
  Using fingers, hands, and arms to bring an object towards oneself, or to move it from place to place, such as when pulling a door closed.

- *d4451 Pushing*
  Using fingers, hands, and arms to move something from oneself, or to move it from place to place, such as when pushing an animal away.

- *d4452 Reaching*
  Using the fingers, hands, and arms to extend outwards and touch and grasp something, such as when reaching across a table or desk for a book.

- *d4453 Turning or Twisting the Hands or Arms*
  Using fingers, hands, and arms to rotate, turn, or bend an object, such as is required to use tools or utensils.

- *d4454 Throwing*
  Using fingers, hands, and arms to lift something and propel it with some force through the air, such as when tossing a ball.

- *d4455 Catching*
  Using fingers, hands, and arms to grasp a moving object in order to bring it to a stop and hold it, such as when catching a ball.

- *d4458 Hand and Arm Use, Other Specified*
- *d4459 Hand and Arm Use, Unspecified*

Problems with hand and arm use can be affected by the conditions described in d440 Fine Hand Use. Evaluation of hand use is the same as the evaluation discussed in d440 Fine Hand Use. To evaluate arm use add additional components looking at joint and bone functions, muscle functions, and movement functions, all of which can be found in b7 Neuro-musculoskeletal and Movement-Related Functions. That chapter also has information on assessment, documentation, treatment, and adaptation of dysfunction in areas affecting hand and arm use.

Recreational therapists document the extent of difficulty a client has with hand and arm use. For example, when assistance is not provided, the client has moderate difficulty throwing a baseball during a league game (d4454._ _ _ 2).

Refer to the chapters on Body Mechanics and Ergonomics and Constraint Induced Movement Therapy in the companion book, *Recreational Therapy Basics, Techniques, and Interventions*, for specific treatment information.

### Cross References

In *Recreational Therapy for Specific Diagnoses and Conditions, First Edition*, ICF code d445 Hand and Arm Use is listed in five chapters: Amputation and Prosthesis, Guillain-Barré Syndrome, Osteoarthritis, Rheumatoid Arthritis, and Spina Bifida.

In *Recreational Therapy Basics, Techniques, and Interventions, First Edition*, treatment for ICF code d445 Hand and Arm Use is discussed in three chapters: Body Mechanics and Ergonomics, Constraint-Induced Movement Therapy, and Neuro-Developmental Treatment.

### d449 Carrying, Moving, and Handling Objects, Other Specified and Unspecified

### Walking and Moving (d450 - d469))

### d450 Walking

Moving along a surface on foot, step by step, so that one foot is always on the ground, such as when strolling, sauntering, walking forwards, backwards, or sideways.

Inclusions: walking short or long distances; walking on different surfaces; walking around obstacles

Exclusions: transferring oneself (d420); moving around (d455)

- *d4500 Walking Short Distances*
  Walking for less than a kilometer, such as walking around rooms or hallways, within a building or for short distances outside.

- *d4501 Walking Long Distances*
  Walking for more than a kilometer, such as across a village or town, between villages, or across open areas.

- *d4502 Walking on Different Surfaces*
  Walking on sloping, uneven, or moving surfaces, such as on grass, gravel, or ice and snow, or walking aboard a ship, train, or other vehicle.

- *d4503 Walking around Obstacles*
  Walking in ways required to avoid moving and immobile objects, people, animals, and vehicles, such as walking around a marketplace or shop, around or through traffic or other crowded areas.

- *d4508 Walking, Other Specified*
- *d4509 Walking, Unspecified*

In the past the term *ambulation* was used to mean *walking* with or without adaptive equipment. While the term ambulation is frequently heard in treatment settings, the World Health Organization has moved away from using the term ambulation and instead uses the easier to understand term walking. When a client uses a method other than walking to get from one place to another the term now used is "moving around." The simplification of this terminology makes translation of concepts into other languages easier and helps demystify healthcare by using words clients are comfortable with.

Before a therapist asks a client to walk, s/he reviews the illness or injury and medical orders. Medical orders provide information on any precautions or parameters that need to be followed. The precautions may include weight-bearing restrictions, heart rate parameters, blood pressure parameters, restrictions to prolonged and direct sunlight, oxygen saturation levels, and range restrictions, along with other possibilities. Recreational therapists next read the latest physical therapy clinical notes and consult with the primary physical therapist working with the client. The clinical notes will inform the recreational therapist of the current walking skills of the client, such as distance allowed, device, level of assistance, and specific gait deviations. Consulting with the physical therapist is helpful when further information is needed, such as specific cueing or guarding technique used by the physical therapist when walking with the client. If the recreational therapist is working with a client who is not being seen (or has not been seen) by a physical therapist, the therapist asks the client and others, such as a caregiver, family, or other healthcare providers, for information on walking skills, makes observation, and does functional testing.

Recreational therapists address functional walking, meaning that walking is addressed within real-life activities that may include walking on outdoor surfaces, walking around obstacles, walking through manual doors, or walking while performing a task. Recreational therapists focus on using learned walking techniques in real-life settings and activities. Consequently, recreational therapists address the skill of walking after the client achieves functional walking skills. Functional skills are usually defined by distance and level of assistance. For distance, walking at least 50' for indoor activities, 250' for short community distances, and greater than 500' for general community activities is considered functional. Regarding level of assistance, the client must require minimal assistance or less by one person. Moderate assistance is typically more than a family member or caregiver can handle, making walking an unrealistic mobility choice for home and community activities. Although this is a general rule of thumb, it is important to note that there are exceptions to the rule that are made on an individual basis.

The best way to enhance community mobility skills is to "just do it." Practice and repetition will enhance the client's confidence and skills, and allow for increased opportunities to find solutions for physical and attitude barriers. The therapist may find it helpful to start out by reviewing the techniques and then practicing outdoor walking and moving techniques on the facility's campus. Do not overwhelm the client by trying everything in one day. Provide positive feedback. Empathize with client's reservations and fears about walking and moving outdoors. The therapist will need to discuss issues related to outdoor and other community tasks and assist the client in problem solving outdoor walking and moving skills. Questions that need to be considered are practical considerations like: How can the client safely use her walker and carry mail from the mailbox? Is it appropriate for the client to walk with a cane while walking his pet poodle?

The therapist may also wish to write up guidelines and give them to the client for reference after discharge. Educate the client's family, friends, and caregivers who will be walking with the client outdoors so they are aware of how to best assist the client.

Clients with impairments often need to keep their hands free for balance or for using mobility aids such as canes and crutches. Adaptation of techniques or equipment can increase the client's walking and moving ability. Some common adaptations and equipment to assist with functional walking and moving include:

- *Baskets*: When the client's hands need to be on the walker, it is hard to carry things. By attaching a basket for carrying items to the front of a walker, a client's hands remain free. Do not put too much weight in the basket or the walker will become front heavy and tip over.
- *Waist packs*: Instead of using a pocket book, encourage clients to use a waist pack so that arms and hands are free to maintain balance and good posture. If the client wants to use a pocket book, use one with a long strap so that it can be slung across the body. This way, it will be more stable and won't slide off the person's shoulder when walking.
- *Ice pick tip*: A retractable ice pick attachment that is available for canes can be very helpful for clients who want to hike on uneven dirt paths.
- *Backpacks*: A backpack is a good alternative for carrying bulky items such as laundry, groceries,

or crafts. Instruct clients in appropriate fitting and weight limits.

- *Cell phone or hand radio*: Cell phones are an important safety device. For example, if a client riding the bus gets off at the wrong stop, s/he can use the cell phone to get assistance. Hand radios (also called "walkie-talkies") are good for short-range communication, such as a person who is gardening in the back yard and needs to contact his spouse who is indoors should he need assistance.

Recreational therapists document the extent of difficulty a client has with walking. For example, when assistance is provided, the client has mild difficulty walking across the grass in his backyard (d4502.1 _ _).

Refer to the chapters on Body Mechanics and Ergonomics, Balance Training, Constraint Induced Movement Therapy, Motor Learning and Training Strategies, and Walking and Gait Training in the companion book, *Recreational Therapy Basics, Techniques, and Interventions*, for specific treatment information.

### Cross References

In *Recreational Therapy for Specific Diagnoses and Conditions, First Edition*, ICF code d450 Walking is listed in 13 chapters: Amputation and Prosthesis, Cerebrovascular Accident, Chronic Obstructive Pulmonary Disease, Diabetes Mellitus, Guillain-Barré Syndrome, Heart Disease, Multiple Sclerosis, Osteoarthritis, Parkinson's Disease, Rheumatoid Arthritis, Spina Bifida, Total Joint Replacement, and Visual Impairments and Blindness.

In *Recreational Therapy Basics, Techniques, and Interventions, First Edition*, treatment for ICF code d450 Walking is discussed in six chapters: Activity Pattern Development, Animal Assisted Therapy, Aquatic Therapy, Constraint-Induced Movement Therapy, Neuro-Developmental Treatment, and Walking and Gait Training.

### d455 Moving Around

Moving the whole body from one place to another by means other than walking, such as climbing over a rock or running down a street, skipping, scampering, jumping, somersaulting, or running around obstacles.

Inclusions: crawling, climbing, running, jogging, jumping, and swimming

Exclusions: transferring oneself (d420), walking (d450)

- *d4550 Crawling*
  Moving the whole body in a prone position from one place to another on hands, or hands and arms, and knees.

- *d4551 Climbing*
  Moving the whole body upwards or downwards, over surfaces or objects, such as climbing steps, rocks, ladders or stairs, curbs, or other objects.

- *d4552 Running*
  Moving with quick steps so that both feet may be simultaneously off the ground.

- *d4553 Jumping*
  Moving up off the ground by bending and extending the legs, such as jumping on one foot, hopping, skipping, and jumping or diving into water.

- *d4554 Swimming*
  Propelling the whole body through water by means of limb and body movements without taking support from the ground underneath.

- *d4558 Moving Around, Other Specified*
- *d4559 Moving Around, Unspecified*

Crawling, climbing, running, and jumping are all developmental skills. Swimming is generally considered a learned skill. Crawling typically begins between six and nine months and is fully developed by nine to 12 months. Climbing stairs with assistance usually occurs around 15-18 months and children usually climb basic household objects, such as chairs and beds, well by the age of two. Small hops are seen in toddlers around 18-24 months and by two years of age a toddler can jump and run.

Ways of moving around other than walking are an important consideration. For instance, a person who has both legs amputated at the hip may be able to use a swing-through gait or a modified crawl as an alternative to a wheelchair to get around in the home. Alternative forms of mobility are also evident in many sports and recreation activities, where running, jogging, swimming, skating, sliding, skipping, hopping, rolling, and climbing are part of the activity. These movements are areas of concern for the recreational therapist who treats a person's involvement in recreation and sport activities.

Like walking, the therapist must first review the physician's notes for the client's mobility-related precautions and parameters and consult with the physical therapist to discuss issues related to moving around in a specific manner. The specific interventions used to work on problems associated with the form of mobility will vary depending on the diagnosis.

Problems with the forms of mobility covered in this code are noted through direct observation, task analysis, and formal testing. Therapists document, at a minimum, the specific form of mobility, the specific problems noted, and the level of assistance required for the activity. For example, "Client requires minimal assistance to maintain dynamic sitting balance in moderate ranges when sliding down a 40° sliding board (d4558._ _ _ 1; sliding)." If the person uses a piece of equipment for mobility, the code d465 Moving Around Using Equipment is referenced in assessment and treatment.

Refer to the chapters on Body Mechanics and Ergonomics, Aquatic Therapy, Constraint Induced Movement Therapy, Motor Learning and Training Strategies, Neuro-Developmental Treatment, and Walking and Gait Training in the companion book, *Recreational Therapy Basics, Techniques, and Interventions*, for specific treatment information on treatment.

### Cross References

In *Recreational Therapy for Specific Diagnoses and Conditions, First Edition*, ICF code d455 Moving Around is listed in two chapters: Amputation and Prosthesis and Heart Disease.

In *Recreational Therapy Basics, Techniques, and Interventions, First Edition*, treatment for ICF code d455 Moving Around is discussed in five chapters: Activity and Task Analysis, Body Mechanics and Ergonomics, Aquatic Therapy, Neuro-Developmental Treatment, and Walking and Gait Training.

### d460 Moving Around in Different Locations

Walking and moving around in various places and situations, such as walking between rooms in a house, within a building, or down the street of a town.

Inclusions: moving around within the home, crawling or climbing within the home; walking or moving within buildings other than the home, and outside the home and other buildings

- *d4600 Moving Around within the Home*
  Walking and moving around in one's home, within a room, between rooms, and around the whole residence or living area.

  Inclusions: moving from floor to floor, on an attached balcony, courtyard, porch, or garden

- *d4601 Moving Around within Buildings Other Than Home*
  Walking and moving around within buildings other than one's residence, such as moving around other people's homes, other private buildings, community and private or public buildings and enclosed areas.

  Inclusions: moving throughout all parts of buildings and enclosed areas, between floors, inside, outside, and around buildings, both public and private

- *d4602 Moving Around outside the Home and Other Buildings*
  Walking and moving around close to or far from one's home and other buildings, without the use of transportation, public or private, such as walking for short or long distances around a town or village.

  Inclusions: walking or moving down streets in the neighborhood, town, village, or city; moving between cities and further distances, without using transportation

- *d4608 Moving Around in Different Locations, Other Specified*
- *d4609 Moving Around in Different Locations, Unspecified*
  Moving around within the home, outdoors, and within other buildings requires different skills than moving around in a clinical setting. There are various environmental factors that have the potential to hinder or facilitate mobility, as discussed in the Environmental Factors section of the ICF. These could be physical objects, the natural and man-made environment, or services, systems, and policies. As reviewed in the walking code set, recreational therapists focus on moving around in real-life settings during activities in the home, outdoors, and in other buildings outside of the home.

  Note that the term "moving around" does not denote a specific way of moving around, although it is limited to moving around *without* equipment and it does not include the use of transportation. If the client uses a piece of equipment, use code d465 Moving Around Using Equipment. If the therapist wants to score the client's ability to move around using transportation, refer to the code set d470 - d489 Moving Around Using Transportation.

Recreational therapists conduct a holistic assessment of the environment, as well as outlining variables that have the potential to hinder or facilitate moving around in different locations. Problems with barriers are solved and facilitators are noted. Depending on the setting, therapists may opt to practice moving around in different locations by simulating the specific environment to build confidence, decrease anxiety, and provide opportunities for problem solving in a safe location. Community integration training in the places the client will be going to after discharge is ideal whenever possible to fully assess, problem solve, and adapt for moving around in the alternative setting.

Recreational therapists document the extent of difficulty a client has with moving around in different locations. For example, when assistance is not provided, the client has moderate difficulty moving around inside the community bowling alley (d4601._ _ _ 2).

Refer to the chapters on Body Mechanics and Ergonomics; Community Participation: Integration, Transitioning, and Inclusion; Community Problem Solving; and Motor Learning and Training Strategies in the companion book, *Recreational Therapy Basics, Techniques, and Interventions*, for specific treatment information.

### Cross References

In *Recreational Therapy for Specific Diagnoses and Conditions, First Edition*, ICF code d460 Moving Around in Different Locations is listed in 10 chapters: Amputation and Prosthesis, Chronic Obstructive Pulmonary Disease, Guillain-Barré Syndrome, Hearing Loss, Intellectual Disability, Multiple Sclerosis, Spina Bifida, Spinal Cord Injury, Traumatic Brain Injury, and Visual Impairments and Blindness.

In *Recreational Therapy Basics, Techniques, and Interventions, First Edition*, treatment for ICF code d460 Moving Around in Different Locations is discussed in three chapters: Adaptive Sports, Animal Assisted Therapy, and Walking and Gait Training.

### d465 Moving Around Using Equipment

Moving the whole body from place to place, on any surface or space, by using specific devices designed to facilitate moving or create other ways of moving around, such as with skates, skis, or scuba equipment, or moving down the street in a wheelchair or a walker.

Exclusions: transferring oneself (d420); walking (d450); moving around (d455); using transportation (d470); driving (d475)

Moving around using equipment includes moving around using any piece of mobility equipment, whether for assistance or sport, on any surface and in any space. This code may be challenging for therapists who work in rehabilitation settings where they assess, treat, document, and adapt for individual mobility skills with a piece of equipment. For example, therapists need to document separately about a person's ability to go up and down stairs, up and down curbs, walk on uneven outdoor surfaces, walk on indoor level surfaces, up and down hills, in and out of manual doors, and in and out of elevators.

Therapists document skills separately because a person's needs and abilities vary from activity to activity. It also allows the therapist a clear way of documenting progress with specific mobility activities. It is unclear at this time how therapists will go about using this code. A therapist might score this code by the average level of difficulty of all the mobility skills that use equipment, choose the lowest score of all the mobility skills that use equipment, or opt to score a specific mobility skill and designate the specific skill scored to the right of the score in the additional notes section. The last choice provides more information to those who read the notes and better documentation to justify the treatment provided.

Recreational therapists document the extent of difficulty a client has with moving around using equipment. For example, when assistance is not provided, the client has mild difficulty roller skating at the community roller skating rink (d465._ _ _ 1).

Refer to the chapters on Body Mechanics and Ergonomics; Balance Training; Community Participation: Integration, Transitioning, and Inclusion; Community Problem Solving; Disability Rights: Education and Advocacy; Energy Conservation Techniques; Motor Learning and Training Strategies;

Transfers; Walking and Gait Training; and Wheel-chair Mobility in the companion book, *Recreational Therapy Basics, Techniques, and Interventions*, for specific treatment information.

### Cross References

In *Recreational Therapy for Specific Diagnoses and Conditions, First Edition*, ICF code d465 Moving Around Using Equipment is listed in eight chapters: Amputation and Prosthesis, Chronic Obstructive Pulmonary Disease, Multiple Sclerosis, Osteoarthritis, Parkinson's Disease, Spina Bifida, Spinal Cord Injury, and Traumatic Brain Injury.

In *Recreational Therapy Basics, Techniques, and Interventions, First Edition*, treatment for ICF code d465 Moving Around Using Equipment is discussed in four chapters: Activity and Task Analysis, Adaptive Sports, Walking and Gait Training, and Wheelchair Mobility.

## d469 Walking and Moving, Other Specified and Unspecified

## Moving Around Using Transportation (d470 - d489)

### d470 Using Transportation

Using transportation to move around as a passenger, such as being driven in a car or on a bus, rickshaw, jitney, animal-powered vehicle, or private or public taxi, bus, train, tram, subway, boat, or aircraft.

Inclusions: using human-powered transportation; using private motorized or public transportation

Exclusions: moving around using equipment (d465); driving (d475)

- *d4700 Using Human-Powered Vehicles*
  Being transported as a passenger by a mode of transportation powered by one or more people, such as riding in a rickshaw or rowboat.

- *d4701 Using Private Motorized Transportation*
  Being transported as passenger by private motorized vehicle over land, sea, or air, such as by a taxi or privately owned aircraft or boat.

- *d4702 Using Public Motorized Transportation*
  Being transported as a passenger by a motorized vehicle over land, sea, or air designed for public transportation, such as being a passenger on a bus, train, subway, or aircraft.

- *d4708 Using Transportation, Other Specified*
- *d4709 Using Transportation, Unspecified*

Transportation equals independence for many clients. It provides clients with the ability to leave their homes and access places in the community that contribute to health maintenance and promotion.

The recreational therapist establishes a baseline of functional travel skills related to using transportation by documenting with this ICF code and others that may also be relevant. For example, walking and moving endurance may be required to get to the transportation; the client may need training to effectively interact with strangers in community; or the client may require assistance to transfer on and off the bus seat. The therapist should also document the purpose of training to use transportation, such as going back and forth to work or to the senior center.

Community integration training is one of the primary focuses of recreational therapy practice. Training for using transportation is a major component. This is a complex process that involves functional skills in all domains. While using private and public transportation is a complex task, the World Health Organization devotes only one category to getting from one place to another using transportation, which emphasizes the movement aspect of transportation. The causes of deficits in using transportation are documented and treated using other ICF codes.

Mobility in the community could be a relatively easy process in which the therapist needs to address dysfunction in only one area for successful integration. For example, a client with a left lower extremity amputation is admitted for prosthetic training. He uses the subway to go back and forth to work and desires to continue using this type of transportation. The client has no cognitive impairments and only needs to address functional skills related to mobility that are discussed in other codes in d4 Mobility: the ability to climb stairs, board the subway train, get on and off the subway seat, use an escalator, and walk to and from the destination prior to and after boarding.

In other situations the therapist may need to address a variety of skills in many domains. For example, a client with a traumatic brain injury who exhibits moderate cognitive and social impairments may need to relearn a broad base of skills. Physically the client has mildly impaired walking and moving endurance. The training is to teach the client how to take a public bus three times a week to a community brain injury program. In this example, the therapist needs to address money management skills, using a bus map and schedule, problem solving skills, safety skills, social interaction skills, and time management skills. The therapist may need to adapt or modify the task to increase client safety and his functional ability to utilize the bus, such as designing a simplified bus map and time schedule, pre-making bus money envelopes, or using cue cards for dealing with common problems.

The therapist must be very adept at evaluating and documenting all of the deficits and needs of the client, as well as being creative with the adaptation or modification of thought processes to enhance function and safety. The therapist may also need to provide education and counseling related to the travel process, such as the client's rights under the Americans with Disabilities Act or community energy conservation techniques, to further enhance traveling skills.

The *Community Integration Program* (Armstrong & Lauzen, 1994) and the *Bus Utilization Skills Assessment* (BUS) (burlingame, 1989) are good resources for more information on transportation training.

Recreational therapists document the extent of difficulty a client has with using transportation. For example, when assistance is not provided, the client has moderate difficulty using the public bus (d4702._ _ _ 2).

### Cross References

In *Recreational Therapy for Specific Diagnoses and Conditions, First Edition*, ICF code d470 Using Transportation is listed in eight chapters: Amputation and Prosthesis, Hearing Loss, Intellectual Disability, Multiple Sclerosis, Pressure Ulcers, Rheumatoid Arthritis, Spina Bifida, and Visual Impairments and Blindness.

In *Recreational Therapy Basics, Techniques, and Interventions, First Edition*, treatment for ICF code d470 Using Transportation is discussed in three chapters: Activity and Task Analysis, Education and Counseling, and Wheelchair Mobility.

### d475 Driving

Being in control of and moving a vehicle or the animal that draws it, traveling under one's own direction or having at one's disposal any form of transportation, such as a car, bicycle, boat, or animal-powered vehicle.

Inclusions: driving human-powered transportation, motorized vehicles, animal-powered vehicles

Exclusions: moving around using equipment (d465); using transportation (d470)

- *d4750 Driving Human-Powered Transportation*
  Driving a human-powered vehicle, such as a bicycle, tricycle, or rowboat.

- *d4751 Driving Motorized Vehicles*
  Driving a vehicle with a motor, such as an automobile, motorcycle, motorboat, or aircraft.

- *d4752 Driving Animal-Powered Vehicles*
  Driving a vehicle powered by an animal, such as a horse-drawn cart or carriage.

- *d4758 Driving, Other Specified*
- *d4759 Driving, Unspecified*

Occupational therapists and recreational therapists may be part of an adaptive driving program at a rehabilitation facility. Generally, further specialized training in adaptive driving is needed before clinical professionals participate in this type of program. Driving plays a vital role in independence and is a valued skill that people do not like to give up. There are many adaptations that allow people with disabilities to drive including:

- A steering wheel knob that allows a person to drive using one hand.
- A push/pull arm next to the steering wheel that allows a person to push for gas and pull for brake with one hand.
- Various switches that can be mounted in various places in a vehicle to operate a variety of vehicle functions, such as tapping a switch with the left elbow to operate the windshield wipers.
- Converted minivans that have a ramp that automatically folds out.
- Converted minivans that have the driver seat removed so that a wheelchair can be manipulated into a driving position and strapped or snapped down to the floor.

In addition to driving an automobile, this code set includes driving human powered transportation, such as a bicycle or rowboat, motorized vehicles besides automobiles, such as motorcycles or riding lawn mowers, and animal-powered vehicles, such as a horse-drawn cart. Clearance is often necessary to operate a vehicle after an injury, for example when neurological injury has occurred and the client desires to return to driving an automobile. However, medical clearance is not always necessary to operate personal modes of transportation such as bicycles, rowboats, or riding lawn mower. The treatment team needs to consider the safety of the person and others and suggest restrictions on kinds of driving when it is appropriate.

Recreational therapists conduct a task analysis and evaluate it against the person's skills for operating vehicles. Unless they are specially certified, recreational therapists should not do evaluations with automobiles.

Therapists document the specific vehicle that the client wants to operate, the level of assistance needed to perform the task, and any other issues that are relevant to the situation. For example "Client requires minimal assistance to maintain dynamic sitting balance to pedal 16" bicycle while wearing right lower extremity prosthesis and using a right pedal clip (d4750.0 _ _ 1; bicycling)."

Therapists assist clients in their desire to operate vehicles through treatment and adaptation. Treatment and adaptation will vary depending on the particular mode of transportation, diagnosis, and abilities and limitations of the client. For example, in one situation a therapist may work with a client to learn alternative ways for steering a powerboat with one hand, while in another case a therapist may work with a client who has had an amputation in teaching her how to ride a bicycle using a lower or upper extremity prosthesis.

### Cross References

In *Recreational Therapy for Specific Diagnoses and Conditions, First Edition*, ICF code d475 Driving is listed in four chapters: Epilepsy, Hearing Loss, Multiple Sclerosis, and Rheumatoid Arthritis.

In *Recreational Therapy Basics, Techniques, and Interventions, First Edition*, treatment for ICF code d475 Driving is discussed in one chapter: Participation.

### d480 Riding Animals for Transportation

Traveling on the back of an animal, such as a horse, ox, camel, or elephant.

Exclusions: driving (d475); recreation and leisure (d920)

In the United States, the most common animal used for transportation is the horse. However, riding a horse for leisure would not be scored under this code. It would be coded under d920 Recreation and Leisure because there is a specific exclusion in this code. This code refers to riding an animal for traveling. Therefore, if a client was riding an animal to get from one place to another for the purpose of transportation, such as riding a horse from camp to the local store, this code could be used.

Recreational therapists who are unfamiliar with the skills involved in riding a particular animal will need to seek out qualified professionals to conduct an appropriate assessment of the client's abilities to ride the animal. Specific deficits identified are addressed as appropriate. Dysfunctions that are identified can be referenced in this book for further guidance on assessment, documentation, treatment, and adaptation for the problem. Adaptations may include a modified saddle, a standing box to assist a person in mounting an animal, and modified steering systems.

Recreational therapists document the extent of difficulty a client has with riding animals for transportation. For example, the client has no difficulty riding a horse to move from one area of the farm to another (d480._ _ _ 0).

### Cross References

In *Recreational Therapy for Specific Diagnoses and Conditions, First Edition*, there are no references for ICF code d480 Riding Animals for Transportation.

In *Recreational Therapy Basics, Techniques, and Interventions, First Edition*, there are no references for ICF code d480 Riding Animals for Transportation.

### d489 Moving Around Using Transportation, Other Specified and Unspecified

### d498 Mobility, Other Specified

### d499 Mobility, Unspecified

### References
Armstrong, M. & Lauzen, S. (1994). *Community integration program*, 2nd ed., Ravensdale, WA: Idyll Arbor.

Balfour, J. L. & Kaplan, G. A. (2002). Neighborhood environment and loss of physical function in older adults: Evidence from the Alameda County study. *American Journal of Epidemiology, 155*(6), 507-15.

Bedini, L. A. (2008). Magic as a therapeutic intervention with older adults with mild cognitive and physical limitation. *Annual in Therapeutic Recreation, XVI*, 159-170.

burlingame, j. (1989). *Bus utilization skills assessment.* Ravensdale, WA: Idyll Arbor.

burlingame, j. & Blaschko, T. (2010). *Assessment tools for recreational therapy and related fields*, fourth edition. Ravensdale, WA: Idyll Arbor.

Chan, L., Beaver, S., Maclehose, R. F., Jha, A., Maciejewski, M., & Doctor, J. N. (2002). Disability and health care costs in the Medicare population. *Archives of Physical Medicine and Rehabilitation, 83*, 1196-1201.

*Dorland's Illustrated Medical Dictionary*, 29th Ed. (2000). Philadelphia: W. B. Saunders.

Duncan, R. P. & Earhart, G. M. (2011). Measuring participation in individuals with Parkinson disease: Relationships with disease severity, quality of life, and mobility. *Disability and Rehabilitation, 33*(15-16), 1440-1446.

Foote, S. M. & Hogan, C. (2001). Disability profile and health care costs of Medicare beneficiaries under age sixty-five. *Health Aff, 20*, 242-253.

Guralnik, J. M., Alecxih, L., Branch, L. G., & Wiener, J. M. (2002). Medical and long-term care costs when older persons become more dependent. *American Journal of Public Health, 92*, 1244-1245.

Kisner, C. & Colby, L. (1990). *Therapeutic exercise: Foundations and techniques*, 2nd ed. Philadelphia, PA: F. A. Davis.

Maynard, C. S., Amari, A., Wieczorek, B., Christensen, J. R., & Slifer, K. (2010). Interdisciplinary behavioral rehabilitation of pediatric pain-associated disability: Retrospective review of an inpatient treatment protocol. *Journal of Pediatric Psychology, 35*(2), 128-137.

Rand, D., Eng, J. J., Liu-Ambrose, T., & Tawashy, A. E. (2010). Feasibility of a 6-month exercise and recreation program to improve executive functioning with memory in individuals with chronic stroke. *Neurorehabilitation and Neural Repair, 24*(8), 722-729.

Snethen, G., McCormick, B. P., Smith, R., & Van Puymbroeck, M., (2011). Independence through community access and navigation in adults with schizophrenia spectrum disorders, Part 2: Treatment planning and implementation. *American Journal of Recreation Therapy, 10*(1), 25-34.

Van Meeteren, J., Roebroeck, M. E., Celen, E., Donkervoort, M., Stam, H. J., & Transition Research Group South West Netherlands. (2008). Functional activities of the upper extremity of young adults with cerebral palsy: A limiting factor for participation. *Disability and Rehabilitation, 30*(5), 387-395.

Wilkie, R., Peat, G., Thomas, E., & Croft, P. (2007). Factors associated with restricted mobility outside the home in community dwelling adults ages fifty years and older with knee pain: An example of use of the international classification of functioning to investigate participation restriction. *Arthritis and Rheumatism, 57*, 1382-1389

# Chapter 5 Self-Care

This chapter is about caring for oneself, washing and drying oneself, caring for one's body and body parts, dressing, eating and drinking, and looking after one's health.

*Sample Scoring for Self-Care*

---

- In an inpatient drug and alcohol program, a client reports that prior to admission all of his leisure activities revolved around drug use, which would be coded in this chapter using d5702 Maintaining One's Health. His family tried to persuade him to avoid such risks, but he never heeded their advice. The correct scoring would look like this: d5702.4 _ _ 4.
- During leisure activities in the hospital, the client is incontinent for urine (d5300 Regulating Urination) approximately 10% of the time. He requires staff reminders at regular intervals to prevent such occurrences. The correct scoring would look like this: d5300._ 0 1 _.

---

Self-care is a necessary and basic component for all life activities. Without good self-care, clients risk their health and jeopardize their quality of life. For example, Kennedy, Rogers, and Bower (2007) note that "[d]isease control and outcomes depend to a significant degree on the effectiveness of self-management" (p. 968). Recreational therapy aims for clients to routinely engage in effective self-care within and through leisure and community engagement for the purpose of health promotion, secondary prevention, and life quality. Recreational therapy also utilizes leisure and community activities as a means to improve self-care, including activities that foster health-promoting behaviors.

## *Assessment of Self-Care*

Recreational therapists assess self-care abilities via review of the medical record, consultation with other healthcare clinicians, client and caregiver interviews, direct requests, and observation. Once baselines are obtained, exploration of needs related to application of self-care in leisure and community activities is completed. Treatment interventions aimed at application of self-care skills in leisure and community settings are implemented. The application of those skills in the context of leisure and community activities is then assessed by direct observation of performance.

## *Treatment of Self-Care*

Since effectiveness of self-care hinges on many variables, such as knowledge, support, ability, motivation, initiation, beliefs, and resources, multiple avenues can be explored to foster effective self-care.

For example, data analysis of 16,754 participants with diabetes found that individuals with minor and major depression were less likely to engage in self-care behaviors, such as leisure time physical activity and routine eye exams. This showed the need to address underlying mental health issues impacting self-care behaviors (Egede, Ellis, & Grubaugh, 2009).

In a study that looked at family influences Dunbar et al. (2008) found that those without family or who lived alone and were socially isolated were highly vulnerable to poor self-care. This indicated the value of social support for self-care behaviors.

The transition of self-care techniques post discharge from healthcare facilities is key, as skills learned in rehabilitation are not always transferable into real-life situations. For example, in regards to stroke rehabilitation, "[r]esearch consistently demonstrates that the transition from rehabilitation to self-care at home is problematic.... Clients frequently report feeling isolated and abandoned in the community after discharge from services… and [face] the need to adapt to changes in their functional abilities and role performance" (Cott, Wiles, & Devitt, 2007, p. 1567).

## *Evidence Review*

Several studies highlight evidence-based practice related to self-care. This is only a sample of the evidence. A thorough review of the literature is needed to identify evidence-based practice interventions that reflect the needs and characteristics of the individual client.

Rao and Gagie (2006) considered the effectiveness of visual aids and supports in teaching multiple skills, including self-care skills, to children with autism, as they are primarily visual learners. Visual supports can provide structure, routine, and sequence to daily activities. Consequently, children with autism respond better to visual activity transitions, such as a picture schedule with times, rather than verbal activity transitions, such as the statement, "Time to get ready for school." When developing visual supports, the authors recommend the following: (1) trial training that involves breaking the desired task or behavior into discrete steps (task analysis), (2) deciding an appropriate visual support for each step, (3) using individual, explicit instruction sessions, (4) prompting and fading procedures as needed to guide and teach children with autism to use the visual supports, and (5) using effective reinforcers as rewards for successful use of the supports according to criterion. In leisure, children with autism are drawn to repetitive routines. To expand leisure skills, experiences, and exploration, and discourage self-stimulating behaviors, a visual organizer can be used to present leisure choices. The child can then decide which s/he would like to do and in what order.

Murphy and Carbone (2008) discussed the benefits of participation in sports for children with disabilities, including reversal of deconditioning, optimizing physical functioning, and maintaining fitness. In order to participate, however, safety considerations must be assessed and addressed. For example, individuals with Down syndrome should avoid activities that involve contact or collision. Children with asthma need to have their medication available and they must be allowed to modify their involvement based on exacerbations and environmental conditions. Individuals with spinal cord injury at risk for autonomic dysreflexia should be allowed to participate in sports only after coaches are trained in recognizing signs and symptoms and demonstrate the ability to remove triggers. There should be no latex products around children with spina bifida because they have high prevalence of latex allergies. Providers should be prepared to deal with hyperthermia in children with neurodevelopmental disabilities due to thermoregulation impairments. Some children may be at a higher risk for musculoskeletal injuries and overuse injuries, such as shoulder injuries in wheelchair athletes. Children with autism might have

difficulties with verbal instruction from coaches. "The child's current health status, the level of competition, the specific sport and position to be played, availability of protective or adaptive equipment, whether the sport can be modified to allow safer participation, and the ability of the child and parent to understand and accept the risk involved must be addressed before participation" (p. 1059).

Roth and Lovell (2007) conducted a study of 735 adult patients admitted and discharged from an urban inpatient rehabilitation program. Data was gathered during admission and at a one-year follow up via telephone. Participants with scores of approximately 80 or greater on the follow-up *Functional Independence Measure*, which includes self-care tasks, had substantially increased scores on the *Frenchay Activities Index*, a brief home and community activity index. The scores indicated that participants at this level of functional independence are more likely to perform community skills.

Driver et al. (2006) conducted a study of 18 adults at least one year post injury at a Rancho Los Amigos level of VI or higher. Participants were randomly assigned to the control group or experimental group. The experimental group participated in aquatic exercise classes for one hour three times a week for eight weeks. The control group participated in an eight-week vocational rehabilitation class. Participants in the experimental group had significant improvements in health responsibility, physical activity, nutrition, spiritual growth, interpersonal relationships, self-esteem, coordination, body fat, strength, flexibility, and endurance. The authors speculate that the following may have contributed to the increase in health promoting behaviors: Improvement in self-esteem and locus of control in the aquatics program may have transferred over to other health behaviors, and/or through participation in the aquatics exercise program, participants may have become more conscious about other healthy lifestyle behaviors.

Wang and Stumbo (2009) evaluated data from the *Behavioral Risk Factor Surveillance System* (BRFSS) on 30,632 older adults representing all 50 states. They looked at physical health, emotional health, and quality of life. Findings indicated that physical activity was especially important for self-rated overall health, physical health, and overall life satisfaction. Emotional support was also important to mental health and overall life satisfaction. Utilization of special equipment was found to negatively affect self-rated overall health. Related to recreational therapy practice, the authors highlight the importance of physical activity for adults with activity limitations, the need for creative physical activity interventions that can meet the needs of older adults with activity limitations who use specialized equipment, educating people about the importance of physical activity engagement prior to older adult years to promote higher degrees of health perception in older adulthood, and access to alternative forms of physical activity for individuals who have difficulty leaving the home.

### Cross References

In *Recreational Therapy for Specific Diagnoses and Conditions, First Edition*, ICF code d5 Self-Care and its subcategories are listed in 37 chapters: Amputation and Prosthesis, Attention-Deficit/Hyperactivity Disorder, Autism Spectrum Disorder, Back Disorders and Back Pain, Borderline Personality Disorder, Burns, Cancer, Cerebral Palsy, Cerebrovascular Accident, Chronic Obstructive Pulmonary Disease, Diabetes Mellitus, Epilepsy, Feeding and Eating Disorders, Fibromyalgia and Juvenile Fibromyalgia, Gambling Disorder, Guillain-Barré Syndrome, Hearing Loss, Heart Disease, Intellectual Disability, Major Depressive Disorder, Multiple Sclerosis, Neurocognitive Disorders, Obesity, Osteoarthritis, Osteoporosis, Parkinson's Disease, Post-Traumatic Stress Disorder, Pressure Ulcers, Rheumatoid Arthritis, Schizophrenia Spectrum and Other Psychotic Disorders, Sickle Cell Disease, Spina Bifida, Spinal Cord Injury, Substance-Related Disorders, Total Joint Replacement, Traumatic Brain Injury, and Visual Impairments and Blindness.

In *Recreational Therapy Basics, Techniques, and Interventions, First Edition*, treatment for ICF code d5 Self-Care and its subcategories are discussed in 26 chapters: Activity and Task Analysis, Adjustment and Response to Disability, Body Mechanics and Ergonomics, Education and Counseling, Parameters and Precautions, Participation, Stress, Activity Pattern Development, Aquatic Therapy, Assertiveness Training, Balance Training, Behavior Strategies and Interventions, Bibliotherapy, Cognitive Behavioral Counseling, Community Problem Solving, Constraint-Induced Movement Therapy, Energy Conser-

vation Techniques, Leisure Education and Counseling, Leisure Resource Awareness, Mind-Body Interventions, Montessori Method, Neuro-Developmental Treatment, Physical Activity, Sexual Well-Being, Social Skills Training, and Values Clarification.

### d510 Washing Oneself

Washing and drying one's whole body, or body parts, using water and appropriate cleaning and drying materials or methods, such as bathing, showering, washing hands and feet, face and hair, and drying with a towel.

Inclusions: washing body parts, the whole body and drying oneself

Exclusions: caring for body parts (d520), toileting (d530)

- *d5100 Washing Body Parts*
  Applying water, soap, and other substances to body parts, such as hands, face, feet, hair, or nails, in order to clean them.

- *d5101 Washing Whole Body*
  Applying water, soap, and other substances to the whole body in order to clean oneself, such as taking a bath or shower.

- *d5102 Drying Oneself*
  Using a towel or other means for drying some part or parts of one's body, or the whole body, such as after washing.

- *d5108 Washing Oneself, Other Specified*
- *d5109 Washing Oneself, Unspecified*
  Washing the whole body is an activity that occurs commonly within the home, although it may also occur in a community setting, such as showering in a locker room at a health club. Washing body parts, such as hand washing, may occur more frequently in community settings for routine hygiene and health. Drying body parts or the whole body accompanies both of these tasks in most situations, although there are exceptions like showering before entering a pool. Recreational therapists holistically evaluate the skills and tasks required to participate in recreational and community activities where washing and drying the whole body or parts of the body may be included. These may include washing hands before dining when eating out, showering before entering a pool,

removing nail polish, washing and drying a residual amputated limb in a community setting when it becomes sweaty with odor, and rinsing sand off of the feet at the beach shower. Washing and drying is much more than the typical morning or evening shower.

In the ICF, recreational therapists document washing and drying skills by level of difficulty. Other ways to document performance include level of assistance required, equipment and techniques utilized, and contraindications followed.

Washing and drying, although sounding quite simple, can require special techniques and equipment, as well as require the individual to follow special instructions, including contraindications. These may include not getting a leg cast wet when bathing, using a long-handled sponge or tub bench, not using oil-based products because it could breed bacteria in a wound, and one-handed techniques for drying hair. Recommendations for washing and drying can come from a variety of health professionals including recreational therapists who identify washing and drying as components of a particular activity.

Recreational therapists document the extent of difficulty a client has with washing oneself in real life environments. For example, at the health club the client has mild difficulty showering due to the confined space and lack of shower bars (d5101._ _ _ 1).

Therapists evaluate the current recommendations for techniques and equipment, as well as contraindications from all sources, and teach a client how to integrate those recommendations into specific activities. In some cases, recommendations cannot easily be transferred to recreational and community activities. Some examples include how to wash and dry a residual limb when out in a community setting, how to operate a pull-cord shower at the beach and wash oneself while only having the use of one hand, or how to shower in a health club locker room when a tub bench is not available. Recreational therapists assist clients in problem solving for these types of situations through the identification of modified techniques and equipment, as well as address related issues that are foreseen as possible barriers to washing and drying during recreational and community activities. For example, at a beach shower, the client could hook one end of a bungee cord to the pull

shower chain and the other end to the top of a water shoe or onto a stationary item like a beach chair to keep tension on the shower cord for continuous water flow. Recreational therapists are expected to find these creative solutions to problems because they are the ones who teach clients how to survive in the real world.

***Cross References***

In *Recreational Therapy for Specific Diagnoses and Conditions, First Edition*, ICF code d510 Washing Oneself is listed in one chapter: Major Depressive Disorder.

In *Recreational Therapy Basics, Techniques, and Interventions, First Edition*, treatment for ICF code d510 Washing Oneself is discussed in two chapters: Activity and Task Analysis and Social Skills Training.

### d520 Caring for Body Parts

Looking after those parts of the body, such as skin, face, teeth, scalp, nails, and genitals, that require more than washing and drying.

Inclusions: caring for skin, teeth, hair, finger and toe nails

Exclusions: washing oneself (d510), toileting (d530)

- *d5200 Caring for Skin*
  Looking after the texture and hydration of one's skin, such as by removing calluses or corns and using moisturizing lotions or cosmetics.

- *d5201 Caring for Teeth*
  Looking after dental hygiene, such as by brushing teeth, flossing, and taking care of a dental prosthesis or orthosis.

- *d5202 Caring for Hair*
  Looking after the hair on the head and face, such as by combing, styling, shaving, or trimming.

- *d5203 Caring for Fingernails*
  Cleaning, trimming, or polishing the nails of the fingers.

- *d5204 Caring for Toenails*
  Cleaning, trimming, or polishing the nails of the toes.

- *d5208 Caring for Body Parts, Other Specified*
- *d5209 Caring for Body Parts, Unspecified*

Caring for skin, teeth, hair, fingernails, and toenails is important for hygiene and prevention of health issues, such as losing teeth, skin cancer due to prolonged, unprotected sun exposure, hair lice, or fingernail infections. Some of these tasks are performed in the client's home, and some are also performed in community and social settings. Therefore, performance of these activities and consequences of not following proper hygiene procedures can affect social relationships, which would be documented in d7 Interpersonal Interactions and Relationships.

In the ICF, recreational therapists document the level of difficulty that a client is having with the task. Other ways to document caring for body parts include the level of assistance required, specific adaptive equipment and techniques utilized, and impact on specific life activities. Recreational therapists document the extent of difficulty a client has with caring for body parts. For example, the client has no difficulty combing his hair at school using a universal cuff (d5202._ _ _ 0).

Recreational therapists are concerned with caring for body parts as it impacts participation in life activities, such as forming social relationships or participating in activities that have a component of body part care such as putting on sunscreen at an outdoor pool. Therapists assist the client in problem solving for specific skills and situations and make recommendations for adaptive equipment, modifications, and techniques. For example a five-year-old boy uses a beige universal cuff to hold a hair comb. The boy is embarrassed to use the adaptive comb at school because his peers make fun of him, but they also make fun of him when his hair is unkempt. Either way, he is teased by his peers. The therapist learns that many of the boys in the class like dinosaurs, so she purchases a small stuffed dinosaur and hot glues it to the top of the universal cuff making the dinosaur appear to be holding the comb. The adaptive comb is now perceived as being "cool" by the boy and his peers.

### Cross References

In *Recreational Therapy for Specific Diagnoses and Conditions, First Edition*, ICF code d520 Caring for Body Parts is listed in four chapters: Amputation and Prosthesis, Diabetes Mellitus, Pressure Ulcers, and Spina Bifida.

In *Recreational Therapy Basics, Techniques, and Interventions, First Edition*, treatment for ICF code d520 Caring for Body Parts is discussed in two chapters: Activity and Task Analysis and Social Skills Training.

### d530 Toileting

Planning and carrying out the elimination of human waste (menstruation, urination, and defecation), and cleaning oneself afterwards.

Inclusions: regulating urination, defecation, and menstrual care

Exclusions: washing oneself (d510), caring for body parts (d520)

- *d5300 Regulating Urination*
  Coordinating and managing urination, such as by indicating need, getting into the proper position, choosing and getting to an appropriate place for urination, manipulating clothing before and after urination, and cleaning oneself after urination.

- *d5301 Regulating Defecation*
  Coordinating and managing defecation such as by indicating need, getting into the proper position, choosing and getting to an appropriate place for defecation, manipulating clothing before and after defecation, and cleaning oneself after defecation.

- *d5302 Menstrual Care*
  Coordinating, planning, and caring for menstruation, such as by anticipating menstruation, and using sanitary towels and napkins.

- *d5308 Toileting, Other Specified*
- *d5309 Toileting, Unspecified*

Regulating urination, defecation, and menstrual care in leisure and community activities can be a complex process for some clients resulting in lack of activity engagement. The client may, for example, fear having an accident when in the community so he chooses to stay home rather than participate.

In the ICF, therapists document the level of difficulty that a client has with each task. Therapists may also document the level of assistance needed, adaptive equipment and techniques, the setting, and activities that are impacted by difficulties in this area.

For example, when assistance is not provided, the client has moderate difficulty using the public restroom to urinate (d5300._ _ _ 2).

Many components are involved in these processes. Body structures and functions, including mental and psychological functions, must be free of deficits or alternatives will need to be sought. This may include the use of medications (e.g., stool softeners, medications to control bladder spasms), adaptive equipment (e.g., use of a digital stimulator, catheter, pads that hold urine), and/or special techniques (e.g., changes in body position, using a toileting time schedule). Urination, defecation, and menstrual care can also be very time consuming, especially if the client requires the use of extensive medications, equipment, and techniques. For example, a client with complete tetraplegia will need to devote about two and a half hours a day to bladder and bowel care. She will need to self-catheterize every four to six hours requiring about one and half hours a day, waiting one hour after taking a suppository for it to loosen the stools and then using other methods to assist in stool release such as a digital stimulator. This does not include the time needed to set-up, undress, dress, and transfer.

If urination, defecation, or menstrual care is not well controlled, severe secondary complications can occur including skin breakdowns and infection. Skin breakdowns can be life threatening, especially for those who have compromised immune systems and severe mobility limitations. From a social perspective, the odor of urine, feces, and menstrual blood, as well as the observation of soiled clothes, deters social interaction from others, affecting social relationships and health.

The chance of accidents, the difficulty in trying to toilet in the community or other people's homes that do not meet the client's accessibility needs, the amount of time required to perform the task, and the level of assistance needed to perform the task are common obstacles to leisure and community activities. The recreational therapist assists the client in problem solving for the identified barriers in the specific real-life situations of the client, and addresses the development of new skills and techniques as appropriate. New skills and techniques are taught when previously learned skills do not transfer well into real-life situations:

For example, a client was taught how to use a transfer board to transfer from the wheelchair to the toilet. This works well for the client in his home bathroom, however it does not work well in a public bathroom because the size of the stall is too small to use the transfer board. The client's caregiver is not able to transfer the client onto the toilet because of back problems. The recreational therapist suggests the use of a Texas catheter for community activities, limiting the amount of liquids consumed prior to going out, and using the bathroom at home before leaving. See b6 Genitourinary and Reproductive Functions for more ideas.

### Cross References

In *Recreational Therapy for Specific Diagnoses and Conditions, First Edition*, ICF code d530 Toileting is listed in two chapters: Cerebrovascular Accident (Stroke) and Sickle Cell Disease.

In *Recreational Therapy Basics, Techniques, and Interventions, First Edition*, treatment for ICF code d530 Toileting is discussed in three chapters: Activity and Task Analysis, Community Problem Solving, and Social Skills Training.

### d540 Dressing

Carrying out the coordinated actions and tasks of putting on and taking off clothes and footwear in sequence and in keeping with climatic and social conditions, such as by putting on, adjusting, and removing shirts, skirts, blouses, pants, undergarments, saris, kimonos, tights, hats, gloves, coats, shoes, boots, sandals, and slippers.

Inclusions: putting on or taking off clothes and footwear and choosing appropriate clothing

- *d5400 Putting on Clothes*
  Carrying out the coordinated tasks of putting clothes on various parts of the body, such as putting clothes on over the head, over the arms and shoulders, and on the lower and upper halves of the body; putting on gloves and headgear.

- *d5401 Taking off Clothes*
  Carrying out the coordinated tasks of taking clothes off various part of the body, such as pulling clothes off and over the head, off the arms and shoulders, and off the lower and upper

halves of the body; taking off gloves and head-gear.

- *d5402 Putting on Footwear*
  Carrying out the coordinated tasks of putting on socks, stockings, and footwear.

- *d5403 Taking off Footwear*
  Carrying out the coordinated tasks of taking off socks, stocking, and footwear.

- *d5404 Choosing Appropriate Clothing*
  Following implicit or explicit dress codes and conventions of one's society or culture and dressing in keeping with climatic conditions.

- *d5408 Dressing, Other Specified*
- *d5409 Dressing, Unspecified*

Dressing is commonly thought about as the domain of occupational therapy, but recreational therapists also play an important role in this code set. Dressing, as described in this ICF code set, is more than just putting on major clothing items such as shirts and pants. It also includes undergarments, gloves, hats, headgear, socks, footwear, including roller skates and water shoes, and jackets used in recreation. This is much more than the dressing skills that are typically considered. This code set also includes the choice of appropriate clothing to follow an explicit or implicit dress code, conventions of one's society or culture, and dressing according to climatic conditions. Difficulty with this skill is often due to disabilities from sensory impairments, mental impairments such as schizophrenia and dementia, and lack of experience, such as young children who choose clothing based on likes or novice hikers who do not understand the danger of alpine weather.

Choosing appropriate clothing for dress codes and conventions of society or culture will also have an impact on other life areas including the development of social relationships, level of group acceptance, and attitudes of others towards the client. This can lead to impaired participation in life activities, which should be documented with other ICF codes. In most cases, people judge others by their appearance and clothing is a major factor. Possibilities include: "She has no respect for God because she is wearing jeans in church." "She wears fancy clothes, so she must be stuck up." "How can his parents allow him to go out of the house dressed like that? They must not be upstanding people."

In the ICF, the recreational therapist documents the level of difficulty that the client has with each task. For example, when assistance is not provided, the client has moderate difficulty donning roller skates at the public roller skating rink (d5402._ _ _ 2).Therapists may also document on discipline-specific forms the level of assistance needed, the specific setting, adaptive equipment, techniques utilized, and activities impacted by difficulties in this area.

Although it is not currently coded this way in the ICF, dressing, in some cases, may be a barrier to a particular life activity. For example, difficulties in choosing appropriate clothing for church may result in difficulties in d9300 Organized Religion.

Recreational therapists evaluate the needs and requirements related to dressing for leisure and community activities that are part of the client's lifestyle, as well as explicit and implicit dress codes and standards for the client's culture and society. If difficulties are noted, therapists seek to reduce or eliminate the dysfunction through the identification of resources, adaptive equipment, such as dressing aids, and techniques, such as how to tie roller skate laces with impaired hand function. The current adaptive equipment and techniques utilized by the client are evaluated for appropriateness in other life situations and recommendations are then suggested. For example a client who was taught how to dress from a supine position, will need another technique when trying on clothes at a store.

### Cross References

In *Recreational Therapy for Specific Diagnoses and Conditions, First Edition*, ICF code d540 Dressing is listed in five chapters: Amputation and Prosthesis, Chronic Obstructive Pulmonary Disease, Osteoarthritis, Rheumatoid Arthritis, and Sickle Cell Disease.

In *Recreational Therapy Basics, Techniques, and Interventions, First Edition*, treatment for ICF code d540 Dressing is discussed in two chapters: Activity and Task Analysis and Social Skills Training.

### d550 Eating

Carrying out the coordinated tasks and actions of eating food that has been served, bringing it to the mouth, and consuming it in culturally acceptable ways, cutting or breaking food into pieces, opening bottles and cans, using eating implements, having meals, feasting, or dining.

Exclusions: drinking (d560)

Eating is more than the act of opening containers, using utensils, breaking or cutting food into pieces, bringing food to the mouth, and swallowing the food. It includes the skill of consuming food in culturally acceptable ways, as well as having meals, feasting, and dining. Culturally acceptable ways of eating will vary depending upon the culture of the client, as well as the culture in which s/he is eating. For example, someone who is Chinese may be expected to use chopsticks and share bowls of food with others at the table when at home, but when out at a fancy restaurant, the client chooses to use utensils and food is not shared. During certain religious holidays or cultural events, manners for food consumption may also change. Usually a higher standard of manners is expected during Christmas dinner than during non-holiday family meals.

This leads into the differences between meals, feasting, and dining. Meals are commonly defined by food that is routinely eaten periodically during the day, such as eating a sandwich at lunchtime or having dinner with the family. Feasting, on the other hand, often indicates a celebration, while dining is often characterized as an elegant meal in a community setting, such as an upscale restaurant.

Food consumption behaviors for each of these differ. For example, during a meal in the home a client may sip the last bit of soup from the bowl and use his sleeve to wipe his mouth without any negative remarks or looks from his family because it is normal eating behavior in his home. However, if the client behaved in the same manner while dining out, it would most likely be perceived as inappropriate. The client realizes that this manner of food consumption is not appropriate for dining out and instead tips the soup bowl and uses a spoon to get the last bit of broth and uses a napkin to blot his mouth clean. Feast behavior can be a bit harder to categorize, but during most celebratory feasts people tend to eat more and socialize more. Food consumption manners may be different with people handing food to other people, sharing plates of food with children, or eating in different locations such as while walking around.

Therapists are aware that food consumption behaviors are influenced by culture, religion, society,

setting, and purpose. They address the expected behaviors. If food consumption behaviors are not appropriate, secondary problems can result that affect other health areas. The client may be rejected by peers and receive fewer invitations to events. Although the ICF does not currently code in this manner, eating impairments can be a barrier to other life activities.

Despite the focus of this discussion on food consumption, recreational therapists are also concerned with the client's ability to perform basic eating skills such as opening containers, using utensils, breaking or cutting food, bringing food to the mouth, and swallowing.

The therapist evaluates the current techniques used by the client and evaluates the functionality of those skills in real-life settings. In the ICF the therapist documents the level of difficulty the client has with each task. For example, when assistance is not provided, the client has mild difficulty eating at a fancy restaurant (d550._ _ _ 1; restaurant dining). Therapists may also document in discipline-specific documentation the level of assistance needed, specific adaptive equipment and techniques utilized, the specific setting, and other activities that are affected by any dysfunction.

The therapist treats problems with d550 Eating by looking at the underlying causes of the dysfunction and finding training or adaptations to reduce the problems. For example, a client may use a special plate that has raised sides like a bowl so that she is able to scoop food easily onto the spoon by sliding it up the side of the plate. This type of bowl is not available at restaurants and the client does not feel comfortable bringing her own bowl because having to move food from the restaurant plate onto her special plate would be difficult for her and she does not feel comfortable asking the waiter or the chef to use the plate. In this situation, the therapist may recommend the use of a plate guard (a piece of plastic that hooks around the outside of standard plate) or the therapist may work with the client to help her be more assertive. What is important is finding a way to allow the client to eat out because it is part of normal social life.

### Cross References

In *Recreational Therapy for Specific Diagnoses and Conditions, First Edition*, ICF code **d550** Eating is listed in two chapters: Feeding and Eating Disorders and Obesity.

In *Recreational Therapy Basics, Techniques, and Interventions, First Edition*, treatment for ICF code d550 Eating is discussed in four chapters: Activity and Task Analysis, Assertiveness Training, Montessori Method, and Social Skills Training.

### d560 Drinking

Taking hold of a drink, bringing it to the mouth, and consuming the drink in culturally acceptable ways, mixing, stirring, and pouring liquids for drinking, opening bottles and cans, drinking through a straw or drinking running water such as from a tap or a spring; feeding from the breast.

Exclusions: eating (d550)

One way to drink something is to open a container, pour the drink, stir or mix it, bring it to the mouth and drink in a culturally acceptable manner. Drinking also includes the use of drinking fountains, breast-feeding, straws, and cupping hands to hold water. There are a variety of adaptive drinking devices such as weighted drinking glasses, cups with specially designed handles and lids, and drinking aids such as cups with special spouts or specially designed straws.

Therapists evaluate the client's current devices used for drinking and determine if they are appropriate to meet the needs of the client in leisure and community activities that are part of the client's lifestyle. In some instances, they will not meet the client's needs and further recommendations will be needed. For example a specialized drinking bottle may not fit in a standard bike water bottle holder or a client may have a specialized cup at home but encounters difficulty when she goes out to eat because she is unable to hold a standard drinking glass at a restaurant.

Drinking also includes the consumption of liquids in a culturally acceptable manner. For example, at home you may drink water from a water bottle, but at a restaurant it is expected that you pour the water from the bottle into a glass. Another example may be that at a restaurant you do not share a drinking glass, but at church everyone takes a sip of wine from the chalice. Recreational therapists are aware of the differences in liquid consumption behaviors that are influenced by culture, religion, society, setting, and

purpose and address the related behaviors. If behaviors are not appropriate, secondary problems can result, including rejection by peers, that can impair the social and mental health of the client. Although the ICF does not currently code in this manner, drinking impairments can be a barrier to other life activities.

In the ICF, recreational therapists document the level of difficulty that a client has with each task. For example, when hiking, client has mild difficulty operating a flip top water bottle (d560._ _ _ 1). Therapists may also document in discipline-specific documentation the level of assistance needed, adaptive equipment or techniques utilized, the setting, and other life activities that are affected by dysfunction in this area.

If an individual is having difficulty with the drinking process itself, the therapist will consult with nursing, speech therapy (for swallowing issues), and occupational therapy to determine if there are particular techniques that the recreational therapist can carry over into treatment sessions, such as tucking in the chin when sucking on straw at a restaurant or cues to purse lips. Current drinking devices are assessed to determine appropriateness of carryover into recreation and community activities. For example, an open cup with a large handle won't be appropriate to take on a hiking trail. Appropriate drinking vessels for particular activities, with adaptations as needed, are determined based on the client's abilities. When determining drinking vessels the therapist also considers the social aspects that surround the particular vessel to make sure it is culturally appropriate and acceptable to the client.

### Cross References

In *Recreational Therapy for Specific Diagnoses and Conditions, First Edition*, ICF code d560 Drinking is listed in one chapter: Feeding and Eating Disorders.

In *Recreational Therapy Basics, Techniques, and Interventions, First Edition*, treatment for ICF code d560 Drinking is discussed in two chapters: Activity and Task Analysis and Social Skills Training.

### d570 Looking After One's Health

Ensuring physical comfort, health, and physical and mental well-being, such as by maintaining a balanced diet, and an appropriate level of physical activity, keeping warm or cool, avoiding harms to health, following safe sex practices, including using condoms, getting immunizations and regular physical examinations.

Inclusions: ensuring one's physical comfort; managing diet and fitness; maintaining one's health

- *d5700 Ensuring One's Physical Comfort*
  Caring for oneself by being aware that one needs to ensure, and ensuring, that one's body is in a comfortable position, that one is not feeling too hot or cold, and that one has adequate lighting.

- *d5701 Managing Diet and Fitness*
  Caring for oneself by being aware of the need and by selecting and consuming nutritious foods and maintaining physical fitness.

- *d5702 Maintaining One's Health*
  Caring for oneself by being aware of the need and doing what is required to look after one's health, both to respond to risks to health and to prevent ill-health, such as by seeking professional assistance; following medical and other health advice; and avoiding risks to heath such as physical injury, communicable diseases, drug-taking, and sexually transmitted diseases.

- *d5708 Looking After One's Health, Other Specified*
- *d5709 Looking After One's Health, Unspecified*
  These are broad codes that encompass a variety of issues included in the scope of recreational therapy practice. Therapists can use the broad code of d570 Looking After One's Health or can be more specific by choosing the descriptive codes under this heading.

### Ensuring One's Physical Comfort

Common issues addressed by recreational therapy that fall under this code include:

- Lack of appropriate use of joint protection techniques, as for rheumatoid arthritis. See b710 Mobility of Joint Functions for information on joint protection techniques.
- Awareness of and making changes for temperatures that affect functioning, as when heat exacerbates multiple sclerosis symptoms or temperature changes are not noticed by someone who has sensory deficits such as a complete spinal cord injury. See b270 Sensory Functions Related to Temperature and Other Stimuli for

more information on how to assess, treat, document, and adapt for dysfunction in this area.

- Awareness and proper positioning of the body including ergonomics and body mechanics. Examples include a client who lacks awareness of a limb as the result of a stroke, a client who is not positioning her body correctly in a device such as a wheelchair or a splint, or a client who needs to learn comfortable ways to use a computer workstation or proper body mechanics in an activity. See Activities and Participation d4 Mobility for information on how to assess, treat, document, and adapt for dysfunction in these areas.
- Education and problem solving to ensure proper lighting. For example, a client who has low vision may benefit from direct white light on a subject to increase visibility of the subject and needs to know where to purchase a light and how to set it up correctly at the work area.

### Managing Diet and Fitness

Common interventions addressed by recreational therapy that fall under this code include issues related to nutrition and physical fitness. Recreational therapists address nutritional needs as they relate to choosing and consuming nutritious foods in real-life situations such as restaurants and eating on the go. The therapist obtains recommendations from the client's nutritionist, physician, and/or speech therapist, if there are dietary restrictions related to swallowing, and evaluates the possible barriers that could hinder the client's ability to follow through with their recommendations. Integration training in settings that pose difficulty for the client can be helpful to reinforce newly learned nutrition behaviors. Recreational therapists also assist clients in incorporating leisure time physical activity into their lifestyle for health and quality of life. Refer to the chapter on Physical Activity in the companion book, *Recreational Therapy Basics, Techniques, and Interventions*, for more information.

### Maintaining One's Health

This code relates to a client's activities and behaviors needed to maintain his/her health. The specific activities and behaviors are determined by each client's needs and will therefore vary from client to client. This code is different from other codes in this chapter because it focuses on "awareness" and "action." It challenges the therapist to ask the questions: "Is the client aware of activities and behavior that impact his/her health?" and, "Is the client able to follow through on what is required for maintaining his/her health by implementing recommendations, carrying over learned skills, and making healthy choices that impact health, level of functioning, independence, and quality of life?" In essence, can the client pull it all together and integrate what s/he needs to do to stay healthy?

Therapists in a rehabilitation setting are able to assess a client's "awareness" through verbalizations and discussions about what needs to be done to stay healthy. A healthy activity pattern for after discharge can be developed.

Evaluating the client's ability to act on a plan can be harder, though. Sometimes the initial phases of the activity plan can be started while the client is still working with the recreational therapist to evaluate how well the client will be able to fulfill the plan. Another way to assess the client's ability to perform required actions is to give out homework assignments and see how well they are carried out. Even if this kind of assessment isn't possible, therapists are typically aware of the client's activities and behaviors during structured and unstructured time through their observations and reports from other health care professionals. Using the available information, the therapist can evaluate the client's ability to follow through with health activities and behaviors and make a guess as to how well the client will be able to maintain his/her health. Ideally, the client will be seen for follow-up evaluations after discharge to get a more accurate picture of health maintenance if there is a concern in this area.

The code does not allow the therapist to delineate between "awareness" and "action," therefore the therapist needs to ask both of these questions:

- To what extent is the client aware of the health activities and behaviors that affect his/her health? (knowledge, measured as a fraction).
- To what extent is the client able to carry over healthy activities and behaviors into his/her daily life? (action, measured as a fraction).

A suggestion on how to score this code is to look at both components that are required for maintaining one's health, awareness and action. To find out how many of the actions a client will actually do to maintain his/her health multiply the awareness fraction times the action fraction. For example, if a client has 60% of the knowledge required to maintain his health and acts on it every time, he still is able to do only 60% of the things required to maintain his health. The 40% difficulty would be scored d570._ _ _ 2. Similarly, if a client knows everything that she needs to do to maintain her health, but acts on it only 60% of the time, she will also be doing 60% of the things required to maintain her health. The 40% difficulty would be scored d570._ _ _ 2. The multiplication is required when a client does not know everything and does not act on everything s/he knows. For example, a client who knows 60% of what is required and acts on it 60% of the time will be doing only 36% of what is required to maintain health (.6 times .6) The 64% difficulty would be scored d570._ _ _ 3. From a treatment perspective it is usually best to work on the component (awareness or action) that is lower.

Recreational therapists put a strong emphasis on maintaining health through client engagement in forms of physical leisure that are safe and appropriate for the client's abilities and limitations. Recreational therapists explore the client's interests to identify forms of physical leisure activity that are attractive to the client.

Once a safe, appropriate, and realistic form of physical leisure is identified and clearance for participation in the activity is given by the client's physician, the therapist addresses the development of functional skills that are necessary for participation. The therapist helps the client to identify resources for participation and problem solves for anticipated barriers. See d175 Solving Problems. Lastly, integration training provides the therapist with the opportunity to assess the client's performance in his/her real-life setting, address unforeseen issues, and provide emotional and professional support. Score the findings under the specific community activity, for example d4702 Using Public Motorized Transportation, d4601 Moving Around within Buildings Other Than Home, d4602 Moving Around outside the Home and Other Buildings, or d9201 Sports.

### Cross References

In *Recreational Therapy for Specific Diagnoses and Conditions, First Edition*, ICF code d570 Looking After One's Health is listed in 33 chapters:

Amputation and Prosthesis, Attention-Deficit/Hyperactivity Disorder, Autism Spectrum Disorder, Back Disorders and Back Pain, Borderline Personality Disorder, Burns, Cancer, Cerebral Palsy, Cerebrovascular Accident, Chronic Obstructive Pulmonary Disease, Diabetes Mellitus, Epilepsy, Feeding and Eating Disorders, Fibromyalgia and Juvenile Fibromyalgia, Gambling Disorder, Guillain-Barré Syndrome, Heart Disease, Intellectual Disability, Major Depressive Disorder, Multiple Sclerosis, Neurocognitive Disorders, Obesity, Osteoarthritis, Parkinson's Disease, Post-Traumatic Stress Disorder, Rheumatoid Arthritis, Sickle Cell Disease, Spina Bifida, Spinal Cord Injury, Substance-Related Disorders, Total Joint Replacement, Traumatic Brain Injury, and Visual Impairments and Blindness.

In *Recreational Therapy Basics, Techniques, and Interventions, First Edition*, treatment for ICF code d570 Looking After One's Health is discussed in 20 chapters: Activity and Task Analysis, Adjustment and Response to Disability, Education and Counseling, Participation, Stress, Activity Pattern Development, Aquatic Therapy, Assertiveness Training, Bibliotherapy, Cognitive Behavioral Counseling, Energy Conservation Techniques, Leisure Education and Counseling, Leisure Resource Awareness, Mind-Body Interventions, Montessori Method, Physical Activity, Sexual Well-Being, Social Skills Training, Therapeutic Relationships, and Values Clarification.

## d598 Self-Care, Other Specified

## d599 Self-Care, Unspecified

### References

Barlow, J., Wright, C., Sheasby, J., Turner, A., & Hainsworth, J. (2002). Self-management approaches for people with chronic conditions: A review. *Pat Educ Couns, 48*,177-187.

Cott, C. A., Wiles, R., & Devitt, R. (2007). Continuity, transition and participation: Preparing clients for life in the community post-stroke. *Disability and Rehabilitation, 29*(20-21), 1566-1574.

Driver, S., Rees, K., O'Connor, J., & Lox, C. (2006). Aquatics, health-promoting self-care behaviors and adults with brain injuries. *Brain Injury, 20*(2), 133-141.

Dunbar, S. B., Clark, P. C., Quinn, C., Gary, R. A., & Kaslow, N. J. (2008). Family influences on heart failure self-care and outcomes. *Journal of Cardiovascular Nursing, 23*(3), 258-265.

Egede, L. E., Ellis, C., & Grubaugh, A. L. (2009). The effect of depression on self-care behaviors and quality of care in a national sample of adults with diabetes. *General Hospital Psychiatry, 31*, 422-427.

Kennedy, A., Rogers, A., & Bower, P. (2007). Support for self-care for patients with chronic disease. *British Medical Journal, 335*, 968-970.

Murphy, N. A. & Carbone, P. S. (2008). Promoting participation of children with disabilities in sports, recreation, and physical activities. *Pediatrics, 121*, 1057-1061.

Rao, S. M. & Gagie, B. (2006). Learning through seeing and doing: Visual supports for children with autism. *Teaching Exceptional Children, 38*(6), 26-33.

Roth, E. J. & Lovell, L. (2007). Community skill performance and its association with the ability to perform everyday tasks by stroke survivors one year following rehabilitation discharge. *Topics in Stroke Rehabilitation, 14*(1), 48-56.

Wang, Y. & Stumbo, N. J. (2009). Factors affecting quality of life for community-dwelling older adults with a disability: Implications for therapeutic recreation practice and research. *Annual in Therapeutic Recreation, XVII*, 18-30.

# Chapter 6 Domestic Life

This chapter is about carrying out domestic and everyday actions and tasks. Areas of domestic life include acquiring a place to live, food, clothing, and other necessities, household cleaning and repairing, caring for personal and other household objects, and assisting others.

*Sample Scoring of Domestic Life*

- A teenager with a mild traumatic brain injury recently began working at the neighborhood ice cream stand. He is saving his money to buy a new skateboard (d6200 Shopping). He is able to independently select the skateboard he wants to purchase (no difficulty = 0), but requires maximum assistance to compare the quality and price to other skateboards (complete difficulty = 4). He has no problems paying for the skateboard (good money skills, no difficulty = 0) but plans on riding it home after he purchases it (two miles on a very busy six-lane boulevard, complete difficulty = 4). To score his shopping skills, the therapist can either use the average of the scores (0, 0, 4, 4 = 8 divided by 4 = 2) or choose the lowest score (4), which is the recommendation of the author. Consequently, the correct scoring would look like this: d6200.4 _ _ 4.

- The parents of a child with a congenital disability adopted a puppy from the local shelter. The child is responsible for helping with pet care (d6506 Taking Care of Animals). She has to feed the puppy every morning and evening, play with the puppy at least one hour a day, and take it for a short walk up and down the block two times a day. The child is physically and cognitively able to perform such tasks, but often "forgets" to complete all of the required tasks. On average, she completes 90% of the required tasks (mild difficulty = 1). With reminders from her parents, she completes all of the tasks (no difficulty = 0). The correct scoring would look like this: d6506.0 _ _ 1.

Domestic life is comprised of common, everyday activities. The degree of engagement in such activities will vary depending on interest, ability, motivation, resources, and living situation. Lack of engagement in domestic life activities, if not met through the actions of others, can jeopardize health and quality of life. For example, if an individual has difficulty doing housework, whether from problems such as hoarding or from physical or psychological impairment, the home can become unsanitary and breed disease. If an individual has trouble caring for his/her children, the children may be taken away by the Department of Human Services. And, if an individual has difficulty preparing meals, nutritional needs might not be met. These are also basic skills that a child or adolescent learns through assisting others with such tasks.

Domestic life activities are not only necessary life tasks. These activities are also vital to our health, well-being, and quality of life. For example, a review of the literature found that people who own and care for a pet dog experience a reduction in the frequency of minor physical ailments; have a decreased risk for coronary heart disease and are more likely to be alive one year after having a heart attack; have lower serum triglycerides, stress, blood pressure, and heart rate; have lower autonomic responses to stressful situations; and ameliorate the effects of stressful life events; engage in more physical activity; have less anxiety, loneliness, and depression; experience feelings of autonomy, competence, and self-esteem; and have increased social interactions with others (Wells, 2007). The author also found that service dogs increase social interactions with others, decrease feelings of isolation, and improve social confidence, self-esteem, independence, and social identity. Residential dogs and animal visits in nursing homes result in happier, more alert, and more responsive residents. In prisons, residential dogs increase self-esteem and improve behavior, respect for authority, social interaction, and leadership. Some dogs were found to have the ability to detect ill health, such as cancer, oncoming epileptic seizures, or hypoglycemia.

In another study, all levels of gardening for older adults were found to enhance relaxation, psychological and physiological functioning, and overall life satisfaction (Cheng et al., 2010).

As a final example, helping and assisting others through volunteer work has also been found to have health benefits. Piliavin and Siegl (2007) found through a longitudinal study that volunteer work has a causal relationship with psychological well-being, particularly feeling good about oneself and feeling of "mattering." Continuous volunteer work for a variety of organizations led to more positive effects on psychological well-being. Psychological well-being is moderated by the level of social integration. Those who are less socially integrated benefit the most psychologically from volunteer experiences.

### Assessment of Domestic Life

Recreational therapists assess domestic life abilities through the medical record, consultation with other healthcare clinicians, client and caregiver interview, direct request, and observation. Once baselines are obtained, exploration of needs related to application of domestic life skills in leisure and community activities is completed. Treatment interventions aimed at using domestic life skills in leisure and community settings are implemented. Then skills in leisure and community activities are assessed by direct observation of performance.

### Treatment of Domestic Life

A client may acquire knowledge and skills related to domestic life from other health professionals, but recreational therapists evaluate and address (1) the impact of domestic life skills on participation in life activities (e.g., difficulty dressing that is impairing ability and motivation to go to the health club), (2) the skills required to complete tasks in various community and recreational settings (e.g., how to propel a wheelchair uphill while walking the dog), (3) adaptive equipment and techniques in addition to those provided by other healthcare professionals to minimize difficulty in real-life settings (e.g., utilizing a bungee cord to hold pants down when self-cathing in a public bathroom), and (4) integration training in the specific area where the client performs the tasks. Recreational therapists who work in independent living and assisted living may additionally address domestic life skills and tasks in the home setting for the purpose of teaching and promoting independence with basic life tasks.

### Evidence Review

Several studies highlight evidence-based practice related to domestic life. This is only a sample of the evidence. A thorough review of the literature is needed to identify evidence-based practice inter-

ventions that reflect the needs and characteristics of the individual client.

Lee and Kim (2007) conducted a study of 23 individuals with dementia in a long-term care facility. The subjects had a sleep disturbance and/or agitation. Participation in a five-week gardening program showed significant improvement in sleep, agitation level, and cognition.

Volicer et al. (2006) conducted an observational study of 90 veterans with dementia on two specialized dementia units in a long-term care facility. The residents were engaged in "continuous activity programming." Traditional activity programming consists of scheduled activities with blocks of open time between activities. Continuous activity programming is different in that it requires the involvement of all staff to continuously involve the residents in meaningful activity throughout the day. The residents might help pick out clothes, deliver a towel to another resident, help with simple meal preparation, gather items for activities, and help to water the plants on the unit. The authors note that apathy and agitation are often outcomes of inability to initiate meaningful activities. Consequently, increased engagement in meaningful activity is needed to prevent apathy and agitation, as well as improve quality of life. Engagement in the continuous activity programming model increased the number of hours involved in activity, decreased the use of psychotropic medication, improved nutrition, increased family satisfaction, decreased agitation, and improved sleep.

Sisirak et al. (2007) conducted a study of 60 adults with moderate to severe intellectual disability. Their challenging behaviors caused them to be relocated from an institutional setting to a community living center (a dispersed group home in a community with non-gated domestic houses) or congregate care facility (a large-scale group home in the community gated off from the surrounding community and run by the government). Measures were recorded prior to relocation, 12 months post relocation, and 24 months post relocation. The community group achieved more domestic skills in cleaning, laundry, table setting, food preparation, routine household chores, and prevocational and vocational skills. They were better at staying on task, task completion, care for equipment, and number and time skills that were developed through counting objects during table setting, meal preparation, and grocery shopping. They also had increased opportunities for socialization with others in the community. The community group also had significantly improved levels of trustworthiness and decreased sexual behavior. They showed more respect for others' property, less taking and damaging of others' property, less lying and cheating, and fewer instances of removing clothes and inappropriate touching. "This indicates reduced maladaptive behavior as a result of living in dispersed community housing as opposed to the larger-scale cluster center where there was more contact with other residents who were perhaps inappropriate role models and little encouragement to modify behavior in these areas" (p. 428). The community group also had increased opportunities for everyday choice making. Both groups showed increased quality of life scores. However the community group accessed more places in the community more frequently, had greater variety and number of daily routines, more input into decisions, and more personal achievements.

### Cross References

In *Recreational Therapy for Specific Diagnoses and Conditions, First Edition*, ICF code d6 Domestic Life and its subcategories are listed in 20 chapters: Amputation and Prosthesis, Cancer, Cerebrovascular Accident, Chronic Obstructive Pulmonary Disease, Feeding and Eating Disorders, Fibromyalgia and Juvenile Fibromyalgia, Hearing Loss, Heart Disease, Intellectual Disability, Neurocognitive Disorders, Obesity, Osteoarthritis, Osteoporosis, Parkinson's Disease, Pressure Ulcers, Rheumatoid Arthritis, Spinal Cord Injury, Substance-Related Disorders, Traumatic Brain Injury, and Visual Impairments and Blindness.

In *Recreational Therapy Basics, Techniques, and Interventions, First Edition*, treatment for ICF code d6 Domestic Life and its subcategories are discussed in 11 chapters: Adjustment and Response to Disability, Body Mechanics and Ergonomics, Activity Pattern Development, Adaptive Sports, Anger Management, Assertiveness Training, Balance Training, Cognitive Behavioral Counseling, Constraint-Induced Movement Therapy, Disability Rights: Education and Advocacy, and Wheelchair Mobility.

## Acquisition of Necessities (d610 - d629)

### d610 Acquiring a Place to Live

Buying, renting, furnishing, and arranging a house, apartment, or other dwelling.

Inclusions: buying or renting a place to live and furnishing a place to live

Exclusions: acquisition of goods and services (d620); caring for household objects (d650)

- *d6100 Buying a Place to Live*
  Acquiring ownership of a house, apartment, or other dwelling.

- *d6101 Renting a Place to Live*
  Acquiring the use of a house, apartment, or other dwelling belonging to another in exchange for payment.

- *d6102 Furnishing a Place to Live*
  Equipping and arranging a living space with furniture, fixtures, and other fittings and decorating rooms.

- *d6108 Acquiring a Place to Live, Other Specified*
- *d6109 Acquiring a Place to Live, Unspecified*
  Recreational therapists who work in community integration settings as clients transition from assisted living to independent living environments are likely to score this code. Situations that arise to necessitate the need of acquiring a place to live include (1) no available pre-established home for the client to return to or move into, (2) desire by the client or client's guardian to live someplace different, (3) a current living situation that is no longer appropriate for the client, such as a home that doesn't meet accessibility needs, or (4) discharge from a residential program. The most common situation for a recreational therapist is assisting a client who is being discharged from a residential treatment setting.

In the ICF, therapists document the level of difficulty that the client has with each task, as well as listing any environmental factors that hinder or facilitate the task. For example, when assistance is not provided, the client has moderate difficulty choosing appropriate furniture that meets his needs (d6102._ _ _ 2). Therapists may also document more specific skills in discipline-specific documentation such as level of assistance, barriers, and facilitators to the activity, issues related to acquiring a place to live, client needs related to a living place, and the impact that it has on other life activities.

Recreational therapists assist clients in identifying their specific living needs such as how much money is available to purchase or rent and maintain a home, proximity to important destinations, ease of travel to other destinations, type of home, accessibility of the home, the surrounding environment, and available resources in the community.

Recreational therapists also assist clients in identifying appropriate furnishings by helping them choose furniture that provides adequate support for the client so that s/he can safely transfer onto and off of the furniture and allows an appropriate amount of space around the furnishings for safe mobility. Common adaptations to standard furnishings will depend on the needs of the client. Touch lights and lever door handles are common adaptations for physical disabilities. Integration training will further facilitate the process to allow the therapist to determine the actual level of accessibility and the ability of the surrounding environment to meet the client's needs.

### Cross References

In *Recreational Therapy for Specific Diagnoses and Conditions, First Edition*, ICF code d610 Acquiring a Place to Live is listed in one chapter: Multiple Sclerosis.

In *Recreational Therapy Basics, Techniques, and Interventions, First Edition*, there are no references for ICF code d610 Acquiring a Place to Live.

### d620 Acquisition of Goods and Services

Selecting, procuring, and transporting all goods and services required for daily living, such as selecting, procuring, transporting, and storing food, drink, clothing, cleaning materials, fuel, household items, utensils, cooking ware, domestic appliance and tools; procuring utilities and other household services.

Inclusions: shopping and gathering daily necessities

Exclusions: acquiring a place to live (d610)

- *d6200 Shopping*
  Obtaining, in exchange for money, goods and services required for daily living (including instructing and supervising an intermediary to do the shopping), such as selecting food, drink, cleaning materials, household items, or clothing

in a shop or market; comparing quality and price of the items required, negotiating and paying for selected goods or services, and transporting goods.

- *d6201 Gathering Daily Necessities*
  Obtaining, without exchange of money, goods and services required for daily living (including instructing and supervising an intermediary to gather daily necessities), such as by harvesting vegetables and fruits, and getting water and fuel.

- *d6208 Acquisition of Goods and Services, Other Specified*
- *d6209 Acquisition of Good and Services, Unspecified*

Recreational therapists, particularly those who work in the independent living movement and rehabilitation settings, address the skills related to acquisition of goods and services. For this ICF code, this includes shopping and gathering necessities. Shopping and gathering daily necessities, although commonly considered things that one has to do, are also things from which one can derive pleasure, satisfaction, and health. The act of shopping, for instance, is more than just buying groceries. It is also an opportunity to get out of the house for exercise, socialization, and cognitive processing.

The skills required for shopping and gathering daily necessities are complex, including mobility skills, cognitive skills, vision, social skills, and physical skills. A person out shopping may have to deal with walking on outdoor and indoor surfaces, car transfers, transfers to the store's electric scooter, toilet transfers, and changing body positions to reach items. The experience can require basic and complex math, attention, memory, problem solving, direction following, reading, and comprehending aisle signs. Social experiences may include interacting with familiar and unfamiliar people, assertion of needs, and requesting assistance from others. The person also needs the strength to lift items, push a store cart, and carry bags, along with balance and endurance.

In the ICF, therapists document the level of difficulty that the client has with the task of shopping and/or gathering daily necessities. For example, when assistance is not provided, the client has moderate difficulty shopping (d6200._ _ _ 2). In discipline-specific documentation, therapists will also document the level of assistance required for each specific skill in the task, recommendations, adaptive equipment, techniques utilized, and the problems that the difficulty with shopping imposes on other life activities and needs.

Due to the number and complexity of the skills required to shop and gather daily necessities, it is recommended that the therapist identify and score all of the codes that lie outside of this code set that are relevant to the client's ability to shop or gather daily necessities. For example, if the client needs to perform car transfers to be able to go shopping, the therapist would score d4200 Transferring Oneself While Sitting. If a client needs to lift grocery items, the therapist would score d4300 Lifting. If a client needs short-term memory skills to recall a shopping list, then b1440 Short-Term Memory would be scored. The skills that are involved in performing any community activity are numerous and it would be a daunting task for the therapist to identify and code every related code, therefore the best approach is to identify the skills in the community task that are difficult for the client and identify and score only those codes. So if a client does not have difficulty with short-term memory, then there is no need to identify and score the code of short-term memory even though it is a skill that occurs with the task of shopping and gathering daily necessities.

Outside of functional skill development, common educational interventions related to shopping and gathering daily necessities may include education about community energy conservation techniques to maximize safety and productivity, community accessibility training about what a community facility has to have in order to meet the accessibility needs of the client, outdoor mobility techniques for walking or using a wheelchair in a community setting, problem solving for community barriers, social skills training, and the Americans with Disabilities Act to know what services clients are entitled to and the level of accessibility to be provided. Family and caregiver training may also need to be a component of training if their assistance is required for task performance.

Recreational therapists will typically begin with functional skill development and education related to the tasks of shopping and gathering daily necessities, followed by community integration training to the specific stores and other locations that the client frequents. Common sites for integration training related to acquiring goods and services include

grocery stores, hardware stores, department stores, drug stores, and clothing stores. The therapist may begin by teaching the client outdoor wheelchair mobility techniques and how to problem solve for community barriers, and then take the client to the client's local grocery store to assess his ability to carry over learned skills into a real-life setting. The community session also provides an opportunity to pose "what if" questions that will assist the client in problem solving unexpected situations in the future.

### Cross References

In *Recreational Therapy for Specific Diagnoses and Conditions, First Edition*, ICF code d620 Acquisition of Goods and Services is listed in nine chapters: Chronic Obstructive Pulmonary Disease, Heart Disease, Intellectual Disability, Multiple Sclerosis, Obesity, Osteoarthritis, Pressure Ulcers, Spinal Cord Injury, and Visual Impairments and Blindness.

In *Recreational Therapy Basics, Techniques, and Interventions, First Edition*, treatment for ICF code d620 Acquisition of Goods and Services is discussed in one chapter: Adaptive Sports.

### d629 Acquisition of Necessities, Other Specified and Unspecified

## Household Tasks (d630 - d649)

### d630 Preparing Meals

Planning, organizing, cooking, and serving simple and complex meals for oneself and others, such as by making a menu, selecting edible food and drink, getting together ingredients for preparing meals, cooking with heat and preparing cold foods and drinks, and serving the food.

Inclusions: preparing simple and complex meals

Exclusions: eating (d550); drinking (d560); acquisition of goods and services (d620); doing housework (d640); caring for household objects (d650); caring for others (d660)

- *d6300 Preparing Simple Meals*
  Organizing, cooking, and serving meals with a small number of ingredients that require easy methods of preparation and serving, such as making a snack or small meal, and transforming food ingredients by cutting and stirring, boiling, and heating food such as rice or potatoes.

- *d6301 Preparing Complex Meals*
  Planning, organizing, cooking, and serving meals with a large number of ingredients that require complex methods of preparation and serving, such as planning a meal with several dishes, and transforming food ingredients by combined actions of peeling, slicing, mixing, kneading, stirring, presenting, and serving food in a manner appropriate to the occasion and culture.

  Exclusions: using household appliances (d6403)

- *d6308 Preparing Meals, Other Specified*
- *d6309 Preparing Meals, Unspecified*

Preparing simple and complex meals is a basic need to sustain life, unless there is another person or service that prepares meals. Preparing meals is often thought of something that is done in the home, although preparation of simple and complex meals is also performed in many other settings including recreational activities such as camping and hiking, work, school, volunteer work at a soup kitchen, and recreational cooking groups. The skill of preparing meals can also be a precursor skill to involvement in other life activities where food is served. The key point is to recognize that, if a client has difficulty preparing simple or complex meals, it could impact involvement in other life activities that provide many benefits.

In the ICF, therapists document the level of difficulty that a client has with each of the tasks in this code set. For example, when assistance is not provided at the campsite, the client has mild difficulty preparing simple meals (d6300._ _ _ 1). Other codes that cause the difficulties should also be scored. In discipline-specific documentation, therapists will additionally document the level of assistance required for each specific skill in the task of meal preparation, recommendations, adaptive equipment, techniques utilized, and the problems that the difficulties with meal preparation impose on other life activities and needs.

A client may acquire knowledge and skills of simple meal preparation from other health professionals. However, it is the recreational therapist who evaluates and addresses the impact of meal preparation skills on participation in life activities, the skills required to prepare simple and complex meals in various community and recreational settings, adaptive equipment and techniques in addition to

those provided by other health care professionals to minimize difficulty with meal preparation in real-life settings, and integration training for the specific area where the client performs meal preparation activities. Recreational therapists who work in independent living and assisted living may additionally address meal preparation in the home setting to promote independence with basic life tasks.

***Cross References***

In *Recreational Therapy for Specific Diagnoses and Conditions, First Edition*, ICF code d630 Preparing Meals is listed in eight chapters: Chronic Obstructive Pulmonary Disease, Feeding and Eating Disorders, Hearing Loss, Intellectual Disability, Multiple Sclerosis, Obesity, Traumatic Brain Injury, and Visual Impairments and Blindness.

In *Recreational Therapy Basics, Techniques, and Interventions, First Edition*, treatment for ICF code d630 Preparing Meals is discussed in one chapter: Assertiveness Training.

### d640 Doing Housework

Managing a household by cleaning the house, washing clothes, using household appliances, storing food, and disposing of garbage, such as by sweeping, mopping, washing counters, walls, and other surfaces; collecting and disposing of household garbage; tidying rooms, closets, and drawers; collecting, washing, drying, folding and ironing clothes; cleaning footwear; using brooms, brushes, and vacuum cleaners; using washing machines, driers, and irons.

Inclusions: washing and drying clothes and garments; cleaning cooking area and utensils; cleaning living area; using household appliances, storing daily necessities, and disposing of garbage

Exclusions: acquiring a place to live (d610); acquisition of goods and services (d620); preparing meals (d630); caring for household objects (d650); caring for others (d660)

- *d6400 Washing and Drying Clothes and Garments*
  Washing clothes and garments by hand and hanging them out to dry in the air.

- *d6401 Cleaning Cooking Area and Utensils*
  Cleaning up after cooking, such as by washing dishes, pans, pots, and cooking utensils, and

cleaning tables and floors around cooking and eating area.

- *d6402 Cleaning Living Area*
  Cleaning the living areas of the household, such as by tidying and dusting, sweeping, swabbing, mopping floors, cleaning windows and walls, cleaning bathrooms and toilets, and cleaning household furnishings.

- *d6403 Using Household Appliances*
  Using all kinds of household appliances, such as washing machines, driers, irons, vacuum cleaners, and dishwashers.

- *d6404 Storing Daily Necessities*
  Storing food, drinks, clothes, and other household goods required for daily living; preparing food for conservation by canning, salting, or refrigerating, keeping food fresh and out of the reach of animals.

- *d6405 Disposing of Garbage*
  Disposing of household garbage such as by collecting trash and rubbish around the house, preparing garbage for disposal, using garbage disposal appliances, burning garbage.

- *d6408 Doing Housework, Other Specified*
- *d6409 Doing Housework, Unspecified*

Housework includes washing and drying clothes, cleaning cooking area and utensils, cleaning living area, using household appliances, storing daily necessities, and disposing of garbage. Housework, although commonly thought of as being performed solely within the client's primary home, occurs in many different settings including camping, vacationing, and visiting others at their residences for an extended period of time. For example, washing and drying clothes may be performed at a campsite. Cleaning a cooking area and utensils may be performed at a picnic. Using household appliances such as a travel iron may be done when vacationing. Storing daily necessities in coolers and suitcases for travel and disposing of garbage while hiking through a park are also part of this code.

If difficulty with housework imposes a barrier to involvement in other life activities, further dysfunction can result. The client may choose to not go on camping trips with her daughter's Girl Scout troop, impacting d7601 Child-Parent Relationships, or the client may limit hikes so he does not have to pack

necessities or worry about disposing of garbage impacting d5701 Managing Diet and Fitness.

In the ICF, therapists document the level of difficulty that a client has with each of the tasks in this code set. For example, when assistance is not provided, the client has moderate difficulty storing daily necessities for a family day trip (d6404._ _ _ 2). ICF codes that cause the difficulty or are also impacted by the deficits are also documented. In discipline-specific documentation, therapists will additionally document the level of assistance required for each specific skill in the task of housework, recommendations, adaptive equipment, techniques utilized, and the problems that difficulty with housework imposes on other life activities and needs.

A client may acquire knowledge and skills of housework from other health professionals. However it is the recreational therapist who evaluates and addresses the impact of housework on participation in other life activities, the skills required of housework in various community and recreational settings, adaptive equipment, techniques in addition to those provided by other health professionals, and integration training to the specific area where the client performs housework activities. Recreational therapists who work in independent living and assisted living may additionally address housework with clients in the residential setting for the purpose of teaching and promoting independence with basic life tasks.

### Cross References

In *Recreational Therapy for Specific Diagnoses and Conditions, First Edition*, ICF code d640 Doing Housework is listed in three chapters: Multiple Sclerosis, Traumatic Brain Injury, and Visual Impairments and Blindness.

In *Recreational Therapy Basics, Techniques, and Interventions, First Edition*, there are no references for ICF code d640 Doing Housework.

### d649 Household Tasks, Other Specified and Unspecified

## Caring for Household Objects and Assisting Others (d650 - d669)

### d650 Caring for Household Objects

Maintaining and repairing household and other personal objects, including house and contents, clothes, vehicles, and assistive devices, and caring for plants and animals, such as painting or wallpapering rooms, fixing furniture, repairing plumbing, ensuring the proper working order of vehicles, watering plants, grooming and feeding pets and domestic animals.

Inclusions: making and repairing clothes; maintaining dwelling, furnishings, and domestic appliances; maintaining vehicles; maintaining assistive devices; taking care of plants (indoor and outdoor) and animals

Exclusions: acquiring a place to live (d610); acquisition of goods and services (d620); doing housework (d640); caring for others (d660); remunerative employment (d850)

- *d6500 Making and Repairing Clothes*
  Making and repairing clothes, such as by sewing, producing, or mending clothes; reattaching buttons and fasteners; ironing clothes, fixing and polishing footwear.

  Exclusions: using household appliances (d6403)

- *d6501 Maintaining Dwelling and Furnishings*
  Repairing and taking care of dwelling, its exterior, interior, and contents, such as by painting, repairing fixtures and furniture, and using required tools for repair work.

- *d6502 Maintaining Domestic Appliances*
  Repairing and taking care of all domestic appliances for cooking, cleaning, and repairing, such as by oiling and repairing tools and maintaining the washing machine.

- *d6503 Maintaining Vehicles*
  Repairing and taking care of motorized and non-motorized vehicles for personal use, including bicycles, carts, automobiles, and boats.

- *d6504 Maintaining Assistive Devices*
  Repairing and taking care of assistive devices, such as prostheses, orthoses, and specialized tools and aids for housekeeping and personal care; maintaining and repairing aids for personal mobility such as canes, walkers, wheelchairs, and scooters; and maintaining communication and recreational aids.

- *d6505 Taking Care of Plants, Indoors and Outdoors*
  Taking care of plants inside and outside the house, such as by planting, watering, and fertilizing plants; gardening and growing foods for personal use.

- *d6506 Taking Care of Animals*
  Taking care of domestic animals and pets, such as by feeding, cleaning, grooming, and exercising pets; watching over the health of animals or pets, planning for the care of animals or pets in one's absence.

- *d6508 Caring for Household Objects, Specified*
- *d6509 Caring for Household Objects, Unspecified*
  Recreational therapists address many of the skills in this section on caring for household objects because they are not only necessities; they are also forms of leisure. Sewing, home remodeling, fixing household appliances, working on cars, maintaining recreation equipment, indoor and outdoor gardening, and caring for pets are all listed under this section. Participation in these tasks, for the most part, is the choice of the individual. For example, one client may choose to buy clothes at the department store rather than making them due to lack of sewing skills or lack of time or interest in the activity, while another client may have the money and means to buy clothing but chooses to make her own clothes because it is enjoyable. The same goes for fixing cars and home remodeling and so on. Many Americans are fortunate to have this choice, but some do not. When these activities are necessities, they are often given priority in the occupational therapy treatment plan. When these activities are primarily leisure driven, they are incorporated into the recreational therapy treatment plan. An exception to this is those recreational therapists who work in settings where part of their role is to assist clients with the development of necessary daily living skills that may not necessarily be leisure driven.

Caring for household objects, although commonly thought of as being performed solely in the client's primary home, occurs in many different settings. A client may mend a button when out in the community, repair a piece of furniture at a friend's home because he has the proper tools, take a household appliance to the repair shop, fix a boat that is docked, repair a skateboard at the skateboard park, grow food at a neighborhood garden, or exercise a pet by going for walks in the park. Consequently, recreational therapists identify and address issues related to caring for household objects in community settings as well as in the home. Impaired ability to care for household objects, especially those that involve community settings, can have an impact on other life activities and areas of health.

In the ICF, therapists document when the client has difficulty with tasks in this code set. For example, when assistance is not provided, the client has moderate difficulty walking the family dog (d6506._ _ _ 2). Other ICF codes that cause or are affected by that difficulty are also documented. In discipline-specific documentation, therapists will additionally document the level of assistance required for each specific skill of caring for household objects, recommendations, adaptive equipment, techniques, and the problems that the difficulty of caring for household objects imposes on other life activities and needs.

A client may acquire knowledge and skills of caring for household objects from other health professionals. However, it is the recreational therapist who evaluates and addresses the impact of caring for household objects on participation in life activities, the skills required to care for household objects in various community and recreational settings, adaptive equipment and techniques in addition to those provided by other health professionals to minimize difficulty with caring for household objects, and integration training to the specific area where the client cares for household objects. Recreational therapists who work in independent living and assisted living may additionally address caring for household objects with clients in the residential setting for the purpose of teaching and promoting independence with basic life tasks.

Tasks in this code set may require the use of adapted tools that are specially designed or are on the general market and techniques that are standard or individualized modifications. When doing an evaluation of these codes, be sure to also check e115 Products and Technology for Personal Use in Daily Living or e140 Products and Technology for Culture, Recreation, and Sport. If one of these is relevant, include it in the documentation. Some of the common adaptations for tasks are provided below.

*Making and repairing clothes*: Adaptations include the repositioning of the sewing machine foot pedal so it can be operated by another body part, needle threaders, direct lighting, hemming clips instead of pins to hold a hem, a rotary cutter instead of scissors, adaptive scissors, and strips of Dycem wrapped around the thumb and index finger to help grip the needle.

*Maintaining dwellings and furnishings*: Adaptive tools and techniques include adaptive cuffs, pole extenders, and adaptive tools with ergonomic design, limited impact, light weight, automatic start, and automatic function. Examples include pole extenders for paintbrush rollers, the use of a clamp to stabilize a piece of broken furniture, putting a piece of putty on a piece of wood and then placing the nail into the putty so that it holds it steady when a client who only has use of one hand is getting the nail started, a lightweight, self-coiling hose to wash the exterior of the home, or a long-handled sponge to wash windows. Adaptive equipment and techniques for dusting, sweeping, swabbing, mopping, cleaning windows and walls, cleaning bathrooms and toilets, and cleaning household furniture include the use of adaptive tools that are either specially designed or on the general market. Some examples include the use of a long-handled duster, an automatic floor vacuum that does not require a human to push it, disposable floor cleaning systems that do not require wringing a mop, a lightweight automatic sweeper instead of a broom, sitting on a chair outside of the tub and cleaning the bathtub with a long-handled scrubby, and the use of spray-on products that do not require scrubbing.

*Maintaining domestic appliances*: Examples include the use of automatic and power tools, homemade items, such as a magnet on the end of a stick to retrieve fallen nails, and individualized techniques.

*Maintaining vehicles*: Examples include the use automatic and power tools, such as an air gun to take off lug nuts instead of using a wrench, a bicycle lift that raises the bike up into the air so that it is easier to work on, placing small parts on a tray or a piece of Dycem so they do not roll away, and built-up tool handles using foam tubing for people who have impaired hand grasp.

*Maintaining assistive devices*: Examples include the use of soft cloth that sticks to a Velcro mitt, the use of electric tools, the use of a palm sander to hold a buffing cloth to care for a sit-ski, or using built-up handles on pliers to tighten a butterfly nut on a pair of adaptive skates.

*Taking care of plants*: Examples include the use of long-handled, lightweight tools, use of raised garden beds and flower boxes, a device that allows a person to raise or lower a hanging flower basket with an automatic release pulley system, a lightweight, self-coiling hose, the use of a wrapping paper tube to slide seeds down to a specific area on the ground, use of a post hole digger instead of a shovel, specially designed gardening tools to maximize joint protection and use larger muscle groups, garden kneelers, and gardening chairs.

*Taking care of animals*: Example include using a long-handled pooper scooper to clean out a kitty litter box, using a basket with a stiff handle to raise and lower animal food to the ground, kitty litter boxes with an automatic cleaning grid, a clothesline to hook a long leash onto so that the dog can get out for exercise in an unfenced yard, modifying a bird cage with a larger door opening to be able to easily access the pet, and adapted pet brushes.

There are many skills needed to participate in the activities of this code set. If deficits are suspected in this area, the therapist conducts a task analysis to determine the specific areas of difficulty. Refer to the code that reflects the area of difficulty for information on assessment, document, treatment, and adaptation.

### Cross References

In *Recreational Therapy for Specific Diagnoses and Conditions, First Edition*, ICF code d650 Caring for Household Objects is listed in two chapters: Amputation and Prosthesis and Multiple Sclerosis.

In *Recreational Therapy Basics, Techniques, and Interventions, First Edition*, there are no references for ICF code d650 Caring for Household Objects.

### d660 Assisting Others

Assisting household members and others with their learning, communicating, self-care, movement, within the house or outside; being concerned about the well-being of household members and others.

Inclusions: assisting others with self-care, movement, communication, interpersonal relations, nutrition, and health maintenance

Exclusion: remunerative employment (d850)

- *d6600 Assisting Others with Self-Care*
  Assisting household members and others in performing self-care, including helping others with eating, bathing, and dressing; taking care of children or members of the household who are sick or have difficulties with basic self-care; helping other with their toileting.

- *d6601 Assisting Others in Movement*
  Assisting household members and others in movements and in moving outside the home, such as in the neighborhood or city, to or from school, place of employment, or other destination.

- *d6602 Assisting Others in Communication*
  Assisting household members and others with their communication, such as by helping with speaking, writing, or reading.

- *d6603 Assisting Others in Interpersonal Relations*
  Assisting household members and others with their interpersonal interactions, such as by helping them to initiate, maintain, or terminate relationships.

- *d6604 Assisting Others in Nutrition*
  Assisting household members and others with their nutrition, such as by helping them to prepare and eat meals.

- *d6605 Assisting Others in Health Maintenance*
  Assisting household members and others with formal and informal health care, such as by ensuring that a child gets regular medical check-ups, or that an elderly relative takes required medication.

- *d6608 Assisting Others, Other Specified*
- *d6609 Assisting Others, Unspecified*

Assisting others, like caring for household objects, can be a necessity or a choice. For example, it is necessary for an adult to assist a child with self-care, but it may not be necessary for a person to assist others with transportation. Like the other codes in this chapter, assisting others occurs in many different contexts and environments, including community settings. Recreational therapists identify and address issues related to assisting others in these settings. Impaired ability to care for others can have an impact on other life activities, thus impacting other areas of health. For example, difficulty caring for an elderly parent requires the client to hire private assistance. This impacts the client's finances and other life activities that require money.

In the ICF, therapists document the level of difficulty that a client has with each of the tasks in this code set. For example, when assistance is not provided, the client has mild difficulty feeding her one-year-old daughter at family functions (d6604._ _ _ 1). Therapists also document other ICF codes that are causing the difficulty and additional difficulties caused by problems with this code set. In discipline-specific documentation, therapists will document the level of assistance required for each specific skill in the task of assisting others, recommendations, adaptive equipment, techniques, and the problems that the difficulty with assisting others imposes on other life activities and needs.

A client may acquire knowledge and skills of assisting others from other health professionals. However, it is the recreational therapist who evaluates and addresses the impact of assisting others on other life activities, the skills required to assist others in various community and recreational settings, adaptive equipment and technique recommendations in addition to those provided by other health professionals, and integration training to the specific area where the client assists others. Treatment involves finding ways to get around the causes of difficulties with assisting others through education, training, or finding suitable adaptations.

### Cross References

In *Recreational Therapy for Specific Diagnoses and Conditions, First Edition*, ICF code d660 Assisting Others is listed in one chapter: Multiple Sclerosis.

In *Recreational Therapy Basics, Techniques, and Interventions, First Edition*, treatment for ICF code d660 Assisting Others is discussed in one chapter: Wheelchair Mobility.

### d669 Caring for Household Objects and Assisting Others, Other Specified and Unspecified

### d698 Domestic Life, Other Specified

### d699 Domestic Life, Unspecified

*References*
Cheng, E. H., Patterson, I., Packer, J., & Pegg, S. (2010). Identifying the satisfactions derived from leisure gardening by older adults. *Annals of Leisure Research, 13*(3), 395-419.
Lee, Y. & Kim, S. (2007). Effects of indoor gardening on sleep, agitation, and cognition in dementia patients: A pilot study. *International Journal of Geriatric Psychiatry, 23*(5), 485-489.
Piliavin, J. A. & Siegl, E. (2007). Health benefits of volunteering in the Wisconsin longitudinal study, *Journal of Health and Social Behavior, 48*(4), 450-464.
Sisirak, J., Marks, B., Heller, T., & Riley, B. B. (2007). Dietary habits of adults with intellectual and developmental disabilities residing in community-based settings. *Intellectual and Developmental Disabilities, 46*(5), 335-345.
Volicer, L., Simard, J., Pupa, J. H., Medrek, R., & Riordan, M. E. (2006). Effects of continuous activity programming on behavioral symptoms of dementia. *Journal of the American Medical Association, 7*(7), 426-431.
Wells, D. L. (2007). Domestic dogs and human health: An overview. *The British Journal of Health Psychology, 12*(1), 145-156.

# Chapter 7 Interpersonal Interactions and Relationships

This chapter is about carrying out the actions and tasks required for basic and complex interactions with people (strangers, friends, relatives, family members, and lovers) in a contextually and socially appropriate manner.

*Sample Scoring of Interpersonal Interactions and Relationships*

- At a summer day program, a 10-year-old girl with autism requires 80% assistance (severe difficulty = 3) to create a friendship with a peer (d7500 Informal Relationships with Friends). With assistance from the therapist, she is able to create a friendship with a peer (no difficulty = 0). The complete scoring for the code would look like this: d7500.0 _ _ 3.
- A 24-year-old male sustained a traumatic brain injury. In rehab, he has difficulty reading social cues (d7104 Social Cues in Relationships) 40% of the time (moderate difficulty = 2). When cued by the therapist, this reduces to 20% difficulty (mild difficulty = 1). During a community integration training session to his local golf range, his difficulty in reading social cues is heightened due to increased distractions. He exhibits 75% difficulty (severe difficulty = 3) reading social cues and this remains unchanged (severe difficulty = 3) even with cues from his girlfriend. The complete scoring for the code would look like this: d7104.3 2 1 3.

Basic and complex interpersonal skills are building blocks in the development of meaningful relationships. These skills are normally developed while growing up, but some conditions limit a person's ability to develop and express appropriate interpersonal interactions. These conditions include developmental disabilities such as autism and mental retardation, psychological disorders such as obsessive-compulsive disorder, schizophrenia, and anxiety disorders, neurological injuries such as brain injury and multiple sclerosis, along with abuse and poor parenting.

Underlying Body Functions that may impair a client's ability to engage in basic interpersonal interactions include b152 Emotional Functions; b1800 Experience of Self; b126 Temperament and Personality Functions; b1 Mental Functions, such as b1142 Orientation to Person; and other impairments such as b230 Hearing Functions and b210 Seeing Functions. Environmental factors may also pose difficulty, including the design of the environment, availability of communication equipment, and barriers that limit social opportunities.

Personal Factors, although not currently coded in the ICF, can also impact interpersonal interactions and relationships. For example, some clients may have proficient basic and complex interpersonal skills and know how to relate to people but they may lack the willingness to interact out of frustration, anger, disrespect, etc. When interacting with others, clients are evaluated on whether they follow the special rules

of their society and culture for treating other people in structured and unstructured situations. Socially appropriate interactions in one culture may be offensive to another culture causing conflict. Beliefs may differ on how relationships should operate. Consequently, the client may feel that s/he doesn't fit in with the currently available peer group or s/he may feel pressured to conform to more dominant social norms, negatively affecting the formation of healthy relationships.

The ability to engage in appropriate interpersonal interactions and create, maintain, and terminate relationships within the context of leisure and community activities is a primary area of concern for recreational therapy. If a client has difficulty with basic and/or complex interpersonal interactions, the formation, maintenance, and quality of relationships will suffer and have negative consequences on the client's health and quality of life.

For example, in a Whitehall study of 10,308 British civil servants, findings indicated that those who reported lower reciprocity in their social relationships with partners, relatives, or workmates had significantly more sleep problems and depression, along with lower physical and mental health scores (Chandola, Marmot, & Siegrist, 2007).

A meta-analytic review of 148 studies (308,849 people followed for an average of 7.5 years) found that individuals who had adequate or good social relationships had a 50% greater likelihood of survival compared to those with poor or insufficient social relationships (Holt-Lunstad, Smith, & Layton, 2010). The authors noted that this statistical finding exceeds many well-know risk factors for mortality including obesity and physical inactivity. They call for the inclusion of social relationship screenings as part of routine medical care, along with the outright promotion of social connections and the facilitation of "naturally occurring social relations and community-based interventions" (p 14).

Social relationships have also been found to positively influence health behavior across the life course (Umberson, Crosnoe, & Reczek, 2010), leisure and recreation participation (King et al., 2010; Sasidharan et al., 2006), and the development of a more positive "biological profile" reducing risk of disease processes (Uchino, 2006).

As a final example, data analyzed from the Behavioral Risk Factor Surveillance System (BRFSS) for over 300,000 people found that lower social and emotional support yielded fair or poor general health, dissatisfaction with life, higher disability, increased days of physical and mental distress, activity limitation, depressive symptoms, anxiety symptoms, insufficient sleep, higher levels of pain, increased smoking, increased obesity, physical inactivity, heavy drinking, and fewer reported days of vitality (Strine et al., 2008).

### Assessment of Interpersonal Interactions and Relationships

Assessment of basic and complex interpersonal interaction skills and relationships is not a simple process. A multi-faceted behavioral approach is recommended, including an interview, multiple observations, and ongoing re-assessment. Because a client's interpersonal interactions may differ by situations and persons, assessment in more than one setting and with a variety of people is warranted. Recreational therapists note and record observed behaviors in the context of naturally occurring and structured leisure and community activities and utilize behavioral checklists or rating scales to record information on social strengths and weaknesses. Standardized tools that the recreational therapist might consider include: *Leisure Social/Sexual Assessment*, the *CERT-Psych/R*, the *FOX*, the *School Social Behavior Scales*, the *Home and Community Social Behavior Scales*, and the *Social Attributes Checklist*.

A full evaluation of difficulties and impairments is also conducted to identify underlying impairments affecting interpersonal interactions and relationships, such as hearing or visual impairment, mood instability, and inability to handle stress. An evaluation of the environment is conducted to determine its conduciveness to interpersonal interactions and creation and maintenance of relationships. The therapist also evaluates personal factors that may influence interactions and relationships, such as attitudes, beliefs, and culture.

When evaluating a client's relationship with others, the others are included in the observation. This can be done, for example, by playing a game together or including the other person in community integration training sessions. A client's account of the relationship should not be the sole determinant, whenever possible. Ideally, observations should take place in the real-life situations to obtain the most accurate data. This is especially true for family and caregiver relationships, as this is a key relationship for client recovery, health, and quality of life.

### Treatment of Interpersonal Interactions and Relationships

Refer to Social Skills Training in the companion book, *Recreational Therapy Basics, Techniques, and Interventions* for specific treatment information.

### Evidence Review

Several studies are provided to highlight evidence-based practice related to interpersonal interactions and relationships. This is only a sample of the evidence. A thorough review of the literature is needed to identify evidence-based practice interventions that reflect the needs and characteristics of the individual client. Therapists can also refer to d3 Communication for evidenced-based interventions related to social skills, as this overlaps with interpersonal interactions and relationships.

Ryan et al. (2008) conducted a study of 17 couples, one of which had a stroke. The couples were living at home and had been discharged from a health facility for at least six months. The couples participated in an eight-week group therapy program that included couple therapy, recreational therapy, leisure education, physiotherapy, exercise therapy, speech therapy, recreation participation with other couples, and informal peer contact. The leisure education consisted of five sessions looking at development of cognitive understanding of leisure, positive attitude towards leisure experiences, participatory and decision-making skills, and knowledge and ability to use resources. It also addressed attitudes, values awareness, interests, barriers, resources, and planning. At the end of the program, couples developed an individualized recreational therapy intervention plan focused on community reintegration. The *Leisure Diagnostic Battery*, along with a self-report of individual and couple leisure pursuits, was utilized to measure leisure functioning at pre-treatment, post treatment, and eight-month follow up. The couples were found to have increased perception for leisure opportunities, increased community engagement, and increased spousal perception of the partner's leisure competence. The participants who had a stroke reported trying a new physical, community-based program (53%), making a new social contact to do "things" (24%), and resuming or continuing a past interest (47%). Spousal relationships were strengthened through the program.

Van Nieuwenhuijzen and Vriens (2012) conducted a study of 79 children age eight to twelve years with mild to moderate borderline intellectual disabilities and behavioral problems that caused limitations in social and adaptive behavior. Findings indicate that participants who had difficulties with emotion recognition, interpretation, working memory, and inhibition skills were more likely to have difficulties processing social information and problem solving. Emotion recognition and working memory help to encode information more thoroughly. Emotion recognition and interpretation skills are predictive of adequate response generation, evaluation, and selection. Although social skills training and behavior regulation training are commonly provided, "it is important for clinicians to examine both social information processing skills and social cognitive skills, in order to unravel the underlying causes of behavior problems and inadequate social information processing.... Understanding social information processing leads to more understanding in parents and teachers and changes their attitude towards the child" (p. 432).

McDonald et al. (2008) conducted a study of 39 people with severe, chronic acquired brain injury. Participants completed a weekly three-hour group session for 12 weeks. The sessions focused on social behaviors, such as greetings, introducing oneself to others, listening, giving compliments, starting a conversation, selecting topics, being assertive, and coping with disagreements. Each session had goals and interventions tailored to client needs. The group structure consisted of warm-up games, review of homework, introduction of a target skill, discussion of potential issues and solutions, therapist modeling of appropriate and inappropriate behavior, and role playing to develop new skills. Immediate feedback and extensive repetition aided learning and memory. There were homework assignments each week. There was an additional one-hour individual session each week that focused on psychological issues, such as mood and self-esteem. Participants improved by reducing self-centered behavior and increasing partner involvement. They were less likely to talk about themselves and more likely to encourage the other person to contribute to the conversation, improving on a key problem for frontal lobe traumatic brain injury.

### Cross References

In *Recreational Therapy for Specific Diagnoses and Conditions, First Edition*, ICF code d7 Interpersonal Interactions and Relationships and its subcategories are listed in 35 chapters: Amputation and Prosthesis, Attention-Deficit/Hyperactivity Disorder, Autism Spectrum Disorder, Back Disorders and Back Pain, Borderline Personality Disorder, Burns, Cancer, Cerebral Palsy, Cerebrovascular Accident, Chronic Obstructive Pulmonary Disease, Epilepsy, Feeding and Eating Disorders, Fibromyalgia and Juvenile Fibromyalgia, Gambling Disorder, Generalized Anxiety Disorder, Guillain-Barré Syndrome, Hearing Loss, Heart Disease, Intellectual Disability, Major Depressive Disorder, Multiple Sclerosis, Neurocognitive Disorders, Obesity, Oppositional Defiant Disorder and Conduct Disorder, Osteoarthritis, Parkinson's Disease, Post-Traumatic Stress Disorder, Rheumatoid Arthritis, Schizophrenia Spectrum and Other Psychotic Disorders, Sickle Cell Disease, Spina Bifida, Spinal Cord Injury, Substance-Related Disorders, Traumatic Brain Injury, and Visual Impairments and Blindness.

In *Recreational Therapy Basics, Techniques, and Interventions, First Edition*, treatment for ICF code d7 Interpersonal Interactions and Relationships and its subcategories are discussed in 32 chapters: Activity and Task Analysis, Adjustment and Response to Disability, Education and Counseling,

Parameters and Precautions, Participation, Stress, Activity Pattern Development, Adaptive Sports, Adventure Therapy, Anger Management, Animal Assisted Therapy, Aquatic Therapy, Assertiveness Training, Behavior Strategies and Interventions, Bibliotherapy, Cognitive Behavioral Counseling, Cognitive Retraining and Rehabilitation, Disability Rights: Education and Advocacy, Group Psychotherapy Techniques, Leisure Education and Counseling, Leisure Resource Awareness, Life Review, Mind-Body Interventions, Montessori Method, Reality Orientation, Reminiscence, Sensory Interventions, Sexual Well-Being, Social Skills Training, Therapeutic Relationships, Therapeutic Thematic Arts Programming, and Values Clarification.

## General Interpersonal Interactions (d710 - d729)

### d710 Basic Interpersonal Interactions

Interacting with people in a contextually and socially appropriate manner, such as by showing consideration and esteem when appropriate, or responding to the feelings of others.

Inclusions: showing respect, warmth, appreciation, and tolerance in relationships; responding to criticism and social cues in relationships; and using appropriate physical contact in relationships

- *d7100 Respect and Warmth in Relationships*
  Showing and responding to consideration and esteem, in a contextually and socially appropriate manner.

- *d7101 Appreciation in Relationships*
  Showing and responding to satisfaction and gratitude, in a contextually and socially appropriate manner.

- *d7102 Tolerance in Relationships*
  Showing and responding to understanding and acceptance of behavior, in a contextually and socially appropriate manner.

- *d7103 Criticism in Relationships*
  Providing and responding to implicit and explicit differences of opinion or disagreement, in a contextually and socially appropriate manner.

- *d7104 Social Cues in Relationships*
  Giving and reacting appropriately to signs and hints that occur in social interactions.

- *d7105 Physical Contact in Relationships*
  Making and responding to bodily contact with others, in a contextually and socially appropriate manner.

- *d7108 Basic Interpersonal Interactions, Other Specified*

- *d7109 Basic Interpersonal Interactions, Unspecified*

There are a set of basic interpersonal skills that are required before a person is able to develop meaningful relationships with others. These skills are normally developed while growing up, but some conditions, such as autism and intellectual/developmental disability, can limit a person's ability to develop interpersonal skills. Psychological disorders, such as obsessive-compulsive disorder and schizophrenia, are often accompanied by deficits in the ability to interact with others appropriately. These skills can also be lost as a result of brain injury. Even mild brain injury may result in some loss of ability to handle interpersonal interactions. Many of the clients that we serve will be working on these prerequisite skills to improve their ability to interact with others.

Some of the underlying skills will be found in Body Functions. The most important ones are b152 Emotional Functions, b1800 Experience of Self, and b126 Temperament and Personality Functions. Without these basic building blocks, it is hard to have interpersonal interactions. Other parts of b1 Mental Functions, such as b1142 Orientation to Person, are important to maintaining interpersonal interactions, but they are not required at this basic level. It is not uncommon to hear stories of clients with dementia who still act appropriately with other people even when they have forgotten most of their own lives and can't remember who the other person is. Clients with dementia do need a basic sense of themselves, though.

Assessment of basic interpersonal interaction skills is not a simple process. It requires a multifaceted approach characterized by pre-treatment assessment, on-going evaluation, and post-treatment assessment. Consistent with behavioral and learning theories, this model assesses interpersonal interactions within a behavioral framework. Ways to assess behaviors were discussed in the introduction to this chapter.

The therapist documents the deficits found and plans the appropriate interventions. For example, when assistance is not provided, the client has moderate difficulty reading social cues when socializing with friends (d7104._ _ _ 2). Assessment and intervention are integrally related when teaching skills in interpersonal interactions. Assessment is ongoing, so that the training changes as an individual's performance changes. The pre-treatment assessment techniques can also be used to evaluate how well the objectives have been met. Progress is measured only in relationship to stated objectives about specific problem areas that have been identified in the ongoing assessments. Treatment involves an ongoing process where the client learns skills or relearns previously understood skills in a developmentally appropriate order.

Adaptations are often required for clients with deficits in interpersonal interactions. Generally it involves working with the caregivers to explain what the client's deficits are and why they happen. This is especially important when the deficits occur in a person who previously had appropriate social skills, such as the result of a brain injury or a stroke. It is often hard for caregivers to understand and accept an interpersonal skill deficit when no or minimal physical deficits are present. Consequently, caregivers are educated on how to best respond to inappropriate social behaviors. The two primary issues are making sure the behaviors of the client do not harm him/her physically, emotionally, or in relationships and re-educating the client in interpersonal skills.

The response of the caregiver to inappropriate social behaviors often comes from a place of love and caring, feelings of upset or fear, or feelings of protection. Caregivers also need to learn about the issues involved in continued interpersonal skill recovery. If inappropriate behavior is allowed to continue, it will become a more ingrained response, making it even more difficult to change later. Also, when considering theories related to neuroplasticity, if faulty connections are allowed to continue, the caregiver is actually fostering the development of the faulty connections and telling the brain that the correct connections are not needed and can therefore be discarded.

The response of the caregiver to inappropriate social behaviors will vary depending on the response it elicits in the client, the situation at hand, and feelings provoked in the caregiver. Teaching the caregiver to respond in an even-toned voice that is non-judgmental is often the best course of action. For example, instead of saying, "Why did you say that to him?" which automatically puts a person on the defensive, the caregiver should say, "Mike is clearly upset after your talk with him. He is crying. What do you think we should do?" or "I know it is hard. We have to remind ourselves that yelling at him does not help him and that what he really needs is for us just to sit and listen to him sometimes." Other approaches may include cueing and, although difficult and not always possible, manipulating the interactions to make them easier.

The role of the caregiver as a teacher can take a major toll on the relationship. For example, the wife of a client may begin to feel more like a parent to her husband than a wife, which can affect other life areas such as emotional closeness, sexual life, and family roles and responsibilities. It is also important for therapists to remember that caregivers have needs as well. They need to feel loved, appreciated, and cared for. If they are not getting this from their loved one, even if they understand the reasons, it can leave the caregiver feeling unfulfilled, lonely, and stressed. Therefore, attention to the needs of the caregiver should also be a priority.

### Cross References

In *Recreational Therapy for Specific Diagnoses and Conditions, First Edition*, ICF code d710 Basic Interpersonal Interactions is listed in 15 chapters: Autism Spectrum Disorder, Cerebrovascular Accident, Feeding and Eating Disorders, Gambling Disorder, Hearing Loss, Intellectual Disability, Major Depressive Disorder, Multiple Sclerosis, Oppositional Defiant Disorder and Conduct Disorder, Post-Traumatic Stress Disorder, Schizophrenia Spectrum and Other Psychotic Disorders, Spina Bifida, Substance-Related Disorders, Traumatic Brain Injury, and Visual Impairments and Blindness.

In *Recreational Therapy Basics, Techniques, and Interventions, First Edition*, treatment for ICF code d710 Basic Interpersonal Interactions is discussed in 16 chapters: Education and Counseling, Participation, Adaptive Sports, Adventure Therapy, Animal Assisted Therapy, Assertiveness Training, Behavior Strategies and Interventions, Bibliotherapy, Cognitive Behavioral Counseling, Group Psychotherapy Techniques, Leisure Education and Counseling, Mind-Body Interventions, Montessori Method,

Sensory Interventions, Social Skills Training, and Values Clarification.

## d720 Complex Interpersonal Interactions

Maintaining and managing interactions with other people, in a contextually and socially appropriate manner, such as by regulating emotions and impulses, controlling verbal and physical aggression, acting independently in social interactions, and acting in accordance with social rules and conventions.

Inclusions: forming and terminating relationships; regulating behaviors within interactions; interacting according to social rules; and maintaining social space

- *d7200 Forming Relationships*
  Beginning and maintaining interactions with others for a short or long period of time, in a contextually and socially appropriate manner, such as by introducing oneself, finding and establishing friendships and professional relationships, starting a relationship that may become permanent, romantic, or intimate.

- *d7201 Terminating Relationships*
  Bringing interactions to a close in a contextually and socially appropriate manner, such as by ending temporary relationships at the end of a visit, ending long-term relationships with friends when moving to a new town, or ending relationships with work colleagues, professional colleagues, and service providers, and ending romantic or intimate relationships.

- *d7202 Regulating Behaviors within Interactions*
  Regulating emotions and impulses, verbal aggression and physical aggression in interactions with others, in a contextually and socially appropriate manner.

- *d7203 Interacting According to Social Rules*
  Acting independently in social interactions and complying with social conventions governing one's role, position, or other social status in interactions with others.

- *d7204 Maintaining Social Space*
  Being aware of and maintaining a distance between oneself and others that is contextually, socially, and culturally appropriate.

- *d7208 Complex Interpersonal Interactions, Other Specified*
- *d7209 Complex Interpersonal Interactions, Unspecified*

The second part of this chapter (d720 Complex Interpersonal Interactions) explores the development of basic social skills related to general interpersonal interactions. The majority of clients who require this level of training will have cognitive impairments that greatly reduce their ability to understand and interpret social rules and interactions. For clients in this category "overlearning" social skills will be needed so that the actions are executed without much thought.

As with the previous section, underlying skills will be found in the body functions chapter, including b152 Emotional Functions, b1800 Experience of Self, and b126 Temperament and Personality Functions. The client will also need skills in b1 Mental Functions, such as b1142 Orientation to Person, to maintain interpersonal interactions. Assessment of complex interpersonal interaction skills is very similar to assessment of basic skills. It also requires a multifaceted approach characterized by pre-treatment assessment, on-going evaluation, and post-treatment assessment. Refer to d710 Basic Interpersonal Interactions for suggestions.

Other methods of assessment include further behavioral observations in a variety of settings. The recreational therapist is especially appropriate for conducting these assessments because s/he is responsible for taking the client into the community where a variety of settings may be found. Teaching a client with a brain injury how to ride the bus can be done with verbal instruction in a medical setting. Some limited role-playing can also help to make sure that the client understands all of the steps required. However, only an actual ride on the bus will demonstrate that the client has the necessary *social* skills to ride the bus successfully. The failure to have appropriate interactions with other riders and the bus driver cause more problems than cognitive deficits (burlingame, 1989). Similar kinds of problems can be assessed and documented in other community settings.

The therapist documents the deficits found and plans the appropriate interventions. For example, when assistance is not provided, the client has moderate difficulty maintaining social space on the public bus (d7204._ _ _ 2). To teach skills in this area the therapist must integrally relate the assessment and intervention. Assessment is ongoing, so that the training changes as an individual's performance changes. The pre-treatment assessment techniques can also be used to evaluate how well the objectives have been met. Progress is only measured in relationship to stated objectives and specific problems areas identified in the ongoing assessments.

Treatment involves an ongoing process where the client learns skills or relearns previously understood skills in a developmentally appropriate order. Participating in activities in the community is strongly tied to appropriate social interactions. Managing emotions can be extremely difficult for someone with a traumatic brain injury or stroke. It is important to explain to clients and caregivers the need to be in calm surroundings as much as possible, that it is all right to take a time out when things become too stressful, and that the emotional overload may become easier to handle as the brain heals. See b152 Emotional Functions for more thoughts on handling emotional issues.

As with the basic interpersonal interaction skills, adaptations are often required for clients with deficits. Adaptations usually involve working with the caregivers of the client to explain what the client's deficits are and why they happen. This is especially important when the deficits occur to a person who previously had appropriate social skills. It is hard to see from the outside that there have been changes. The inside is very different, though, and caregivers and others who come in contact with the client need to understand how to handle situations so that the client can be successful.

Some specific requirements are accepting the social deficits of the client, giving very specific, concrete statements about inappropriate behavior to halt the behavior, minimizing adverse consequences of the behavior, encouraging awareness of social deficits, and making it clear to the client that loved ones understand and accept his/her social deficits and are willing and able to provide needed assistance.

### Cross References

In *Recreational Therapy for Specific Diagnoses and Conditions, First Edition*, ICF code d720 Complex Interpersonal Interactions is listed in 13 chapters: Attention-Deficit/Hyperactivity Disorder, Autism Spectrum Disorder, Cerebrovascular Acci-

dent, Feeding and Eating Disorders, Gambling Disorder, Hearing Loss, Intellectual Disability, Multiple Sclerosis, Oppositional Defiant Disorder and Conduct Disorder, Schizophrenia Spectrum and Other Psychotic Disorders, Spina Bifida, Substance-Related Disorders, and Traumatic Brain Injury.

In *Recreational Therapy Basics, Techniques, and Interventions, First Edition*, treatment for ICF code d720 Complex Interpersonal Interactions is discussed in eight chapters: Activity and Task Analysis, Education and Counseling, Animal Assisted Therapy, Group Psychotherapy Techniques, Montessori Method, Reality Orientation, Sensory Interventions, and Social Skills Training.

### d729 General Interpersonal Interactions, Other Specified and Unspecified

### Particular Interpersonal Relationships (d730 - d779)

### d730 Relating with Strangers

Engaging in temporary contacts and links with strangers for specific purposes, such as when asking for directions or making a purchase.

Relating to strangers, for most clients, involves the application of the basic and complex interpersonal skills already described. Sometimes there are psychosocial issues, such as shyness, or psychological issues, including autism, anxiety disorders, and psychoses, that make it difficult to make contact with any other person. These will show up in most interpersonal interactions and can be handled using the techniques in d710 Basic Interpersonal Interactions and d720 Complex Interpersonal Interactions.

There is one set of clients who need to have special consideration when dealing with strangers, clients with intellectual/developmental disability. Clients who have intellectual/developmental disability often do not have a good understanding of what a stranger is and will follow the instructions of anyone who appears friendly. They may not be able to distinguish between helpers, such as clerks in stores, and people who wish to do them harm. Recreational therapists need to assess the client's ability to recognize helpers and other strangers. Then they need to teach the clients appropriate ways to interact with strangers.

Recreational therapists document the extent of difficulty a client has with relating with strangers. For example, when assistance is not provided, the client has moderate difficulty relating appropriately with strangers at the community swim club (d730._ _ _ 2).

### Cross References

In *Recreational Therapy for Specific Diagnoses and Conditions, First Edition*, ICF code d730 Relating with Strangers is listed in four chapters: Multiple Sclerosis, Spinal Cord Injury, Traumatic Brain Injury, and Visual Impairments and Blindness.

In *Recreational Therapy Basics, Techniques, and Interventions, First Edition*, treatment for ICF code d730 Relating with Strangers is discussed in three chapters: Activity and Task Analysis, Animal Assisted Therapy, and Social Skills Training.

### d740 Formal Relationships

Creating and maintaining specific relationships in formal settings, such as with employers, professionals, or service providers.

Inclusions: relating with persons in authority, with subordinates, and with equals

- *d7400 Relating with Persons in Authority*
  Creating and maintaining formal relations with people in positions of power or of a higher rank or prestige relative to one's own social position, such as an employer.

- *d7401 Relating with Subordinates*
  Creating and maintaining formal relations with people in positions of lower rank or prestige relative to one's own social position, such as an employee or servant.

- *d7402 Relating with Equals*
  Creating and maintaining formal relations with people in the same position of authority, rank, or prestige relative to one's own social position.

- *d7408 Formal Relationships, Other Specified*
- *d7409 Formal Relationships, Other Unspecified*
  Formal relationships add a layer of complexity to the relationship skills covered in d710 Basic Interpersonal Interactions and d720 Complex Interpersonal Interactions. These relationships require the client to follow the special rules of his/her society in the way s/he treats other people in structured situations. In North America formal relationships are most likely to

be seen in the workplace, including the military, which probably has the most formal structure found in Western society. Prisons are also highly formalized. For teenagers and children, these relationships will occur at school and when playing team sports. In a medical setting, problems with the relationship between the medical personnel, clients, and people associated with clients would probably be scored with this code.

Deficits in this area can be caused by many diagnoses. Clients with intellectual/developmental disability may not have learned the relationships yet. Inability to function in formal relationships is a defining characteristic of some psychological diagnoses, and it is present in many others. Clients with brain injuries may have lost the understanding of how to act in formal situations or they may not be able to tolerate having to follow authority figures. Some clients may be in denial or simply fed up with a frustrating medical condition and are, therefore, unwilling to follow medical prescriptions.

Measuring deficits in formal relationships is usually done through observation. There are some formal tools used to record the observations including the *CERT-Psych/R*, the *School Social Behavior Scales*, and the *Home and Community Social Behavior Scales*. Recreational therapists document the extent of difficulty a client has with formal relationships. For example, when assistance is not provided, the client has moderate difficulty relating to peers at school, often bossing them around and demanding they engage in particular activities (d7402._ _ _ 2).

Treatment depends on the cause of the deficit. Clients will fail in these relationships because of cognitive issues, such as not being able to accomplish the task required, and/or emotional issues, such as anger. Many of the aspects of b1 Mental Functions or other parts of the A&P chapters may come into play. If the deficits are treated or adaptations for them are found, the problems documented with this code should be resolved.

### Cross References

In *Recreational Therapy for Specific Diagnoses and Conditions, First Edition*, ICF code d740 Formal Relationships is listed in six chapters: Autism Spectrum Disorder, Burns, Multiple Sclerosis, Oppositional Defiant Disorder and Conduct Disorder, Traumatic Brain Injury, and Visual Impairments and Blindness.

In *Recreational Therapy Basics, Techniques, and Interventions, First Edition*, treatment for ICF code d740 Formal Relationships is discussed in four chapters: Education and Counseling, Animal Assisted Therapy, Social Skills Training, and Therapeutic Relationships.

### d750 Informal Social Relationships

Entering into relationships with others, such as casual relationships with people living in the same community or residence, or with co-workers, students, playmates, or people with similar backgrounds or professions.

Inclusions: informal relationships with friends, neighbors, acquaintances, co-inhabitants, and peers

- *d7500 Informal Relationships with Friends*
  Creating and maintaining friendship relationships that are characterized by mutual esteem and common interests.

- *d7501 Informal Relationships with Neighbors*
  Creating and maintaining informal relationship with people who live in nearby dwellings or living areas.

- *d7502 Informal Relationships with Acquaintances*
  Creating and maintaining informal relationships with people whom one knows but who are not close friends.

- *d7503 Informal Relationships with Co-inhabitants*
  Creating and maintaining informal relationships with people who are co-inhabitants of a house or other dwelling, privately or publicly run, for any purpose.

- *d7504 Informal Relationships with Peers*
  Creating and maintaining informal relationships with people who share the same age, interest, or other common feature.

- *d7508 Informal Social Relationships, Other Specified*
- *d7509 Informal Social Relationships, Unspecified*
  Informal social relationships are based on the relationship skills covered in d710 Basic Interpersonal Interactions and d720 Complex Interpersonal Interactions. These relationships require the client to maintain appropriate interactions with people the client knows.

Deficits in this area can be caused by many diagnoses. Clients with intellectual/developmental disability may not have learned the relationships yet. Inability to function in casual relationships can be part of many psychological diagnoses. Clients with brain injuries may have lost the understanding of how to act in these situations. They may be unable to function in these situations because they can no longer process the subtle social cues that are required to act appropriately or they may not be able to tolerate dealing with the frustrations that interacting with other people often brings.

Measuring deficits in informal relationships is usually done through observation or formal tools. It is important to document the type of deficit and the particular situation where the deficit occurs, so that treatment can be planned appropriately and progress can be measured. For example, when assistance is not provided, the client has moderate difficulty maintaining friendships due to difficulties reciprocating needs (d7500._ _ _ 2).

Measurement can be difficult in some situations. For example, a client in a long-term care facility may not interact with other clients because s/he can't hear what they are saying. This would be a deficit in b230 Hearing Functions, not in relationships. Other clients may be in situations where there are few opportunities for informal social relationships, even if the client is able to participate in them. Clients in psychiatric facilities and clients in medical isolation are in two possible situations where it might be difficult to create and maintain informal social relationships.

Treatment depends on the cause of the deficit. Clients with intellectual/developmental disability need to learn the basic concepts behind these relationships. Other clients will usually fail in these relationships because of cognitive issues, such as not being able to accomplish the task required, and/or emotional issues, such as fear or anger. Many of the aspects of b1 Mental Functions or other parts of the A&P chapters may come into play. If the deficits are treated or adaptations for them are found, the problems documented with this code should be resolved.

### Cross References

In *Recreational Therapy for Specific Diagnoses and Conditions, First Edition*, ICF code d750 Informal Social Relationships is listed in 11 chapters:

Autism Spectrum Disorder, Cerebrovascular Accident, Feeding and Eating Disorders, Fibromyalgia and Juvenile Fibromyalgia, Intellectual Disability, Major Depressive Disorder, Multiple Sclerosis, Neurocognitive Disorders, Obesity, Spina Bifida, and Traumatic Brain Injury.

In *Recreational Therapy Basics, Techniques, and Interventions, First Edition*, treatment for ICF code d750 Informal Social Relationships is discussed in two chapters: Animal Assisted Therapy and Social Skills Training.

### d760 Family Relationships

Creating and maintaining kinship relations, such as with members of the nuclear family, extended family, foster and adopted family and step-relationships, more distant relationships such as second cousins, or legal guardians.

Inclusions: parent-child and child-parent relationships, sibling and extended family relationships

- *d7600 Parent-Child Relationships*
  Becoming and being a parent, both natural and adoptive, such as by having a child and relating to it as a parent or creating and maintaining a parental relationship with an adoptive child, and providing physical, intellectual, and emotional nurture to one's natural or adoptive child.

- *d7601 Child-Parent Relationships*
  Creating and maintaining relationships with one's parent, such as a young child obeying his or her parents or an adult child taking care of his or her elderly parents.

- *d7602 Sibling Relationships*
  Creating and maintaining a brotherly or sisterly relationship with a person who shares one or both parents by birth, adoption, or marriage.

- *d7603 Extended Family Relationships*
  Creating and maintaining a family relationship with members of one's extended family, such as with cousins, aunts and uncles, and grandparents.

- *d7608 Family Relationships, Other Specified*
- *d7609 Family Relationships, Unspecified*
  Family relationships are based on the relationship skills covered in d710 Basic Interpersonal Interactions and d720 Complex Interpersonal Interactions. These relationships require the client to maintain appropriate interactions with people the client knows well. Sorting out and modifying family relationships can be one of the most difficult tasks for any medical professional. If significant changes are required, the deficits should usually be handled by a psychologist or other professional trained to deal with family dynamics. Recreational therapists may be involved when the basic family relationship is sound, but some changes in the client's condition require the family to change how they relate to the client. Serious illnesses, significant physical disabilities, and brain injuries are areas where the recreational therapist may be able to provide services.

Measuring deficits in family relationships is usually done through observation in both hospital and community settings. There are some formal tools used to record the observations including the *Home and Community Social Behavior Scales* and the *Family APGAR*. Recreational therapists document the extent of difficulty a client has with family relationships. For example, when assistance is not provided, the client has complete difficulty maintaining a relationship with his parents and as a result often runs away from home (d7601._ _ _ 4).

Often the behavior will be recorded as a chart note. It is important to document the type of deficit and the particular situation where the deficit occurs, so that treatment can be planned appropriately and progress can be measured. Note that the deficits recorded may be deficits that the client has or they may be deficits with members of the family. Sometimes the most significant problem is that the family has not figured out how to deal with the new condition of the client and/or the client has not adjusted to his/her new role in the family. For example, consider a client who is a single parent of a fifteen-year-old daughter. Due to a physical disability, the client now requires physical assistance from the daughter who willingly provides the needed assistance. The client is now struggling with maintaining a parent-child relationship with her daughter because the family roles have changed. She reports that it is difficult to reprimand her daughter for poor behavior because she fears that the daughter may not provide her with the physical assistance that she needs.

Treatment depends on the cause of the deficit. For clients with intellectual/developmental disability the client may need to learn more about these relationships. Many of the aspects of b1 Mental Functions or other parts of the A&P chapters may come into play for other clients. Family issues are often treated by providing accurate information about how the client's abilities have changed. If the deficits are treated or adaptations for them are found, the problems documented with this code should be resolved.

### Cross References

In *Recreational Therapy for Specific Diagnoses and Conditions, First Edition*, ICF code d760 Family Relationships is listed in 17 chapters: Attention-Deficit/Hyperactivity Disorder, Autism Spectrum Disorder, Back Disorders and Back Pain, Borderline Personality Disorder, Feeding and Eating Disorders, Fibromyalgia and Juvenile Fibromyalgia, Gambling Disorder, Heart Disease, Intellectual Disability, Major Depressive Disorder, Multiple Sclerosis, Obesity, Post-Traumatic Stress Disorder, Spina Bifida, Spinal Cord Injury, Substance-Related Disorders, and Traumatic Brain Injury.

In *Recreational Therapy Basics, Techniques, and Interventions, First Edition*, treatment for ICF code d760 Family Relationships is discussed in four chapters: Participation, Animal Assisted Therapy, Mind-Body Interventions, and Social Skills Training.

### *d770 Intimate Relationships*

Creating and maintaining close or romantic relationships between individuals, such as husband and wife, lovers, or sexual partners.

Inclusions: romantic, spousal, and sexual relationships

- *d7700 Romantic Relationships*
  Creating and maintaining a relationship based on emotional and physical attraction, potentially leading to long-term intimate relationships.

- *d7701 Spousal Relationships*
  Creating and maintaining an intimate relationship of a legal nature with another person, such as in a legal marriage, including becoming and being a legally married wife or husband or an unmarried spouse.

- *d7702 Sexual Relationships*
  Creating and maintaining a relationship of a sexual nature, with a spouse or other partner.

- *d7708 Intimate Relationships, Other Specified*
- *d7709 Intimate Relationships, Unspecified*

This section of the chapter looks at skills related to intimacy and its appropriate expression, regulation, and range. Intimate relationships are based on the relationship skills covered in d710 Basic Interpersonal Interactions and d720 Complex Interpersonal Interactions. These relationships require the client to maintain appropriate interactions with people the client is extremely close to. Sorting out and modifying intimate relationships can be as difficult as sorting out family relationships. If significant changes are required, the deficits should usually be handled by a psychologist or other professional trained to deal with these dynamics.

Recreational therapists may be involved when the basic relationship is sound, but some changes in the client's condition require a change in the relationship. Serious illnesses, significant physical disabilities, and brain injuries are areas where the recreational therapist may be able to provide services. The recreational therapist will also be involved in teaching the skills required for intimate relationships to clients with intellectual/developmental disability.

The client's expression of sexuality is often uncomfortable for staff. In too many settings the client's sexuality is avoided or discouraged. Since, in most situations, an individual's development and expression of intimate relationships, including his/her expression of sexuality, is most appropriate in non-work settings, the recreational therapist should be prepared to work with a client on his/her appropriate expression of social skills, including ones related to intimate relationships and sexuality. See b640 Sexual Functions for specific information on how recreational therapists address sexuality with clients.

Assessment of deficits in intimate relationships is almost always the result of the client or someone who knows the client presenting the information to the treatment team. For example, despite having assistance from his partner, the client reports having moderate difficulty maintaining a sexual relationship (d7702.2 _ _ _). The one major exception to this is with clients who have intellectual/developmental disability where the therapist uses a tool such as the *Leisure Social/Sexual Assessment* to measure the client's knowledge about intimate relationships. The interview part of that assessment is a useful tool for gathering information about the client's social behavior, which will aid in selection, grouping, and development of objectives. In order to develop an appropriate individualized program for gaining leisure and social/sexual knowledge and skills it is necessary to obtain information about the client's present use of time, knowledge, skills, and interests. If conducted by a professional trained in assessment techniques, the interview has a high degree of validity and reliability for broad assessment.

For all clients, the development of a client's social skills, especially related to his/her expression of intimate relationship skills, is a difficult area of treatment. The therapist needs to help the client develop intimate skills without creating a sexually charged atmosphere during treatment and without the client developing intimate feelings for the therapist. This is especially challenging when working with clients who have cognitive impairments. Refer to the Sexual Well-Being chapter in the companion book, *Recreational Therapy Basics, Techniques, and Interventions*, for specific treatment instructions.

Treatment for other clients depends on the underlying cause of the deficit. See b640 Sexual Functions for a discussion of how to treat physical and emotional issues related to sexuality. Psychological issues, with their intricate interactions with family relationships, are probably best handled by a psychologist specifically trained to deal with sexual and relationship issues.

### Cross References

In *Recreational Therapy for Specific Diagnoses and Conditions, First Edition*, ICF code d770 Intimate Relationships is listed in 12 chapters: Back Disorders and Back Pain, Feeding and Eating Disorders, Gambling Disorder, Heart Disease, Intellectual Disability, Major Depressive Disorder, Multiple Sclerosis, Osteoarthritis, Post-Traumatic Stress Disorder, Rheumatoid Arthritis, Spina Bifida, and Traumatic Brain Injury.

In *Recreational Therapy Basics, Techniques, and Interventions, First Edition*, treatment for ICF code d770 Intimate Relationships is discussed in four chapters: Participation, Animal Assisted Therapy, Sexual Well-Being, and Social Skills Training.

### *d779 Particular Interpersonal Relationships, Other Specified and Unspecified*

### *d798 Interpersonal Interactions and Relationships, Other Specified*

### *d799 Interpersonal Interactions and Relationships, Unspecified*

### Reference

burlingame, j. (1989). *Bus utilization skills assessment*. Ravensdale, WA: Idyll Arbor.

Chandola, T., Marmot, M., & Siegrist, J. (2007). Failed reciprocity in close social relationships and health: Findings from the Whitehall II study. *Journal of Psychosomatic Research, 63*(4), 403-411.

Holt-Lunstad, J., Smith, T. B., & Layton, B. (2010). Social relationships and mortality risk: A meta-analytic review. *PLoS Medicine, 7*(7), 1-20.

King, G., Law, M., Hanna, S., King, S., Hurley, P., Rosenbaum, P., Kertoy, M., & Petrenchik, T. (2006). Predictors of the leisure and recreation participation of children with physical disabilities: A structural equation modeling analysis. *Children's Health Care, 35*(3), 209-234.

McDonald, S., Tate, R., Togher, L., Bornhofen, C., Long, E., Gertler, P., & Bowen, R. (2008). Social skills treatment for people with severe, chronic acquired brain injuries: A multicenter trial. *Archives of Physical Medicine and Rehabilitation, 89*(9), 1648-1659.

Ryan, C. A., Stiell, K. M., Gailey, G. F., & Makinen, J. A. (2008). Evaluating a family centered approach to leisure education and community integration following a stroke. *Therapeutic Recreation Journal, XLII*(2), 119-131.

Sasidharan, V., Payne, L., Orsega-Smith, & Godbey, G. (2006). Older adults' physical activity participation and perceptions of wellbeing: Examining the role of social support for leisure. *Managing Leisure, 11*(3), 164-185.

Strine, T. W., Chapman, D. P., Balluz, L., & Mokdad, A. H. (2008). Health-related quality of life and health behaviors by social and emotional support. *Social Psychiatry and Psychiatric Epidemiology, 43*, 151-159.

Uchino, B. N. (2006). Social support and health: A review of physiological processes potentially underlying links to disease outcomes. *Journal of Behavioral Medicine, 29*(4), 377-387.

Umberson, D., Crosnoe, R., & Reczek, C. (2010). Social relationships and health behavior across life course. *Annual Review of Sociology, 36*, 139-157.

Van Nieuwenhuijzen, M. & Vriens, A. (2012). (Social) cognitive skills and social information processing in children with mild to borderline intellectual disabilities. *Research in Developmental Disabilities, 33*, 426-434.

# Chapter 8 Major Life Areas

This chapter is about carrying out the tasks and actions required to engage in education, work, and employment and to conduct economic transactions.

*Sample Scoring of Major Life Areas*

- A young adult is transitioning from living at home with her parents to living on her own. To help her with this transition, her father is teaching her how to cook (d810 Informal Education). When her father provides assistance with measuring ingredients she has no difficulty. If her father does not provide assistance with measuring ingredients she has moderate difficulty. The complete scoring would look like this: d810.0 _ _ 2.
- A teenager with a history of behavioral problems volunteers at a local horse farm (d855 Non-Remunerative Employment). About 50% of the time he is scheduled to volunteer at the farm, he doesn't show up. If his mom is home, she makes sure he wakes up on time and gets to the farm on his assigned days. The complete scoring would look like this: d855.0 _ _ 3.

This chapter is divided into three significantly different sections: Education, Work and Employment, and Economic Life.

Many tasks and actions are required to engage in informal or formal education. These include learning, gaining admission, engaging in school-related responsibilities and privileges, attending, working cooperatively with others, organizing, studying, completing tasks and projects, and advancing to other stages of education. Many different skill sets, such as d7202 Regulating Behaviors within Interactions, d140 Learning to Read, and b144 Memory Functions are required for success in education tasks.

The ability to engage in meaningful life work has a direct impact on health and quality of life. For example, a longitudinal study of older adults found that volunteering is related to increased happiness (Dulin et al., 2012). In another longitudinal study of older adults, those who volunteered for other-oriented reasons had a lower mortality risk four years later, especially those who volunteered more regularly and frequently. Those who volunteered for self-oriented reasons had a higher mortality risk similar to those who did not volunteer (Konrath et al., 2012). As a final example, a study of 271,642 individuals aged 15 and up from 139 countries found that self-rated health was significantly associated with having social support from friends and relatives and volunteering.

Play is part of a child's education. It is a necessary component for healthy development, as well as a human right (United Nations, 2006). Play develops imagination; develops dexterity and physical, cognitive, and emotional strength; contributes to healthy brain development; provides a context to engage, create, explore, and interact with the world; provides a context for conquering fears while practicing adult roles; helps to develop new competencies that enhance confidence and resilience to face future challenges; helps children learn how to work in groups, to share, to negotiate, to resolve conflicts, and learn self-advocacy skills; provides opportunities to practice decision-making skills, move at one's own pace and discover areas of interest leading to full engagement in passionate interests; builds active, healthy bodies; creates feelings of joy; provides a context to express views, experiences, and frustrations; helps with adjustment to school and enhances learning readiness, learning behaviors, and problem solving skills; and fosters development of social-emotional learning (Ginsburg, 2007).

Economic skills of basic and complex economic transactions and economic self-sufficiency are skills required for independent living, unless another person, such as a guardian carries the responsibility for the individual.

*Assessment of Major Life Areas*

Recreational therapists utilize various methods to assess the three aspects of major life areas including but not limited to interview, observation, functional testing, and standardized assessments. Assessments for education include the *Home and Community Social Behavior Scales*, the *Play Assessment Scale* (PAS), *Transdisciplinary Play-Based Assessment* (TPBA), the *Play in Early Childhood Evaluation System* (PIECES), the *Play Observation Scale*, the

*Preschool Play Scale* (PPS), *Test of Playfulness*, Play History, the *Leisure Diagnostic Battery* (section E: Playfulness), the *General Recreation Screening Tool* (GRST), the *Recreation Early Development Screening Tool* (REDS) (Steger, Dik & Duffy, 2012; Kelly-Vance & Ryalls, 2008; Rubin, 2001; burlingame & Blaschko, 2010), as well as developmental assessment tools that include play behavior, such as the *Developmental Assessment of Young Children, Version 2* (DAYC-2), *Ages and Stages Questionnaire* (ASQ), and *Hawaii Early Learning Profile* (HELP). Work and employment assessments include the Work and Meaning Inventory (WAMI) and client discussions. Economic life is usually assessed based on client discussions.

### Treatment of Major Life Areas

Treatment for Major Life Areas will vary depending upon the underlying causes of difficulty. Underlying causes are determined through clinical interview, functional assessment, observation, and standardized assessment tools. For example, if a client has difficulty engaging in volunteer work due to deficits in social skills, the therapist would refer to d7 Interactions and Relationships for treatment direction, as well as Social Skills Training in the companion book, *Recreational Therapy Basics, Techniques, and Interventions.*

### Evidence Review

Reviews of several studies are provided below to highlight evidence-based practice related to major life areas. This is only a sample of the evidence. A thorough review of the literature is needed to identify evidence-based practice interventions that reflect the needs and characteristics of the individual client.

In October 1999, immediately following Hurricane Floyd, recreational therapy professionals and pre-professionals provided services to address disaster-related behavior problems to 450 fourth and fifth grade students from the Pattillo Elementary School (Russoniello et al., 2002). They delivered a five week stress management program to teachers and students using the I'm in Charge of Me (I-C Me) program, a biopsychosocial program strategy that utilizes cognitive behavior stress control to aid in managing stress and increase self-concept. The intervention improved behavior, and attentiveness, assertiveness; decreased hyperactive behavior; and improved academic grades.

Moore and Russ's 2006 review of the literature indicated that pretend play is effective in inpatient and outpatient settings for preventing and reducing anxiety and distress, as well positively impacting pain, externalizing behavior, and increasing adaptation to chronic illness.

Smith and Van Puymbroeck (2011) provided a framework for exploring play in children who have autism using a strengths-based recovery model. Recreational therapists are encouraged to evaluate the strengths of current play skills, although they are not developmentally traditional, and build upon those strengthens to foster development. For example, the therapist could build on stereotypic play behavior of flipping through picture books and use it to create picture books that help the child navigate through his day. "By starting from the child's play preferences, professional are able to use high interest areas and activities to help holistically improve the child's well-being" (p. 21).

Fegan (2012) investigated how people with serious mental illness experienced volunteering at a mental health agency where they received prior care. The following themes were identified: (1) rehearsing for a new direction, (2) treading carefully at first, (3) discovering a new self, and (4) using my experiences and extending relationships. Supported volunteering using a framework comprised of these themes helped with recovery because it fostered positive risk taking and development of a valued identity that integrated their mental health experience.

Steger, Dik, and Duffy, (2012) reviewed the *Work and Meaning Inventory* (WAMI) as a way to measure the extent of meaning experienced in work. The areas measured included experiencing positive meaning in work, work as a context for meaning making, and work benefits for the greater good. They also proposed a multidimensional model of work that can be helpful to healthcare professionals.

Trainor and colleagues (2011) found through a review of the literature that only about 17% of adolescents with disabilities work during the summer. They also found that, according to parents, 30% of adolescents with disabilities spend much of their free time socializing with others and 50% spend their free summer months watching television. Engagement in summer employment has been found to be "positively associated with development of self-determination, high school completion, strong connections with the community, and securing postsecondary employment" (p. 157). For adolescents with disabilities, "summer employment and community involvement [helps] to develop attitudes, knowledge, and skills that can enhance their postsecondary transition goals" (p. 157). As a result of these concerns, the authors conducted three focus groups consisting of 16 adolescents with various disabilities (e.g., learning disability, emotional-behavioral disability, autism spectrum disorder, cognitive disability) to better understand their perspectives on summer employment (economic life) and summer activities. Reasons cited for summer employment and/or community activity engagement included an opportunity to earn money, to learn something (e.g., summer enrichment activities such as Drivers Education, unpaid internship), and to relax and recreate (having free time from school and work). They identified that having assistance from teachers and parents was helpful to find employment and activities and identified "volunteering as valuable experiences that lead to additional employment opportunities" (p. 164). Identified barriers to employment included lack of response to applications, mismatched interests and work opportunities, workplace skills and expectations, and getting along with coworkers and supervisors. The authors concluded that professionals must be cognizant that adolescents with disabilities (1) may have different motivations to work, which must be understood, (2) value independence and self-determination but need guidance from adults in finding and maintaining employment, and (3) development of social connections and peer relationships are pivotal to the development of transition-related knowledge and skills. They recommended that professionals provide planning and guidance to align motivation and interests, balance self-determination and adult support, and provide support to address interpersonal skills and social network development during summer employment and activities.

### Cross References

In *Recreational Therapy for Specific Diagnoses and Conditions, First Edition*, ICF code d8 Major Life Areas and its subcategories are listed in 28 chapters: Amputation and Prosthesis, Attention-Deficit/Hyperactivity Disorder, Autism Spectrum Disorder, Back Disorders and Back Pain, Borderline Personality Disorder, Burns, Cancer, Cerebral Palsy,

Cerebrovascular Accident, Chronic Obstructive Pulmonary Disease, Epilepsy, Fibromyalgia and Juvenile Fibromyalgia, Gambling Disorder, Hearing Loss, Heart Disease, Intellectual Disability, Major Depressive Disorder, Multiple Sclerosis, Osteoarthritis, Osteoporosis, Parkinson's Disease, Post-Traumatic Stress Disorder, Rheumatoid Arthritis, Schizophrenia Spectrum and Other Psychotic Disorders, Sickle Cell Disease, Spina Bifida, Spinal Cord Injury, and Substance-Related Disorders.

In *Recreational Therapy Basics, Techniques, and Interventions, First Edition*, treatment for ICF code d8 Major Life Areas and its subcategories are discussed in 11 chapters: Activity and Task Analysis, Adjustment and Response to Disability, Body Mechanics and Ergonomics, Participation, Stress, Activity Pattern Development, Anger Management, Behavior Strategies and Interventions, Cognitive Retraining and Rehabilitation, Disability Rights: Education and Advocacy, and Social Skills Training.

## Education (d810 - d839)

### d810 Informal Education

Learning at home or in some other non-institutional settings, such as learning crafts and other skills from parents or family members, or home schooling.

See the discussion at the end of this section.

### Cross References

In *Recreational Therapy for Specific Diagnoses and Conditions, First Edition*, ICF code d810 Informal Education is listed in five chapters: Attention-Deficit/Hyperactivity Disorder, Fibromyalgia and Juvenile Fibromyalgia, Multiple Sclerosis, Post-Traumatic Stress Disorder, and Traumatic Brain Injury.

In *Recreational Therapy Basics, Techniques, and Interventions, First Edition*, there are no references for ICF code d810 Informal Education.

### d815 Preschool Education

Learning at an initial level of organized instruction, designed primarily to introduce a child to the school-type environment and prepare it for compulsory education, such as by acquiring skills in a day-care or similar setting as preparation for advancement to school.

See the discussion at the end of this section.

*Cross References*

In *Recreational Therapy for Specific Diagnoses and Conditions, First Edition*, there are no references for ICF code d815 Preschool Education.

In *Recreational Therapy Basics, Techniques, and Interventions, First Edition*, treatment for ICF code d815 Preschool Education is discussed in one chapter: Social Skills Training.

## d820 School Education

Gaining admission to school, engaging in all school-related responsibilities and privileges; learning the course material, subjects, and other curriculum requirements in a primary or secondary education program, including attending school regularly; working cooperatively with other students, taking direction from teachers, organizing, studying, and completing assigned tasks and projects, and advancing to other stages of education.

See the discussion at the end of this section.

*Cross References*

In *Recreational Therapy for Specific Diagnoses and Conditions, First Edition*, ICF code d820 School Education is listed in five chapters: Attention-Deficit/Hyperactivity Disorder, Fibromyalgia and Juvenile Fibromyalgia, Multiple Sclerosis, Post-Traumatic Stress Disorder, and Traumatic Brain Injury.

In *Recreational Therapy Basics, Techniques, and Interventions, First Edition*, treatment for ICF code d820 School Education is discussed in one chapter: Social Skills Training.

## d825 Vocational Training

Engaging in all activities of a vocational program and learning the curriculum material in preparation for employment in a trade, job, or profession.

See the discussion at the end of this section.

*Cross References*

In *Recreational Therapy for Specific Diagnoses and Conditions, First Edition*, ICF code d825 Vocational Training is listed in five chapters: Attention-Deficit/Hyperactivity Disorder, Fibromyalgia and Juvenile Fibromyalgia, Multiple Sclerosis, Post-Traumatic Stress Disorder, and Traumatic Brain Injury.

In *Recreational Therapy Basics, Techniques, and Interventions, First Edition*, there are no references for ICF code d825 Vocational Training.

## d830 Higher Education

Engaging in the activities of advanced educational programs in universities, colleges, and professional schools and learning all aspects of the curriculum required for degrees, diplomas, certificates, and other accreditations, such as completing a university bachelor's or master's course of study, medical school, or other professional school.

See the discussion at the end of this section.

*Cross References*

In *Recreational Therapy for Specific Diagnoses and Conditions, First Edition*, ICF code d830 Higher Education is listed in five chapters: Attention-Deficit/Hyperactivity Disorder, Fibromyalgia and Juvenile Fibromyalgia, Multiple Sclerosis, Post-Traumatic Stress Disorder, and Traumatic Brain Injury.

In *Recreational Therapy Basics, Techniques, and Interventions, First Edition*, there are no references for ICF code d830 Higher Education.

## d839 Education, Other Specified and Unspecified

Recreational therapists who work in school settings regularly address barriers to education. Recreational therapists who work in rehabilitation settings also address barriers to education, including problem solving for architectural barriers, developing peer social skills, and assertiveness training. They integrate the client into the specific educational setting whether it is the client's home, recreation center, elementary school, or somewhere else.

In the ICF the therapist documents the client's overall level of difficulty. For example, when assistance is provided, the client has mild difficulty engaging in vocational training (d825.1 _ _ _). In discipline-specific documentation, the therapist makes additional notes about the level of assistance required with the subtasks of school participation, recommendations for the level of assistance needed, adaptive equipment, techniques utilized, and the problems that the difficulty of education imposes on other life activities and needs.

During treatment it is important to note that informal education can also occur in a variety of settings. Informal, as well as formal, education can be related to recreation and leisure, including play (as described later in this code), pursuing a new hobby, or advancing education for personal pleasure versus career gain. Additionally, engaging in school-life and related activities includes such things as sports rallies, plays, and other social and recreational activities outside of the standard formal curriculum. If a recreation activity takes place in an educational setting the therapist will need to decide if it fits best under d820 School Education, as part of "engaging in all school-related responsibilities and privileges," or a more specific d920 Recreation and Leisure code.

Recreational therapists assist clients of all ages in evaluating school activities, barriers, and facilitators. Active problem solving, leisure education and counseling, functional skill development, and community integration training are commonly implemented to minimize barriers, identify further facilitators, and maintain and improve participation and functioning in school activities, including structured school activities, such as sports and clubs, and unstructured school activities, such as socializing in the lunchroom and engaging in activity with others outside the classroom. Engagement in these activities is an integral part of health and quality of life.

Outside of client evaluation, recreational therapists talk with relevant school staff and makes recommendations as needed for appropriate assistance.

### Play

Engagement in play is an important part of what recreational therapists do. It was added as part of this chapter in the Child and Youth version of the ICF before the decision was made to revert to a single version of the ICF. It is unclear at this time if the engagement in play codes from the Child and Youth version of the ICF have been deleted or if they have not yet been transferred into the single version of the ICF. Engagement in play codes were part of this section because "play is a child's work." It is through play that children learn. Because play is vital for a child's learning process, the best place to score children's deficits in play at this time may be here as part of d810 Informal Education. Individuals who are developmentally impaired may be an adult chronologically, but function as a child. Consequently,

chronological age should not be the sole determinant for where deficits in play should be documented. Adults who have deficits in play that affect their lives might also be scored with this code, especially when an adult has a deficit in playing with his/her children. Recreational therapist should also consider, given the situation, if d9200 Play (engaging in games with rules or unstructured or organized games and spontaneous recreation, such as playing chess or cards or children's play) is a more appropriate code. The code d9200 Play is more reflective of the client's ability to play, rather than playing to learn (d810 Informal Education).

Play can be defined in many ways: (1) it is self-chosen, self-initiated, and self-directed, (2) the means are more important then the ends (in other words, play is the most important, not the outcome of the play), (3) it has structure and rules that are created by the imagination of the players, (4) it is imaginative and allows the player to move outside of his/her current real life, (5) it is an activity of the mind where the mind is deeply engrossed, alert, and active, as part of a process of investigation, exploration, and inquiry (Gray, 2008; Mayesky, 2009).

Recreational therapists may further describe play via interaction patterns, play patterns, and specific play-type.

Interaction patterns include (Farrell & Lundegren, 1991):

- *Intra-individual*: Action taking place within the mind or action involving the mind and a part of the body, such as daydreaming; requires no contact with another person or external object.
- *Extra-individual*: Action directed by a person toward an object, such as making a craft; requires no contact with another person.
- *Aggregate*: Action directed by a person toward an object while in the company of other persons who are also directing action towards objects, such as making a craft activity within a craft group, but not interacting with anyone else in the group; action is not directed toward each other; no interaction between participants is required or necessary.
- *Inter-individual*: Action of a competitive nature directed by one person toward another person, such as playing a board game.
- *Unilateral*: Action of a competitive nature among three or more person, one of whom is an

antagonist or "it," such as playing a game of tag; interaction is in simultaneous competitive relationship.

- *Multi-lateral*: Action of a competitive nature among three or more persons with no one person as an antagonist, such as running a race.
- *Intra-group*: Action of a cooperative nature by two or more persons intent upon reaching a mutual goal, such as working together as a team to get a soccer ball in the goal; action requires positive verbal or nonverbal interaction.
- *Inter-group*: Action of a competitive nature between two or more intra-groups, such as playing a competitive volleyball game.

Play patterns include (National Institute for Play, 2009):

- *Attunement play*: infant responds to eye contact with parent with smiles and babbling; both experience surge of joy.
- *Body play and movement*: exploring body movements and abilities, playing with vocal sounds.
- *Object play*: manipulating objects.
- *Social play*: playing with another person or animal, such as wresting, tickling, and imitating.
- *Imaginative and pretend play*.
- *Storytelling-narrative play*.
- *Transformative-integrative and creative play*: shape or re-shape ideas.

Recreational therapists may also choose to further describe the specific type of play in which the client is engaged, such as playing alone with blocks, or highlight a particular type of play that is a concern.

Treatment for play will vary depending upon underlying impairments, difficulties, and barriers. Through observation, clinical interview, functional assessment, and standardized assessment tools, areas of dysfunction are identified and then addressed. Deficits can be based in Body Functions and Body Structures, such as difficulty with sight impacting ability to engage with play materials, Activities and Participation, such as difficulty moving around impacting the ability to engage in active cooperative play activities, and/or Environmental Factors including lack of adaptive play toys.

In *Recreational Therapy for Specific Diagnoses and Conditions*, removed ICF-CY code d880 Engagement in Play is listed in eight chapters:

Amputation and Prosthesis, Attention-Deficit/Hyperactivity Disorder, Autism Spectrum Disorder, Cancer, Cerebral Palsy, Fibromyalgia and Juvenile Fibromyalgia, Hearing Loss, and Intellectual Disability.

## Work and Employment (d840 - d859)

### d840 Apprenticeship (Work Preparation)

Engaging in programs related to preparation for employment, such as performing the tasks required of an apprenticeship, internship, articling, and in-service training.

Exclusions: vocational training (d825)

See the discussion at the end of the section.

#### Cross References
In *Recreational Therapy for Specific Diagnoses and Conditions, First Edition*, ICF code d840 Apprenticeship (Work Preparation) is listed in eight chapters: Cancer, Chronic Obstructive Pulmonary Disease, Hearing Loss, Multiple Sclerosis, Neurocognitive Disorders, Obesity, Substance-Related Disorders, and Traumatic Brain Injury.

In *Recreational Therapy Basics, Techniques, and Interventions, First Edition*, there are no references for ICF code d840 Apprenticeship (Work Preparation).

### d845 Acquiring, Keeping, and Terminating a Job

Seeking, finding and choosing employment, being hired and accepting employment, maintaining and advancing through a job, trade, occupation, or profession, and leaving a job in an appropriate manner.

Inclusions: seeking employment; preparing a resume or curriculum vitae; contacting employers and preparing interviews; maintaining a job; maintaining one's own work performance; giving notice; and terminating a job

- *d8450 Seeking Employment*
  Locating and choosing a job, in a trade, profession, or other form of employment, and performing the required tasks to get hired, such as showing up at the place of employment or participating in a job interview.

- *d8451 Maintaining a Job*
  Performing job-related tasks to keep an occupation, trade, profession, or other form of employment, and obtaining promotion and other advancements in employment.

- *d8452 Terminating a Job*
  Leaving or quitting a job in the appropriate manner.

- *d8458 Acquiring, Keeping, and Terminating a Job, Other Specified*

- *d8459 Acquiring, Keeping, and Terminating a Job, Unspecified*
  See the discussion at the end of the section.

### Cross References

In *Recreational Therapy for Specific Diagnoses and Conditions, First Edition*, ICF code d845 Acquiring, Keeping, and Terminating a Job is listed in 14 chapters: Attention-Deficit/Hyperactivity Disorder, Back Disorders and Back Pain, Borderline Personality Disorder, Cancer, Cerebral Palsy, Chronic Obstructive Pulmonary Disease, Hearing Loss, Major Depressive Disorder, Multiple Sclerosis, Neurocognitive Disorders, Obesity, Post-Traumatic Stress Disorder, Substance-Related Disorders, and Traumatic Brain Injury.

In *Recreational Therapy Basics, Techniques, and Interventions, First Edition*, treatment for ICF code d845 Acquiring, Keeping, and Terminating a Job is discussed in one chapter: Participation.

### d850 Remunerative Employment

Engaging in all aspects of work, as an occupation, trade, profession, or other form of employment, for payment, as an employee, full or part time, or self-employed, such as seeking employment and getting a job, doing the required tasks of the job, attending work on time as required, supervising other workers or being supervised, and performing required tasks alone or in groups.

Inclusions: self-employment, part-time and full-time employment

- *d8500 Self-Employment*
  Engaging in remunerative work sought or generated by the individual, or contracted from others without a formal employment relationship, such as migratory agricultural work, working as a freelance writer or consultant, short-term contract

work, working as an artist or crafts person, owning and running a shop or other business.

Exclusions: part-time and full-time employment (d8501, d8502)

- *d8501 Part-Time Employment*
  Engaging in all aspects of work for payment on a part-time basis, as an employee, such as seeking employment and getting a job, doing the tasks required of the job, attending work on time as required, supervising other workers or being supervised, and performing required tasks alone or in groups.

- *d8502 Full-Time Employment*
  Engaging in all aspects of work for payment on a full-time basis, as an employee, such as seeking employment and getting a job, doing the required tasks of the job, attending work on time as required, supervising other workers or being supervised, and performing required tasks alone or in groups.

- *d8508 Remunerative Employment, Other Specified*

- *d8509 Remunerative Employment, Unspecified*
  See the discussion at the end of the section.

### Cross References

In *Recreational Therapy for Specific Diagnoses and Conditions, First Edition*, ICF code d850 Remunerative Employment is listed in 11 chapters: Back Disorders and Back Pain, Cancer, Chronic Obstructive Pulmonary Disease, Hearing Loss, Heart Disease, Multiple Sclerosis, Neurocognitive Disorders, Obesity, Rheumatoid Arthritis, Substance-Related Disorders, and Traumatic Brain Injury.

In *Recreational Therapy Basics, Techniques, and Interventions, First Edition*, there are no references for ICF code d850 Remunerative Employment.

### d855 Non-Remunerative Employment

Engaging in all aspects of work in which pay is not provided, full-time or part-time, including organized work activities, doing the required tasks of the job, attending work on time as required, supervising other workers or being supervised, and performing required tasks alone or in groups, such as volunteer work, charity work, working for a community or religious group without remuneration, working around the home without remuneration.

Exclusions: Chapter 6 Domestic Life

See the discussion at the end of the section.

### Cross References

In *Recreational Therapy for Specific Diagnoses and Conditions, First Edition*, ICF code d855 Non-Remunerative Employment is listed in eight chapters: Cancer, Chronic Obstructive Pulmonary Disease, Hearing Loss, Multiple Sclerosis, Neurocognitive Disorders, Obesity, Substance-Related Disorders, and Traumatic Brain Injury.

In *Recreational Therapy Basics, Techniques, and Interventions, First Edition*, there are no references for ICF code d855 Non-Remunerative Employment.

### d859 Work and Employment, Other Specified and Unspecified

Employment is actively addressed by a variety of health and welfare disciplines including recreational therapy. Other professionals include the office of vocational rehabilitation, work readiness programs, trade teachers, therapists, and job facilitators.

Examples of recreational therapists addressing employment include:

Recreational therapists who work with troubled youth may assist them in developing life skills, including the skills needed to acquire, keep, and terminate a job. These skills might include interviewing skills, developing a resume, choosing appropriate clothing, communicating with superiors, and time management.

Recreational therapists who work in a developmentally disabled job program assist clients during job performance to facilitate use of job skills, such as task performance, utilizing adaptive techniques, asking for assistance when needed, managing time, and working in a group.

Recreational therapists who work in long-term care may assist residents in identifying and engaging in volunteer opportunities inside or outside of the residential setting as non-remunerative employment. Recreational therapists who work in physical rehabilitation may incorporate worksite evaluations and job analysis into community integration training sessions. Recreational therapists who work in psychiatric care may assist clients with the development of coping mechanisms for stressful situations, including situations that occur at work.

Employment, whether paid or unpaid, provides many health benefits outside of monetary compensation or required obligations. For example, a 65-year-old client who works part time at the local hardware store as remunerative employment doesn't work only because he needs money. He also works for the socialization it provides, such as talking with all the "guys" who come in for supplies. In another example, a 35-year-old woman whose mother died of breast cancer finds that raising money in breast cancer campaigns makes her feel like she is doing something to help other people who are going through what her mom went through, ultimately working as a coping strategy. As a final example, an adolescent who writes articles and poems and submits them to a teen magazine may be paid for the pieces that are accepted (and the money is appreciated), but the adolescent states that acknowledgement of her ideas and thoughts is more rewarding. Recreational therapists understand that work for some people is not just work. It can have a deeper meaning and purpose that, if not pursued, could cause dysfunction in other life areas, such as social and emotional health.

In the ICF therapists score the level of difficulty a client has with work and employment. For example, without assistance, the client has mild difficulty volunteering at the animal shelter (d855._ _ _ 1). In discipline-specific documentation, therapists will additionally document the level of assistance required with each subtask of the work or employment activity, adaptive equipment, techniques, recommendations given, education provided, and the impact that dysfunction in work or employment has on other life tasks, such as d9205 Socializing or d610 Acquiring a Place to Live.

It is important to note that employment can occur in a variety of settings, all with individual characteristics, and that it can be related to recreation and leisure. Volunteering at a local nursing home for pleasure rather than for fulfilling a duty or working part time at the ice cream shop for the purpose of socialization rather than for monetary gain are two examples. Additionally, engaging in employment tasks and projects may also be recreation or sports related. If a recreation or sports activity takes place in an employment setting, the therapist would score one of these codes rather than the recreation and leisure codes in d9 Community, Social, and Civic Life.

Once the therapist identifies that work and employment are areas that need to be addressed in treatment, the recreational therapist assists clients in:

- Developing needed skills (e.g., social skills, direction following, relating to superiors).
- Minimizing barriers (e.g., changing attitudes of others, educating the client about his/her rights to employment under the Americans with Disabilities Act, educating other people as appropriate to the client's needs and abilities).
- Identifying and promoting facilitators (e.g., attitudes of people in positions of authority, products and technology).
- Evaluating the client's performance in the work environment and making recommendations.

### Cross References

In *Recreational Therapy for Specific Diagnoses and Conditions, First Edition*, ICF code d859 Work and Employment, Other Specified and Unspecified is listed in eight chapters: Cancer, Chronic Obstructive Pulmonary Disease, Hearing Loss, Multiple Sclerosis, Neurocognitive Disorders, Obesity, Substance-Related Disorders, and Traumatic Brain Injury.

In *Recreational Therapy Basics, Techniques, and Interventions, First Edition*, there are no references for ICF code d859 Work and Employment, Other Specified and Unspecified.

## Economic Life (d860 - d879)

### d860 Basic Economic Transactions

Engaging in any form of simple economic transaction, such as using money to purchase food or bartering, exchanging goods or services; or saving money.

See the discussion at the end of the section.

### Cross References

In *Recreational Therapy for Specific Diagnoses and Conditions, First Edition*, ICF code d860 Basic Economic Transactions is listed in three chapters: Hearing Loss, Intellectual Disability, and Neurocognitive Disorders.

In *Recreational Therapy Basics, Techniques, and Interventions, First Edition*, treatment for ICF code d860 Basic Economic Transactions is discussed in one chapter: Activity and Task Analysis.

### d865 Complex Economic Transactions

Engaging in any form of complex economic transaction that involves the exchange of capital or property, and the creation of profit or economic value, such as buying a business, factory, or equipment, maintaining a bank account, or trading in commodities.

See the discussion at the end of the section.

### Cross References

In *Recreational Therapy for Specific Diagnoses and Conditions, First Edition*, ICF code d865 Complex Economic Transactions is listed in two chapters: Hearing Loss and Neurocognitive Disorders.

In *Recreational Therapy Basics, Techniques, and Interventions, First Edition*, there are no references for ICF code d865 Complex Economic Transactions.

### d870 Economic Self-Sufficiency

Having command over economic resources, from private or public sources, in order to ensure economic security for present and future needs.

Inclusions: personal economic resources and public economic entitlements

- d8700 Personal Economic Resources
  Having command over personal or private economic resources, in order to ensure economic security for present and future needs.

- d8701 Public Economic Entitlements
  Having command over public economic resources, in order to ensure economic security for present and future needs.

- d8708 Economic Self-Sufficiency, Other Specified
- d8709 Economic Self-Sufficiency, Unspecified
  See the discussion at the end of the section.

### Cross References

In *Recreational Therapy for Specific Diagnoses and Conditions, First Edition*, ICF code d870 Economic Self-Sufficiency is listed in three chapters: Hearing Loss, Neurocognitive Disorders, and Spinal Cord Injury.

In *Recreational Therapy Basics, Techniques, and Interventions, First Edition*, there are no references for ICF code d870 Economic Self-Sufficiency.

## d879 Economic Life, Other Specified and Unspecified

In the ICF recreational therapists document the client's level of difficulty. In discipline-specific documentation, recreational therapists document the level of assistance required with each of the subtasks of the skill, adaptive equipment, techniques, recommendations, and impact of the dysfunction on other life tasks including relationships with the spouse, participation in activities, and nutrition.

Recreational therapists who work in rehabilitation and residential programs regularly address barriers to economic life and promote facilitators, especially with clients who are cognitively impaired or are striving to reach developmental milestones, such as teaching a seven-year-old how to perform basic economic transactions at the toy store with her birthday gift card.

Economic transactions are needed for many recreation and leisure activities and are commonly addressed in the clinic, as well as in real-life environments. Addressing economic self-sufficiency is not commonly included in inpatient rehabilitation programs. However, it is often a component of the recreational therapy treatment plan when working with clients in an independent living program as part of learning basic life skills.

Economic issues have the potential to affect the basic human needs of shelter and food in either a positive or a negative way. They also affect participation in other life activities. If a problem is suspected with economic life, the therapist conducts a task analysis to identify the specific areas of dysfunction, such as d172 Calculating, d177 Making Decisions, or d4402 Manipulating.

## d898 Major Life Areas, Other Specified

## d899 Major Life Areas, Unspecified

### References

burlingame, j. & Blaschko, T. M. (2010). *Assessment tools for recreational therapy and related fields*, 4th edition. Enumclaw, WA: Idyll Arbor, Inc.

Dulin, P. L., Gavala, J., Stephens, C., Kostick, M., & McDonald, J. (2012). Volunteering predicts happiness among older Maori and non-Maori in the New Zealand health, work, and retirement longitudinal study. *Aging and Mental Health, 16*(5), 617-624.

Farrell, P. & Lundegren, H. M. (1991). *The process of recreation programming: Theory and technique*. State College, PA: Venture Publishing.

Fegan, C. (2012). Experiences of volunteering: A partnership between service users and a mental health service in the UK. *Work: A Journal of Prevention, Assessment, & Rehabilitation, 43*(1), 13-21.

Ginsburg, K. (2007). The importance of play in promoting healthy child development and maintaining strong parent-child bonds. *Pediatrics, 119*(1), 182-191.

Gray, P. (2008). Freedom to learn: The roles of play and curiosity as foundations for learning. Freedom to Learn, a blog by *Psychology Today.*

Kelly-Vance, L. & Ryalls, B. O. (2008). Best practices in play assessment and intervention, chapter 33, p 549-560. In *Best Practices in School Psychology V*, Thomas, A. & Grimes. J. (Eds.). Bethesda, MD: NASP.

Konrath, S., Fuhrel-Forbis, A., Lou, A., & Brown, S. (2012). Motives for volunteering are associated with mortality risk in older adults. *Health Psychology, 31*(1), 87-96

Mayesky, M. (2009). *Creative activities for young children.* Independence, KY: Cengage Learning,

Moore, M. & Russ, S. (2006). Pretend play as a resource for children: Implications for pediatricians and health professionals. *Journal of Developmental and Behavioral Pediatrics, 27*(3), 237-248.

*Mosby's Medical Dictionary*, 8th edition. (2009). Associative play. Maryland Heights, MO: Elsevier.

National Institutes for Play. (2009). Play science: The patterns of play. Accessed via website http://www.nifplay.org/states_play.html.

Rubin, K. H. (2001). The play observation scale (POS). Accessed via website http://www.rubin-lab.umd.edu/Coding%20Schemes/POS%20Coding%20Scheme%202001.pdf.

Russoniello, C.V., Skalko, T. K., Beatly, J., & Alexander, D. B. (2002). New paradigms for therapeutic recreation and recreation and leisure service delivery: The Pattillo A+ Elementary School disaster relief project. *Parks and Recreation, 37*(2), 74-81.

Smith, R. L. & Van Puymbroeck, M. (2011). A strengths-based approach to play in children with autism. *American Journal of Recreation Therapy, 10*(1), 17-24.

Stagnitti, K. (2004). Understanding play: The implications of assessment. *Australian Occupational Therapy Journal, 51*, 3-12.

Steger, M. F., Dik, B. J., & Duffy, R. D. (2012). Measuring meaningful work: The work and meaning inventory (WAMI). *Journal of Career Assessment*, 20(3), 322-337.

Trainor, A. A., Carter, E. W., Sweeden, B., Owens, L., Cole, O., & Smith, S. (2011). Perspectives of adolescents with disabilities on summer employment and community experiences. *The Journal of Special Education, 45*(3), 157-170.

United Nations. (2006). Convention on the rights of a child. Accessed via website http://www2.ohchr.org/english/bodies/crc/docs/AdvanceVersions/GeneralComment7Rev1.pdf

# Chapter 9 Community, Social, and Civic Life

This chapter is about the actions and tasks required to engage in organized social life outside the family, in community, social, and civic areas of life.

*Sample Scoring of Community, Social and Civic Life*

- A client wishes to return to her local senior center to participate in various activities, including card playing (d9200 Play) and line dancing (d9202 Arts and Culture). During a community integration training session, the client exhibited no difficulty playing cards (no difficulty = 0), but exhibited a range of mild to moderate difficulty (mild difficulty = 1, moderate difficulty = 2) with line dancing depending on the complexity of movements and level of fatigue. When line dancing, the group leader does not provide any physical assistance to the participants. The complete scoring for code d9202 Arts and Culture would look like this:

  d9202._ _ _ 0 (card playing) Dehn level +3: Active Participation.
  d9202._ _ _ 2 (line dancing) Dehn level +3: Active Participation.

- A client meditates daily at home to commune with his higher power (d930 Religion and Spirituality). He desires to move from a standing position to a sitting position on the floor, get into a cross-legged position, rest the back of his palms on his knees, and hold this position for 30 minutes. Following the meditation session, he will need to resume an upright position. d930 Religion and Spirituality is scored because the meditation is done for this reason. The therapist could also additionally score the specific movements associated with the activity, such as d4103 Sitting, d4153 Maintaining a Sitting Position, etc. In the clinic setting, the client had mild difficulty getting into, maintaining, and getting out of the required movements (mild difficulty = 1). With assistance from the recreational therapist there was no residual difficultly (no difficulty = 0). Despite occasional cues from the recreational therapist, he also had mild difficulty meditating due to attention and concentration difficulties (mild difficulty = 1). Notice that when assistance was provided the client had no difficulty with movements, but continued to have mild difficulty with attention and concentration. Consequently, the third qualifier "capacity, with assistance" was scored a "1" for mild difficulty. Choose the score that reflects the highest level of difficulty. The complete scoring for code d930 Religion and Spirituality would look like this:

  d930._ 1 1 _, (meditating in seated position) Dehn level +3: Active Participation.

Scoring the codes in this chapter can be challenging for a recreational therapist. There are two major concerns: the definition of the term "engaging" and the limited set of available codes. These issues and how to score this chapter in a consistent way are described below.

The word "engaging" is used in each of the definitions in this chapter (e.g., engaging in pastimes, engaging in needlecrafts). The problem is that engaging is not a therapeutic term commonly used in recreational therapy practice and could therefore cause difficulties in scoring if it is not interpreted the same way by all therapists. Since the ICF is based on health (functionality or ability) rather than on disability (problem definitions), the best assumption is that engaging means healthy participation in the activity.

There are two ways to look at healthy participation. The first looks at the ability of the client to perform the actions required in the activity. The second looks at whether the client is participating in a healthy way, an unhealthy way, or merely going through the motions. Going through the motions is not truly engaging in the activity. Both aspects of activities, skills and level of participation, need to be scored to give an accurate picture of the client's ability to engage in the activity.

Scoring the skill level is something recreational therapists do well. The harder part of the scoring arises because engaging in the activities does not always have a positive outcome. Engaging may be unhealthy and negatively impact health and quality of life. For example, a client may have no difficulty in engaging with a gang, yet the gang activities themselves are dangerous to the client and others. In this example, the therapist might think it was appropriate to score all qualifiers of d9100 Informal Associations with a 0 for no difficulty. Someone reviewing the client's chart would think that the client was participating in healthy informal associations without any difficulty. This scoring would lead to an incorrect interpretation of the client's situation.

One way to resolve this problem is to write the name of the activity to the right of the code followed by the Dehn's (1995) level of participation to indicate the health of engagement — "Neighborhood Gang: Dehn level -2 Harm to Others." Dehn levels range from +4 (plus four) for creative participation through 0 (zero) for going through the motions down to -2 (minus two) for harm to others. When the Dehn level is provided after the code, others reading the score of 0 in the qualifiers understand that the client is fully independent in the activity, and they are also alerted that engaging in this informal association is harmful to the client's health or the health of others. With that method a recreational therapist can score both the ability to perform the task and whether the participation is healthy or not.

The second problem is that that there are very few codes covering broad areas of activities. The recreational therapist must be careful to score in a way that gives a true reflection of the client's performance in a specific task.

With this in mind, let's look at one of the recreation and leisure codes.

d9202 Arts and Culture: Engaging in, or appreciating, fine arts or cultural events, such as going to the theater, cinema, museum, or art gallery, or acting in a play, reading for enjoyment, or playing a musical instrument.

Notice that the code includes many activities. The concern is that the skill of appreciating fine art such as looking through a museum catalog is very different from the more physically active task of playing a violin. This causes a problem for the field of recreational therapy because the skill sets for these tasks are quite different and a client may participate in a variety of Arts and Culture activities. One therapist may score the client as having no difficulty with d9202 Arts and Culture because she is only considering the client's ability to look through a collection of museum catalogs. Another therapist may

score the client as having moderate difficulty because he is only considering the client's ability to play the violin. When scoring the codes in this area, the most accurate and helpful way is to use the same code multiple times, once for each activity. For example, a client who engages in three different sports and has varying levels of difficulty would be accurately described if the therapist scored the code three times.

d9201.2 _ _ 3 (basketball)
d9201.3 _ _ 4 (soccer)
d9201.1 _ _ 2 (baseball)

The best solution to the two problems discussed seems to be to add additional information to codes in this section so that they accurately reflect the client's status. Here is one way to do that:

- Identify one specific activity, such as playing baseball.
- Hold the mental picture of "healthy participation" in your mind. Measure how much difficulty the client has in performing the tasks required for this level of healthy participation and choose the appropriate score. If the client has different levels of difficulty with particular tasks associated with the activity, the therapist should take the score that reflects the greatest difficulty.
- After scoring the code, write the name of the specific activity to the right of the code.
- Following the name of the activity, add a description of the participation level (e.g., Dehn level +3: Active Participation).
- Full coding example: d9201.0 2 3 4 (Little League baseball), Dehn level +3: Active Participation

One final concern is that the ICF does not currently allow the therapist to code Body Functions, Body Structures, or Activities and Participation as barriers or facilitators of other activities. Let's look at an example of a client who has maximal difficulty throwing a baseball, no difficulty in keeping score, and minimal difficulty taking turns. These observations are important. They would be scored in the appropriate categories of Body Functions and Activities and Participation. The problem is that there is no way in the current ICF scoring to link, for example, d4454 Throwing with d9201 Sports. Recreational therapists need to keep track of these connections in documentation outside of the ICF to be able to look at the holistic interaction of variables affecting a client's level of health.

It is important to find a way of scoring the ICF so that the value of engagement in community life, recreation and leisure, and religion and spirituality, along with the enjoyment of human rights and citizenship, is accurately documented. We know that healthy engagement contributes to health and well-being, along with quality of life. In one study, 1,246 older adults age 65-95 were followed for 12 years (Agahi & Parker, 2008). Participants were asked to indicate if they participated in specific activities. Findings indicated that those who participated the least had the highest mortality risk. For example, participants who participated in none or one activity tripled their mortality risk when compared to those who participated in six or more activities. Those who participated in two activities had double the mortality risk. Interestingly, social activities had the strongest association with survival among women, while men had stronger associations with survival when participating in "solitary, voluntary, and creative/productive [activities] … independent of other people or the keeping of schedules" (p. 866).

In another longitudinal study, 8,000 middle-aged adults were followed for 20 years (Hyyppa et al., 2006). Findings indicated that "people who are actively engaged in clubs, voluntary societies, hobbies, or in cultural, recreational, and civic activities… live longer than people with moderate leisure participation, and people with no or little leisure participation live the shortest life" (p. 9). Those who had abundant leisure participation decreased their relative risk of death by two thirds when compared to those with little leisure participation.

In addition to longitudinal studies, literature reviews have also found health and quality of life benefits from leisure engagement. For example, a literature review over an 18-year period by Heintzman (2009) found that leisure activities can provide spiritual experiences, contribute to spiritual well-being, and serve as a context for spiritual coping with stress. In a literature review by Iwasaki (2008) leisure activities were found to provide "a context or space for creating meanings which then help to promote the quality of people's lives" (p. 233). A literature review by Porter, Iwasaki, and Shank (2011) identified the specific meanings experienced in leisure activity engagement including a sense of connection and belonging, identity, freedom and autonomy, power and control, and competence and mastery.

Research has also shown that community participation has health and quality of life benefits. For example, a study by Geurtsen et al. (2011) found that a residential community reintegration program for individuals with brain injury improved independent living, societal participation, emotional well-being, and quality of life. Improvements were maintained at one-year follow up. Additionally, a study by Youngkhill et al. (2008) found that community integration significantly contributes to physical, psychological, social, and environmental quality of life and noted that "successful community integration is clearly an important and worthwhile goal for individuals with illness and disability and should be an important priority for recreational therapists" (p. 223).

### Assessment of Community, Social, and Civic Life

Recreational therapists utilize various methods to assess community, social and civic life including interview, observation, functional testing, and standardized assessments such as the *Community Integration Questionnaire* (CIQ), *Craig Handicap Assessment and Reporting Technique* (CHART), *Reintegration to Normal Living Index* (RNLI), *Sydney Psychosocial Reintegration Scale* (SPRS), the *Community Integration Measure* (CIM), and the *Community Integration Program* (CIP).

### Treatment of Community, Social, and Civic Life

Interventions aimed at improving and enhancing community, social, and civic life will vary depending upon identified client needs, abilities, and resources. Interventions might include leisure education and counseling, leisure interest exploration, functional skill development, community integration training, resource awareness and education, human rights education, problem solving, and/or activity adaptations for barriers. Interventions from standardized programs, such as the *Community Integration Program* (Armstrong & Lauzen, 1994), might also be utilized.

### Evidence Review

Reviews of several studies are provided below to highlight evidence-based practice related to community, social, and civic life. This is only a sample of the evidence. A thorough review of the literature is needed to identify evidence-based practice interventions that reflect the needs and characteristics of the individual client.

Dermatis, Galanter, and Bunt (2010) conducted a study of approximately 209 adults in an Alcoholics Anonymous program to determine spiritual orientation and treatment outcomes using the *Spirituality Self-Rating Scale* (SSRS). Findings indicated that spiritual orientation was positively correlated with greater clinical progress and acceptance of program principles. "It was demonstrated that the SSRS, a measure of spiritual orientation consistent with the conceptualization of spirituality in the 12-Step group model, has potential value as a predictor of clinical outcomes" (p. 312).

White, Drechsel, and Johnson (2006) reviewed a faith-based community wellness program called Faithfully Fit Forever. Each class is divided into three components (mind, body, and spirit). For mind there is a 10-minute session on a health topic, such as dealing with stress or managing blood pressure. For body the participants engage in 60 minutes of group exercise. Spirit has an undetermined time for spiritual readings and discussion. The authors note that holding programs at faith-based community settings provides many benefits:

- It brings health promotion to people who need it within a safe, supportive, and familiar setting, while helping combat insufficient access to wellness programs.
- A spiritual setting is a good place for making "changes."
- "The supportive and trusting environment found within these relationships helps influence and encourage people to strive for healthier lifestyles" (p. 131).

Winkler, Unsworth, and Sloan (2006) conducted a study of 40 participants with severe traumatic brain injury, an average of 8.8 years post injury, to identify predictive factors of community integration. Findings indicated that severity of injury, age at time of injury, level of disability, and challenging behavior were predictive of the level of community integration. The authors recommend that "interventions that minimize challenging behavior and disability may make a significant difference to the level of community integration experienced by people with severe traumatic brain injury" (p. 8).

A systematic review of the literature by Verdonschot et al. (2009) showed that the following environmental factors that affect human rights had a positive impact on community participation for individuals with intellectual disability: opportunities to make choices, variety and stimulation of the environment of facilities, opportunities for resident involvement in policy making, small residential facilities, opportunities for autonomy, vocational services, social support, family involvement, assistive technology, and positive staff attitudes. Environmental factors that negatively impacted community participation for individuals with intellectual disability included lack of transportation and not feeling accepted.

Barker et al. (2009) conducted a study of 270 individuals with spinal cord injury. The presence of secondary conditions was the single most important predictor of quality of life, followed by the extent of societal participation. "Of concern, however, is that many rehabilitation services continue to focus their day-to-day service delivery on impairments and activity limitations with less emphasis on participation. These findings prompt the need for both hospital and community rehabilitation services to place greater emphasis on assessment and intervention related to social participation, particularly on enhancing factors that facilitate participation and overcoming barriers that impede participation" (p. 154).

Conti, Voelkl, and McGuire (2009) conducted a review of the literature related to leisure and prevention of dementia (39 articles). Findings indicate that higher frequency and variety of activities in a person's life has a relationship with deterrence of dementia and mental decline. Higher levels of physical activity are associated with better scores on cognitive tests and lowered risk of developing dementia. Higher amounts and quality of social interactions has a positive relationship with cognition. Increased participation in intellectually challenging activities was associated with lower cognitive decline. Because causality was not proven, caution must be used when stating that such leisure can prevent cognitive decline. The authors recommend that recreational therapists (1) test and document outcomes of their programs concerning prevention of cognitive decline, (2) provide clients with a wide variety of leisure opportunities that are both physically and cognitively challenging, (3) provide passive activities that build social relationships, and (4) educate clients about the relationship of leisure engagement and cognitive decline, but caution that there is no guarantee.

### Cross References

In *Recreational Therapy for Specific Diagnoses and Conditions, First Edition*, ICF code d9 Community, Social, and Civic Life and its subcategories are listed in 38 chapters: Amputation and Prosthesis, Attention-Deficit/Hyperactivity Disorder, Autism Spectrum Disorder, Back Disorders and Back Pain, Borderline Personality Disorder, Burns, Cancer, Cerebral Palsy, Cerebrovascular Accident, Chronic Obstructive Pulmonary Disease, Diabetes Mellitus, Epilepsy, Feeding and Eating Disorders, Fibromyalgia and Juvenile Fibromyalgia, Gambling Disorder, Generalized Anxiety Disorder, Guillain-Barré Syndrome, Hearing Loss, Heart Disease, Intellectual Disability, Major Depressive Disorder, Multiple Sclerosis, Neurocognitive Disorders, Obesity, Oppositional Defiant Disorder and Conduct Disorder, Osteoarthritis, Osteoporosis, Parkinson's Disease, Post-Traumatic Stress Disorder, Pressure Ulcers, Rheumatoid Arthritis, Sickle Cell Disease, Spina Bifida, Spinal Cord Injury, Substance-Related Disorders, Total Joint Replacement, Traumatic Brain Injury, and Visual Impairments and Blindness.

In *Recreational Therapy Basics, Techniques, and Interventions, First Edition*, treatment for ICF code d9 Community, Social, and Civic Life and its subcategories are discussed in 23 chapters: Adjustment and Response to Disability, Body Mechanics and Ergonomics, Parameters and Precautions, Participation, Stress, Activity Pattern Development, Adaptive Sports, Anger Management, Animal Assisted Therapy, Aquatic Therapy, Balance Training, Bibliotherapy, Cognitive Behavioral Counseling, Disability Rights: Education and Advocacy, Energy Conservation Techniques, Group Psychotherapy Techniques, Leisure Education and Counseling, Leisure Resource Awareness, Mind-Body Interventions, Montessori Method, Physical Activity, Social Skills Training, and Therapeutic Thematic Arts Programming.

### d910 Community Life

Engaging in all aspects of community social life, such as engaging in charitable organizations, service clubs, or professional social organizations.

Inclusions: informal and formal associations; ceremonies

Exclusions: non-remunerative employment (d855); recreation and leisure (d920); religion and spirituality (d930); political life and citizenship (d950)

- *d9100 Informal Associations*
  Engaging in social or community associations organized by people with common interests, such as local social clubs or ethnic groups.

- *d9101 Formal Associations*
  Engaging in professional or other exclusive social groups, such as associations of lawyers, physicians, or academics.

- *d9102 Ceremonies*
  Engaging in non-religious rites or social ceremonies, such as marriages, funerals, or initiation ceremonies.

- *d9108 Community Life, Other Specified*
- *d9109 Community Life, Unspecified*

Community life can best be described as engaging in community groups and clubs with specific people joining together for a specific interest. Notice that this code excludes recreation and leisure, religion and spirituality, and political life. However the groups and clubs can be related to recreation, leisure, religion, spirituality, or politics. There is a distinction, although it is subtle.

The community life code set is about engaging in community groups and clubs, whereas d920 Recreation and Leisure, d930 Religion and Spirituality, and d950 Political Life and Citizenship are about engaging in the specific activity. For example, if a client belonged to a senior citizen social club, the therapist would score d9100 Informal Associations related to the level of difficulty that he has engaging in the construct of a club. This would include group membership skills such as calling people to action, voting, following group rules, expressing opinions within a group, and following unstated social rules. This same client, while at the social club, engages in card playing. Card playing is a specific recreation activity, so the therapist would score his level of difficulty with card playing under the Recreation and Leisure code set (d9200 Play).

Engaging in community groups and clubs is one of the major areas of recreational therapy practice. The result of engaging in community life can directly affect a person's health in a positive or negative way. For example, a client who participates in a community group that raises money for children in need may reap the positive benefits of having a social network, getting exercise through physical challenges that raise money, and raising her sense of self-esteem in being part of an organization that gives to the community. On the other hand, another client may belong to a neighborhood gang (d9100 Informal Associations) that is involved with illegal activities, such as selling illegal drugs and destroying other's property. The client may state the same benefits as our previous client such as the benefits of having a social network, getting physical exercise by fighting with other gangs, and raising his sense of pride in being a part of a gang that accepts only a select few. This is another example of the need to use Dehn's (1995) participation levels in addition to the standard ICF scoring.

### Assessment of Community Life

For this code recreational therapists evaluate the health of a client's community life as part of the total lifestyle. The difficulties that a client may have with engagement in community life may include lack of awareness of:

- Resources.
- Human rights (d940 Human Rights).
- Community barriers.
- Energy conservation.
- Adaptations for engagement.

The client may also have difficulty with specific skills, such as:

- Social skills (d7 Interpersonal Interactions and Relationships).
- Time management (d230 Carrying Out Daily Routine).
- Mobility (d4 Mobility).
- Anger management (b126 Temperament and Personality Functions, and d710 Basic Interpersonal Interactions).
- Adjustment to disability (b126 Temperament and Personality Functions).

Therapists should score these and other codes, as appropriate, in addition to the community life code.

Through observation, clinical interview, functional assessment, and standardized assessment tools, areas of dysfunction are identified. Deficits can be based in Body Functions and Body Structures (e.g., difficulty with speech impacting ability to verbally participate in group meetings), Activities and Participation (e.g., difficulty with social skills impacting ability to follow group rules), and/or Environmental Factors (e.g., lack of accessibility to enter the building).

Recreational therapists document the extent of difficulty a client has with community life. For example, despite having assistance from his wife, the client has moderate difficulty engaging at the senior center (d910.2 _ _ _ Following rules; Dehn level +3: Active Participation).

### Treatment of Community Life

Treatment for Community Life will vary depending on underlying impairments, difficulties, and barriers. For example, if a client has difficulty engaging in informal associations due to deficits in getting to locations where meetings are held, the therapist would refer to d4 Mobility for treatment direction, as well as the companion book, *Recreational Therapy Basics, Techniques, and Interventions* for information on Walking and Gait Training, Wheelchair Mobility, and other chapters related to getting around in the community.

### Cross References

In *Recreational Therapy for Specific Diagnoses and Conditions, First Edition*, ICF code d910 Community Life is listed in 19 chapters: Amputation and Prosthesis, Back Disorders and Back Pain, Borderline Personality Disorder, Cerebrovascular Accident, Chronic Obstructive Pulmonary Disease, Diabetes Mellitus, Epilepsy, Gambling Disorder, Intellectual Disability, Major Depressive Disorder, Multiple Sclerosis, Oppositional Defiant Disorder and Conduct Disorder, Post-Traumatic Stress Disorder, Rheumatoid Arthritis, Spina Bifida, Spinal Cord Injury, Substance-Related Disorders, Traumatic Brain Injury, and Visual Impairments and Blindness.

In *Recreational Therapy Basics, Techniques, and Interventions, First Edition*, treatment for ICF code d910 Community Life is discussed in eight chapters: Adjustment and Response to Disability, Participation,

Aquatic Therapy, Cognitive Behavioral Counseling, Group Psychotherapy Techniques, Leisure Education and Counseling, Social Skills Training, and Therapeutic Thematic Arts Programming.

## d920 Recreation and Leisure

Engaging in any form of play, recreational, or leisure activity, such as informal or organized play and sports, programs of physical fitness, relaxation, amusement or diversion, going to art galleries, museums, cinemas, or theaters; engaging in crafts or hobbies, reading for enjoyment, playing musical instruments; sightseeing, tourism, and traveling for pleasure.

Inclusions: play, sports, arts and culture, crafts, hobbies, and socializing

Exclusions: riding animals for transportation (d480); remunerative and non-remunerative work (d850 and d855); religion and spirituality (d930); political life and citizenship (d950)

- *d9200 Play*
  Engaging in games with rules or unstructured or unorganized games and spontaneous recreation, such as playing chess or cards, or children's play.

- *d9201 Sports*
  Engaging in competitive and informal or formally organized games or athletic events, performed alone or in a group, such as bowling, gymnastics, or soccer.

- *d9202 Arts and Culture*
  Engaging in, or appreciating, fine arts or cultural events, such as going to the theater, cinema, museum, or art gallery, or acting in a play, reading for enjoyment, or playing a musical instrument.

- *d9203 Crafts*
  Engaging in handicrafts, such as pottery or knitting.

- *d9204 Hobbies*
  Engaging in pastimes such as collecting stamps, coins, or antiques.

- *d9205 Socializing*
  Engaging in informal or casual gatherings with others, such as visiting friends or relatives or meeting informally in public places.

- *d9208 Recreation and Leisure, Other Specified*
- *d9209 Recreation and Leisure, Unspecified*

Recreation and leisure in the ICF are related to specific categories of activities that are commonly performed for pleasure and enjoyment. For example, playing an instrument falls under d9202 Arts and Culture. If a client plays an instrument for pleasure and enjoyment, the therapist would use this code. If the client plays an instrument for any other reason, such as work, the therapist would code the appropriate code instead. For work it would be d850 Remunerative Employment.

The terms recreation and leisure are often used synonymously. The field of recreational therapy, however, often divides the terms. Recreation is commonly defined as activity, compared to leisure that is defined as a state of mind. Looking at this code set, it is obvious that it is activity focused. Leisure, however, as a state of mind, can be reflected in many of the ICF codes, such as d9100 Informal Associations, d6200 Shopping, d630 Preparing Meals, d6500 Making and Repairing Clothes, d6501 Maintaining Dwelling and Furnishings, d6503 Maintaining Vehicles, and d6506 Taking Care of Animals.

It could be argued that the other codes in the ICF, as mentioned above, are related to tasks that *need* to be done rather than tasks that are done for pleasure and enjoyment. However, to say that would mean that pleasure and enjoyment are absent from all activities outside of those categorized in the recreation and leisure code set. This is simply not true. Consequently, recreational therapists must decide if it is more appropriate to score an activity done for pleasure as a recreation and leisure code or to use a code that better reflects the specific activity. Here are some examples: If a client has the hobby of gardening, the therapist can use the code d6505 Taking Care of Plants, Indoors and Outdoors or d9204 Hobbies. If a client builds hot rod cars for fun, the therapist can use the code d6503 Maintaining Vehicles or d9204 Hobbies.

Therapists must also be careful when choosing codes for physical activities. For example, in d4 Mobility there are a variety of codes that reflect a type of movement that is also a sport, including d4551 Climbing, d4552 Running, and d4554 Swimming. If the therapist desires to score a type of movement, the mobility codes would be used (e.g., d4554 Swimming). However, if the therapist wants to score swimming as a sport (from a more holistic view), d9201 Sports would be used.

Recreational therapists conduct a detailed recreation and leisure assessment through the use of clinical interview, observation, functional assessment, and standardized assessment. The aim is to identify a person's strengths and weaknesses related to recreation and leisure engagement; explore leisure attitudes, motivations, and interests; assess the health of the person's leisure lifestyle as it pertains to achieving optimal development, health, and quality of life; determine recreation and leisure engagement patterns; identify barriers and facilitators to leisure engagement; and identify the client's recreation and leisure goals. As discussed in the introduction to the chapter, the best way to score this set of codes is to include the specific activity and level of participation.

When treating these codes, very often a therapist will need to begin with education about the consequences of an inappropriate leisure lifestyle and the benefits of recreation and leisure participation as it pertains to the current needs of the client, whether it is a lack of physical exercise, mental stimulation, or emotional engagement.

To reduce deficiencies found in these codes, the client may require leisure interest testing and exploration. Inaccurate information may need to be corrected, such as educating a client about adaptive equipment, techniques, and resources to engage in an activity that the client thought was only for able-bodied people. Counseling interventions may be employed followed by functional skill development related to activity participation. The specific functional skills addressed will depend on the activity and the needs of the client. Therapists can refer to the specific skill in other ICF codes for information on how to assess, document, treat, and adapt for any deficits. Integration training typically follows, allowing the therapist to address issues that arise in a real-life setting and further assess the client's ability to integrate skills into his life.

Recreational therapists document the extent of difficulty a client has with recreation and leisure. For example, without assistance the client has moderate difficulty knitting baby doll clothes (d9203._ _ _2 Knitting baby doll clothes; Dehn level +3: Active Participation).

### Cross References

In *Recreational Therapy for Specific Diagnoses and Conditions, First Edition*, ICF code d920 Recreation and Leisure is listed in 34 chapters: Amputation and Prosthesis, Attention-Deficit/Hyperactivity Disorder, Autism Spectrum Disorder, Back Disorders and Back Pain, Burns, Cancer, Cerebral Palsy, Cerebrovascular Accident, Chronic Obstructive Pulmonary Disease, Diabetes Mellitus, Epilepsy, Feeding and Eating Disorders, Gambling Disorder, Generalized Anxiety Disorder, Guillain-Barré Syndrome, Hearing Loss, Intellectual Disability, Major Depressive Disorder, Multiple Sclerosis, Neurocognitive Disorders, Obesity, Oppositional Defiant Disorder and Conduct Disorder, Osteoarthritis, Osteoporosis, Parkinson's Disease, Post-Traumatic Stress Disorder, Pressure Ulcers, Rheumatoid Arthritis, Spina Bifida, Spinal Cord Injury, Substance-Related Disorders, Total Joint Replacement, Traumatic Brain Injury, and Visual Impairments and Blindness.

In *Recreational Therapy Basics, Techniques, and Interventions, First Edition*, treatment for ICF code d920 Recreation and Leisure is discussed in 13 chapters: Education and Counseling, Participation, Activity Pattern Development, Animal Assisted Therapy, Aquatic Therapy, Balance Training, Community Participation: Integration, Transitioning, and Inclusion, Group Psychotherapy Techniques, Leisure Education and Counseling, Leisure Resource Awareness, Mind-Body Interventions, Physical Activity, and Social Skills Training.

### d930 Religion and Spirituality

Engaging in religious or spiritual activities, organizations and practices for self-fulfillment, finding meaning, religious or spiritual value, and establishing connection with a divine power, such as is involved in attending a church, temple, mosque, or synagogue, praying or chanting for a religious purpose, and spiritual contemplation.

Inclusions: organized religion and spirituality

- *d9300 Organized Religion*
  Engaging in organized religious ceremonies, activities, and events.

- *d9301 Spirituality*
  Engaging in spiritual activities or events, outside an organized religion.

- *d9308 Religion and Spirituality, Other Specified*
- *d9309 Religion and Spirituality, Unspecified*

The terms religion and spirituality are often used interchangeably, however there are distinct differences between the two. Religion is an external expression of faith in God or a higher being. There are specific beliefs, values, and practices that unite a person with a religious community. Spirituality, on the other hand, is an intrinsic quality, as in "She is a spiritual person." It is a feeling of connectedness with oneself, nature, the world, and/or a higher spirit. The ability to "stand outside of his/her immediate sense of time and place and to view life from a larger, more detached perspective" describes a common component of spirituality called spiritual transcendence (Rowe & Allen, 2004, p. 1). Spirituality can arise from the practice of religion, but the practice of a religion is not necessary to be spiritual.

Ninety to 95% of people in the United States say that they believe in God or a higher being (Miller & Thoresen, 2003), yet religion and spirituality are rarely addressed in a healthcare setting. This is mostly due to fears of invading a person's privacy and overstepping the client-therapist boundary. Spirituality, however, whether obtained through religious or non-religious activities, is becoming increasingly recognized as being a benefit for health that needs to be addressed in the healthcare setting. (It is already a requirement for facilities operating under OBRA regulations as described in Tag 248: Activities.)

Seaward (1997) theorizes that there are four specific internal processes that nurture spiritual health — centering, emptying, grounding, and connecting.

*Centering*: Centering is a process of turning inwards and exploring personal thoughts, feelings, attitudes, and perceptions to gain a greater sense of the self. Activities such a meditation and yoga and rhythmic exercises such as running, walking, and swimming are common interventions to facilitate centering.

*Emptying*: Emptying is a process of letting go of destructive thoughts, feelings, and actions that inhibit spiritual growth. Expressive writing (Pennebaker & Evans, 2015) can be helpful to increase awareness of thoughts, feelings, attitudes, values, and perceptions that inhibit a person from reaching his/her full life potential and satisfaction. Destructive traits that inhibit this growth often come to light and can then be released (emptied). Once the consciousness is cleared, the spirit (soul, core) is ready to receive new insights and move on to grounding.

*Grounding*: In grounding a person reflects inward to find inner resources to face the challenges that lie before him/her and sharpens coping skills to manage stressful encounters in a healthy and self-fulfilling way. Meditation or prayer can be helpful to find inner strength and peace. Stress management and relaxation training strengthen coping skills. Problem solving and communication skills can also prove helpful in the development and tuning of healthy coping skills. Seaward recommends the additional modalities of paying attention to nature, participating in rituals, reading, discussing ideas and values with others, and simply paying attention to life as ways that help with grounding the spirit.

*Connecting*: In the first three processes (centering, empting, grounding), the person focuses on connecting with the self. In the final process, the person focuses on connecting with others, nature, and with a higher power or spirit. Seaward states, "Those people who engage fully in the connecting process, without the influence of judgment, greed, or fear, show an undeniable enthusiasm for life" (Seaward, 1997, p. 153).

Much of the literature about spirituality reports that meaning in one's life, connecting with a higher power, feeling connected to the world, having a nurturing relationship with oneself, having a strong personal value system, and having a meaningful purpose in the world affect health in a positive way.

"Spirituality is one of several known psychosocial variables that influence the course of health over an individual's lifetime...[and] it may play an independent role in helping individuals attend to positive elements in their life" (Bartlett et al, 2003, p. 780). It has been linked with happiness and positive health perceptions (Daaleman, Perera, & Studenski, 2004), positive affect and outlook (Myers, 2000; Diener, 2000; Rowe & Allen, 2004), decreased vulnerability to depression, even in the face of grief and loss (Ellison & Levin, 1998; McIntosh, Silver, & Wortman, 1993), enhanced immune functioning, enhanced ability to adapt and cope with illness or disability (Bartlett et al, 2003; Rowe & Allen, 2004), and an increased ability to look at things from different perspectives along with creative problem solving (Ashby, Isen, & Turken, 1999).

Interestingly, a significant positive correlation between spirituality and age has been reported (Rowe & Allen, 2004), perhaps because increased spirituality is required to cope with the realization of mortality (Reed, 1991).

Although spirituality may have a significant correlation with age, health care professionals must not forget about the spiritual needs of a child. Elkins and Cavendish (2004) remind health professionals that attitudes and values expressed by a child are often influenced by the family's spiritual ideas and beliefs. Children have spiritual lives that deserve to be continued and fostered in a healthcare setting. Spirituality is a growth process and, although people's development of spirituality varies, basic building blocks of spirituality often begin in childhood. Therapists should interview the parents, as discussed below, to determine any specific spiritual or religious needs that should be implemented in the hospital setting and pay attention to signs of spiritual needs in the child. Elkins and Cavendish (2004) report that "children may use humor, poetry, stories, spiritual readings, religious artifacts, pictures, and art to send cues related to spiritual needs" (p. 181).

Healthcare professionals who provide education and counseling, teach disease management, or conduct client/family support groups should incorporate the development of spirituality whenever possible (Rowe & Allen, 2004). Although religion and spirituality are not totally neglected in clinical practice, Hathaway, Scott, and Garver (2004) found that they do not receive an adequate level of clinical attention in everyday practice. They recommend that professionals incorporate an assessment of religious and spiritual health into clinical practice. Clinicians can begin by asking simple preliminary questions that probe the faith and spirituality of a client and expand exploration of the issues as relevant and appropriate. Therapists should also educate the client on the health benefits of spirituality and explain that it is an element of health that is routinely addressed in practice in order to provide the best services possible, as well as to respect the client's beliefs. A common line of questioning might look like this:

- Ask the client if s/he is affiliated with a specific religion. If yes, what religion? Does the client consider himself/herself to be a spiritual person? What does being spiritual mean to the client? Has this helped the client navigate through life's challenges? The client may be wondering why you are asking these questions and possibly feeling a little uncomfortable because religion and spirituality have typically been kept private. Explain to the client that you are asking these questions because spirituality is an area of health that is gaining more attention since it has been found to have health benefits and a positive effect on the client's condition. Ask if it is okay to continue with a few more questions.

- Ask the client if s/he participates regularly in specific rituals to meet his/her spiritual needs and if there are specific restrictions that staff should be aware of such as no meat on Fridays during Lent or no one is allowed to see the client's hair except her husband.

- Develop a spiritual health treatment plan that meets the needs of the client and fosters spiritual growth.

If the client is not affiliated with a specific religion and s/he states no spirituality in his/her life, the client may be briefly educated on why spirituality is assessed in therapy and that there is no intention to offend. However, because spirituality is recognized as an aspect of health, it should not be disregarded due to the client's verbalizations of lack of spirituality. Clients should be given experiences to grow and the word "spirituality" does not necessarily have to be used, especially if the client isn't able to grasp the difference between religion and spirituality and feels that the therapist is pushing religion. For example, a client can be encouraged to sit outside in the fresh air before therapy begins or be given a journal. These techniques are not modalities only for spiritual growth. They are also aids to help decrease stress, open the mind to new ideas, and induce relaxation.

"Spiritual health is a dynamic and flexible dimension of health, one that can be enhanced as a result of prolonged and conscientious effort" (McGee, Nagel, & Moore, 2003). Interventions that foster centering, emptying, grounding, and connecting can deepen spirituality. Therapists should keep an open mind, ask open-ended questions, and validate the importance of the individual's spirituality. Additionally, therapists who work with terminally ill children or adults may find that "spiritual care may be the only source of comfort when a cure is not possible" (Elkins & Cavendish, 2004, p. 184).

Recreational therapists document the extent of difficulty a client has with religion and spirituality. For example, when assistance is not provided, the client reports having mild difficulty saying prayers at night due to word finding problems (d9301._ _ _ 1 Saying prayers; Dehn level +3: Active Participation).

### Cross References

In *Recreational Therapy for Specific Diagnoses and Conditions, First Edition*, ICF code d930 Religion and Spirituality is listed in five chapters: Cancer, Major Depressive Disorder, Post-Traumatic Stress Disorder, Traumatic Brain Injury, and Visual Impairments and Blindness.

In *Recreational Therapy Basics, Techniques, and Interventions, First Edition*, treatment for ICF code d930 Religion and Spirituality is discussed in two chapters: Participation and Leisure Resource Awareness.

### d940 Human Rights

Enjoying all nationally and internationally recognized rights that are accorded to people by virtue of their humanity alone, such as human rights as recognized by the United Nations Universal Declaration of Human Rights (1948) and the United Nations Standard Rules for the Equalization of Opportunities for Persons with Disabilities (1993); the right to self-determination or autonomy; and the right to control over one's destiny.

Exclusions: political life and citizenship (d950)

The term "enjoying" is different from "engaging" which is used for the other parts of this chapter's code set. Enjoying means that a client benefits fully from, profits from, and takes advantage of his/her human rights. Difficulty with enjoying human rights can be due to a number of things including:

- The client is unaware of his/her rights.
- The client does not know how to achieve his/her rights.
- The client lacks the appropriate skills, such as assertiveness, to achieve his/her rights.
- The client has been overpowered and stripped of his/her rights. This can be seen in as a result of childhood abuse and in cases where the client was held as a prisoner.
- The client is being denied his/her human rights. Examples include: A public facility refuses to build a wheelchair ramp although is required to

do so under the Americans with Disabilities Act. A woman is forced to wear a religious garb by her caretaker when she is afforded the right within her country not to wear it if she so chooses. A child is kept in a basement without food or clothing.

- Organization, facilities, and other people are unaware of human rights they are to be providing, such as a company that is unaware of requirements to make accommodations for someone who has a disability.

In the ICF, therapists document the level of difficulty that a client has with enjoying his/her human rights. It is recommended that along with documenting specific rights that are not available, therapists compare the percent of rights enjoyed to the total afforded to determine the level of difficulty. In discipline-specific documentation, therapists make additional notations about the specific human rights that are not being enjoyed, barriers that hinder enjoyment, recommendations for change, related skill development, and level of assistance required from another person to enjoy human rights. If a client is being denied his/her basic human rights and it poses a danger to the client, as with an abused child or elder, it is the responsibility of the therapist to report it immediately to appropriate authorities including police, social workers, and the child welfare office.

Recreational therapists are knowledgeable about basic disability law and general human rights, teach clients about their rights and how to access those rights, assist clients in developing skills to achieve their rights, and educate others that are affecting the client's ability to fully enjoy his/her human rights.

Common environmental factors affecting human rights include products and technology, support and relationships, attitudes, and services, systems, and policies. Refer to the Environmental Factors ICF codes for information on assessing and treating these areas.

Recreational therapists document the extent of difficulty a client has with enjoying human rights. For example, despite having available assistance from family, the client has complete difficulty enjoying human rights, as client is currently forced to practice a religion, is not permitted to leave the house, and is severely neglected (no bed, tattered clothes, limited food) (d940.4 _ _).

In *Recreational Therapy for Specific Diagnoses and Conditions, First Edition*, ICF code d940 Human Rights is listed in four chapters: Cerebral Palsy, Spina Bifida, Spinal Cord Injury, and Total Joint Replacement.

In *Recreational Therapy Basics, Techniques, and Interventions, First Edition*, treatment for ICF code d940 Human Rights is discussed in three chapters: Bibliotherapy, Disability Rights: Education and Advocacy, and Leisure Education and Counseling.

## d950 Political Life and Citizenship

Engaging in the social, political, and governmental life of a citizen, having legal status as a citizen and enjoying the rights, protections, privileges, and duties associated with that role, such as the right to vote and run for political office, to form political associations; enjoying the rights and freedoms associated with citizenship (e.g., the rights of freedom of speech, association, religion, protection against unreasonable search and seizure, the right to counsel, to a trial, and other legal rights and protection against discrimination); having legal standing as a citizen.

Exclusion: human rights (d940)

The code measures the degree to which the client engages in life as a citizen and how fully the client enjoys the rights, protections, privileges, and duties associated with citizenship. In the United States people have freedom to vote, run for office, form political associations, and enjoy freedom of speech, freedom of religion, freedom of association, protection against unreasonable search and seizure, the right to counsel and to a fair trial, and protection from discrimination. However, despite having these rights and freedoms there are instances when these rights and freedoms are not fully afforded. One common example is not providing clients with ways to vote.

In the ICF, therapists document the level of difficulty that a client has with enjoying his/her political life and citizenship. For example, without assistance, the client has complete difficulty voting in an election (d950. _ _ _ 4 Voting; Dehn level +2: Spectator). It is recommended that therapists, along with documenting specific rights that are not available, compare the percent of rights enjoyed to the total that should be available. In discipline-specific documentation, therapists make additional

notations about the specific rights of citizenship that are not being enjoyed, barriers that hinder enjoyment, recommendations for change, related skill development, and level of assistance required for enjoying citizenship rights. If a client is being denied his/her basic political or citizenship rights and danger to the client is possible, such as a client who is being harassed because of her religion, it is the responsibility of the therapist to encourage the client to make a police report. If the client refuses, and danger is believed to be imminent, the therapist must report it to appropriate authorities.

Recreational therapists are knowledgeable about basic rights, protections, and privileges that correlate with citizenship. They teach clients about their rights, such as informing a recent immigrant to the United States that he has freedom to practice religion, and educate others that are affecting the client's ability to enjoy the rights and privileges of citizenship, such as having a discussion with the activity leader about non-discrimination laws.

Common environmental factors affecting a client's ability to enjoy rights, privileges, and freedoms of citizenship include attitudes and the lack of appropriate services, systems, and policies. Refer to the Environmental Factors ICF codes for information on assessing and treating these areas.

In *Recreational Therapy for Specific Diagnoses and Conditions, First Edition*, ICF code d950 Political Life and Citizenship is listed in two chapters: Spina Bifida and Spinal Cord Injury.

In *Recreational Therapy Basics, Techniques, and Interventions, First Edition*, treatment for ICF code d950 Political Life and Citizenship is discussed in one chapter: Disability Rights: Education and Advocacy.

## d998 Community, Social, and Civic Life, Other Specified

## d999 Community, Social, and Civic Life, Unspecified

### References

Agahi, N. & Parker, M. G. (2008). Leisure activities and mortality: Does gender matter? *Journal of Aging and Health, 20*(7), 855-871.

Armstrong, M. & Lauzen, S. (1994). *Community Integration Program*. Ravensdale, WA: Idyll Arbor.

Ashby, F. G., Isen, A. M., & Turken, A. U. (1999). A neuropsychological theory of positive affect and its influence on cognition. *Psychol Rev, 106*(3), 529-550.

Barker, R. N., Kendall, M. D., Amsters, D. I., Pershouse, K. J., Haines, T. P., & Kuipers, P. (2009). The relationship between quality of life and disability across the lifespan for people with spinal cord injury. *Spinal Cord, 47*, 149-155.

Bartlett, S. J., Piedmont, R., Bilderback, A., Matsumoto, A. K., & Bathon, J. M. (2003). Spirituality, well-being and quality of life in people with rheumatoid arthritis. *Arthritis Rheum 49*(6):778-783.

Conti, A., Voelkl, J. E., & McGuire, D. (2009). The potential role of leisure in the prevention of dementia. *Annual in Therapeutic Recreation, XVII*, 31-45.

Daaleman, T., Perera, S., & Studenski, S. (2004). Religion, spirituality, and health status in geriatric outpatients. *Annuals of Family Medicine, 2*(1).

Dehn, D. (1995). *Leisure Step Up.* Ravensdale, WA: Idyll Arbor.

Dermatis, H., James, T., Galanter, M., & Bunt, G. (2010). An exploratory study of spiritual orientation and adaptation to therapeutic community treatment. *Journal of Addictive Diseases, 29*, 306-313.

Diener, E. (2000). Subjective well-being: The science of happiness and a proposal for a national index. *American Psychology, 55*:34-43.

Elkins, M. & Cavendish, R. (2004). Developing a plan for pediatric spiritual care. *Holistic Nurse Practitioner, 18*(4):179-184.

Ellison, C. & Levin, J. (1998). The religion-health connection: Evidence, theory, and future directions. *Health Education Behavior, 25*:700-20.

Geurtsen, G. J., van Heugten, C. M., Martina, J. D., Rietveld, A. C., Meijer, R. M., & Geurts, A. C. (2011). A prospective study to evaluate a residential community reintegration program for patients with chronic acquired brain injury. *Archives of Physical Medicine and Rehabilitation, 92*, 696-704.

Hathaway, W., Scott, S., & Garver, S. (2004). Assessing religious/spiritual functioning: A neglected domain in clinical practice? *Professional Psychology: Research and Practice, 35*(1).

Heintzman, P. (2009). The spiritual benefits of leisure. *Leisure/Loisir, 33*(1), 419-445.

Hyyppa, M. T., Maki, J., Impivaara, O., & Aromaa, A. (2006). Leisure participation predicts survival: A population-based study in Finland. *Health Promotion International, 21*(1), 5-12.

Iwasaki, Y. (2008). Leisure and quality of life in an international and multicultural context: What are major pathways linking leisure to quality of life? *Social Indicators Research, 82*(2), 233-264.

McGee, M., Nagel, L., Moore, M. (2003). A study of university classroom strategies aimed at increasing spiritual health. *College Student Journal, 37*(4).

McIntosh, D., Silver, R., & Wortman, C. (1993). Religion's role in adjustment to a negative life event: Coping with the loss of a child. *Journal of Personal Social Psychology.* 65:812-21.

Miller, W. R. & Thoresen, C. E. (2003). Spirituality, religion, and health: An emerging research field. *American Psychologist, 58*(1), 24-35.

Myers, D. (2000). The funds, friends, and faith of happy people. *American Psychology, 55*, 56-67.

Pennebaker, J. & Evans, J. (2015). *Expressive writing: words that heal.* Enumclaw, WA: Idyll Arbor.

Porter, H., Iwasaki, Y. & Shank, J. (2011). Conceptualizing meaning-making through leisure experiences. Society & Leisure, 33(2), 167-194.

Reed, P. G. (1991). Self-transcendence and mental health in oldest-old adults. *Nursing Research, 40*(1), 5-11.

Rowe, M. & Allen, R. (2004). Spirituality as a means of coping with chronic illness. *American Journal of Health Studies, 19*(1).

Seaward, B. (1997). *Stand like mountain, flow like water: Reflections on stress and human spirituality.* Deerfield Beach, FL: Health Communications, Inc.

Verdonschot, M. M. L., deWitte, L. P., Reichrath, E., Buntinx, W. H. E., & Curfs, L. M. G. (2009). Impact of environmental factors on community participation of persons with an intellectual disability: A systematic review. *Journal of Intellectual Disability Research, 53*(1), 54-64.

White, J. A., Drechsel, J., & Johnson, J. (2006). Faithfully fit forever: A holistic exercise and wellness program for faith communities. *Journal of Holistic Nursing, 24*(2), 127-131.

Winkler, D., Unsworth, C., & Sloan, S. (2006). Factors that lead to successful community integration following severe traumatic brain injury. *Journal of Head Trauma Rehabilitation, 21*(1), 8-21.

Youngkhill, S. C., Lundberg, N., McCormick, B., & Heo, J. (2008). Contribution of community integration to quality of life for participants of community-based adaptive sports. *Therapeutic Recreation Journal, XLII*(4), 217-226.

# Environmental Factors

*Heather R. Porter*

Environmental Factors are things in the environment that facilitate or present barriers for the client. It is divided into five chapters.

## Scoring

Recreational therapists score environmental factors codes (e-codes) in many practice settings.

*Environmental factors* make up the physical, social, and attitudinal environment in which people live and conduct their lives.

The ICF lists 74 three-digit codes for environmental factors. Each has the potential to influence a client's level of impairment and difficulty. They are referred to as e-codes. E-codes are on a positive-negative Likert scale. The therapist can use a negative score with only the decimal point to show that an environmental factor is a barrier. To show that a deficit in e1650 Financial Assets is a moderate barrier to paying for involvement in d920 Recreation and Leisure the therapist would use this notation e1650.2. Environmental factors can also be a positive facilitator, which can be shown by using a plus sign before the score instead of a period. For example, showing that e350 Domesticated Animals is a mild facilitator to d2401 Handling Stress would be scored as e350+1.

To score environmental factors the therapist first identifies the appropriate code to score as described in General Coding Guidelines shown below.

## General Coding Guidelines (WHO, 2001)

- Choose the appropriate codes that best reflect the client's functioning as it relates to the purpose of the encounter.
- Only choose codes that are relevant to the context of the health condition. It is unrealistic to think that a health professional has the time to assess the extent that each environmental factor is a barrier or facilitator for every client. Health professionals should evaluate and assess environmental factors as barriers or facilitators for the specific impairment, activity, or life situation that is being addressed in the encounter.

- Do not make inferences about other environmental factors based on ones that have already been identified. Meaning, (1) just because an e-code is a barrier or facilitator for one activity does not mean that it is a barrier for other activities and (2) just because an e-code has been identified as a barrier or facilitator does not mean that environmental codes that are typically related are barriers or facilitators as well. For example, although e1650 Financial Assets may be a barrier for participation in an activity, it cannot be assumed that lack of money results in lack of needed assistive devices.
- Only choose codes that reflect the specific predefined timeframe. Environmental factors that relate to a timeframe outside of the predefined timeframe should not be coded.
- Use the most specific code whenever possible. For example, if light intensity is identified as a facilitator for d9203 Crafts, score the specific code of e2400 Light Intensity rather than the broader code of e240 Light.

The code is written down in its entirety. This includes the letter and number. All environmental factor codes begin with an e. If the environmental factor is a barrier, a decimal point is placed after the code. After the decimal point the extent of the barrier is recorded. If the environmental code is a facilitator, a + sign is placed after the code. After the + sign the extent of the facilitator is recorded. The scoring scale for environmental factors is shown in Table 13. The e___ is the specific environmental code and the number after the decimal point or + sign denotes the extent the code acts as a barrier or facilitator.

## Table 13: Scoring for Environmental Factors (WHO, 2001)

Scoring for Each Qualifier

e___.0: NO barrier, 0-4% (none, absent, negligible…)

e___.1: MILD barrier, 5-24% (slight, low…)

e___.2: MODERATE barrier, 25-49% (medium, fair…)

e___.3: SEVERE barrier, 50-95% (high, extreme…)

e___.4: COMPLETE barrier, 96-100% (total…)

e___+0: NO facilitator, 0-4% (none, absent, negligible…)

e___+1 MILD facilitator, 5-24% (slight, low…)

e___+2 MODERATE facilitator, 25-49% (medium, fair…)

e___+3 SUBSTANTIAL facilitator, 50-95% (high, extreme…)

e___+4 COMPLETE facilitator, 96-100% (total…)

e___.8 barrier, not specified

e___+8 facilitator, not specified

e___.9 not applicable

There are a variety of options to document e-codes. E-codes can be written:

*After each ICF component*: Therapists can make a list of e-codes that affect one ICF component. For example, the therapist may identify six e-codes as barriers and four e-codes as facilitators for Body Functions as a whole.

*After each code*: Therapists can attach e-codes after each code for which a barrier or facilitator is identified. For example, if a client's pet dog (e350 **Domesticated Animals**) is a moderate facilitator for handling stress (d2401 **Handling Stress**), the observation could be written as: d2401.1 _ _ 3; e350+2.

*As a separate entry*: Therapists can list e-codes as a separate group unrelated to a specific ICF component or specific ICF code.

The recreational therapist will most likely find it helpful to note e-codes after each specific ICF code. This reflects the recreational therapy clinical process and provides the reader with a better understanding of the barriers and facilitators as they relate to a specific impairment or difficulty.

### Environmental Factors Assessment

A major question in using e-codes is how to decide if an environmental factor is mild, moderate, severe, or complete? The ICF does not tell us clearly how to delineate among the levels, so it appears that

it is left to the judgment of the clinician to determine the level of barrier or facilitator. To reduce the subjectivity of the scores, we propose that recreational therapists use the following formula.

E-codes as facilitators: If the environmental factor is taken away, how many levels of impairment or difficulty does the client drop down? If the client's level of impairment or difficulty does not change when the facilitator is removed, then it is a +0 (no facilitator). If the client's level of impairment or difficulty drops by one level when the facilitator is removed (e.g., mild difficulty to moderate difficulty), then it is a +1 (mild facilitator). If the client's level of impairment or difficulty drops by two levels when the facilitator is removed, then it is a +2 (moderate facilitator). If the client's level of impairment or difficulty drops by three levels when the facilitator is removed, then it is a +3 (substantial facilitator). If the client's level of impairment or difficulty drops by four levels, then it is a +4 (complete facilitator).

E-codes as barriers: If the environmental factor is taken away (the barrier is removed), how many levels of impairment or difficulty does the client improve? If the client's level of impairment or difficulty does not change when the barrier is removed, then it is a .0 (no barrier). If the client's performance improves by one level when the barrier is removed (e.g., complete difficulty to severe difficulty), then it is a .1 (mild barrier). If the client's performance improves by two levels when the barrier is removed, then it is a .2 (moderate barrier). If the client's performance improves by three levels when the barrier is removed, then it is a .3 (severe barrier). If the client's performance improves by four levels (complete difficulty to no difficulty), then it is a .4 (complete barrier).

Of course there will be times when using the formula will be difficult, especially when the e-code is just one of several environmental variables, or the ability to assess the outcome of taking away a facilitator or barrier is not appropriate or feasible. If this is the case, best clinical judgment will need to be used.

### E-code as Barrier and Facilitator

In some situations, an e-code can be scored as both a facilitator and a barrier. Example from e1 **Products and Technology**: A client who lives in a long-term care facility only attends entertainment events when food is provided. When food is not provided, the client does not attend. This is an example of how e1100 Food can be a facilitator to d9202 Arts and Culture. The scoring of d9202 Arts and Culture that reflects the impact of e1100 Food could look like this: d9202.0 _ _ 4; e1100+4 OR like this d9202.0 _ _ 4; e1100.4. The first d-code qualifier reflects the level of difficulty that the client has in a real-life setting with assistance (performance) and the fourth qualifier reflects his level of difficulty in a real-life setting when assistance is not provided (performance without assistance). The e-code could be rated a +4 or a .4 because when food is provided the client's level of difficulty reduces by four levels, but in the same sense when food is not provided the client's level of difficulty increases by four levels. The ICF does not provide the therapist with direction on how to resolve this problem.

This book recommends that therapists score the e-code as a facilitator rather than a barrier in this type of situation. Barriers are often thought of as being always or almost always present and facilitators are often thought of as something that can be introduced to increase or improve action or task performance. This helps the therapist in teaching others about the use of facilitators to decrease the level of difficulty a client has with a specific action, task, or activity. The identified facilitator is also already in the client's environment. It is usually easier to keep something already present in an environment than to try to remove something or add something.

### E-code is Qualifier Specific

In some situations, the e-code is qualifier specific. We can see from e4 Attitudes: a 23-year-old client with tetraplegia attends college and lives off campus. He has a personal care attendant with him at all times to assist with overcoming barriers, self-care, and schoolwork. When the client tries to strike up a conversation with other students outside of class, the attendant rushes him along and says, "We don't have time for this." When the attendant is not present (e.g., takes a break to use the bathroom), the client has no difficulty with d9205 Socializing. When the attendant is present, the client has total difficulty socializing. The scoring of d9205 Socializing that reflects the impact of e440 Individual Attitudes of Personal Care Providers and Personal Assistants would look like this: d9205.4 _ _ 0; e440.4. The first qualifier reflects the level of difficulty that the client has in a real-life setting with assistance (performance) and the fourth qualifier reflects his level of difficulty in a real-life

setting when assistance is not provided (performance without assistance). The e-code was rated a .4 because it increased his level of difficulty with the task by four levels. The same attendant, however, facilitates the client's socialization in therapy sessions by cueing the client to strike up conversations. The question of how to score the level of barrier or facilitator of the attendant related to socialization is now difficult. The therapist has two choices for scoring. First, the therapist can score the average. Is the attendant, on average, more of a facilitator or more of a barrier to socialization for the client? If the attendant is more of a barrier than a facilitator, the therapist would score the average negative impact that he has on the client's engagement in socialization. A plus score would be used if the attendant is more of a facilitator. Second, if there is no average, which is probably the case in this example because the attendant just has different attitudes that are reflected differently in capacity versus performance environments, then the therapist should designate this after the e-code. For example, d9205.4 0 4 0; e440.4 (performance) e440+4 (capacity).

### The Use of .0 and +0

In some situations, the .0 or +0 should be used. The therapist may identify a specific barrier or facilitator to engagement in an activity or life situation with a very small overall impact. In this situation, the therapist should still score the e-code rather than delete it because it alerts the people who will be evaluating the data that there is something to consider. If barriers, even if they are slight, do not gain attention, they can easily become larger, making them more difficult to eliminate or reduce. Likewise, if facilitators, even if they are slight, are brought to the attention of data reviewers, they may be able to be encouraged within our society.

Example from e1 Products and Technology: A client has moderate difficulty walking on uneven surfaces. He would like to go for walks at the local park but the paths are unpaved, hilly, and full of tree roots making it dangerous and unrealistic. This is an example of how e1603 Products and Technology of Parks, Conservation, and Wildlife Areas can be a barrier to d4602 Moving Around outside the Home and Other Buildings. The scoring of d4602 Moving Around outside the Home and Other Buildings that reflects the impact of e1603 Products and

Technology of Parks, Conservation, and Wildlife Areas as a barrier would look like this: d4602.2 _ _ 2; e1603.0. The first qualifier reflects the client's average level of difficulty moving around outside the home in his current life situation given supports and constraints as a whole (not just in the park). The e-code is rated a .0 because it was determined by the therapist that if the park trails were paved, it would not change (or negligibly change) the overall level of difficulty that the client has with all of the aspects of d4602 Moving Around outside the Home and Other Buildings.

### Environmental Factors Treatment

Recreational therapists seek to reduce or elimi-nate barriers, as well as strengthen and support facilitators, as they pertain to play, leisure, recreation, and community engagement. The specific methods will vary depending upon the barrier or facilitator. For example, if a family member's attitude is impeding leisure engagement ("She can't do that, so there is no use in even trying it."), the therapist might employ an educational or experiential approach to aid in changing the family member's perception. If adaptive recreation equipment is a barrier, the therapist might educate the person on where to obtain the adaptive device or the therapist might adapt the device for the person. If direct lighting is a facilitator for a resident in long-term care for engaging in craft activities, the therapist might have a conversation with the activity leader at the nursing home to make sure direct lighting continues to be provided for the individual during these activities.

# Chapter 1 Products and Technology

This chapter is about the natural or human-made products or systems of products, equipment, and technology in an individual's immediate environment that are gathered, created, produced, or manufactured. The ISO 9999 classification of technical aids defines these as "any product, instrument, equipment, or technical system used by a disabled person, especially produced or generally available, preventing, compensating, monitoring, relieving, or neutralizing" disability. It is recognized that any product or technology can be assistive. (See ISO 9999: Technical aids for disabled persons — Classification (second version); ISO/TC 173/SC 2, ISO/IDS 9999 (rev.)) For the purposes of this classification of environmental factors, however, assistive products and technology are defined more narrowly as any product, instrument, equipment, or technology adapted or specially designed for improving functioning of a disabled person.

### *Sample Scoring for Products and Technology for Communication as a Barrier*

- A client who is deaf has complete difficulty using a standard telephone in the clinic. This is an example of how e1250 General Products and Technology for Communication can be a barrier to d3600 Using Telecommunication Devices. The scoring of d3600 Using Telecommunication Devices that reflects the impact of e1250 General Products and Technology for Communication as a barrier would look like this: d3600._ 4 _ _; e1250.4. The second qualifier reflects complete difficulty in using a standard telephone in a clinic setting without assistance (capacity without assistance). It is the clinical judgment of the therapist that the use of an adaptive telephone (TTY) would result in the client having no difficulty in using the telephone. The e-code is rated a .4 because the standard telephone (when compared to a TTY) increases the client's level of difficulty by four levels from no difficulty to complete difficulty.

### *Sample Scoring for Products and Technology for Communication as a Facilitator*

- The same client in the previous example is given and shown how to use an adaptive telephone (TTY). She has mild difficulty using the TTY, but with assistance from the therapist, there is no residual difficulty. This is an example of how e1251 Assistive Products and Technology for Communication can be a facilitator for d3600 Using Telecommunication Devices. The scoring of d3600 Using Telecommunication Devices that reflects the impact of e1251 Assistive Products and Technology for Communication as a facilitator would look like this: d3600._ 4 0 _; e1251+4. The second qualifier reflects complete difficulty using a standard telephone without assistance in the clinic (capacity without assistance). The third qualifier reflects no difficulty using a TTY with assistance of the therapist in the clinic (capacity with assistance). The e-code was rated a +4 because the communication product improved her level of difficulty by four levels from complete difficulty to no difficulty.

The availability, appropriateness, quality, and effectiveness of products and technology will determine the extent to which they are a facilitator or barrier to a person's functioning, life participation, and quality of life. For example, Henderson, Skelton, and Rosenbaum (2008) reviewed 54 studies and found that the utilization of assistive devices for children with functional impairments increased their capacity for activities and participation. The authors also noted that prior to prescribing assistive devices, clinicians must consider cost, accessibility to community environments, adaptability of the device to growth, and social acceptance of the device.

The cost of devices, especially adaptive recreation devices, can severely hinder engagement in activity. For example, adolescents with disabilities cited the cost of specialized equipment as the most common reason for non-participation in sports (Murphy & Carbone, 2008). In another study of 427 parent-child pairs where the child had a disability, parents reported that environmental barriers, such as accessibility, limited their children's recreational, community, and social participation (Law et al., 2007). The authors note that this is a major concern because participation has a major influence on child development. They further recommend that we should aim to "enhance participation by minimizing disabling gaps between a child's capabilities and the social and physical demands of the environments in which children live, learn, play, and develop" (p. 1641).

The environment also plays a vital role in our health. For example, the percentage of green space in a person's living environment has a positive correlation with perceived general health, highlighting the importance of allocating green space in spatial planning (Maas et al., 2006).

### Assessment of Products and Technology

Recreational therapists assess the needs of clients related to products and technology, as well as prescribe and evaluate the effectiveness of products and technology, especially as it pertains to community participation and leisure engagement. Methods utilized in the assessment will vary depending on the individual client. Interview, observation, standardized assessment tools, and functional performance are most common.

### Treatment of Products and Technology

Recreational therapists educate clients about products and technology that will enhance play, leisure, recreation, and community engagement. Education consists several parts including obtaining the products and technology and its use. The therapist starts with where to purchase products and technology and ideas on how to fund purchases. Once the products or technology is obtained, the therapist teaches the client how to use it, how to care for it, and how to make adaptations to meet the client's individual needs, such as attaching a cuff to a handle. If required, the therapist may also work with the client to create simple products, such as making a card holder out of a phone book.

### Evidence Review

Reviews of several studies are provided to highlight evidence-based practice related to products and technology. This is only a sample of the evidence. A thorough review of the literature is needed to identify evidence-based practice interventions that reflect the needs and characteristics of the individual client.

Sizsmith et al. (2006) explained an inter-disciplinary project called INDEPENDENT to explore the potential of technology and design solutions to enhance the quality of life for people with dementia and to help them live independently. The project entailed interviews with clients and caregivers, as well as a series of workshops aimed at assisting the identification of technology that could be helpful, such as using a simple music player containing a single play button for easy operation or using a "photo phone" that allows a person to contact the person depicted without using a conventional telephone. The authors suggested that healthcare professionals consider using this project as a model for practice.

Johnson et al. (2007) conducted a study of 84 individuals with spina bifida aged 13 to 27 years. Of the participants, 72% reported limited participation in structured activities. The authors note that underutilization of assistive technology could delay successful transitions to independent living and community participation.

Lawson (2011) conducted a qualitative study of 12 adults who sustained a stroke several years prior. Participants identified adjustment to disability, support, finances, and resources as impacting their ability to engage in productive activity and maintain community involvement. The level of activity affected their quality of life. The author provided specific suggestions to address these areas including teaching communication skills for handling unwanted help; providing support during new activities in rehabilitation, community integration, and inclusive recreation; providing leisure education services; adapting activities; and answering sexuality issues.

Tortosa-Martinez, Zoerink, and Yoder (2011) conducted a systematic review of evidence-based practice literature over the last 10 years related to therapeutic activity for dementia or Alzheimer's disease. Evidence supports the positive relationship between engagement in meaningful therapeutic recreation experiences and amelioration of Alzheimer's disease symptoms. Improvements included more positive affect, fewer days of dementia behavior, reduced depression, improved sleep, higher levels of activity engagement, improved physical health, decreased restlessness, decreased agitation, slower decline in activities of daily living, and improved cognition. "Within non-pharmacological interventions, the careful use of therapeutic recreation activities seems to be feasible for delaying the onset of the disease and controlling the symptoms associated with the disease" (p. 63).

*Cross References*

In *Recreational Therapy for Specific Diagnoses and Conditions, First Edition*, ICF code e1 Products and Technology and its subcategories are listed in 18 chapters: Amputation and Prosthesis, Borderline Personality Disorder, Cancer, Cerebral Palsy, Cerebrovascular Accident, Chronic Obstructive Pulmonary Disease, Feeding and Eating Disorders, Hearing Loss, Heart Disease, Obesity, Osteoarthritis, Parkinson's Disease, Rheumatoid Arthritis, Spina Bifida, Spinal Cord Injury, Total Joint Replacement, Traumatic Brain Injury, and Visual Impairments and Blindness.

In *Recreational Therapy Basics, Techniques, and Interventions, First Edition*, treatment for ICF code e1 Products and Technology and its subcategories are discussed in four chapters: Education and Counseling, Adaptive Sports, Disability Rights: Education and Advocacy, and Reality Orientation.

### *e110 Products or Substances for Personal Consumption*

Any natural or human-made object or substance gathered, processed, or manufactured for ingestion.

Inclusions: food, drink, and drugs

- *e1100 Food*
  Any natural or human-made object or substance gathered, processed, or manufactured to be eaten, such as raw, processed, and prepared food and liquids of different consistencies, herbs and minerals (vitamin and other supplements).

- *e1101 Drugs*
  Any natural or human-made object or substance gathered, processed, or manufactured for medicinal purposes, such as allopathic and naturopathic medication.

- *e1108 Products or Substances for Personal Consumption, Other Specified*
- *e1109 Products or Substances for Personal Consumption, Unspecified*

The discussion of this code looks at each of the subheadings separately.

### *Food*

Food is a basic human need. Without a healthy, balanced diet of enough food and proper kinds of food, body structures and functions are harmed, ultimately affecting life activities. Severe nutritional deficiencies, whether caused by the environment (e.g., famine) or from personal choice (e.g., anorexia), can also result in death. Lack of proper nutrition can be caused by lack of food availability, impaired access to healthy foods, behavioral issues, loss of appetite from a health condition, difficulties attaining healthy food items, or general lack of self-care. Consequently, food can be a barrier to the health of a specific body structure or function, as well as a barrier to life activities, such as d5701 Managing Diet and Fitness and d630 Preparing Meals. Lack of food, caused by any means, may also affect other life activities, specifically activities that are closely tied to food.

In Western culture, food has become more than just a basic human need. It has also become closely linked with social activities, thus making food a possible barrier or facilitator of social and recreational activities. Some examples include: Lack of food in the home may be a barrier for a client to invite someone over to his home to visit, thus impacting d7200 Forming Relationships. The need to have pureed food is embarrassing for a client at a restaurant, so the client then chooses to limit her engagement in d9100 Informal Associations. The lack of healthy food options at school is hindering a child with diabetes from maintaining a proper diet as documented by b5401 Carbohydrate Metabolism.

Food as a facilitator can be described in much the same way. For example, food can contribute to the health of a specific body structure or function, as well as facilitate involvement in social, community, and recreational activities. Interestingly, the pairing of food with recreational activities often yields higher attendance rates in residential facilities. For example: The availability of free food on a college campus increases a client's participation in d9205 Socializing. The offering of healthy snacks at an exercise class in a long-term care setting increases a client's participation in exercise — d5701 Managing Diet and Fitness.

Recreational therapists consider the role of food in hindering or facilitating engagement in leisure and community activities and design appropriate interventions to either:

- Reduce or eliminate the negative effect of food on a particular life activity. The therapist might problem solve for d6201 Gathering Daily Necessities because it is a barrier for the client to inviting people over to socialize or identify pureed foods offered by the restaurant that will not draw attention to the client so that she continues to engage in dining out with friends for maintaining relationships — d7200 Forming Relationships.

- Maintain or further facilitate the positive impact of food on life activities. The therapist might ensure that healthy snacks continue to be offered at exercise class to increase engagement in d5701 Managing Diet and Fitness or talk with the client's social worker to make sure that the client is still eligible for food stamps so that he feels comfortable in his availability of food to invite others over for d9205 Socializing.

### Example of Food as a Facilitator and Barrier

A client who lives in a long-term care facility only engages art and culture events when food is provided. This is an example of how e1100 Food can be a facilitator to d9202 Arts and Culture. At the facility, the client has no difficulty (0) engaging in Arts and Culture. However, if food is not provided the client does not engage in Arts and Culture resulting in complete difficulty (4). The scoring of d9202 Arts and Culture that reflects the impact of e1100 Food would look like this d9202.0 _ _ 4; e1100+4. The score of a +4 for e1100 Food was chosen because food, as a facilitator, reduced his level of difficulty by four levels. On the other hand, the therapist could also score e1100 Food as a barrier to d9202 Arts and Culture because lack of food poses a barrier to engagement in arts and culture. Consequently, the therapist could alternatively score e1100 Food as a barrier: d9202.0 _ _ 4; e1100.4. The c-code score of a .4 was chosen because food, when not provided, reduced the client's level of engagement by four levels. When deciding to score an e-code as a facilitator or a barrier, choosing the positive and scoring it as a facilitator is usually preferred.

### Drugs

The use of prescription and non-prescription drugs in Western culture is quite common and often relied on as a primary means of treating illness or disease. Medication, therefore, can be a major facilitator in the health of a body structure or function, supporting greater performance in life activities. However, side effects of medications can have devastating effects on life activities as well. For example, medication that causes severe drowsiness

impacts the ability to engage in d910 Community Life.

There are also drugs that are manufactured and sold illegally. Use of illegal substances can lead to substance dependence, impacting not only specific body structures and functions, but significantly impairing life activities, such as d845 Acquiring, Keeping, and Terminating a Job and d760 Family Relationships. Outside of ingesting drugs, whether legal or illegal, the presence of drugs in a neighborhood can also impact activity levels. A child may not be allowed outside to play due to fear of drug peddlers impacting d9200 Play. A client who refuses to walk to the local store due to fear of drug peddlers impacts d5701 Managing Diet and Fitness.

Recreational therapists consider the role of drugs in hindering or facilitating engagement in life activities and design appropriate interventions to either:

- Reduce or eliminate the negative effect of drugs on a particular life activity. The therapist might identify safe places to exercise where the client does not feel threatened by neighborhood drugs or discuss with the client's physician the negative effect that a drug is having on a client's participation in community activities to problem solve for other approaches or medications.
- Maintain or further facilitate the positive impact of drugs on life activities. The recreational therapist, as a clinical team member, reinforces the importance of taking needed medication that positively affects engagement in healthy life activities.

### Example of Drugs as a Barrier

A client is addicted to cocaine (e1101 Drugs). In the treatment facility, he exhibits complete difficulty (4) maintaining relationships with family members (d760 Family Relationships) when they come to visit. The family reports that he had no problem with this skill before he started using drugs. This is an example of how e1101 Drugs can be a barrier to d760 Family Relationships. The scoring of d760 Family Relationships that reflects the impact of e1101 Drugs as a barrier would look like this: d760._4 _ _; e1101.4. The second qualifier (capacity without assistance) reflects complete difficulty with creating and maintaining relationships with people who visit while in the standardized environment of a treatment facility. The e-code is rated a .4 because drugs increase the client's level of difficulty with maintaining relationships by four levels from no difficulty as reported by the family to complete difficulty as observed in the facility.

***Example of Drugs as a Facilitator***

A client has a mood disorder that causes a moderate impairment (2) in b1521 Regulation of Emotion. A prescription medication (e1101 Drugs) helps her to regulate her emotions but she still has a residual, mild impairment (1). This is an example of how e1101 Drugs can be a facilitator for b1521 Regulation of Emotion. The scoring of b1521 Regulation of Emotion that reflects the impact of e1101 Drugs as a facilitator would look like this: b1521.1; e1101+1. The qualifier reflects the client's current level of mild impairment with regulation of emotion. The e-code is rated a +1 because the prescription medication improves her level of impairment by one level from moderate impairment to mild impairment.

***Cross References***

In *Recreational Therapy for Specific Diagnoses and Conditions, First Edition*, ICF code e110 Products or Substances for Personal Consumption is listed in one chapter: Heart Disease.

In *Recreational Therapy Basics, Techniques, and Interventions, First Edition*, there are no references for ICF code e110 Products or Substances for Personal Consumption.

## e115 Products and Technology for Personal Use in Daily Living

Equipment, products, and technologies used by people in daily activities, including those adapted or specially designed, located in, on or near the person using them.

Inclusions: general and assistive products and technology for personal use

- *e1150 General Products and Technology for Personal Use in Daily Living*
  Equipment, products, and technologies used by people in daily activities, such as clothes, textiles, furniture, appliances, cleaning products, and tools, not adapted or specially designed.

- *e1151 Assistive Products and Technology for Personal Use in Daily Living*
  Adapted or specially designed equipment, products, and technologies that assist people in daily living, such as prosthetic and orthotic devices, neural prostheses (e.g., functional stimulation devices that control bowels, bladder, breathing, and heart rate), and environmental control units aimed at facilitating individuals' control over their indoor setting (scanners, remote control systems, voice-controlled systems, timer switches).

- *e1158 Products and Technology for Personal Use in Daily Living, Other Specified*
- *e1159 Products and Technology for Personal Use in Daily Living, Unspecified*

Products and technology for daily activities whether general or adapted can a barrier or a facilitator to body structures, body functions, and life activities. It is quite easy for therapists to understand how products and technology can be a facilitator. For example, a switch to operate the electronic dog food feeder enables d6506 Taking Care of Animals. It is through continued exploration of products and technology by reading catalogs, researching on the Internet, talking with other professionals, designing and trying out devices, and attending professional conferences and workshops that the therapist's awareness and skills related to making devices grows and flourishes.

Technology however, is not always a good thing. In some situations, extensive adaptations may inhibit health maintenance or promotion. For example, a client may use extensive switches and timers to perform tasks so he never has to move from his chair, thus getting no exercise during the day. Also, common everyday items, such as clothes and furniture can pose a barrier, especially if they impede abilities. For example, clothes with small buttons can be a barrier to d540 Dressing and furniture that is too low can be a barrier to d4103 Sitting.

Recreational therapists consider the role products and technology for personal use in daily living play in hindering or facilitating engagement in life activities and design appropriate interventions to either:

- Reduce or eliminate the negative effect of technology for daily living on a particular life activity. The therapist might identify bathing suit options that are easier to put on and take off to increase engagement in an adult water exercise class or arrange for higher chairs in the craft room.

- Maintain or further facilitate the positive impact of technology for daily living on life activities. The therapist might assess current technology to determine if newer technology would further benefit the client and encourage appropriate use of technology for daily living.

### Example of Products and Technology for Personal Use in Daily Living as a Barrier

At home, a client has complete difficulty putting on clothes due to poor hand and arm function. This is an example of how e1150 General Products and Technology for Personal Use in Daily Living (clothing) can be a barrier for d5400 Putting on Clothes. The scoring for d5400 Putting on Clothes that reflects the impact of e1150 General Products and Technology for Personal Use in Daily Living as a barrier would look like this: d5400._ _ _ 4; e1150.4. The fourth qualifier reflects complete difficulty in his current life situation with putting on clothing without assistance (performance without assistance). In the therapist's clinical judgment, the client would have no difficulty putting on clothes if adaptive clothing were provided, thus the Products and Technology for Personal Use in Daily Living (specifically clothing) is believed to be increasing his level of difficulty by four levels from no difficulty to complete difficulty. Thus, the e-code is rated a .4.

### Example of Products and Technology for Personal Use in Daily Living as a Facilitator

In a clinic setting, a client with multiple sclerosis has severe difficulty (3) holding a hairbrush. However, when using a cuff to hold the brush, she has no difficulty brushing her hair, d5202 Caring for Hair. This is an example of how e1151 Assistive Products and Technology for Personal Use in Daily Living can be a facilitator for d5202 Caring for Hair. The scoring for d5202 Caring for Hair that reflects the impact of e1151 Assistive Products and Technology for Personal Use in Daily Living as a facilitator would look like this: d5202._ 3 0 _; e1151+3. The second qualifier reflects severe difficulty caring for hair in a clinic setting without assistance of the cuff (capacity without assistance). The third qualifier reflects her ability to brush her hair in a clinic setting

with assistance of the cuff (capacity with assistance). The e-code was rated a +3 because it improved her level of difficulty by three levels from severe difficulty to no difficulty.

### Cross References

In *Recreational Therapy for Specific Diagnoses and Conditions, First Edition*, ICF code e115 Products and Technology for Personal Use in Daily Living is listed in eight chapters: Osteoarthritis, Parkinson's Disease, Rheumatoid Arthritis, Spina Bifida, Spinal Cord Injury, Total Joint Replacement, Traumatic Brain Injury, and Visual Impairments and Blindness.

In *Recreational Therapy Basics, Techniques, and Interventions, First Edition*, there are no references for ICF code e115 Products and Technology for Personal Use in Daily Living.

## e120 Products and Technology for Personal Indoor and Outdoor Mobility and Transportation

Equipment, products, and technologies used by people in activities of moving inside and outside buildings, including those adapted or specially designed, located in, on, or near the person using them.

Inclusions: general and assistive products and technology for personal indoor and outdoor mobility and transportation

- *e1200 General Products and Technologies for Personal Indoor and Outdoor Mobility and Transportation*
  Equipment, products, and technologies used by people in activities of moving inside and outside buildings, such as motorized and non-motorized vehicles used for the transportation of people over ground, water, and air (e.g., buses, cars, vans, other motor-powered vehicles and animal-powered transporters), not adapted or specially designed.

- *e1201 Assistive Products and Technology for Personal Indoor and Outdoor Mobility and Transportation*
  Adapted or specially designed equipment, products, and technologies that assist people to move inside and outside buildings, such as walking devices, special cars and vans, adaptations to

vehicles, wheelchairs, scooters, and transfer devices.

- *e1208 Products and Technology for Personal Indoor and Outdoor Mobility and Transportation, Other Specified*
- *e1209 Products and Technology for Personal Indoor and Outdoor Mobility and Transportation, Unspecified*

Products and technology, whether general or assistive, for personal indoor and outdoor mobility and transportation can be a barrier or facilitator to body structures, body functions, and life activities. To determine if it is a barrier or a facilitator, the therapist must first identify the products and technology for mobility and transportation that are pertinent to the client by asking what is currently being used, what is desired, what problems are identified, and what is needed. There are many products for personal indoor and outdoor mobility and transportation. Planes, trains, wheelchairs, and canes would all be on the list. Therapists must also be aware of non-traditional forms of mobility and transportation used by a client, such as roller skates, bicycles, skateboards, and Segways. See e140 Products and Technology for Culture, Recreation, and Sport if mobility devices are used for recreation or sport.

Products and technology for mobility and transportation can be facilitators or barriers to engagement in life activities such as d6200 Shopping, d9202 Arts and Culture, d450 Walking. For example, a client needs a rolling walker for outdoor mobility but her insurance does not cover the full cost of the walker so she does not have one. Not having a walker is a barrier under e1201 Assistive Products and Technology for Personal Indoor and Outdoor Mobility and Transportation, and lacking proper equipment coverage identifies e5802 Health Policies as an additional barrier.

Impaired engagement or lack of engagement in life activities as a result of a barrier to personal indoor and outdoor mobility and transportation can directly or indirectly affect body functions, body structures, and life activities. For example, lack of transportation in a rural environment limits the client's d9205 Socializing that negatively impacts d2401 Handling Stress and b1265 Optimism. Improperly prescribed or unprescribed use of adaptive mobility or transportation equipment can hinder health maintenance and promotion, as well. A client might use an electric scooter for community activities when she could walk without injury or harm. The currently used form of general or assistive transportation may not meet the needs of the client, such as a client using a public bus for transportation, even though the first step into the bus is rather high. Several times the client has lost her balance and fallen.

Recreational therapists consider the role of products and technology for outdoor mobility and transportation in hindering or facilitating engagement in life activities and design appropriate interventions to either:

- Reduce or eliminate the negative effect of outdoor mobility and transportation on a particular life activity. For example, a client with a lower extremity prosthetic is having difficulty riding a bicycle for transportation because the prosthetic foot keeps sliding off the pedal. The recreational therapist prescribes a toe clip to hold the prosthetic foot on the pedal.
- Maintain or further facilitate the positive impact of outdoor mobility and transportation on life activities. For example the therapist assesses current mobility and transportation options to determine if newer products or technology would further benefit the client and encourages continued use of products and technology for mobility and transportation.

### Example of Products and Technology for Personal Mobility and Transportation as a Barrier

A client uses the public bus system (d4702 Using Public Motorized Transportation) for transportation. She has advanced rheumatoid arthritis that causes her to have severe difficulty (3) lifting her foot onto the first step of the bus. It is about an 18-inch high step with a rail. The client is able to step up and down an eight-inch step with a rail with no difficulty (0). Consequently, if the bus on her route was a "kneeling bus" (the front right air shock lowers the bus step height), she would have no difficulty boarding the bus. This is an example of how e1200 General Products and Technology for Personal Indoor and Outdoor Mobility and Transportation can be a barrier for d4702 Using Public Motorized Transportation. The scoring of d4702 Using Public Motorized Transportation that reflects the impact of e1200 General Products and Technology for

Personal Indoor and Outdoor Mobility and Transportation as a barrier would look like this: d4702._ _ _ 3; e1200.3. The fourth qualifier (performance without assistance) reflects severe difficulty with using public motorized transportation in a life situation without assistance. The e-code was rated a .3 because the height of the bus step increases the client's level of difficulty to board the bus by three levels from no difficulty stepping up an eight-inch step with a rail to severe difficulty stepping up an eighteen-inch bus step with a rail.

### Example of Products and Technology for Personal Mobility and Transportation as a Facilitator

An adolescent client with congenital lower extremity and upper extremity malformations has complete difficulty (4) propelling her manual wheelchair long distances at the mall (d4601 Moving Around within Buildings Other Than Home). When going to the mall with her friends, she doesn't want her friends to push her in the wheelchair, as she prefers to be fully independent. Consequently, she uses the electric scooter provided by the mall when she is with her friends. This is an example of how e1201 Assistive Products and Technology for Personal Indoor and Outdoor Mobility and Transportation can be a facilitator for d4601 Moving Around within Buildings Other Than Home. The scoring of d4601 Moving Around within Buildings Other Than Home that reflects the impact of e1201 Assistive Products and Technology for Personal Indoor and Outdoor Mobility and Transportation as a facilitator would look like this: d4601.0 _ _ 4; e1210+4. The first qualifier (performance with assistance) reflects no difficulty with mobility in a life situation with assistance (due to the use of the electric scooter). The fourth qualifier (performance without assistance) reflects complete difficulty with mobility in a life situation without assistance. The e-code was rated a +4 because it reduced her level of difficulty by four levels from complete difficulty to no difficulty.

### Cross References

In *Recreational Therapy for Specific Diagnoses and Conditions, First Edition*, ICF code e120 Products and Technology for Personal Indoor and Outdoor Mobility and Transportation is listed in two chapters: Spinal Cord Injury and Total Joint Replacement.

In *Recreational Therapy Basics, Techniques, and Interventions, First Edition*, there are no references for ICF code e120 Products and Technology for Personal Indoor and Outdoor Mobility and Transportation.

### e125 Products and Technology for Communication

Equipment, products, and technologies used by people in activities of sending and receiving information, including those adapted or specially designed, located in, on, or near the person using them.

Inclusions: general and assistive products and technology for communication

- *e1250 General Products and Technology for Communication*
  Equipment, products, and technology used by people in activities of sending and receiving information, such as optical and auditory devices, audio recorders and receivers, television and video equipment, telephone devices, sound transmission systems, and face-to-face communication devices, not adapted or specially designed.

- *e1251 Assistive Products and Technology for Communication*
  Adapted or specially designed equipment, products, and technologies that assist people to send and receive information, such as specialized vision devices, electro-optical devices, specialized writing devices, drawing or handwriting devices, signaling systems and special computer software and hardware, cochlear implants, hearing aids, FM auditory trainers, voice prostheses, communication boards, glasses, and contact lenses.

- *e1258 Products and Technology for Communication, Other Specified*
- *e1259 Products and Technology for Communication, Unspecified*
  Products and technology for communication can be a barrier or facilitator. For example, a television, radio, instant messaging on the computer, and video conference calls can be a facilitator for many life activities including d6200 Shopping, d7200 Forming Relationships, and d8451 Maintaining a Job. The same technology can also be a barrier when

the client uses it in an addictive or escapist way by watching too much television, playing too many computer games, or becoming addicted to gambling or pornography on the Internet. Products and technology for communication can also be a barrier when they hinder participation in life activities, as when a client is unable to operate a computer or telephone.

Adaptive communication products and technology are usually facilitators when general products and technology are not sufficient, for example a telephone that has a flashing light when it rings is a facilitator for d3600 Using Telecommunication Devices. Assistive products and technology that are misprescribed or unprescribed can prove to be a barrier in situations where the piece of equipment does not perform in the manner expected or desired. One example is a mouth stick a client ordered through a catalog that does not have the correct bend on it to easily access computer keyboard keys, resulting in neck pain and ineffective communication.

Recreational therapists consider the role of products and technology for communication in hindering or facilitating engagement in life activities and design appropriate interventions to either:

- Reduce or eliminate the negative effect of products and technology for communication on a particular life activity. For example, a client with a hearing impairment does not hear the high pitch of a telephone ring. The therapist prescribes a special light for the telephone that flashes when it rings.
- Maintain or further facilitate the positive impact of products and technology for communication on life activities. The therapist assesses current products and technology for communication to determine if newer products or technology would further benefit the client and encourages continued appropriate use of products and technology for communication.

### Example of Products and Technology for Communication as a Barrier

A client who is deaf has complete difficulty using a standard telephone in the clinic. This is an example of how e1250 General Products and Technology for Communication can be a barrier to d3600 Using Telecommunication Devices. The scoring of d3600 Using Telecommunication Devices

that reflects the impact of e1250 General Products and Technology for Communication as a barrier would look like this: d3600._ 4 _ _; e1250.4. The second qualifier reflects complete difficulty in ability to use a standard telephone in a clinic setting without assistance (capacity without assistance). It is the clinical judgment of the therapist that the use of an adaptive telephone (TTY) would result in the client having no difficulty in using the telephone. The e-code is rated a .4 because the standard telephone, when compared to a TTY, increases the client's level of difficulty by four levels from no difficulty to complete difficulty.

### Example of Products and Technology for Communication as a Facilitator

The same client in the previous example is given and shown how to use an adaptive telephone (TTY). She has mild difficulty using the TTY, but with assistance from the therapist, there is no residual difficulty. This is an example of how e1251 Assistive Products and Technology for Communication can be a facilitator for d3600 Using Telecommunication Devices. The scoring of d3600 Using Telecommunication Devices that reflects the impact of e1251 Assistive Products and Technology for Communication as a facilitator would look like this: d3600._ 4 0 _; e1251+4. The second qualifier reflects complete difficulty using a standard telephone without assistance in the clinic (capacity without assistance). The third qualifier reflects no difficulty using a TTY with assistance of the therapist in the clinic (capacity with assistance). The e-code was rated a +4 because the communication technology improved her level of difficulty by four levels from complete difficulty to no difficulty.

### Cross References

In *Recreational Therapy for Specific Diagnoses and Conditions, First Edition*, there are no references for ICF code e125 Products and Technology for Communication.

In *Recreational Therapy Basics, Techniques, and Interventions, First Edition*, there are no references for ICF code e125 Products and Technology for Communication.

### e130 Products and Technology for Education

Equipment, products, processes, methods, and technology used for acquisition of knowledge, expertise or skill, including those adapted or specially designed.

Inclusions: general or assistive products and technology for education

- *e1300 General Products and Technology for Education*
  Equipment, products, processes, methods, and technology used for acquisition of knowledge, expertise, or skill at any level, such as books, manuals, educational toys, computer hardware or software, not adapted or specially designed.

- *e1301 Assistive Products and Technology for Education*
  Adapted and specially designed equipment, products, processes, methods, and technology used for acquisition of knowledge, expertise, or skill, such as specialized computer technology.

- *e1308 Products and Technology for Education, Other Specified*
- *e1309 Products and Technology for Education, Unspecified*

Products and technology for education can be a barrier or facilitator. General products such as books, educational toys, and computer programs can assist with learning (a facilitator). Likewise, adaptive products and technology such as adaptive learning toys, Braille books, or voice activated computer programs can also facilitate education. Products and technology, whether general or adapted, can be a barrier for education when it is not affordable, accessible, acceptable, and appropriate to promote the acquisition of knowledge, expertise, or skill. This may include products and technology that are inappropriate for the specific age, learning style, educational level, or knowledge and skill desired.

Recreational therapists consider the role of products and technology for education in hindering or facilitating engagement in life activities and design appropriate interventions to either:

- Reduce or eliminate the negative effect of products and technology for education on a particular life activity. For example a client with low vision is unable to see textbook materials. The therapist prescribes a specialized magnification device to allow the client to see textbook print.
- Maintain or further facilitate the positive impact of products and technology for education on life

activities. The therapist assesses current products and technology for education to determine if newer products or technology would further benefit the client and encourages continued use of products and technology for education.

### Example of Products and Technology for Education as a Barrier

A four-year-old girl with a mild developmental disability attends a mainstream pre-school. The school does not have adaptive learning toys and the teaching methods are not geared for children who have disabilities. The parents and teacher agree that the child is not progressing in this type of environment and is only engaging in about 40% of the learning activities. This is an example of how e1300 General Products and Technology for Education can be a barrier to d815 Preschool Education. The scoring of d815 Preschool Education that reflects the impact of e1300 General Products and Technology for Education as a barrier would look like this: d815.-_ _ _ 3; e1300.3. The fourth qualifier reflects severe difficulty with engaging in preschool learning activities in the client's current life situation given available supports. This is calculated by the level of difficulty determined through amount of non-engagement in learning activities even with the assistance of the teachers and current devices (performance with assistance). The therapist anticipates that the child would have no difficulty engaging in learning activities if placed in a pre-school program specially designed for children with a mild developmental disability. Consequently, the e-code is rated a .3 because the current teaching toys and methods are believed to be increasing her level of difficulty with engagement in learning activities by three levels from no difficulty to severe difficulty.

### Example of Products and Technology for Education as a Facilitator

The same child in the previous example now attends a pre-school program that is specially designed for children who have a mild developmental disability. She exhibits no difficulty in engaging in learning activities. This is an example of how e1301 Assistive Products and Technology for Education can be a facilitator for d815 Preschool Education. The scoring of d815 Preschool Education that reflects the impact of e1301 Assistive Products and Technology for Education as a facilitator would look like this: d815.0 _ _ 3; e1301+3. The first qualifier reflects no difficulty with preschool in her current life situation with all available supports and constraints, which includes the assistive products and technology available in her new classroom (performance). The fourth qualifier reflects severe difficulty with preschool if assistance is removed as shown in the previous example (performance without assistance). The e-code is rated a +3 because the assistive products and technology for education improve her level of difficulty by three levels from severe difficulty to no difficulty.

### Cross References

In *Recreational Therapy for Specific Diagnoses and Conditions, First Edition*, ICF code e130 Products and Technology for Education is listed in one chapter: Visual Impairments and Blindness.

In *Recreational Therapy Basics, Techniques, and Interventions, First Edition*, there are no references for ICF code e130 Products and Technology for Education.

### e135 Products and Technology for Employment

Equipment, products, and technology used for employment to facilitate work activities.

Inclusions: general and assistive products and technology for employment

- *e1350 General Products and Technology for Employment*
  Equipment, products, and technology used for employment to facilitate work activities, such as tools, machines, and office equipment, not adapted or specially designed.

- *e1351 Assistive Products and Technology for Employment*
  Adapted or specially designed equipment, products, and technology used for employment to facilitate work activities, such as adjustable tables, desks, and filing cabinets; remote control entry and exit of office doors; computer hardware, software, accessories, and environmental control units aimed at facilitating an individual's conduct of work-related tasks and aimed at control of the work environment (e.g., scanners, remote control systems, voice-controlled systems, and timer switches).

- *e1358 Products and Technology for Employment, Other Specified*
- *e1359 Products and Technology for Employment, Unspecified*

Products and technology for employment, whether general or assistive, can be a barrier or a facilitator to body structures, body functions, and activities and participation. For example, if a client operates a computer at work and has carpal tunnel syndrome, lack of an ergonomically correct computer station could be a barrier for pain management in the hands (e.g., b28016 Pain in Joints) as well as impair specific body structures of the hand muscles. Consequently, the lack of a proper computer set-up could impact her ability to maintain her job (d8451 Maintaining a Job) and also affect her financial security (e.g., d870 Economic Self-Sufficiency). On the other hand, if an ergonomic computer station was provided, it could act as a facilitator for b28016 Pain in Joints, d8451 Maintaining a Job, and d870 Economic Self-Sufficiency.

Products and technology for employment may also be a barrier if improperly prescribed, resulting in dysfunction. Another kind of barrier occurs if they do not meet the needs of the client, such as a client who is provided with a manual screwdriver when he really needs a cordless power screwdriver. Any product or technology must also be available, affordable, acceptable, and accessible in order to be a facilitator. In some instances, this is not the case and further environmental factors may need to be identified as the underlying causes of difficulty. This may include e430 Individual Attitudes of People in Positions of Authority or e590 Labor and Employment Services, Systems, and Policies.

Employment and work-related tasks are commonly addressed by occupational therapy. However, recreational therapy may address issues related to employment and work if it is not done primarily for financial compensation but for leisure enjoyment, such as a retired person working part time at the local day care center because she enjoys helping the children.

Recreational therapists consider the role of products and technology for employment in hindering or facilitating engagement in life activities and design appropriate interventions to either:

- Reduce or eliminate the negative effect of products and technology for employment on a particular life activity. For example, a client works part time at the local hardware store. He has multiple herniated discs and needs to change his body position often throughout the day to alleviate sensations of pain. The therapist prescribes a stool for periodic sitting and floor blocks to periodically place one foot on to shift body weight.

- Maintain or further facilitate the positive impact of products and technology for employment on life activities. The therapist assesses current products and technology for employment to determine if newer products or technology would further benefit the client and encourage continued use of products and technology for employment.

### *Example of Products and Technology for Employment as a Barrier*

A client has carpal tunnel syndrome in both hands. She is a typist. Using a standard keyboard she is unable to perform 45% of her typing responsibilities (2) due to wrist pain. Her boss told her that if she does not increase her productivity to 80% she will be terminated (d8451 Maintaining a Job). The client has no other difficulties at work affecting her ability to maintain her job. This is an example of how e1350 General Products and Technology for Employment can be a barrier for d8451 Maintaining a Job. The scoring of d8451 Maintaining a Job that reflects the impact of e1350 General Products and Technology for Employment as a barrier would look like this: d8451._ _ _ 2; e1350.2. The last qualifier (performance without assistance) reflects severe difficulty with maintaining a job in her current real-life work situation given all available supports and constraints. If adaptive computer equipment was provided and utilized, it is anticipated the client would have no difficulties (0). The e-code is rated a .2 because her current computer equipment is believed to be increasing her level of difficulty in maintaining her job by two levels from no difficulty with assistive equipment to moderate difficulty without equipment.

### *Example of Products and Technology for Employment as a Facilitator*

The client in the previous example is prescribed mobile wrist supports and an ergonomic keyboard. The use of the adaptive devices raises her productivity to 80% (20% difficulty remaining) and she is able to keep her job. This is an example of how e1351 Assistive Products and Technology for Employment can be a facilitator for d8451 Maintaining a Job. The scoring of d8451 Maintaining a Job that reflects the impact of e1351 Assistive Products and Technology for Employment as a facilitator would look like this: d8451.0 _ _ 2; e1351+2. The first qualifier (performance with assistance) reflects no difficulty maintaining her job in her current life situation with all available supports and constraints that now includes adaptive computer equipment. The score of no difficulty (0) was chosen because her boss asked her to reach a level of 80% to keep her job. The fourth qualifier reflects moderate difficulty with maintaining her job without the use of the adaptive equipment (performance without assistance), as explained in the previous example. The e-code is rated a +2 because the adaptive computer equipment improved her level of difficulty by two levels from moderate difficulty to no difficulty.

### *Cross References*

In *Recreational Therapy for Specific Diagnoses and Conditions, First Edition*, ICF code e135 Products and Technology for Employment is listed in one chapter: Obesity.

In *Recreational Therapy Basics, Techniques, and Interventions, First Edition*, there are no references for ICF code e135 Products and Technology for Employment.

## e140 Products and Technology for Culture, Recreation, and Sport

Equipment, products, and technology used for the conduct and enhancement of cultural, recreational, and sporting activities, including those adapted or specially designed.

Inclusions: general and assistive products and technology for culture, recreation, and sport

- *e1400 General Products and Technology for Culture, Recreation, and Sport*
  Equipment, products, and technology used for the conduct and enhancement of cultural, recreational, and sporting activities, such as toys, skis, tennis balls, and musical instruments, not adapted or specially designed.

- *e1401 Assistive Products and Technology for Culture, Recreation, and Sport*
  Adapted or specially designed equipment, products, and technology used for the conduct and enhancement of cultural, recreational, and sporting activities, such as modified mobility devices for sports, adaptations for musical and other artistic performance.

- *e1408 Products and Technology for Culture, Recreation, and Sport, Other Specified*

- *e1409 Products and Technology for Culture, Recreation, and Sport, Unspecified*

Products and technology for culture, recreation, and sport, whether general or assistive, can be a barrier or a facilitator to body structures, body functions, and activities and participation. For example, if a client engages in the sport of skiing and owns his own skis, then general products for culture, recreation, and sport would be a facilitator for d9201 Sports. Likewise, if a client has a spinal cord injury and uses an adaptive sit-ski to engage in skiing, then e1401 Assistive Products and Technology for Culture, Recreation, and Sport would be a facilitator for d9201 Sports.

Products and technology for culture, recreation, and sport can also be a barrier to participation if they are not available, accessible, affordable, or acceptable. Also, if it is improperly prescribed, dysfunction can occur or it may not meet the needs of the client, such as a child who is given an adult size guitar instead of a junior size guitar. In some instances, further environmental factors may need to be identified as the underlying causes of difficulty. For example there may be policy issues at the school for giving out instruments — e585 Education and Training Services, Systems, and Policies.

Recreational therapists consider the role of products and technology for culture, recreation, and sport in hindering or facilitating engagement in life activities and design appropriate interventions to either:

- Reduce or eliminate the negative effect of products and technology for culture, recreation, and sport on a particular life activity. For example, a client wants to participate in wheelchair racing but lacks the appropriate equipment of a racing wheelchair. The therapist assists the client in problem solving and identifying available resources to obtain a racing wheelchair.

- Maintain or further facilitate the positive impact of products and technology for culture, recreation, and sport on life activities. The therapist assesses current products and technology for culture, recreation, and sport to determine if newer products or technology would further benefit the client and encourage continued use of products and technology for culture, recreation, and sport.

### Example of Products and Technology for Culture, Recreation, and Sport as a Barrier

A 15-year-old boy with major depressive disorder in an inpatient psychiatric facility indicated that he would like to learn how to play the guitar (d810 Informal Education). (Note that the code d810 Informal Education is used instead of code d9202 Arts and Culture because d9202 Arts and Culture reflects playing the guitar, while d810 Informal Education reflects learning how to play the guitar.) The recreational therapist planned to teach him some of the basics and then refer him for further lessons post discharge. His mother, who is addicted to drugs, bought him a pink guitar because *she* liked it. The boy refuses to take lessons because he is embarrassed by the color of the guitar. This is an example of how e1400 General Products and Technology for Culture, Recreation, and Sport can be a barrier to d810 Informal Education. The scoring of d810 Informal Education that reflects the impact of e1400 General Products and Technology for Culture, Recreation, and Sport as a barrier would look like this: d810._ 4 4 _; e1400.4. The second qualifier (capacity without assistance) indicates complete difficulty in learning how to play the guitar because he lacked a guitar. The third qualifier (capacity with assistance) is also a 4 because the color of the guitar served as a complete barrier to learning how to play the guitar. The e-code was rated a .4 because it resulted in complete difficulty in learning how to play the guitar

### Example of Products and Technology for Culture, Recreation, and Sport as a Facilitator

A 32-year-old client with traumatic bilateral above-knee amputations desires to engage in wheelchair tennis (d9201 Sports). With his current wheelchair (a lightweight, rigid frame wheelchair) he is unable to make the sharp turns required to play the sport and lacks a stable base of support (4). His family ran a fundraiser and was able to purchase a tennis wheelchair for the client. He is now able to play wheelchair tennis without difficulty (0). This is an example of how e1401 Assistive Products and Technology for Culture, Recreation, and Sport can be a facilitator for d9201 Sports. The scoring of d9201 Sports that reflects the impact of e1401 Assistive Products and Technology for Culture, Recreation, and Sport as a facilitator would look like this: d9201.0 _ _ 4; e1401+4. The first qualifier (performance with assistance) reflects no difficulty playing wheelchair tennis in his current life situation given all available supports and constraints including the tennis wheelchair. The fourth qualifier (performance without assistance) reflects complete difficulty with the skill of playing tennis in his current environment if all available supports were removed. The e-code was rated a +4 because the tennis wheelchair improved his ability to play tennis by four levels (complete difficulty to no difficulty).

### Cross References

In *Recreational Therapy for Specific Diagnoses and Conditions, First Edition*, ICF code e140 Products and Technology for Culture, Recreation, and Sport is listed in six chapters: Cancer, Chronic Obstructive Pulmonary Disease, Heart Disease, Spinal Cord Injury, Total Joint Replacement, and Traumatic Brain Injury.

In *Recreational Therapy Basics, Techniques, and Interventions, First Edition*, treatment for ICF code e140 Products and Technology for Culture, Recreation, and Sport is discussed in two chapters: Education and Counseling and Community Participation: Integration, Transitioning, and Inclusion.

### e145 Products and Technology for the Practice of Religion or Spirituality

Products and technology, unique or mass-produced, that are given or take on a symbolic meaning in the context of the practice of religion or spirituality, including those adapted or specially designed.

Inclusions: general and assistive products and technology for the practice of religion and spirituality

*   *e1450 General Products and Technology for the Practice of Religion or Spirituality*
    Products and technology, unique or mass-produced, that are given or take on a symbolic

meaning in the context of the practice of religion or spirituality, such as spirit houses, maypoles, headdresses, masks, crucifixes, menorahs, and prayer mats, not adapted or specially designed.

*   *e1451 Assistive Products and Technology for the Practice of Religion or Spirituality*
    Adapted or specially designed products and technology that are given, or take on a symbolic meaning in the context of the practice of religion or spirituality, such as Braille religious books, Braille tarot cards, and special protection for wheelchair wheels when entering temples.

*   *e1458 Products and Technology for the Practice of Religion or Spirituality, Other Specified*
*   *e1459 Products and Technology for the Practice of Religion or Spirituality, Unspecified*

Products and technology for the practice of religion or spirituality, whether general or assistive, can be a barrier or a facilitator to body structures, body functions, and activities and participation. For example, if wearing a cross necklace makes a client feel protected and helps her manage stressful situations, then e1450 General Products and Technology for the Practice of Religion or Spirituality would be a facilitator for d2401 Handling Stress. Likewise, if a client has a special prayer written for him by his pastor that he finds helpful in managing feelings of anxiety, then e1451 Assistive Products and Technology for the Practice of Religion or Spirituality would be a facilitator for b152 Emotional Functions.

Products and technology for the practice of religion and spirituality can also be barriers to participation in activities if they are not available, accessible, affordable, or acceptable. Also, if it is improperly prescribed, dysfunction can occur or it may not meet the needs of the client. Products and technology for religion or spirituality may also impact life activities in a negative way if they cause the client or others harm. For example, a negative impact might be a belief in a product or technology that affects a client's judgment, such as "I can jump off this six-story building and I will not be injured because I am wearing a special religious medal that keeps me from harm." In this example, if the medal was not adapted or specially designed, e1450 General Products and Technology for the Practice of

Religion or Spirituality would be a barrier to b1645 Judgment.

Recreational therapists consider the role of products and technology for the practice of religion and spirituality in hindering or facilitating engagement in life activities and design appropriate interventions to either:

- Reduce or eliminate the negative effect of products and technology for the practice of religion and spirituality on a particular life activity. For example, a client wants to participate in a specific spiritual dance but lacks hair due to chemotherapy. This means that the headdress will not stay on her head. The therapist researches and identifies a product to hold the headdress on.

- Maintain or further facilitate the positive impact of products and technology for the practice of religion and spirituality on life activities. The therapist assesses current products and technology for the practice of religion and spirituality to determine if newer products or technology would further benefit the client and encourages continued use of products and technology for the practice of religion and spirituality.

### *Example of Products and Technology for the Practice of Religion and Spirituality as a Barrier*

A client believes that a religious medal that she wears on a necklace keeps her from harm. She has attempted several times (an average of 25%) while at the clinic to engage in unsafe activities, such as walking without needed assistance, stating that the religious medal will keep her from falling. This is an example of how e1450 General Products and Technology for the Practice of Religion or Spirituality can be a barrier to b1645 Judgment. The scoring of b1645 Judgment that reflects the impact of e1450 General Products and Technology for the Practice of Religion or Spirituality as a barrier would look like this: b1645.3; e1450.2. The qualifier on b1645 Judgment reflects severe judgment impairment. The level of judgment impairment (3) was determined through testing and observation including the observation of the unsafe incidents. The e-code was rated a .2 (moderate barrier) because the therapist determined through testing that the client's belief in the religious medal appears to account for 25% of her judgment impairment while the other 75% appears to be related to other cognitive impairments.

### *Example of Products and Technology for the Practice of Religion and Spirituality as a Facilitator*

A client is currently experiencing many life changes and unfortunate situations causing a high level of stress. In the hospital, the client finds comfort in her spiritual beliefs that a higher power is guiding and helping her. She carries a small carved stone dove in her pocket as a physical reminder. With the emotional comfort of staff, her spiritual beliefs, and the stone dove, she is able to handle stress with minimal difficulty. This is an example of how e1450 General Products and Technology for the Practice of Religion or Spirituality can be a facilitator for d2401 Handling Stress. The scoring of d2401 Handling Stress that reflects the impact of e1450 General Products and Technology for the Practice of Religion or Spirituality as a facilitator would look like this: d2401._ _ 1 _; e1450+1. The third qualifier (capacity with assistance) reflects mild difficulty in handling stress with assistance in the hospital. It would not be appropriate to take away the stone dove to determine the extent of its facilitation. The extent could be estimated by the frequency the client reaches into her pocket and grasps the dove, talks about the dove, and carries the dove. In this situation, the therapist rated the e-code a +1 because it was her clinical judgment that the dove is a mild facilitator in the larger set of coping mechanisms used by the client.

### *Cross References*

In *Recreational Therapy for Specific Diagnoses and Conditions, First Edition*, there are no references for ICF code e145 Products and Technology for the Practice of Religion or Spirituality.

In *Recreational Therapy Basics, Techniques, and Interventions, First Edition*, there are no references for ICF code e145 Products and Technology for the Practice of Religion or Spirituality.

### *e150 Design, Construction, and Building Products and Technology of Buildings for Public Use*

Products and technology that constitute an individual's indoor and outdoor human-made environment that is planned, designed, and constructed for public use, including those adapted or specially designed.

Inclusion: design, construction and building products and technology of entrances and exits, facilities, and routing

- *e1500 Design, Construction, and Building Products and Technology for Entering and Exiting Buildings for Public Use*
  Products and technology of entry and exit from the human-made environment that is planned, designed, and constructed for public use, such as design, building, and construction of entries and exits to buildings for public use (e.g., workplaces, shops, and theater), public buildings, portable and stationary ramps, power-assisted doors, lever doors handles, and level door thresholds.

- *e1501 Design, Construction, and Building Products and Technology for Gaining Access to Facilities inside Buildings for Pubic Use*
  Products and technology of indoor facilities in design, building, and construction for public use, such as washroom facilities, telephones, audio loops, lifts or elevators, escalators, thermostats (for temperature regulation), and dispersed accessible seating in auditoriums or stadiums.

- *e1502 Design, Construction, and Building Products and Technology for Way Finding, Path Routing, and Designation of Locations in Buildings for Public Use*
  Indoor and outdoor products and technology in design, building, and construction for public use to assist people to find their way inside and immediately outside buildings and locate the places they want to go to, such as signage, in Braille or writing, size of corridors, floor surfaces, accessible kiosks, and other forms of directories.

- *e1508 Design, Construction, and Building Products and Technology of Buildings for Public Use, Other Specified*
- *e1509 Design, Construction, and Building Products and Technology of Buildings for Public Use, Unspecified*

Design, construction, and building products and technology of buildings for public use can be a barrier or a facilitator to body structures, body functions, and life activities. For example, the construction of a ramp to enter a public building (e1500 Design, Construction, and Building Products and Technology for Entering and Exiting Buildings for Public Use) could be a facilitator for d9300

Organized Religion (entering a church). In another example, wheelchair accessible seating (e1501 Design, Construction, and Building Products and Technology for Gaining Access to Facilities inside Buildings for Pubic Use) in a theater could be a facilitator for d9202 Arts and Culture. A final example would be large print signage (e1502 Design, Construction, and Building Products and Technology for Way Finding, Path Routing, and Designation of Locations in Buildings for Public Use) in a building as a facilitator for d6200 Shopping (reading grocery aisle signs) for someone with a vision impairment.

Design, construction, and building products and technology of buildings for public use can also be a barrier to participation in activities if it is not available, accessible, affordable, or acceptable. Also, if it is improperly prescribed, dysfunction can occur, such as a ramp that is too steep causing the client to lose control of her wheelchair, or it may not meet the needs of the client, such as a wheelchair accessible bathroom on the second floor but no elevator to get to the second floor.

Recreational therapists consider the role of design, construction, and building products and technology of buildings for public use in hindering or facilitating engagement in life activities and design appropriate interventions to either:

- Reduce or eliminate the negative effect of products and technology of buildings for public use on a particular life activity. For example, a client wants to attend his granddaughter's dance recital in a school auditorium. He requires the use of a wheelchair. Wheelchair accessible seating is at the back of the auditorium. However, it is not feasible for him to sit there because he also has a visual impairment that hinders his ability to see the stage from a distance. So, although wheelchair accessible seating is provided, it does not meet his needs. The therapist educates the client about the Americans with Disabilities Act and the school's requirement to accommodate his needs in a way that is reasonable. The client calls the school and discusses his situation. The school identifies a safe area in front of the stage for the client to sit in his wheelchair for the recital.

- Maintain or further facilitate the positive impact of products and technology of buildings for public use on life activities. The therapist assesses current products and technology of buildings for public use to determine if newer products or technology would further benefit the client and encourages continued use of products and technology of buildings for public use.

### Example of Design, Construction, and Building Products and Technology of Buildings for Public Use as a Barrier

A client who uses a manual wheelchair reports having difficulty getting into buildings that provide opportunities for social and community associations because there are steps at the entrances and no ramps. This is an example of how e1500 Design, Construction, and Building Products and Technology for Entering and Exiting Buildings for Public Use can be a barrier for d9100 Informal Associations. The scoring of d9100 Informal Associations that reflects the impact of e1500 Design, Construction, and Building Products and Technology for Entering and Exiting Buildings for Public Use as a barrier would look like this: d9100.2 _ _ _; e1500.1. The first qualifier (performance with assistance) reflects moderate difficulty with overall engagement in informal associations in his current life situation given all currently available supports and constraints. This qualifier was scored a 2 from testing and observation that showed difficulty with 40% of the task due to multiple issues, including poor communication skills and lack of self-confidence in abilities. As determined by the therapist, the inaccessible entrances account, on average, for one level of the difficulty with engagement in informal associations. If the barrier were removed by installing ramps, the client would still have a residual mild difficulty with engagement in informal associations. This is why the e-code was rated a .1 to account for one level of difficulty with engagement in informal associations.

### Example of Design, Construction, and Building Products and Technology of Buildings for Public Use as a Facilitator

The same client in the previous example learns about portable ramps. He educates the workers at the places he likes to go about where they can be purchased. Some of the places purchase a portable ramp and now place them over the steps when he visits. He also keeps one in his car trunk and requests assistance from the workers at the site to help him set it up if they do not have one. This is an example of how e1500 Design, Construction, and Building Products and Technology for Entering and Exiting Buildings for Public Use can be a facilitator for d9100 Informal Associations. The scoring of d9100 Informal Associations that reflects the impact of e1500 Design, Construction, and Building Products and Technology for Entering and Exiting Buildings for Public Use as a facilitator would look like this: d9100.1 _ _ 2; e1500+1. The first qualifier (performance with assistance) reflects mild difficulty engaging in informal associations in his current life situation given all available supports and constraints. This score reflects the one level positive change due to the use of portable ramps as discussed in the previous example. The fourth qualifier (performance without assistance) reflects moderate difficulty engaging in informal associations in his current life situation when supports are removed. See the previous example for an explanation of this score. The e-code was rated a +1 because the portable ramps improved his ability to engage in informal associations by one level.

### Cross References

In *Recreational Therapy for Specific Diagnoses and Conditions, First Edition*, ICF code e150 Design, Construction, and Building Products and Technology of Buildings for Public Use is listed in four chapters: Borderline Personality Disorder, Osteoarthritis, Spina Bifida, and Spinal Cord Injury.

In *Recreational Therapy Basics, Techniques, and Interventions, First Edition*, treatment for ICF code e150 Design, Construction, and Building Products and Technology of Buildings for Public Use is discussed in one chapter: Adaptive Sports.

### e155 Design, Construction, and Building Products and Technology of Buildings for Private Use

Products and technology that constitute an individual's indoor and outdoor human-made environment that is planned, designed, and constructed for private use, including those adapted or specially designed.

Inclusions: design, construction, and building products and technology of entrances and exits, facilities, and routing

- *e1550 Design, Construction, and Building Products and Technology for Entering and Exiting of Buildings for Private Use*
  Products and technology of entry and exit from the human-made environment that is planned, designed, and constructed for private use, such as entries and exits to private homes, portable and stationary ramps, power-assisted doors, lever door handles, and level door thresholds.

- *e1551 Design, Construction, and Building Products and Technology for Gaining Access to Facilities inside Buildings for Private Use*
  Products and technology related to design, building, and construction inside buildings for private use, such as washroom facilities, telephones, audio loops, kitchen cabinets, appliances, and electronic controls in private homes.

- *e1552 Design, Construction, and Building Products and Technology for Way Finding, Path Routing, and Designation of Locations in Buildings for Private Use*
  Indoor and outdoor products and technology in design, building, and construction of path routing, for private use, to assist people to find their way inside and immediately outside buildings and locate the places they want to go to, such as signage, in Braille or writing, size of corridors, and floor surfaces

- *e1558 Design, Construction, and Building Products and Technology of Buildings for Private Use, Other Specified*
- *e1559 Design, Construction, and Building Products and Technology of Buildings for Private Use, Unspecified*
  See e150 Design, Construction, and Building Products and Technology of Buildings for Public Use. The only difference is that this code set refers to buildings for private use.

### Cross References

In *Recreational Therapy for Specific Diagnoses and Conditions, First Edition*, there are no references for ICF code e155 Design, Construction, and Building Products and Technology of Buildings for Private Use.

In *Recreational Therapy Basics, Techniques, and Interventions, First Edition*, there are no references for ICF code e155 Design, Construction, and Building Products and Technology of Buildings for Private Use.

### e160 Products and Technology of Land Development

Products and technology of land areas, as they affect an individual's outdoor environment through the implementation of land use policies, design, planning, and development of space, including those adapted or specially designed.

Inclusions: products and technology of land areas that have been organized by the implementation of land use policies, such as rural areas, suburban areas, urban areas, parks, conservation areas, and wildlife reserves

- *e1600 Products and Technology of Rural Land Development*
  Products and technology in rural land areas, as they affect an individual's outdoor environment through the implementation of rural land use policies, design, planning, and development of space, such as farm lands, pathways, and signposting.

- *e1601 Products and Technology of Suburban Land Development*
  Products and technology in suburban land areas, as they affect an individual's outdoor environment through the implementation of suburban land use policies, design, planning, and development of space, such as curb cuts, pathways, signposting, and street lighting.

- *e1602 Products and Technology of Urban Land Development*
  Products and technology in urban land areas as they affect an individual's outdoor environment through the implementation of urban land use policies, design, planning, and development of space, such as curb cuts, ramps, signposting, and street lighting.

- *e1603 Products and Technology of Parks, Conservation, and Wildlife Areas*
  Products and technology in land areas making up parks, conservation, and wildlife areas, as they affect an individual's outdoor environment through the implementation of land use policies and design, planning, and development of space, such as park signage and wildlife trails.

- *e1608 Products and Technology of Land Development, Other Specified*
- *e1609 Products and Technology of Land Development, Unspecified*

Products and technology of land development can be a barrier or a facilitator to body structures, body functions, and life activities. For example, changes in street lighting (e1601 Products and Technology of Suburban Land Development) could be a facilitator to evening activities d9205 Socializing in an area that has been previous unlit. Another example would be the development of land in rural areas (e1600 Products and Technology of Rural Land Development) for a shopping center as a facilitator to d6200 Shopping.

Products and technology of land development can also be a barrier to activity participation if it is improperly designed, such as not meeting ADA accessibility guidelines, or doesn't meet the needs of the client, such as pathways that do not have curb cuts or that have a gravel surface making them inaccessible for people who use manual wheelchairs.

Recreational therapists consider the role of products and technology of land development in life activities and design appropriate interventions to either:

- Reduce or eliminate the negative effect of products and technology of land development on a particular life activity. For example a client wants to walk a three-mile path in a park. The paths in the park are paved, but they are not marked, making it difficult for the client to find her way back. The client and therapist call their local representative and identify the process to install appropriate park path markers.
- Maintain or further facilitate the positive impact of products and technology of land development on life activities. The therapist assesses current products and technology of land development to determine if newer products or technology would further benefit the client and encourage continued use of products and technology of land development.

### Example of Products and Technology of Land Development as a Barrier

A client has moderate difficulty (2) walking on uneven surfaces. He would like to go for walks at the local park but the paths are unpaved making it

unsafe. This is an example of how e1603 Products and Technology of Parks, Conservation, and Wildlife Areas can be a barrier to d4602 Moving Around outside the Home and Other Buildings. The scoring of d4602 Moving Around outside the Home and Other Buildings that reflects the impact of e1603 Products and Technology of Parks, Conservation, and Wildlife Areas as a barrier would look like this: d4602.2 _ _ 2; e1603.2. The first qualifier (performance with assistance) indicates moderate difficulty walking at the park with currently available supports and constraints. The fourth qualifier (performance without assistance) is also a 2 because there are no supports or constraints that could be taken away that would change his ability to walk at the park, consequently the score remains the same. The e-code was rated a .2 because it is anticipated that if the trails were paved the client's level of difficulty walking at the park would change from moderate difficulty to no difficulty, a two level change.

### Example of Products and Technology of Land Development as a Facilitator

A client recently moved from the city to a rural farm area. There is no street signage. His friends, who live in the city, do not come to visit him because they get lost easily. This affects his ability to socialize with his city friends (d9205 Socializing). The client has mild difficulty socializing with peers in his new neighborhood for various reasons. He petitioned the county to put up street signs. Once the street signs were posted, his friends from the city visited more often since they did not fear getting lost. This is an example of how e1600 Products and Technology of Rural Land Development can be a facilitator for d9205 Socializing. The scoring of d9205 Socializing that reflects the impact of e1600 Products and Technology of Rural Land Development would look like this: d9205.1 _ _ _; e1600+0. The first qualifier (performance with assistance) reflects mild difficulty socializing in his current life situation given supports and constraints. The mild difficulty with socializing is due to a variety of issues related to the move including feeling uncomfortable around new peers. Even though the street signs were hung, he continues to exhibit mild difficulty socializing in his new environment. Consequently, the signage did not make enough of an impact to warrant a level change.

*Cross References*

In *Recreational Therapy for Specific Diagnoses and Conditions, First Edition*, there are no references for ICF code e160 Products and Technology of Land Development.

In *Recreational Therapy Basics, Techniques, and Interventions, First Edition*, there are no references for ICF code e160 Products and Technology of Land Development.

### e165 Assets

Products or objects of economic exchange such as money, goods, property, and other valuables that an individual owns or of which he or she has rights of use.

Inclusions: tangible and intangible products and goods, financial assets

- *e1650 Financial Assets*
  Products, such as money and other financial instruments, which serve as a medium of exchange for labor, capital goods, and services.

- *e1651 Tangible Assets*
  Products or objects, such as houses and land, clothing, food, and technical goods, which serve as a medium of exchange for labor, capital goods, and services.

- *e1652 Intangible Assets*
  Products, such as intellectual property, knowledge, and skills, which serve as a medium of exchange for labor, capital good, and services.

- *e1658 Assets, Other Specified*
- *e1659 Assets, Unspecified*

Assets can be a barrier or a facilitator to body structures, body functions, and life activities. For example, financial assets could be a facilitator to participate in d9204 Hobbies. It could also be a barrier to participation in d9204 Hobbies if the client lacks the financial assets to pay for needed hobby materials. The exchange of tangible assets, such as clothing or food, for labor, goods, and services, as well as the exchange of intangible assets such as knowledge and skills for labor, goods, and services is also part of Western culture. It is commonly used for informal trade (bartering) instead of a formalized exchange. For example, an elderly neighbor does not like to cook, so a client agrees to make her a casserole each week in exchange for her teaching him how

to play the piano (intangible asset). Another example would be helping a family member build a shed in the backyard in exchange for help in hanging a new front door.

Recreational therapists consider the role of assets in life activities and design appropriate interventions to either:

- Reduce or eliminate the negative effect of assets on a particular life activity. For example, a client wants to exercise at the local YMCA but does not have the financial assets to pay for membership. The client and therapist contact the YMCA to see if there are scholarship funds available or the possibility of the client providing other assets in exchange for the membership, such as helping at the front desk.

- Maintain or further facilitate the positive impact of assets on life activities. The therapist assesses current assets to determine if other assets would further benefit the client and encourage continued use of current assets.

*Example of Assets as a Barrier*

A client desires to learn how to play the piano. She does not have enough money to pay for lessons. This is an example of how e1650 Financial Assets can be a barrier to d810 Informal Education. (Note that the code d810 Informal Education is used instead of code d9202 Arts and Culture because d9202 Arts and Culture reflects playing the piano, while d810 Informal Education reflects learning how to play the piano.) The scoring of d810 Informal Education that reflects the impact of e1650 Financial Assets as a barrier would look like this: d810._ _ _ 4; e1650.4. The fourth qualifier (performance without assistance) indicates complete difficulty in learning how to play the piano without assistance from anyone. The e-code is rated a .4 because lack of finances causes a complete barrier to learning how to play the piano.

*Example of Assets as a Facilitator*

A client's neighbor agreed to give her free piano lessons if she would take her dog for a walk two times a week. The client agreed. This is an example of how e1652 Intangible Assets can be a facilitator for d810 Informal Education. The scoring of d810 Informal Education that reflects the impact of e1652 Intangible Assets as a facilitator would look like this: d810.0 _ _ 4; e1652+4. The first qualifier (performance with assistance) indicates that she has no difficulty learning how to play the piano with assistance. The fourth qualifier (performance without assistance) indicates complete difficulty learning how to play the piano without assistance from others. The e-code was rated a +4 because it increased her ability to learn how to play the piano by four levels from complete difficulty to no difficulty.

### Cross References

In *Recreational Therapy for Specific Diagnoses and Conditions, First Edition*, ICF code e165 Assets is listed in one chapter: Feeding and Eating Disorders.

In *Recreational Therapy Basics, Techniques, and Interventions, First Edition*, there are no references for ICF code e165 Assets.

## e198 Products and Technology, Other Specified

## e199 Products and Technology, Unspecified

### References

Henderson, S., Skelton, H., & Rosenbaum, P. (2008). Assistive devices for children with functional impairments: Impact on child and caregiver function. *Developmental Medicine & Child Neurology, 50*, 89-98.

Johnson, K. L., Dudgeon, B., Kuehn, C., & Walker, W. (2007). Assistive technology use among adolescents and young adults with spina bifida. *American Journal of Public Health, 97*(2), 330-336.

Law, M., Petrenchik, T., King, G., & Hurley, P. (2007). Perceived environmental barriers to recreational, community, and school participation for children and youth with physical disabilities. *Archives of Physical Medicine and Rehabilitation, 88*, 1636-1642.

Lawson, L. M. (2011). Stroke survivor's perceptions of community participation and quality of life. *Annual in Therapeutic Recreation, 19*, 39-51.

Maas, J., Verheij, R. A., Groenewegen, P. P., Vries, S., & Spreeuwenberg, P. (2006). Green space, urbanity and health: How strong is the relation? *Journal of Epidemiology and Community Health, 60*(7), 587-592.

Murphy, N. A. & Carbone, P. S. (2008). Promoting the participation of children with disabilities in sports, recreation, and physical activities. *Pediatrics, 121*, 1057-1061.

Sizsmith, A. J., Gibson, G., Orpwood, R. D., & Torrington, J. M. (2006). Developing a technology "wish-list" to enhance the quality of life of people with dementia. *Gerontechnology, 6*(1), 2-19

Tortosa-Martinez, J., Zoerink, D. A., & Yoder, D. G. (2011). The benefits of therapeutic recreation experiences for people with Alzheimer's disease. *Annual in Therapeutic Recreation, 19*, 52-65

# Chapter 2 Natural Environment and Human-Made Changes to Environment

This chapter is about animate and inanimate elements of the natural or physical environment, and components of that environment that have been modified by people, as well as characteristics of human populations within that environment.

*Sample Scoring of Natural Environment and Human-Made Changes to Environment*

- An 11-year-old girl with severe asthma lives in an urban city. The outdoor air quality is poor making it difficult for her to breathe outdoors. This limits the amount of time she can play outdoors with peers to about 60% of the time. This is an example of how e2601 Outdoor Air Quality can be a barrier to d9205 Socializing, d9200 Play, d7200 Forming Relationships, and b440 Respiration Functions. Let's look at how to score one of these codes. The scoring of b440 Respiration Functions to reflect the impact of e2601 Outdoor Air Quality as a barrier would look like this: b440.2 e2601.2. The qualifier reflects her current level of respiration function impairment. The e-code was rated a .2 because poor outdoor air quality increases her level of difficulty with respiration functions by two levels to moderate impairment. If the outdoor air quality was good, then e2601 Outdoor Air Quality would be a facilitator to all of the activities and functions listed above.

The environment that surrounds a person can facilitate or hinder functioning, health, and quality of life. Consequently, recreational therapists are particularly attentive to the environment in which the client lives and functions. They seek to maximize its benefits and reduce its negative effects. For example, a meta-synthesis of the literature found that "between 13% and 37% of the countries' disease burden could be prevented by environmental improvements, resulting globally in about 13 million deaths per year" (Pruss-Ustun, Bonjour, & Corvalan, 2008). Exposure to high amounts of green space has also been found to lower mortality (Mitchell & Popham, 2008). As a final example, a literature review by van den Berg (2007) found that people perceive natural environments as more restorative and beautiful than urban environments. He also found that they provide restorative properties, such as stress recovery, reduced blood pressure, improved attention and concentration, increased positive affect, decreased anger, fewer health problems, less required pain medication, and shorter hospital stays. They also noted that green space may stimulate physical activity and social contact, as well as expose people to better air quality and reduced noise.

*Assessment of Natural Environment and Human-Made Changes to Environment*

Recreational therapists practice from a holistic perspective. They routinely evaluate the environment in which the client lives through interview, direct observation and evaluation, standardized assessments, and on-site research, particularly if the area is far away or information obtained about the environment is unreliable.

*Treatment of Natural Environment and Human-Made Changes to Environment*

Recreational therapists identify and address the environmental factors identified through the assessment that facilitate or hinder a client's health, engagement in leisure and community tasks, and quality of life.

*Evidence Review*

Reviews of several studies highlight evidence-based practice related to the natural environment and human-made changes to environment. This is only a sample of the evidence. A thorough review of the literature is needed to identify evidence-based practice interventions that reflect the needs and characteristics of the individual client.

Bergman-Evans (2004) conducted a quasi-experimental study with 21 cognitively intact older adults in a state veterans long-term care facility. Post implementation of the Eden Alternative Model, the residents had lower levels of distress, decreased boredom, and decreased helplessness.

Dijkstra, Pieterse, and Pruyn (2006) conducted a review of the literature to explore the effects of the physical environment in healthcare settings on the health and well-being of patients. They found that sunlight, windows, pleasant odor, and chosen seating arrangements had positive effects. They found inconsistent effects for sound, nature, spatial layout, television, and multiple stimuli interventions. The effects were also found to be highly dependent on the characteristics of the patient population and the healthcare setting.

Salem et al. (2011) conducted a study of 11 adults with multiple sclerosis participating in a multi-disciplinary community aquatic program for five weeks, twice a week for 60 minutes. Participants showed improved gait speed, balance, speed, and grip strength. No adverse effects related to the program were reported. The authors note that such a program should be considered "to augment... rehabilitation [and] provide a viable model for a community-based wellness programme for people with disability including individuals with multiple sclerosis." (p. 720)

### Cross References

In *Recreational Therapy for Specific Diagnoses and Conditions, First Edition*, ICF code e2 Natural Environment and Human-Made Changes to Environment and its subcategories are listed in eight chapters: Amputation and Prosthesis, Cerebral Palsy, Cerebrovascular Accident, Epilepsy, Multiple Sclerosis, Neurocognitive Disorders, Obesity, and Visual Impairments and Blindness.

In *Recreational Therapy Basics, Techniques, and Interventions, First Edition*, treatment for ICF code e2 Natural Environment and Human-Made Changes to Environment and its subcategories are discussed in one chapter: Education and Counseling.

### e210 Physical Geography

Features of land forms and bodies of water.

Inclusions: features of geography included within orography (relief, quality, and expanse of land and land forms, including altitude) and hydrography (bodies of water such as lakes, rivers, sea)

- *e2100 Land Forms*
  Features of land forms, such as mountains, hills, valleys, and plains.

- *e2101 Bodies of Water*
  Features of bodies of water, such as lakes, dams, rivers, and streams.

- *e2108 Physical Geography, Other Specified*
- *e2109 Physical Geography, Unspecified*

Physical geography can be a barrier or facilitator to life activities and functions. Recreational therapists consider the role of physical geography in life activities and design appropriate interventions to either:

- Reduce or eliminate the negative effect of physical geography on a particular life activity. In some cases, changing the physical geography of the client's home may be possible, such as leveling out the driveway and paving it to make it easier to walk. However, in most cases the client will need to be taught how to compensate for the barriers. Examples include putting a specialized ice pick end on the bottom of a standard cane to help with walking on uneven surfaces or changing the type of food being grown to one that will thrive in poor soil. In some situations, it might be best for the client to consider moving to a new location that is more geographically favorable.

- Maintain or further facilitate the positive impact of physical geography on life activities. If the physical geography of the client's area is a facilitator for life activities and functioning, therapists bring this to the attention of the client and encourage the client to consider physical geography when making any life changes.

### Example of Bodies of Water as a Barrier

A client desires to grow a vegetable garden. He finds that a small pond bordering his property is contaminated and cannot be used for irrigation. This is an example of how e2101 Bodies of Water can be a barrier to d6505 Taking Care of Plants, Indoors and Outdoors. The scoring of d6505 Taking Care of Plants, Indoors and Outdoors that reflects the impact of e2101 Bodies of Water as a barrier would look like this: d6505.4 _ _ _; e2101.4. The first qualifier reflects complete difficulty in being able to care for plants in his current life situation given supports and constraints (performance). If the water was not contaminated, it is the clinical judgment of the therapist that the client would have no difficulty caring for plants. The e-code is rated a .4 because the water contamination increases the client's level of difficulty by four levels from no difficulty to complete difficulty.

### Example of Bodies of Water as a Facilitator

A client engages in fishing during the summer months. He lives in an area where lakes are prevalent. This is an example of how e2101 Bodies of Water can be a facilitator for d9201 Sports. The scoring of d9201 Sports that reflects the impact of e2101 Bodies of Water would look like this: d9201.0 _ _ 0 (fishing, Dehn Level +3: Active Participation); e2101+0. The first qualifier reflects no difficulty overall with engagement in sports (fishing) in his current life situation given supports and constraints (performance). The fourth qualifier reflects the client's level of difficulty with fishing in his current life situation if supports were removed (performance without assistance). Since the client is independent with engaging in sports, the fourth qualifier is the same as the first qualifier. The e-code is rated a +0 because although it has an impact on the sport of fishing, his level of difficulty with engaging in sports would not change overall.

### Example of Land Forms as a Barrier

A client lives in a hilly neighborhood. He sustained an injury that now requires him to use a manual wheelchair. He does not drive. He used to walk to the stores to do his shopping. Now he lacks the strength and mobility to propel the wheelchair and carry supplies up and down steep hills. This is an example of how e2100 Land Forms can be a barrier to d6200 Shopping. The scoring of d6200 Shopping that reflects the impact of e2100 Land Forms would look like this: d6200.0 _ _ 4; e2100.1. The first qualifier reflects no difficulty shopping in his current life situation if assistance is provided by someone who pushes him in the wheelchair or if he orders supplies by internet or telephone (performance with assistance). The fourth qualifier reflects complete difficulty if assistance is not provided (performance without assistance). The e-code is rated a .1 because it only slightly hinders the client's ability to shop, since he can still shop by phone or internet.

### Cross References

In *Recreational Therapy for Specific Diagnoses and Conditions, First Edition*, there are no references for ICF code e210 Physical Geography.

In *Recreational Therapy Basics, Techniques, and Interventions, First Edition*, there are no references for ICF code e210 Physical Geography.

## e215 Population

Groups of people living in a given environment who share the same pattern of environmental adaptation.

Inclusions: demographic change; population density

- *e2150 Demographic Change*
  Changes occurring within groups of people, such as the composition and variation in the total number of individuals in an area caused by birth, death, ageing of a population, and migration.

- *e2151 Population Density*
  Number of people per unit of land area, including features such as high and low density.

- *e2158 Population, Other Specified*
- *e2159 Population, Unspecified*
  The population that a client is part of can be a facilitator or barrier to life activities and functioning. Recreational therapists consider the role of population in life activities and design appropriate interventions to either:

- Reduce or eliminate the negative effect of population on a particular life activity. In some cases, changing the population of the client's living area may be possible, such as moving into a larger apartment. However, in most cases the client will need to be taught how to compensate for the barriers. For example, if a client is having difficulty adapting to the change of population in the neighborhood, the recreational therapist might assist the client in identifying new sources of social support that meet the client's needs. Instead of conversing so much with neighbors, the client may benefit from participation in a private club that caters to a group that is similar to the client.

- Maintain or further facilitate the positive impact of population on life activities. If the population of the client's area is a facilitator for life activities and functioning of the client, the therapist brings this to the attention of the client and encourages the client to consider population when making any life changes.

### Example of Population as a Barrier and Facilitator

An 85-year-old client reports that many of his neighborhood friends have passed away. Young families are purchasing the homes and there aren't many older people left in his neighborhood to socialize with. He finds it difficult to relate to the younger generation and has difficulty forming relationships with them. This is an example of how e2150 Demographic Change can be a barrier to d7200 Forming Relationships. The scoring of d7200 Forming Relationships to reflect the impact of e2150 Demographic Change as a barrier would look like this: d7200.3 _ _ _; e2150.3. The first qualifier reflects severe difficulty in forming relationships in his current life situation given available supports and constraints (performance with assistance). This score was determined through conversation and observation by the therapist. In the clinical opinion of the therapist, if the demographic change in his neighborhood added more people similar to the client, his level of difficulty with forming relationships would improve to no difficulty (improvement by three levels). Given this premise, the e-code is rated a .3 because demographic change is believed to be the cause of increasing his level of difficulty with socializing by three levels. Note that if the neighborhood was changing so that new people moving in were more similar to the client, then e2150 Demographic Change could be a facilitator to d7200 Forming Relationships. Having other people to talk with might also be a facilitator for d2401 Handling Stress.

### Cross References

In *Recreational Therapy for Specific Diagnoses and Conditions, First Edition*, there are no references for ICF code e215 Population.

In *Recreational Therapy Basics, Techniques, and Interventions, First Edition*, there are no references for ICF code e215 Population.

### e220 Flora and Fauna

Plants and animals.

Exclusions: domesticated animals (e350); population (e215)

- *e2200 Plants*
  Any of various photosynthetic, eukaryotic, multicellular organisms of the kingdom Plantae characteristically producing embryos, containing chloroplasts, having cellulose cell walls, and lacking the power of locomotion, such as trees, flowers, shrubs, and vines.

- *e2201 Animals*
  Multicellular organisms of the kingdom Animalia, differing from plants in certain typical characteristics such as capacity for locomotion, non-photosynthetic metabolism, pronounced response to stimuli, restricted growth, and fixed bodily structure, such as wild or farm animals, reptiles, birds, fish, and mammals.

  Exclusions: assets (e165); domesticated animals (e350)

- *e2208 Fauna and Flora, Other Specified*
- *e2209 Fauna and Flora, Unspecified*
  Plants and animals can be facilitators or barriers to life activities and functions. Recreational therapists consider the role of plants and animals in life activities and design appropriate interventions to either:

- Reduce or eliminate the negative effect of plants and animals on a particular life activity. In some cases, changing the flora and fauna of the client's areas of functioning may be possible, such as planting or cutting down trees and taking out plants that cause allergies. If a client benefits from shaded areas, then it would be beneficial to explore the possibility of planting shade trees in the client's environment. In most cases the client will need to be taught how to compensate for the barriers. For example, if a client is having allergic reactions to plants when outdoors, allergy medications may need to be explored.

- Maintain or further facilitate the positive impact of plants and animals on life activities. If flora and fauna in the client's areas are facilitators to life activities and functioning, the therapist brings this to the attention of the client and encourages the client to consider flora and fauna when making any life changes.

### Example of Plants as a Barrier

An eight-year-old girl has severe allergic reactions to pollen. Consequently her outdoor play activities are restricted during the spring. This is an example of how e2200 Plants, as well as e2255 Seasonal Variation, can be a barrier to d9200 Play. The scoring of d9200 Play to reflect the impact of e2200 Plants and e2255 Seasonal Variation as barriers would look like this: d9200.1 _ _ 3; e2200.1, e2255.1. The first qualifier reflects mild difficulty engaging in play in the client's current life situation given available supports and constraints (performance with assistance). This score was determined through client observation not shared in this example. The fourth qualifier reflects severe difficulty engaging in play in her current life situation should assistance be removed (performance without assistance). This would include removal of allergy medication and assistance from her caregivers. This is not safe or ethical, so this score reflects the clinical judgment of the therapist. Both e-codes are rated a .1 because plants and seasonal variation affect her engagement in play only during one season and, when looking at all of the difficulties that the client has engaging in play, which are not shared in this example, the therapist determined that the plants and seasonal variation only account for one level of change in difficulty.

### Example of Plants as a Facilitator

A 34-year-old female with multiple sclerosis needs to stay out of the sun to avoid fatigue. Her backyard is shaded by trees and this allows her to participate in activities with her children outdoors without experiencing extreme fatigue. This is an example of how e2200 Plants can be a facilitator for d920 Recreation and Leisure. The scoring of d920 Recreation and Leisure to reflect the impact of e2200 Plants as a facilitator would look like this: d920.1 _ _ 3; e2200+1. The first qualifier reflects mild difficulty engaging in recreation and leisure in her current life situation given available supports and constraints (performance with assistance). The fourth qualifier reflects severe difficulty engaging in recreation and leisure in her current life situation without assistance (performance without assistance). The scores chosen were based on the average level of difficulty within a broad range of recreational activities, not just summer activities. The e-code was rated a +1. This was determined through clinical judgment by evaluating the impact of shade on the client's engagement in recreational activity as a whole. The percent of recreational activities affected by shade was limited since it was only a benefit during the hot summer months. Consequently, it is only a minimal facilitator to engagement in recreational activities.

### Example of Animals as a Barrier

A client with osteoporosis has a history of falls. Many of her falls (80%) are related to tripping over her pet cat in her home. This is an example of how e2201 Animals can be a barrier to d4600 Moving Around within the Home. The scoring of d4600 Moving Around within the Home to reflect the impact of e2201 Animals as a barrier would look like this: d4600.3 _ _ _; e2201.3. The first qualifier reflects severe difficulty moving around the house in her current life situation given available supports and constraints (performance with assistance). The e-code is rated a .3 because it is the pet cat that is causing 80% of her falls (severe barrier).

### Example of Animals as a Facilitator

A client had her right knee replaced. She is able to walk short distances in the community without a device and exhibits good balance. She has a pet dog that requires walking every day. She reports that her pet dog is a motivator for her to go outside for a walk every day. This is an example of how e2201 Animals can be facilitator to d5701 Managing Diet and Fitness. The scoring of d5701 Managing Diet and Fitness to reflect the impact of e2201 Animals as a facilitator would look like this: d5701.0 _ _ 2; e2201+2. The first qualifier reflects that she has no difficulty going for a walk in her current life situation given supports and constraints (performance with assistance). The fourth qualifier reflects that while she has no difficulty going for a walk in her current life situation without assistance, the client states that if she didn't have the dog, she would probably only go for walks about half of the time, reducing her attention to appropriate management of fitness by 45% (performance without assistance). Therefore the e-code is rated a +2 (a 45% facilitator). If the client had a large unruly dog that could not be left at home alone, it is possible that the dog would hinder her ability to go for a walk. In this example, e2201 Animals could be a barrier to d5701 Managing Diet and Fitness and d4500 Walking Short Distances.

### Cross References

In *Recreational Therapy for Specific Diagnoses and Conditions, First Edition*, ICF code e220 Flora and Fauna is listed in one chapter: Visual Impairments and Blindness.

In *Recreational Therapy Basics, Techniques, and Interventions, First Edition*, there are no references for ICF code e220 Flora and Fauna.

## e225 Climate

Meteorological features and events, such as the weather.

Inclusions: temperature, humidity, atmospheric pressure, precipitation, wind, and seasonal variations

- *e2250 Temperature*
  Degree of heat or cold, such as high and low temperature, normal or extreme temperature.

- *e2251 Humidity*
  Level of moisture in the air, such as high or low humidity.

- *e2252 Atmospheric Pressure*
  Pressure of the surrounding air, such as pressure related to height above sea level or meteorological conditions.

- *e2253 Precipitation*
  Falling of moisture, such as rain, dew, snow, sleet, and hail.

- *e2254 Wind*
  Air in more or less rapid natural motion, such as a breeze, gale, or gust.

- *e2255 Seasonal Variation*
  Natural, regular, and predictable changes from one season to the next, such as summer, autumn, winter, and spring.

- *e2258 Climate, Other Specified*
- *e2259 Climate, Unspecified*
  Climate can be a barrier or facilitator to life activities and functions. Recreational therapists consider the role of climate on life activities and design appropriate interventions to either:

- Reduce or eliminate the negative effect of climate on a particular life activity. It might not be possible to change the climate of the client's areas of living, so the client will need to be taught how to compensate for the barriers. For example, if a client with multiple sclerosis fatigues easily with heat, then she would be encouraged to keep her core body temperature as low as possible by drinking cold water, wearing a brimmed hat, wearing breathable clothing such as cotton, and using a portable battery-operated fan. Another example would be for the client who is unable to go to church during the winter months to consider other acceptable ways to engage in religious activities.

- Maintain or further facilitate the positive impact of climate on life activities. If the climate in the client's areas of living is a facilitator to life activities and functioning, the therapist brings this to the attention of the client and encourages the client to consider the climate when making any life changes.

### *Example of Temperature and Humidity as a Barrier*

A client has multiple sclerosis. On average she is able to engage in the task of shopping with moderate difficulty. When the humidity and/or temperature are high, it affects her level of functioning. She experiences greater fatigue and weakness and this affects her ability to go shopping in the community, resulting in severe difficulty. This is an example of how e2250 Temperature and e2251 Humidity can be a barrier to d6200 Shopping. The scoring of d6200 Shopping that reflects the impact of e2250 Temperature and e2251 Humidity would look like this: d6200.2 _ _ 4; e2250.2, e2251.2. The first qualifier reflects her average level of difficulty (moderate difficulty) with shopping in her current life situation given support and constraints (performance with assistance). The fourth qualifier reflects complete difficulty to engage in the task of shopping in her current life situation when assistance is not provided (performance without assistance). This score was chosen based on clinical observation and testing by the therapist that is not shared in this example. Both e-codes are rated a .2 because the change in temperature and humidity causes a two-level change in her ability to engage in shopping. Note that if the temperature and humidity were low, e2250 Temperature and e2251 Humidity could be facilitators to d6200 Shopping. As reviewed in Issues Related to E-Codes in ICF Scoring, it may be better to score e-codes as a facilitator rather than as a barrier when they can be both a barrier and a facilitator.

### *Example of Temperature as a Facilitator*

A 10-year-old boy with a developmental disability loves to swim in his backyard outdoor pool. He lives in California where it is often hot enough to swim outdoors. This is an example of how e2250 Temperature can be a facilitator for d4554 Swimming. The scoring of d4554 Swimming to reflect the impact of e2250 Temperature as a facilitator would look like this: d4554.0 _ _ 4; e2250+4. The first qualifier reflects the client's level of difficulty with swimming in his current life situation given supports and constraints (performance with assistance). The fourth qualifier reflects his level of difficulty with swimming if assistance is removed. The e-code was rated a +4 because if the temperature is not hot enough it would completely limit his ability to swim, if indoor swimming was not available.

### Example of Seasonal Variation as a Barrier

A client has a complete spinal cord injury and requires the use of a manual wheelchair for mobility. He lives in an area where it snows and sleets heavily for three months out of the year. During these months, he does not attend church because it is too dangerous to go outside. This is an example of how e2255 Seasonal Variation can be a barrier to d9300 Organized Religion. The scoring of d9300 Organized Religion to reflect the impact of e2255 Seasonal Variation as a barrier would look like this: d9300.1 _ _ 0; e2255.1. The first qualifier reflects that on average he has mild difficulty engaging in organized religion in his current life situation given usual supports and constraints (performance with assistance). This score reflects the average amount of difficulty (no difficulty nine months out of the year and complete difficulty three months out of the year). The e-code is rated a .1 because it causes a one level change in a negative direction (no difficulty to mild difficulty).

### Cross References

In *Recreational Therapy for Specific Diagnoses and Conditions, First Edition*, ICF code e225 Climate is listed in one chapter: Multiple Sclerosis.

In *Recreational Therapy Basics, Techniques, and Interventions, First Edition*, there are no references for ICF code e225 Climate.

### e230 Natural Events

Geographic and atmospheric changes that cause disruption in an individual's physical environment, occurring regularly or irregularly, such as earthquakes and severe or violent weather conditions, e.g., tornadoes, hurricanes, typhoons, floods, forest fires, and ice-storms.

Natural events will most likely be coded only as barriers to activities. Except for people such as firefighters who are employed (d8451 Maintaining a Job) because of natural events, it is hard to think of a situation when an earthquake, flood, forest fire, or ice storm could be a facilitator to life activities or functions. These codes will most likely be barriers to codes in d2 General Tasks and Demands, d4 Mobility, d6 Domestic Life, d8 Major Life Areas, and d9 Community, Social, and Civic Life.

Recreational therapists consider the role of natural events on life activities and design appropriate interventions to reduce or eliminate the negative effect of natural events on a particular life activity. Therapists working with clients who have experienced a natural event recognize that further counseling and assistance may be needed. Therapists assist clients in coping with the disaster and identifying appropriate resources to initiate needed support, such as referring the client to the social worker. If the client lives in an area where natural events are common and lives are regularly disrupted, the client may need to consider relocation to a more stable area, especially if recovery from the natural event requires more skills and abilities than the client has available. For example, the client may not be able to go up on the roof and make repairs each storm season like he did before he was injured.

### Example of Natural Events as a Barrier

A client's home was destroyed in a tornado. She is now having trouble finding a new place to live in the area because many of the homes were destroyed. This is an example of how e230 Natural Events can be a barrier to d610 Acquiring a Place to Live. The scoring of d610 Acquiring a Place to Live to reflect the impact of e230 Natural Events as a barrier would look like this: d610.4 _ _ _; e230.4. The first qualifier reflects the client's complete difficulty in acquiring a place to live in her current life situation given usual supports and constraints (performance with assistance). The e-code is rated a .4 because it causes a four level change in a negative direction (no difficulty to complete difficulty).

### Cross References

In *Recreational Therapy for Specific Diagnoses and Conditions, First Edition*, there are no references for ICF code e230 Natural Events.

In *Recreational Therapy Basics, Techniques, and Interventions, First Edition*, there are no references for ICF code e230 Natural Events.

### e235 Human-Caused Events

Alterations or disturbances in the natural environment, caused by humans, that may result in the disruption of people's day-to-day lives, including events or conditions linked to conflict and wars, such as the displacement of people, destruction of social infrastructure, homes, and lands, environmental disasters, and land, water, or air pollution (e.g., toxic spills).

Human-caused events will most likely be coded as barriers to life activities and functions. It is hard to imagine how a human-caused event such as displacement of people, wars, destruction of social infrastructure, and environmental disasters could be a facilitator to life activities, except for the few employed because of the event.

Therapists working with clients who have experienced a human-caused event recognize that further counseling and assistance may be needed. Therapists assist clients in identifying appropriate resources to initiate needed support, such as referring the client to the social worker. If the client lives in an area where human-caused events are common and lives are regularly disrupted, the client may need to consider relocation to a more stable area, especially if recovery from the human-caused event requires more skills and abilities than the client has available. For example, the client is not able to quickly hide in the home when fighting breaks out on the street.

### Example of Human-Caused Events as a Barrier

A 23-year-old male is sent to war. He returns home two years later. He has recurrent night terrors from PTSD and is unable to successfully cope with daily stressors. This is an example of how e235 Human-Caused Events can be a barrier to d2401 Handling Stress. The scoring of d2401 Handling Stress to reflect the impact of e235 Human-Caused Events as a barrier would look like this: d2401.3 _ _ 4; e235.4. The first qualifier reflects the client's severe difficulty in coping with stress in his current life situation given usual supports and constraints (performance with assistance). The fourth qualifier reflects the client's complete difficulty in coping with stress when assistance is not provided. The e-code is rated a .4 because it is anticipated based upon testing, discussion, and observation that if the human-caused event of war did not occur, the client's ability to cope with stress would rise by four levels.

### Cross References

In *Recreational Therapy for Specific Diagnoses and Conditions, First Edition*, there are no references for ICF code e235 Human-Caused Events.

In *Recreational Therapy Basics, Techniques, and Interventions, First Edition*, there are no references for ICF code e235 Human-Caused Events.

### e240 Light

Electromagnetic radiation by which things are made visible by either sunlight or artificial lighting (e.g., candles, oil, or paraffin lamps, fires, and electricity), and which may provide useful or distracting information about the world.

Inclusions: light intensity; light quality; color contrasts

- *e2400 Light Intensity*
  Level or amount of energy being emitted by either a natural (e.g., sun) or an artificial source of light.

- *e2401 Light Quality*
  The nature of the light being provided and related color contrasts created in the visual surroundings, and which may provide useful information about the world (e.g., visual information on the presence of stairs or a door) or distractions (e.g., too many visual images).

- *e2408 Light, Other Specified*
- *e2409 Light, Unspecified*
  Light can be a barrier or facilitator to life activities and functioning. Recreational therapists consider the role of light on life activities and design appropriate interventions to either:

- Reduce or eliminate the negative effect of light on a particular life activity. In most cases, changes in light in the client's areas of living may be possible through the use of artificial light or shading sunlight. However, in some cases the client will need to be taught how to compensate for the barriers. For example, if a client is having difficulty seeing a task clearly due to problems with light intensity or quality, adaptations need to be sought. Such adaptations include the use of direct light and high intensity light, increased time, such as walking slowly and carefully when walking up a flight of stairs when the edge of the steps are difficult to see due to limited light, and using items with high contrast.

- Maintain or further facilitate the positive impact of light on life activities. If the light in the client's areas of living is a facilitator to life activities and functioning, the therapist brings this to the attention of the client and encourages the client to consider light when making any life or activity changes.

### *Example of Light Intensity and Light Quality as Facilitator and Barrier*

A client has impaired vision. She reports that she has not engaged in making dried flower crafts for several years because she is unable to see the items and craft clearly. Using a high intensity, artificial white light the client is able to see the items and craft clearly. This is an example of how e2400 Light Intensity and e2401 Light Quality can be facilitators for d9203 Crafts. The scoring of d9203 Crafts to reflect the impact of e2400 Light Intensity and e2401 Light Quality as facilitators would look like this: d9203.0 _ _ 4; e2400+4, e2401+4. The first qualifier reflects no difficulty with crafts in her current life situation given usual supports and constraints, including the adaptive light (performance with assistance). The fourth qualifier reflects complete difficulty in her current life situation when assistance from the light is not provided (performance without assistance). Both e-codes are rated a +4 because without them the client's level of difficulty would fall four levels. Prior to the adaptation, e2400 Light Intensity and e2401 Light Quality would have been a barrier to d9203 Crafts.

### *Cross References*

In *Recreational Therapy for Specific Diagnoses and Conditions, First Edition*, ICF code e240 Light is listed in two chapters: Epilepsy and Visual Impairments and Blindness.

In *Recreational Therapy Basics, Techniques, and Interventions, First Edition*, there are no references for ICF code e240 Light.

### *e245 Time-Related Changes*

Natural, regular, or predictable temporal change.

Inclusions: day/night and lunar cycles

- *e2450 Day/Night Cycles*
  Natural, regular, and predictable changes from day through to night and back to day, such as day, night, dawn, and dusk.

- *e2451 Lunar Cycles*
  Natural, regular, and predictable changes of the moon's position in relation to the earth.

- *e2458 Time-Related Changes, Other Specified*
- *e2459 Time-Related Changes, Unspecified*
  Time-related changes can be a barrier or facilitator to life activities and functions. Some suggest lunar cycles are correlated with behavior, even if it is just because the client believes it.

Day/night and lunar cycles cannot be changed. If they present a barrier for life activities and functioning, the client will need to learn to compensate and adapt for the barriers.

### *Example of Day/Night Cycles as a Barrier and Facilitator*

A five-year-old girl has a rare condition of extreme photosensitivity. Sunlight, whether direct or indirect, may not touch her skin. If it does, severe burns occur. She plays outside after the sun goes down and if she needs to go outside during the day, she has to wear a special protective hat, gown, and gloves that cover her entire body. This is an example of how e2450 Day/Night Cycles can be both a barrier and facilitator to d9200 Play. The scoring of d9200 Play to reflect the impact of e2450 Day/Night Cycles as a barrier would look like this: d9200.0 _ _ 4; e2450.4. The first qualifier reflects no difficulty with play in her current life situation with the current supports and constraints of a gown, playing outdoors after sunset, and playing indoors with shades drawn during the day (performance with assistance). The fourth qualifier reflects complete difficulty when assistance is not provided (performance without assistance). The e-code is rated a .4 because day/night cycles can result in a change of four levels if adaptations and assistance is not provided. In this same example, the inability of the child to attend a normal public school and participate in daytime peer activities is another example of how e2450 Day/Night Cycles could be a barrier to d9205 Socializing and d7200 Forming Relationships.

### *Cross References*

In *Recreational Therapy for Specific Diagnoses and Conditions, First Edition*, there are no references for ICF code e245 Time-Related Changes.

In *Recreational Therapy Basics, Techniques, and Interventions, First Edition*, there are no references for ICF code e245 Time-Related Changes.

### *e250 Sound*

A phenomenon that is or may be heard, such as banging, ringing, thumping, singing, whistling, yelling, or buzzing, in any volume, timbre, or tone, and that may provide useful or distracting information about the world.

Inclusions: sound intensity; sound quality

- *e2500 Sound Intensity*
  Level or volume of auditory phenomenon determined by the amount of energy being generated, where high energy levels are perceived as loud sounds and low energy levels as soft sounds.

- *e2501 Sound Quality*
  Nature of a sound as determined by the wavelength and wave pattern of the sound and perceived as the timbre and tone, such as harshness or melodiousness, and which may provide useful information about the world (e.g., sound of dog barking versus a cat meowing) or distractions (e.g., background noise).

- *e2508 Sound, Other Specified*
- *e2509 Sound, Unspecified*
  Sound can be a barrier or facilitator to life activities and functions. Recreational therapists consider the role of sound on life activities and design appropriate interventions to either:

- Reduce or eliminate the negative effect of sound on a particular life activity. In many cases, changes in sound in the client's areas of living may be possible, such as changing the sound intensity and quality of alarm clocks. In some cases the client will need to be taught how to compensate for the barriers. For example, if a client is very sensitive to loud noises, then it might be helpful to explore wearing earplugs when others are using loud equipment nearby. If the client is having difficulty hearing because of the sound intensity or quality, then auditory devices may be explored.

- Maintain or further facilitate the positive impact of sound on life activities. If sounds in the client's living environment are facilitators to life activities and functioning, the therapist brings this to the attention of the client and encourages the client to consider sound when making any life or activity changes.

### *Example of Sound as a Facilitator*

A client is legally blind. She has learned how to use her sense of hearing to identify sounds that give her information she used to get from vision when walking in the community. For example, she listens for the clicking noise that denotes traffic light changes. This is an example of how e250 Sound can be a facilitator for d4602 Moving Around outside the Home and Other Buildings. The scoring of d4602 Moving Around outside the Home and Other Buildings that reflects the impact of e250 Sound as a facilitator would look like this: d4602.0 _ _ 2; e250+2. The first qualifier reflects that she has no difficulty moving around outside the home and other buildings in her current life situation with all available supports and constraints (performance with assistance). The fourth qualifier reflects that she would have moderate difficulty with this task if assistance were removed (performance without assistance). The e-code was rated a +2 because without sound, it is anticipated through clinical judgment that her ability to move around outside would reduce by two levels.

### *Example of Sound Intensity as a Barrier and Facilitator*

A client who had a traumatic brain injury is very sensitive to noise. Loud noises cause him to become agitated. This is an example of how e2500 Sound Intensity can be a barrier to b1263 Psychic Stability. The scoring of b1263 Psychic Stability to reflect the impact of e2500 Sound Intensity as a barrier would look like this: b1263.2; e2500.2. The qualifier reflects the client's moderate impairment with psychic stability as determined through testing and observation. The e-code was rated a .2 because, when loud noises are present, they increase the client's level of difficulty by two levels. If soft sounds surrounded the client's living areas, then e2500 Sound Intensity could be a facilitator to b1263 Psychic Stability.

### *Cross References*

In *Recreational Therapy for Specific Diagnoses and Conditions, First Edition*, ICF code e250 Sound is listed in one chapter: Visual Impairments and Blindness.

In *Recreational Therapy Basics, Techniques, and Interventions, First Edition*, there are no references for ICF code e250 Sound.

### e255 Vibration

Regular or irregular to and fro motion of an object or an individual caused by a physical disturbance, such as shaking, quivering, quick jerky movements of things, buildings, or people caused by small or large equipment, aircraft, and explosions.

Exclusions: natural events (e230), such as vibrations or shaking of the earth caused by earthquake

Vibration can be a barrier or facilitator to life activities and functions. Recreational therapists consider the role of vibration on life activities and design appropriate interventions to either:

- Reduce or eliminate the negative effect of vibration on a particular life activity. In some cases, changes in vibration in the client's areas of living may be possible, such as in the example below. However, in many cases the client will need to be taught how to compensate for the barriers. For example, if a client's spasms are heightened by vibration and there is a lot of vibration in the client's environment, anti-spasm medications may be an area to explore or the client may benefit from moving to another location, such as sleeping in another room farther from the source of vibration.
- Maintain or further facilitate the positive impact of vibration on life activities. If vibrations in the client's living environment are facilitators to life activities and functioning, the therapist brings this to the attention of the client and encourages the client to consider vibrations when making any life or activity changes.

#### Example of Vibration as a Barrier

For a 37-year-old-male with a developmental disability, vibrations cause increased leg spasms with pain and discomfort. The path through the local park is full of tree roots making it a very bumpy ride in a wheelchair. This is an example of how e255 Vibration can be a barrier to d920 Recreation and Leisure. The scoring of d920 Recreation and Leisure to reflect the impact of e255 Vibration as a barrier would look like this: d920.2 _ _ 4; e255.1. The first qualifier reflects the client's moderate difficulty with all recreational activities in his current life setting with all available supports and constraints (performance with assistance). The fourth qualifier reflects the client's level of difficulty with recreational activities

if no assistance, including wheelchairs and medicine, was provided. The qualifier scores are an average of all skills in the blended activity of recreation and leisure as determined by the therapist through testing and observation. The e-code is rated a .1 because, although it completely limits his ability to go through the park, vibration affects only a minimal percentage of his overall recreational activities, therefore it only changes his overall difficulty with recreational activities by one level.

#### Example of Vibration as a Facilitator

An eight-week-old infant is very colicky at night. She cries through most of the night. The mother found a device that attaches to the crib and vibrates the mattress. The vibration relaxes the infant and lets her sleep for longer periods of time during the night. This is an example of how e255 Vibration can be a facilitator to b134 Sleep Functions. The scoring of b134 Sleep Functions to reflect the impact of e255 Vibration as a facilitator would look like this: b134.0; e255+4. The qualifier reflects that the client has no difficulty with sleep functions and that the e-code is a complete facilitator in achieving this level of difficulty. If the vibration was removed, it is anticipated that her level of impairment would increase by four levels, thus reflecting the change of four levels. If the infant cried because of vibrations, for example because she sleeps above a vibrating generator, then e255 Vibration would be a barrier to b134 Sleep Functions.

#### Cross References

In *Recreational Therapy for Specific Diagnoses and Conditions, First Edition*, there are no references for ICF code e255 Vibration.

In *Recreational Therapy Basics, Techniques, and Interventions, First Edition*, there are no references for ICF code e255 Vibration.

### e260 Air Quality

Characteristics of the atmosphere (outside buildings) or enclosed areas of air (inside buildings), and which may provide useful or distracting information about the world.

Inclusions: indoor and outdoor air quality

- *e2600 Indoor Air Quality*
  Nature of the air inside buildings or enclosed areas, as determined by odor, smoke, humidity,

air conditioning (controlled air quality), or uncontrolled air quality, and which may provide useful information about the world (e.g., smell of leaking gas) or distractions (e.g., overpowering smell of perfume).

- *e2601 Outdoor Air Quality*
  Nature of the air outside buildings or enclosed areas, as determined by odor, smoke, humidity, ozone levels, and other features of the atmosphere, and which may provide useful information about the world (e.g., smell of rain) or distractions (e.g., toxic smells).

- *e2608 Air Quality, Other Specified*
- *e2609 Air Quality, Unspecified*

Air quality can be a barrier or facilitator to life activities and functions. Recreational therapists consider the role of air quality on life activities and design appropriate interventions to either:

- Reduce or eliminate the negative effect of air quality on a particular life activity. In some cases, changes in air quality in the client's areas of living may be possible, however in most cases the client will need to be taught how to compensate for the barriers. For example, if a client has difficulty breathing outdoors due to poor air quality, then the client may need to limit the amount of time spent outdoors, use an inhaler when breathing difficulty occurs, or avoid certain activities that contribute to poor air quality.

- Maintain or further facilitate the positive impact of air quality on life activities. If air quality in the client's living environments is a facilitator to life activities and functioning, the therapist brings this to the attention of the client and encourages the client to consider air quality when making any life or activity changes.

### Example of Outdoor Air Quality as a Barrier and Facilitator

An 11-year-old girl with severe asthma lives in an urban city. The outdoor air quality is poor making it difficult for her to breathe outdoors. This limits the amount of time she can play outdoors with peers. This is an example of how e2601 Outdoor Air Quality can be a barrier to d9205 Socializing, d9200 Play, d7200 Forming Relationships, and b440 Respiration Functions. Let's look at how to score one of these codes. The scoring of b440 Respiration Functions to reflect the impact of e2601 Outdoor Air

Quality as a barrier would look like this: b440.2; e2601.2. The qualifier reflects her current level of respiration function impairment. The e-code was rated a .2 because outdoor air quality can increase her level of difficulty with respiration functions by two levels to moderate impairment. If the outdoor air quality was good, then e2601 Outdoor Air Quality would be a facilitator to all of the activities and functions listed above.

### Example of Indoor Air Quality as a Barrier

A client lives in a retirement community. She becomes ill and is transferred to the skilled nursing unit in the retirement community. The skilled care center has a strong odor of urine. The woman's friend is very sensitive to smells and cannot tolerate the odor, so she does not visit her best friend while she is there and the relationship deteriorates. This is an example of how e2600 Indoor Air Quality can be a barrier to maintaining a friendship (d7500 Informal Relationships with Friends). The scoring of d7500 Informal Relationships with Friends to reflect the impact of e2600 Indoor Air Quality as a barrier would look like this: d7500.3 _ _ 4; e2600.3. The first qualifier reflects her severe difficulty in maintaining relationships in her current living environment. This is due to a variety of reasons, not just related to the issue going on with her best friend (performance with assistance). Remember, this is an overall score, not just a score related to this particular situation. The fourth qualifier reflects that there would be a complete difficulty with maintaining relationships without assistance if there was no initiation of conversation by staff and no encouragement by staff to come out of her room (performance without assistance). The e-code was rated a .3 because the indoor air quality is severely limiting her ability to maintain her previous friendships. It is anticipated that if the indoor air quality was good, her friends would visit and she would have no difficulty in maintaining her friendships, thus reflecting a change in three levels.

### Cross References

In *Recreational Therapy for Specific Diagnoses and Conditions, First Edition*, there are no references for ICF code e260 Air Quality.

In *Recreational Therapy Basics, Techniques, and Interventions, First Edition*, there are no references for ICF code e260 Air Quality.

### e298 Natural Environment and Human-Made Changes to Environment, Other Specified

### e299 Natural Environment and Human-Made Changes to Environment, Unspecified

#### References

Bergman-Evans, B. (2004). Beyond the basics: Effects of the Eden alternative model on quality of life issues. *Journal of Gerontological Nursing, 30*(6), 27-34.

Dijkstra, K., Pieterse, M., & Pruyn, A. (2006). Physical environmental stimuli that turn healthcare facilities into healing environments through psychologically mediated effects: Systematic review. *Journal of Advanced Nursing, 56*(2), 166-181

Mitchell, R. & Popham, F. (2008). Effect of exposure to natural environment on health inequalities: An observational population study. *The Lancet, 372*(9650), 1655-1660.

Pruss-Ustun, A., Bonjour, S., & Corvalan, C. (2008). The impact of the environment on health by country: A meta-synthesis. *Environmental Health, 7*(7).

Salem, Y., Scott, A. H., Karpatkin, H., Concert, G., Haller, L., Kaminsky, E., Weisbrot, R., & Spatz, E. (2011). Community-based group aquatic programme for individuals with multiple sclerosis: A pilot study. *Disability and Rehabilitation, 33*(9), 720-728.

van den Berg, A. E. (2007). Preference for nature in urbanized societies: Stress, restoration, and the pursuit of sustainability. *Journal of Social Issues, 63*(1), 79-96.

# Chapter 3 Support and Relationships

This chapter is about people or animals that provide practical physical or emotional support, nurturing, protection, assistance, and relationships to other persons, in their home, place of work, school, or at play or in other aspects of their daily activities. The chapter does not encompass the attitudes of the person or people that are providing the support. The environmental factor being described is not the person or animal, but the amount of physical and emotional support the person or animal provides.

*Sample Scoring for Support and Relationships*

- A client has moderate difficulty with d7200 Forming Relationships. When in social situations her friend gives her non-verbal cues when she begins to say something that is not appropriate. This support decreases the level of difficulty that the client has with d7200 Forming Relationships to mild difficulty. The scoring of d7200 Forming Relationships that reflects the impact of e320 Friends would look like this: d7200.1 _ _ 2; e320+1. The first qualifier of d7200 Forming Relationships is the level of difficulty that the client has in her current life situation with all available supports and constraints (performance with assistance). The fourth qualifier reflects her level of difficulty in a real-life setting when support is not provided (performance without assistance). The e-code was rated a +1 because it lowered her level of difficulty by one level.

Therapists use the codes in this chapter to reflect the amount of physical and emotional support that a person or animal provides to the client. Recreational therapists consider the role of support and relationships on life activities. They design appropriate interventions to either reduce or eliminate the negative effect of support and relationships on a particular life activity. They also maintain or further facilitate the positive impact of support and relationships on life activities. Being aware of supports and relationships that facilitate or hinder the level of difficulty with a function, task, or activity is necessary to improve and enhance client functioning. It highlights the possible need for training, such as training caregivers on how to best provide appropriate physical or emotional support. It also cues the therapist to remind clients that appropriate support increases functioning and health, making it worthwhile to seek out or change support to optimize functioning. For example, in a sample of veterans with multiple sclerosis, greater perceived social support, particularly greater positive social interaction, greater emotional and informational support, and greater affective support, were associated with less depression (Bambara et al., 2011).

*Assessment of Support and Relationships*

Support and relationships are commonly assessed via interview with the client and/or others who know the client well. Notations about support and relationships might also be found in the medical chart. Exploratory questions might include: who are the important people in your life, what is it about these relationships that you value and why, what relationships are most challenging to you and why, etc. Outside of interviewing techniques, the recreational therapist might utilize other tools such as the *Family APGAR*, to measure a client's perception of his/her social system (A = adaptation, P = partnership, G = growth, A = affection, R = resolve).

*Treatment of Support and Relationships*

After determining the client's current relationships and their value, recreational therapists seek to maintain, strengthen, and create relationships that have the potential to positively impact health and quality of life. Likewise, the recreational therapist aims to reduce or change unhealthy relationships that have the potential to negatively impact health and quality of life, such as gang involvement or friends that support addictions.

The development of strong, healthy relationships are born over time as individuals get to know each other, find common interests, and explore attributes of the other person. Important aspects of these relationships include trustworthiness, concern, reciprocity, and mutual respect. Engagement in leisure and community activities provides a context for forming and maintaining relationships, but the activity itself is not the only catalyst. Individual characteristics such as psychic stability, cognitive skills, social skills, motivation, desire, and initiation all play a role. Environmental characteristics such as opportunity, attitudes of others, and accessibility are also important. Because recreational therapists thoroughly embrace the value of support and relationships for health and quality of life, they identify and address underlying variables to foster its development.

### Evidence Review

Reviews of several studies are provided below to highlight evidence-based practice related to support and relationships. This is only a sample of the evidence. A thorough review of the literature is needed to identify evidence-based practice interventions that reflect the needs and characteristics of the individual client.

Benyamini, Medalion, and Garfinkel (2007) conducted a study of 50 couples age 65+ of which one had a form of coronary artery disease. Their findings indicated that if the spouse and client attributed the disease to stress, greater support was provided and felt. The support happened because both people understood that stress doesn't carry blame and requires support from the spouse to cope. If the spouse attributed the disease to lifestyle choices, however, there was more undermining along with the support. The clients reported feeling less supported because criticism of lifestyle was interpreted as being less supportive. Spouses reported less undermining behavior if they perceived low control while the client perceived high control. Clients perceived less support when they perceived their disease to be chronic while their spouses believed it was a short-term health condition. Spousal minimization may create a feeling of not being taken seriously. Undermining by spouses significantly increased when they perceived severe consequences and the clients did not, whereas undermining significantly decreased when both the spouse and client perceived low consequences. The authors advocate for assessing and addressing spouse and client perceptions of disease or illness "because both patient/spouse incongruence and support/undermining have been found to affect medical, functional, and emotional outcomes … [and that] dissimilarities in partners' illness perceptions are often related to patient and/or spouse distress or well-being…. These findings underscore the importance of attending to both partners' perceptions when planning interventions aimed at improving recovery from, and adjustment to, illness" (p. 781).

Orsmond, Krauss, and Seltzer (2004) conducted a study of 235 adolescents and adults with autism who lived at home. Many of the study participants reported no peer relationships outside of pre-arranged settings. The researchers' findings of low rates of friendship indicate that problems developing and maintaining friendships continue through adulthood. It is uncertain if individuals with autism desire or are motivated to form friendships, but studies on higher functioning individuals with autism indicate greater feelings of loneliness and lower quality friendships. Taking a walk and exercising were the most common recreational activities of engagement and they do not require social interaction. Second was engaging in a hobby where the participants had highly intense interests and pre-occupations. Third was attending religious services. Socializing with others was least common, and even that may have been organized by parents or guardians. Younger individuals with fewer social impairments had more peer relationships and more participation in social and recreational activities. Environmental factors however, were not predictive of peer relationships. "This pattern of individual but not environmental predictors points to the durability of the core social deficit of autism throughout the life course" (p. 253). Although not predictive, the extent to which their mothers engaged in similar activities, greater functional independence, less social impairment, and internalizing behavior problems were associated with greater participation in social and recreational activities. "It may be that internalizing behavior (such as being withdrawn) may even facilitate participation [because]… individuals who are withdrawn may be able to be taken to social activities without active resistance, whereas other individuals with autism may more actively avoid social contexts" (p. 254). Additionally, a greater number of community services received and being in or having been in an inclusive school program were associated with greater participation in social and recreational activities indicating that the inclusive environments may "set the stage" for greater participation in non-school based activities.

Lippold and Burns (2009) conducted a study of 30 adults with mild intellectual disability (ID) and 17 adults with physical disabilities (PD). Findings indicated that adults with ID had more restricted social networks, usually limited to family, friends with ID, and staff. They had fewer people in their social circle compared to the PD group, even though the ID group participated in more activities then the individuals with PD. "This finding demonstrates that it is possible to be very present and active in the community while developing and maintaining few relationships other than with staff who accompany such activities" (p. 470). The authors suggest that interventions aimed to improve quality social relationships in the ID population should consider "a focus not on increasing opportunities but on identifying existing or potential critical relationships and ensuring these are fostered" (p. 471).

*Cross References*

In *Recreational Therapy for Specific Diagnoses and Conditions, First Edition*, ICF code e3 Support and Relationships and its subcategories are listed in 28 chapters: Amputation and Prosthesis, Attention-Deficit/Hyperactivity Disorder, Autism Spectrum Disorder, Back Disorders and Back Pain, Borderline Personality Disorder, Burns, Cerebral Palsy, Cerebrovascular Accident, Epilepsy, Feeding and Eating Disorders, Fibromyalgia and Juvenile Fibromyalgia, Hearing Loss, Heart Disease, Intellectual Disability, Neurocognitive Disorders, Obesity, Oppositional Defiant Disorder and Conduct Disorder, Osteoarthritis, Post-Traumatic Stress Disorder, Pressure Ulcers, Rheumatoid Arthritis, Schizophrenia Spectrum and Other Psychotic Disorders, Spina Bifida, Spinal Cord Injury, Substance-Related Disorders, Total Joint Replacement, Traumatic Brain Injury, and Visual Impairments and Blindness.

In *Recreational Therapy Basics, Techniques, and Interventions, First Edition*, treatment for ICF code e3 Support and Relationships and its subcategories are discussed in eight chapters: Education and Counseling, Adaptive Sports, Bibliotherapy, Community Participation: Integration, Transitioning, and Inclusion, Disability Rights: Education and Advocacy, Medical Play and Preparation, Reality Orientation, and Therapeutic Relationships.

### e310 Immediate Family

Individuals related by birth, marriage, and other relationship recognized by the culture as immediate family, such as spouses, partners, parents, siblings, children, foster parents, adoptive parents, and grandparents.

Exclusions: extended family (e315); personal care providers and personal assistants (e340)

How to measure this group's level of support and relationships is discussed at the end of the chapter.

*Cross References*

In *Recreational Therapy for Specific Diagnoses and Conditions, First Edition*, ICF code e310 Immediate Family is listed in six chapters: Autism Spectrum Disorder, Heart Disease, Obesity, Osteoarthritis, Post-Traumatic Stress Disorder, and Rheumatoid Arthritis.

In *Recreational Therapy Basics, Techniques, and Interventions, First Edition*, treatment for ICF code e310 Immediate Family is discussed in two chapters: Medical Play and Preparation and Reality Orientation.

### e315 Extended Family

Individuals related through family or marriage or other relationships recognized by the culture as extended family, such as aunts, uncles, nephew, and nieces.

Exclusions: immediate family (e310)

How to measure this group's level of support and relationships is discussed at the end of the chapter.

*Cross References*

In *Recreational Therapy for Specific Diagnoses and Conditions, First Edition*, ICF code e315 Extended Family is listed in one chapter: Post-Traumatic Stress Disorder.

In *Recreational Therapy Basics, Techniques, and Interventions, First Edition*, there are no references for ICF code e315 Extended Family.

### e320 Friends

Individuals who are close and ongoing participants in relationships characterized by trust and mutual support.

How to measure this group's level of support and relationships is discussed at the end of the chapter.

*Cross References*

In *Recreational Therapy for Specific Diagnoses and Conditions, First Edition*, ICF code e320 Friends is listed in four chapters: Autism Spectrum Disorder,

Heart Disease, Obesity, and Schizophrenia Spectrum and Other Psychotic Disorders.

In *Recreational Therapy Basics, Techniques, and Interventions, First Edition*, there are no references for ICF code e320 Friends.

### e325 Acquaintances, Peers, Colleagues, Neighbors, and Community Members

Individuals who are familiar to each other as acquaintances, peers, colleagues, neighbors, and community members, in situations of work, school, recreation, or other aspects of life, and who share demographic features such as age, gender, religious creed, or ethnicity or pursue common interests.

Exclusions: associations and organizational services (e5550)

How to measure this group's level of support and relationships is discussed at the end of the chapter.

#### Cross References

In *Recreational Therapy for Specific Diagnoses and Conditions, First Edition*, ICF code e325 Acquaintances, Peers, Colleagues, Neighbors, and Community Members is listed in one chapter: Heart Disease.

In *Recreational Therapy Basics, Techniques, and Interventions, First Edition*, there are no references for ICF code e325 Acquaintances, Peers, Colleagues, Neighbors, and Community Members.

### e330 People in Positions of Authority

Individuals who have decision-making responsibilities for others and who have socially defined influence or power based on their social, economic, cultural, or religious roles in society, such as teachers, employers, supervisors, religious leaders, substitute decision-makers, guardians, or trustees.

How to measure this group's level of support and relationships is discussed at the end of the chapter.

#### Cross References

In *Recreational Therapy for Specific Diagnoses and Conditions, First Edition*, ICF code e330 People in Positions of Authority is listed in one chapter: Cerebral Palsy.

In *Recreational Therapy Basics, Techniques, and Interventions, First Edition*, there are no references for ICF code e330 People in Positions of Authority.

### e335 People in Subordinate Positions

Individuals whose day-to-day life is influenced by people in positions of authority in work, school, or other settings, such as students, workers, and members of a religious group.

Exclusions: immediate family (e310)

How to measure this group's level of support and relationships is discussed at the end of the chapter.

#### Cross References

In *Recreational Therapy for Specific Diagnoses and Conditions, First Edition*, there are no references for ICF code e335 People in Subordinate Positions.

In *Recreational Therapy Basics, Techniques, and Interventions, First Edition*, there are no references for ICF code e335 People in Subordinate Positions.

### e340 Personal Care Providers and Personal Assistants

Individuals who provide services as required to support individuals in their daily activities and maintenance of performance at work, education, or other life situation, provided either through public or private funds, or else on a voluntary basis, such as providers of support for home-making and maintenance, personal assistants, transport assistants, paid help, nannies, and others who function as primary caregivers.

Exclusions: immediate family (e310); extended family (e315); friends (e320); general social; support services (e5750); health professionals (e355)

How to measure this group's level of support and relationships is discussed at the end of the chapter.

#### Cross References

In *Recreational Therapy for Specific Diagnoses and Conditions, First Edition*, ICF code e340 Personal Care Providers and Personal Assistants is listed in five chapters: Autism Spectrum Disorder, Borderline Personality Disorder, Hearing Loss, Pressure Ulcers, and Total Joint Replacement.

In *Recreational Therapy Basics, Techniques, and Interventions, First Edition*, treatment for ICF code e340 Personal Care Providers and Personal Assistants is discussed in one chapter: Therapeutic Relationships.

### e345 Strangers

Individuals who are unfamiliar and unrelated, or those who have not yet established a relationship or association, including persons unknown to the individual but who are sharing a life situation with them, such as substitute teachers, co-workers, or care providers.

How to measure this group's level of support and relationships is discussed at the end of the chapter.

*Cross References*

In *Recreational Therapy for Specific Diagnoses and Conditions, First Edition*, there are no references for ICF code e345 Strangers.

In *Recreational Therapy Basics, Techniques, and Interventions, First Edition*, there are no references for ICF code e345 Strangers.

### e350 Domesticated Animals

Animals that provide physical, emotional, or psychological support, such as pets (dogs, cats, birds, fish, etc.) and animals for personal mobility and transportation.

Exclusions: animals (e2201); assets (e165)

How to measure this group's level of support and relationships is discussed at the end of the chapter.

*Cross References*

In *Recreational Therapy for Specific Diagnoses and Conditions, First Edition*, there are no references for ICF code e350 Domesticated Animals.

In *Recreational Therapy Basics, Techniques, and Interventions, First Edition*, there are no references for ICF code e350 Domesticated Animals.

### e355 Health Professionals

All service providers working within the context of the health system, such as doctors, nurses, physiotherapists, occupational therapists, speech therapists, audiologists, orthotist-prosthetists, and medical social workers.

Exclusions: other professionals (e360)

How to measure this group's level of support and relationships is discussed at the end of the chapter.

*Cross References*

In *Recreational Therapy for Specific Diagnoses and Conditions, First Edition*, ICF code e355 Health

Professionals is listed in eight chapters: Amputation and Prosthesis, Borderline Personality Disorder, Hearing Loss, Heart Disease, Intellectual Disability, Pressure Ulcers, Rheumatoid Arthritis, and Visual Impairments and Blindness.

In *Recreational Therapy Basics, Techniques, and Interventions, First Edition*, treatment for ICF code e355 Health Professionals is discussed in two chapters: Community Participation: Integration, Transitioning, and Inclusion and Reality Orientation.

### e360 Other Professionals

All service providers working outside the health system, including lawyers, social workers, teachers, architects, and designers.

Exclusions: health professionals (e355)

How to measure this group's level of support and relationships is discussed at the end of the chapter.

*Cross References*

In *Recreational Therapy for Specific Diagnoses and Conditions, First Edition*, there are no references for ICF code e360 Other Professionals.

In *Recreational Therapy Basics, Techniques, and Interventions, First Edition*, there are no references for ICF code e360 Other Professionals.

### e398 Support and Relationships, Other Specified

### e399 Support and Relationships, Unspecified

Each of these groups has its own type of relationship with the client. The question therapists ask is how much the support acts as a facilitator for or barrier to the client. In the following discussion the type of support is divided into physical or emotional and psychological.

*Physical Support*

Physical support refers to hands-on physical assistance provided to the client such as helping the client to walk, transfer, dress, or bathe. It also refers to physical support beyond physical assistance, which does not require physical contact with the client, such as help with carrying shopping bags, providing transportation, picking up tennis balls after play, putting down the kneeler at church, or running errands.

Hands-on and non-hands-on physical support can greatly affect a client's ability to engage in activities. In some cases, physical support can be a facilitator because it contributes in a positive manner to the level of difficulty that a client has with an activity. In other cases it can be a barrier because it contributes in a negative manner to the level of difficulty that a client has with an activity. Examples are provided below.

### Example of Physical Support as a Facilitator

A client has moderate difficulty with d7200 Forming Relationships. When in social situations her friend gives her non-verbal cues when she begins to say something that is not appropriate. This support decreases the level of difficulty that the client has with d7200 Forming Relationships to mild difficulty. The scoring of d7200 Forming Relationships that reflects the impact of e320 Friends would look like this: d7200.1 _ _ 2; e320+1. The first qualifier of d7200 Forming Relationships is the level of difficulty that the client has in her current life situation with all available supports and constraints (performance with assistance). The fourth qualifier reflects her level of difficulty in a real-life setting when support is not provided (performance without assistance). The e-code was rated a +1 because it lowered her level of difficulty by one level. Thinking of this as emotional and psychological support would also be acceptable. The scoring here reflects the preference to look at the physical nature of the cues. The scoring is the same in either case.

### Example of Physical Support as a Barrier

A client has minimal difficulty with walking outdoors (d465 Moving Around Using Equipment). His wife is very anxious about him walking outdoors because she is afraid that he will fall. Consequently, she holds tightly onto his arm when they walk outside. This gets in the way of him being able to correctly hold onto the walker and actually increases the level of difficulty that he has with d465 Moving Around Using Equipment to moderate difficulty. The scoring of d465 Moving Around Using Equipment that reflects the impact of e310 Immediate Family would look like this: d465.2 _ _ 1; e310.1. The first qualifier of d465 Moving Around Using Equipment is the level of difficulty that the client has in his current life situation with all available supports and constraints (performance with assistance). The fourth

qualifier reflects his level of difficulty in his current life situation when support is not provided (performance without assistance). The e-code was rated a .1 because it increased his level of difficulty with the task by one level.

### Emotional and Psychological Support

Emotional and psychological support can contribute just as much as physical support to level of difficulty. This includes verbal support such as encouraging words, motivational speeches, and guidance without judgment, as well as non-verbal support such as listening, a smile, a pat on the shoulder, sitting with someone, holding hands, and embracing. Animals (e350 Domesticated Animals) provide emotional and psychological support through unconditional love, physical contact, and dependency. Positive feelings about oneself can occur from being needed and being able to provide needed care.

### Example of Emotional and Psychological Support as a Facilitator

A client is shy in peer group play in the hospital, which limits her level of engagement to severe difficulty. When the therapist provides encouraging words and gently guides her into group play, her level of difficulty with engagement decreases to mild difficulty. The scoring of d9200 Play that reflects the impact e355 Health Professionals would look like this: d9200._ 3 1 _; e355+2. The second qualifier is the level of difficulty that a client has in a standard clinic environment without support from the therapist (capacity without assistance). The third qualifier reflects the client's level of difficulty in a standard clinic environment when support is provided by the therapist (capacity with assistance). The e-code was rated a +2 because it decreases her level of difficulty by two levels.

### Example of Emotional and Psychological Support as a Barrier

A client with a progressive chronic illness is struggling to cope with the rapid changes in her life. Her aunt, although believing that she is being helpful, forces the client to problem solve and account for all of her activities. She asks questions like "How are you going to care for your children?" or "Why are you doing so much?" When her aunt is not at the hospital, her level of difficulty with coping is mild. When her aunt comes to the hospital and offers unwanted input, her level of difficulty with coping becomes severe. The scoring of d2401 Handling Stress that reflects the impact of e315 Extended Family would look like this: d2401._ 1 3 _; e315.2. The second qualifier is the client's current level of difficulty handling stress in a standard clinic environment without support (capacity without assistance). The third qualifier reflects her level of difficulty in a standard clinic environment when support is provided (capacity with assistance). The e-code is rated a .2 because it increases the client's level of difficulty by two levels.

### References

Bambara, J. K., Turner, A. P., Williams, R. M., & Haselkorn, J. K. (2011). Perceived social support and depression among veterans with multiple sclerosis. *Disability and Rehabilitation, 33*(1), 1-8.

Benyamini, Y., Medalion, B., & Garfinkel, D. (2007). Patient and spouse perceptions of the patient's heart disease and their associations with received and provided social support and undermining. *Psychology and Health, 22*(7), 765-785.

Lippold, T. & Burns, J. (2009). Social support and intellectual disabilities: A comparison between social networks with intellectual disability and those with physical disability. *Journal of Intellectual Disability Research, 53*(5), 463-473.

Orsmond, G. I., Krauss, M. W., & Seltzer, M. M. (2004). Peer relationships and social and recreational activities among adolescents and adults with autism. *Journal of Autism and Developmental Disorders, 34*(3), 245-256.

# Chapter 4 Attitudes

This chapter is about the attitudes that are the observable consequences of customs, practices, ideologies, values, norms, factual beliefs, and religious beliefs. These attitudes influence individual behavior and social life at all levels, from interpersonal relationships and community associations to political, economic, and legal structures; for example, individual or societal attitudes about a person's trustworthiness and value as a human being that may motivate positive, honorific practices or negative and discriminatory practices (e.g., stigmatizing, stereotyping, and marginalizing or neglect of the person). The attitudes classified are those of people external to the person whose situation is being described. They are not those of the person themselves. The individual attitudes are categorized according to the kinds of relationships listed in e3 Support and Relationships. Values and beliefs are not coded separately from attitudes as they are assumed to be the driving forces behind the attitudes.

## Sample Scoring for Attitudes

- A client's motivation for engagement in therapy is poor (severe impairment = 3). When her sister attends therapy sessions, the client's motivation improves to mild impairment (1). The scoring of b1301 Motivation to reflect the impact of e410 Individual Attitudes of Immediate Family Members as a facilitator would look like this: b1301.3; e410+2. The qualifier for motivation reflects the client's average level of impairment for motivation (severe impairment = 3). The e-code is rated a +2 because the positive attitude of the client's sister improves the client's motivation impairment by two levels from a 3 to a 1.

This chapter is about the attitudes of others as they impact the level of impairment or difficulty that a client has with a particular function or activity. It is not about the attitudes of the client.

In the code descriptions, the term attitude is described using the words "opinion," "belief," and "value." The chapter description notes that beliefs and values are among the driving force of attitudes. Consequently, this chapter incorporates a broad spectrum of beliefs, values, and opinions from individuals and groups, including customs, practices, rules, abstract systems of values and normative beliefs, moral philosophies, moral and religious behavior or etiquette, religious doctrine and resulting norms and practices, and norms governing rituals or social gatherings. Although it is not reflected in the ICF, there are differences in the meaning of attitudes, beliefs, and values.

Looking at the number of individuals and groups listed in this chapter, as well as the descriptions of each code, brings an awareness of the number of people and groups that can facilitate or hinder impairment and task difficulty. Addressing attitudinal barriers has been a long-standing component of recreational therapy practice in both community and treatment settings.

## Assessment of Attitudes

Basic information related to possible sources of attitudinal influence is obtained during the intake and initial assessment. Knowing and synthesizing this information provides the therapist with a springboard for identifying attitudinal influences. This includes the client's:

- *Religion*: Knowing a client's religion and the extent to which the client practices religious beliefs helps the therapist understand the actions and behaviors of the client. It also helps the therapist to identify possible sources of influence.
- *Culture*: Knowing the culture that the client lives in helps the therapist understand the actions and behaviors of the client. A therapist cannot assume that a client of a particular cultural descent practices that culture. For example, a client may be of Chinese descent, but live an Americanized life. Identifying the client's culture of practice will help the therapist to identify possible sources of influence.
- *Living situation*: Knowing who lives with the client tells the therapist possible people of influence.
- *Age*: Knowing the client's age helps the therapist identify who is likely to have the most influence

over the client. For children, parental attitudes are more influential than peers. For adolescents, attitudes of classmates are more influential than parents, although parental attitudes still weigh in heavily. And in the college years, peers' attitudes far outweigh parental attitudes.

Healthcare facilities, although non-discriminatory, often predominantly serve a particular group of people because of their locations. Through hands-on experience and their own research, therapists become aware of particular norms related to the population they serve, including religion, culture, and age. For example, African-American women typically have a strong spirituality. Since they are adults, self-esteem theories say that their likely group of influence is similar peers, especially other members of the church. Consequently, a therapist who is assigned to work with an African-American adult woman should plan to explore the effect of religion (e465 Social Norms, Practices, and Ideologies) and friends (e420 Individual Attitudes of Friends) on impairments and difficulties.

Therapists additionally explore attitudinal influences by listening closely to verbalizations, observing behavior, and asking exploratory questions to better understand sources of influence. If a source of influence can be identified, then there is a chance that it can be used. For example, a client is out at a mall for community integration training with his therapist. He is normally a very talkative and assertive person. The therapist notices that he is avoiding asking questions of people in the community (e.g., "I'll just figure it out myself.", "She looks too busy.", "No, I really just don't want to.") and seems withdrawn. The therapist brings this change in behavior to the attention of the client and prompts the client to analyze the variables influencing his behavior (e.g., "Joe, it seems that you are trying to avoid talking to the people in the stores? This isn't like you. You are usually very talkative and outgoing. Do you notice this? What do you think is causing this change?"). The therapist finds out that the client has had several recent bad experiences with store employees talking down to him. The client says that he would rather just avoid the interactions altogether than feel like a "little kid." This is an example of how e445 Individual Attitudes of Strangers can be a barrier to using assertion and social interactions for getting needs met.

### Treatment of Attitudes

It is important to note that the attitudes that are being discussed are not the attitudes of the client, but those of people interacting with the client. Therefore, the focus of the treatment is not necessarily the attitudes, which the therapist may not be able to influence. What the therapist can do is assist the client in learning skills to maximize benefits and minimize limitations that come with attitudes of those around them.

If the identified attitude is negatively contributing to an impairment or engagement in a life activity, the therapist seeks to decrease the extent of the barrier and/or increase the client's coping skills for the barrier to positively increase functioning. For example, the therapist might educate people at the facility about proper etiquette when talking to a client who uses a wheelchair. A therapist can also teach a client coping skills for dealing with the actions of others that would provide a better outcome, such as how to view behaviors of others from different viewpoints and how to use simple, non-aggressive remarks to change the behavior of others or, at least, increase their awareness of their behavior.

On the other hand, if attitudes of specific individuals or groups are facilitators, the therapist may find it helpful to incorporate the specific people in the client's treatment to further facilitate progress. For example, if the positive attitude of the client's sister is a facilitator for motivation, then asking her to attend therapy sessions could be beneficial. Highlighting the positive influences of a person or group to the client can also be helpful so that the client and therapist can discuss how to maintain involvement with the person or group for continued benefits. Finally, clients are encouraged to consider the impact of life changes on these resources. For example, the client may lose the positive influences of neighbors if the individual moves to another neighborhood.

### Evidence Review

Reviews of several studies are provided below to highlight evidence-based practice related to attitudes. This is only a sample of the evidence. A thorough review of the literature is needed to identify evidence-based practice interventions that reflect the needs and characteristics of the individual client.

Bellin and Rice (2009) conducted a cross-sectional sample of 224 siblings of youths with spina bifida ages 11 to 18 to identify key factors associated with the quality of sibling relationships. They found that that siblings who felt supported in their family were able to express themselves. They felt included and valued when there was shared decision making and open communication. These siblings reported more positive relationships with their brothers or sisters who had spina bifida, as compared to the siblings who did not attain these personal needs in their families.

Ison et al. (2010) conducted a disability awareness program for 147 school students in Australia aged nine to 11 consisting of two ninety-minute sessions held one to two weeks apart. The program used a cognitive behavioral approach. Some of the most popular parts of the program included disability simulation activities, meeting and interacting with people who have disabilities, learning about different disabilities, practicing sign language, and learning about achievements of a Paralympian. The program yielded significant improvements in disability knowledge, attitudes, and acceptance of people with disabilities.

Verdonschot et al. (2009) conducted a systematic review of the literature. Out of 236 initial hits, nine quantitative studies and two qualitative studies met the selection criteria. The researchers found that opportunities to make choices, variety and stimulation in facilities, opportunities for involvement in policy making, small facilities, opportunities for autonomy, vocational services, family involvement and social support, assistive technology, and positive staff attitude had a positive impact on community leisure participation. They also found that lack of transportation and negative attitude of people in the community had a negative impact on community leisure participation.

### Cross References

In *Recreational Therapy for Specific Diagnoses and Conditions, First Edition*, ICF code e4 Attitudes and its subcategories are listed in 11 chapters: Amputation and Prosthesis, Attention-Deficit/Hyperactivity Disorder, Borderline Personality Disorder, Cerebral Palsy, Cerebrovascular Accident, Epilepsy, Obesity, Oppositional Defiant Disorder and Conduct Disorder, Schizophrenia Spectrum and Other Psychotic Disorders, Spinal Cord Injury, and Visual Impairments and Blindness.

In *Recreational Therapy Basics, Techniques, and Interventions, First Edition*, treatment for ICF code

e4 Attitudes and its subcategories are discussed in four chapters: Education and Counseling, Adaptive Sports, Disability Rights: Education and Advocacy, and Leisure Education and Counseling.

### e410 Individual Attitudes of Immediate Family Members

General or specific opinions and beliefs of immediate family members about the person or about other matters (e.g., social, political, and economic issues), that influence individual behavior and actions.

How to score this group's attitudes is discussed at the end of the chapter.

### Cross References

In *Recreational Therapy for Specific Diagnoses and Conditions, First Edition*, ICF code e410 Individual Attitudes of Immediate Family Members is listed in one chapter: Cerebrovascular Accident (Stroke).

In *Recreational Therapy Basics, Techniques, and Interventions, First Edition*, there are no references for ICF code e410 Individual Attitudes of Immediate Family Members.

### e415 Individual Attitudes of Extended Family Members

General or specific opinions and beliefs of extended family members about the person or about other matters (e.g., social, political, and economic issues), that influence individual behavior and actions.

How to score this group's attitudes is discussed at the end of the chapter.

### Cross References

In *Recreational Therapy for Specific Diagnoses and Conditions, First Edition*, ICF code e415 Individual Attitudes of Extended Family Members is listed in one chapter: Attention-Deficit/Hyperactivity Disorder.

In *Recreational Therapy Basics, Techniques, and Interventions, First Edition*, there are no references for ICF code e415 Individual Attitudes of Extended Family Members.

### e420 Individual Attitudes of Friends

General or specific opinions and beliefs of friends about the person or about other matters (e.g., social, political, and economic issues), that influence individual behavior and actions.

How to score this group's attitudes is discussed at the end of the chapter.

***Cross References***

In *Recreational Therapy for Specific Diagnoses and Conditions, First Edition*, there are no references for ICF code e420 Individual Attitudes of Friends.

In *Recreational Therapy Basics, Techniques, and Interventions, First Edition*, there are no references for ICF code e420 Individual Attitudes of Friends.

### e425 Individual Attitudes of Acquaintances, Peers, Colleagues, Neighbors, and Community Members

General or specific opinions and beliefs of acquaintances, peers, colleagues, neighbors, and community members about the person or about other matters (e.g., social, political, and economic issues), that influence individual behavior and actions.

How to score this group's attitudes is discussed at the end of the chapter.

***Cross References***

In *Recreational Therapy for Specific Diagnoses and Conditions, First Edition*, ICF code e425 Individual Attitudes of Acquaintances, Peers, Colleagues, Neighbors, and Community Members is listed in one chapter: Attention-Deficit/Hyperactivity Disorder.

In *Recreational Therapy Basics, Techniques, and Interventions, First Edition*, there are no references for ICF code e425 Individual Attitudes of Acquaintances, Peers, Colleagues, Neighbors, and Community Members.

### e430 Individual Attitudes of People in Positions of Authority

General or specific opinions and beliefs of people in positions of authority about the person or about other matters (e.g., social, political, and economic issues), that influence individual behavior and actions.

How to score this group's attitudes is discussed at the end of the chapter.

***Cross References***

In *Recreational Therapy for Specific Diagnoses and Conditions, First Edition*, there are no references

for ICF code e430 Individual Attitudes of People in Positions of Authority.

In *Recreational Therapy Basics, Techniques, and Interventions, First Edition*, there are no references for ICF code e430 Individual Attitudes of People in Positions of Authority.

### e435 Individual Attitudes of People in Subordinate Positions

General or specific opinions and beliefs of people in subordinate positions about the person or about other matters (e.g., social, political, and economic issues), that influence individual behavior and actions.

How to score this group's attitudes is discussed at the end of the chapter.

***Cross References***

In *Recreational Therapy for Specific Diagnoses and Conditions, First Edition*, there are no references for ICF code e435 Individual Attitudes of People in Subordinate Positions.

In *Recreational Therapy Basics, Techniques, and Interventions, First Edition*, there are no references for ICF code e435 Individual Attitudes of People in Subordinate Positions.

### e440 Individual Attitudes of Personal Care Providers and Personal Assistants

General or specific opinions and beliefs of personal care providers and personal assistants about the person or about other matters (e.g., social, political, and economic issues), that influence individual behavior and actions.

How to score this group's attitudes is discussed at the end of the chapter.

***Cross References***

In *Recreational Therapy for Specific Diagnoses and Conditions, First Edition*, there are no references for ICF code e440 Individual Attitudes of Personal Care Providers and Personal Assistants.

In *Recreational Therapy Basics, Techniques, and Interventions, First Edition*, there are no references for ICF code e440 Individual Attitudes of Personal Care Providers and Personal Assistants.

### e445 Individual Attitudes of Strangers

General or specific opinions and beliefs of strangers about the person or about other matters (e.g., social, political, and economic issues), that influence individual behavior and actions.

How to score this group's attitudes is discussed at the end of the chapter.

*Cross References*

In *Recreational Therapy for Specific Diagnoses and Conditions, First Edition*, there are no references for ICF code e445 Individual Attitudes of Strangers.

In *Recreational Therapy Basics, Techniques, and Interventions, First Edition*, there are no references for ICF code e445 Individual Attitudes of Strangers.

### e450 Individual Attitudes of Health Professionals

General or specific opinions and beliefs of health professionals about the person or about other matters (e.g., social, political, and economic issues), that influence individual behavior and actions.

How to score this group's attitudes is discussed at the end of the chapter.

*Cross References*

In *Recreational Therapy for Specific Diagnoses and Conditions, First Edition*, ICF code e450 Individual Attitudes of Health Professionals is listed in two chapters: Borderline Personality Disorder and Visual Impairments and Blindness.

In *Recreational Therapy Basics, Techniques, and Interventions, First Edition*, there are no references for ICF code e450 Individual Attitudes of Health Professionals.

### e455 Individual Attitudes of Health-Related Professionals

General or specific opinions and beliefs of health-related professionals about the person or about other matters (e.g., social, political, and economic issues), that influence individual behavior and actions.

How to score this group's attitudes is discussed at the end of the chapter.

*Cross References*

In *Recreational Therapy for Specific Diagnoses and Conditions, First Edition*, there are no references for ICF code e455 Individual Attitudes of Health-Related Professionals.

In *Recreational Therapy Basics, Techniques, and Interventions, First Edition*, there are no references

for ICF code e455 Individual Attitudes of Health-Related Professionals.

### e460 Societal Attitudes

General or specific opinions and beliefs generally held by people of a culture, society, subcultural, or other social group about other individuals or about other social, political, and economic issues, that influence group or individual behavior and actions.

How to score societal attitudes is discussed at the end of the chapter.

*Cross References*

In *Recreational Therapy for Specific Diagnoses and Conditions, First Edition*, ICF code e460 Societal Attitudes is listed in one chapter: Schizophrenia Spectrum and Other Psychotic Disorders.

In *Recreational Therapy Basics, Techniques, and Interventions, First Edition*, there are no references for ICF code e460 Societal Attitudes.

### e465 Social Norms, Practices, and Ideologies

Customs, practices, rules, and abstract systems of values and normative beliefs (e.g., ideologies, normative world views, and moral philosophies) that arise within social contexts and that affect or create societal and individual practices and behaviors, such as social norms of moral and religious behavior or etiquette; religious doctrine and resulting norms and practices, norms governing rituals or social gathering.

How to score social aspects of attitudes is discussed at the end of the chapter.

*Cross References*

In *Recreational Therapy for Specific Diagnoses and Conditions, First Edition*, there are no references for ICF code e465 Social Norms, Practices, and Ideologies.

In *Recreational Therapy Basics, Techniques, and Interventions, First Edition*, there are no references for ICF code e465 Social Norms, Practices, and Ideologies.

### e498 Attitudes, Other Specified

### e499 Attitudes, Unspecified

Scoring attitudes as barriers or facilitators to impairment and life activities can be done as shown in these examples.

### Example of Attitudes as a Barrier

A 23-year-old client with tetraplegia attends college. When attending classes, he has a personal care attendant with him at all times to assist with overcoming barriers, self-care, and schoolwork. When the client tries to strike up a conversation with other students outside of class, the attendant rushes him along and says, "We don't have time for this." When the attendant is not present, for example taking a break to use the bathroom, the client has no difficulty d9205 Socializing. When the attendant is present, the client has complete difficulty socializing. The scoring of d9205 Socializing that reflects the impact of e440 Individual Attitudes of Personal Care Providers and Personal Assistants as a barrier would look like this: d9205.4 _ _ 0; e440.4. The first qualifier reflects the level of difficulty that the client has in his current life situations given all available supports and constraints (performance with assistance). The fourth qualifier reflects his level of difficulty in his current life situation when assistance is not provided (performance without assistance). The e-code was rated a .4 because the personal care assistant increased the student's level of difficulty with socializing by four levels.

### Example of Attitudes as a Facilitator

A client's motivation for engagement in therapy is poor (severe impairment = 3). When her sister attends therapy sessions, the client's motivation improves to mild impairment (1). The scoring of b1301 Motivation to reflect the impact of e410 Individual Attitudes of Immediate Family Members as a facilitator would look like this: b1301.3; e410+2. The qualifier for motivation reflects the client's average level of impairment for motivation (severe impairment = 3). The e-code is rated a +2 because the positive attitude of the client's sister improves the client's motivation impairment by two levels.

### References

Bellin, M. H. & Rice, K. M. (2009). Individual, family, and peer factors associated with quality of sibling relationships in families of youths with spinal bifida. *Journal of Family Psychology, 23*(1), 39-47.

Ison, N., McIntyre, S., Rothery, S., Smithers-Sheedy, H., Goldsmith, S., Parsonage, S., & Foy, L. (2010). "Just like you": A disability awareness programme for children that enhanced knowledge, attitudes, and acceptance: Pilot study findings. *Developmental Neurorehabilitation, 13*(5), 360-368.

Verdonschot, M. M. L., deWitte, L. P., Reichrath, E., Buntinx, W. H. E., & Curfs, L. M. G. (2009). Impact of environmental factors on community participation of persons with intellectual disability: A systematic review. *Journal of Intellectual Disability Research, 53*(1), 54-64.

# Chapter 5 Services, Systems, and Policies

This chapter is about:

1. Services that provide benefits, structured programs, and operations, in various sectors of society, designed to meet the needs of individuals. (Included in services are the people who provide them). Services may be public, private, or voluntary, and may be established at a local, community, regional, state, provincial, national, or international level by individuals, associations, organizations, agencies, or governments. The goods provided by these services may be general or adapted and specially designed.

2. Systems that are administrative control and organizational mechanisms, and are established by governments at the local, regional, national, and international levels, or by other recognized authorities. These systems are designed to organize, control, and monitor services that provide benefits, structured programs and operations in various sectors of society.

3. Policies constituted by rules, regulations, conventions, and standards established by governments at the local, regional, national, and international levels, or by other recognized authorities. Policies govern and regulate the systems that organize, control, and monitor services, structured programs, and operations in various sectors of society.

### *Sample Scoring of Services, Systems, and Policies*

- A client who lives in a rural area does not have access to transportation (e5400 Transportation Services). Consequently, this completely impedes his ability to socialize with friends (d9205 Socializing). If someone drives him to see his friends he has no difficulty. Since the lack of transportation increases his level of difficulty socializing by four levels from a 0 to a 4, it is coded as a .4. The correct scoring of d9205 Socializing would look like this: d9205.4 _ _ 0; e5400.4

- A client wants to volunteer at a local pet rescue facility (d855 Non-Remunerative Employment). The entrance to the facility is not accessible. The recreational therapist educated the client about the Americans with Disabilities Act (ADA) and then encouraged the client to contact the facility to see if they would be able to make the entrance accessible (e5452 Civil Protection Policies). The owners of the facility agreed to put a portable ramp outside when she comes to volunteer. Due to the ADA, the client now has no difficulties accessing the building and volunteering. If the ADA did not exist, the facility would most likely not make the change and the client would not be able to volunteer. Consequently, the ADA improved her ability to volunteer at the facility by four levels (improved from a 4 to a 0). The correct scoring of d855 Non-Remunerative Employment would look like this: d855.0 _ _ 4; e5452+4

Recreational therapists are aware of and educate clients about services, systems, and policies as they relate to participation in leisure and community life. They routinely advocate for services, systems, and policies that enhance disability rights, quality of life, and full participation in leisure and community life. When services, systems, and policies (whether absent or ill devised) impact participation in life, resultant dysfunction can occur.

### *Assessment of Services, Systems, and Policies*

During the recreational therapy assessment, the therapist analyzes the client's current, past, and future engagement in leisure and community activities. Part of this process involves the assessment of environ-

mental factors that facilitate and/or hinder participation. These include services, systems, and policies.

### *Treatment of Services, Systems, and Policies*

If a service, system, or policy is identified as a barrier to engagement in a life activity, recreational therapists provide the client with relevant information, such as information on the Americans with Disabilities Act, review the basics of the information provided, and practice application of the information to real-life situations. If a service, system, or policy is outside of the scope of the therapist's knowledge, the therapist finds other professionals, such as a social worker or case manager, who can intervene and provide the client with further guidance.

*Evidence Review*

A review of one study is provided below to highlight evidence-based practice related to services, systems, and policies. This is only a sample of the evidence. A thorough review of the literature is needed to identify evidence-based practice interventions that reflect the needs and characteristics of the individual client.

Hammel et al. (2006) conducted a participatory action research study with 20 adults who had a stroke. The study aimed at identifying barriers and supports to community living and participation. The researchers found "environmental and system level barriers, as well as effective strategies for promoting participation via environmental modification and systems level changes" (p. 43). In regards to system level barriers specifically, the participants reported issues related to policies on community accessibility, lack of enforcement of the Americans with Disabilities Act, lack of guidelines in policies for cognitive and communication access, and lack of programs offering discounted or free participation benefits. Participants additionally noted that transportation policies and services provided by community facilities were helpful. These included preplanning access needs and being responsive to recommendations to improve access. The authors went on to say that lack of community participation is a major concern for people with disabilities because it impairs function, as well as limits freedom, control, societal inclusion, community membership, and civil rights.

*Cross References*

In *Recreational Therapy for Specific Diagnoses and Conditions, First Edition*, ICF code e5 Services, Systems, and Policies and its subcategories are listed in 13 chapters: Amputation and Prosthesis, Borderline Personality Disorder, Burns, Cerebral Palsy, Epilepsy, Hearing Loss, Obesity, Osteoarthritis, Rheumatoid Arthritis, Schizophrenia Spectrum and Other Psychotic Disorders, Spinal Cord Injury, Substance-Related Disorders, and Visual Impairments and Blindness.

In *Recreational Therapy Basics, Techniques, and Interventions, First Edition*, treatment for ICF code e5 Services, Systems, and Policies and its subcategories are discussed in three chapters: Education and Counseling, Adaptive Sports, and Disability Rights: Education and Advocacy.

## e510 Services, Systems, and Policies for the Production of Consumer Goods

Services, systems, and policies that govern and provide for the production of objects and products consumed or used by people.

- *e5100 Services for the Production of Consumer Goods*
  Services and programs for the collection, creation, production, and manufacturing of consumer goods and products, such as for products and technology used for mobility, communication, education, transportation, employment, and housework, including those who provide these services.

  Exclusions: education and training services (e5850); communication services (e5350); e1 Products and Technology

- *e5101 Systems for the Production of Consumer Goods*
  Administrative control and monitoring mechanisms, such as regional, national, or international organizations that set standards (e.g., International Organization for Standardization) and consumer bodies, that govern the collection, creation, production, and manufacturing of consumer goods and products.

- *e5102 Policies for the Production of Consumer Goods*
  Legislation, regulations, and standards for the collection, creation, production, and manufacturing of consumer goods and products, such as food and drug regulations.

- *e5108 Services, Systems, and Policies for the Production of Consumer Goods, Other Specified*
- *e5109 Services, Systems, and Policies for the Production of Consumer Goods, Unspecified*
  Recreational therapists advocate for services, systems, and policies related to the production of consumer goods, such as adaptive equipment, mostly through support and involvement in professional organizations. If a service, system, or policy is identified as a barrier to engagement in a life activity, recreational therapists provide the client with relevant information that might be used to make a change. They also work with other health professionals who can intervene and provide further guidance. Both recreational therapists and other health professionals use

these e-codes as descriptors. If the service barrier is on a local level and pertains directly to engagement in a specific activity, the recreational therapist will commonly intervene, such as talking to the paratransit driver to clarify a scheduling policy that is troubling a client.

***Cross References***

In *Recreational Therapy for Specific Diagnoses and Conditions, First Edition*, there are no references for ICF code e510 Services, Systems, and Policies for the Production of Consumer Goods.

In *Recreational Therapy Basics, Techniques, and Interventions, First Edition*, there are no references for ICF code e510 Services, Systems, and Policies for the Production of Consumer Goods.

### *e515 Architecture and Construction Services, Systems, and Policies*

Services, systems, and policies for the design and construction of buildings, public and private.

Exclusions: open space planning services, systems, and policies (e520)

- *e5150 Architecture and Construction Services*
  Services and programs for design, construction, and maintenance of residential, commercial, industrial, and public buildings, such as house-building, the operationalization of design principles, building codes, regulations, and standards, including those who provide these services.

- *e5151 Architecture and Construction Systems*
  Administrative control and monitoring mechanisms that govern the planning, design, construction, and maintenance of residential, commercial, industrial, and public buildings, such as for implementing and monitoring building codes, construction standards, and fire and life safety standards.

- *e5152 Architecture and Construction Policies*
  Legislation, regulation, and standards that govern the planning, design, construction, and maintenance of residential, commercial, industrial, and public buildings, such as policies on building codes, construction standards, and fire and life safety standards.

- *e5158 Architecture and Construction Services, Systems, and Policies, Other Specified*
- *e5159 Architecture and Construction Services, Systems, and Policies, Unspecified*

Recreational therapists advocate for services, systems, and policies related to architecture and construction, such as accessibility issues, mostly through support and involvement in professional organizations. If a service, system, or policy is identified as a barrier to engagement in a life activity, recreational therapists provide the client with relevant information that might be used to make a change, including information about the Americans with Disabilities Act. They also work with other health professionals who can intervene and provide further guidance. Both recreational therapists and other health professionals use these e-codes as descriptors. If the service barrier is on a local level and pertains directly to engagement in a specific activity, the recreational therapist will commonly intervene, such as educating the supervisor at the recreation center about reasonable accommodations under the Americans with Disabilities Act to reduce or eliminate barriers at the center for the client.

***Cross References***

In *Recreational Therapy for Specific Diagnoses and Conditions, First Edition*, there are no references for ICF code *e515 Architecture and Construction Services, Systems, and Policies*.

In *Recreational Therapy Basics, Techniques, and Interventions, First Edition*, there are no references for ICF code *e515 Architecture and Construction Services, Systems, and Policies*.

### *e520 Open Space Planning Services, Systems, and Policies*

Services, systems, and policies for the planning, design, development, and maintenance of public lands (e.g., parks, forests, shorelines, wetlands) and private lands in the rural, suburban, and urban context.

Exclusions: architecture and construction services, systems, and policies (e515)

- *e5200 Open Space Planning Services*
  Service and programs aimed at planning, creating, and maintaining urban, suburban, rural, recreational, conservation, and environmental space, meeting and commercial open spaces

(plazas, open-air markets), and pedestrian and vehicular transportation routes for intended uses, including those who provide these services.

Exclusions: products for design, building, and construction for public (e150) and private (e155) use; products of land development (e160)

- *e5201 Open Space Planning Systems*
Administrative control and monitoring mechanisms, such as for the implementation of local, regional, or national planning acts, design codes, heritage or conservation policies, and environmental planning policy, that govern the planning, design, development, and maintenance of open space, including rural, suburban, and urban land, parks, conservation areas, and wildlife reserves.

- *e5202 Open Space Planning Policies*
Legislation, regulations, and standards that govern the planning, design, development, and maintenance of open space, including rural land, suburban land, urban land, parks, conservation areas, and wildlife reserves, such as local, regional, or national planning acts, design codes, heritage or conservation policies, and environmental planning policies.

- *e5208 Open Space Planning Services, Systems, and Policies, Other Specified*
- *e5209 Open Space Planning Services, Systems, and Policies, Unspecified*

Recreational therapists advocate for services, systems, and policies related to open space planning, such as park trails, through direct discussions with local planning offices and support and involvement in professional organizations. If a service, system, or policy is identified as a barrier to engagement in a life activity, recreational therapists provide the client with relevant information that might be used to make a change, including information about the Americans with Disabilities Act. They also work with other health professionals who can intervene and provide further guidance. Both recreational therapists and other health professionals use these e-codes as descriptors. If the service barrier is on a local level and pertains directly to engagement in a specific activity, the recreational therapist will commonly intervene, such as educating the park supervisor about reasonable accommodations under the Americans with Disabilities Act to reduce or eliminate barriers at the park for the client.

*Cross References*

In *Recreational Therapy for Specific Diagnoses and Conditions, First Edition*, ICF code e520 Open Space Planning Services, Systems, and Policies is listed in one chapter: Obesity.

In *Recreational Therapy Basics, Techniques, and Interventions, First Edition*, there are no references for ICF code e520 Open Space Planning Services, Systems, and Policies.

### e525 Housing Services, Systems, and Policies

Services, systems, and policies for the provision of shelters, dwellings, or lodging for people.

- *e5250 Housing Services*
Services and programs aimed at locating, providing, and maintaining houses or shelters for persons to live in, such as estate agencies, housing organizations, shelters for homeless people, including those who provide these services.

- *e5251 Housing Systems*
Administrative control and monitoring mechanisms that govern housing or sheltering of people, such as systems for implementing and monitoring housing policies.

- *e5252 Housing Policies*
Legislation, regulations, and standards that govern housing or sheltering of people, such as legislation and policies for determination of eligibility for housing or shelter, policies concerning government involvement in developing and maintaining housing, and policies concerning how and where housing is developed.

- *e5258 Housing Services, Systems, and Policies, Other Specified*
- *e5259 Housing Services, Systems, and Policies, Unspecified*

Recreational therapists do not typically address services, systems, and policies related to housing. However, there may be times when certain groups of recreational therapists are a part of housing advocacy, such as in the independent living movement. If a service, system, or policy is identified as a barrier to engagement in a life activity, recreational therapists provide the client with relevant information that might be used to make a change, including information about the Americans with Disabilities Act. They also work with other health professionals who can intervene and provide further guidance. Both recreational therapists and other health professionals use these e-codes as descriptors. If the service barrier is on a local level and pertains directly to engagement in a specific activity, the recreational therapist will commonly intervene. For example, a recreational therapist working in the independent living movement might advocate for a handicap parking space in front of the client's apartment by educating the apartment manager about the Americans with Disabilities Act.

### Cross References

In *Recreational Therapy for Specific Diagnoses and Conditions, First Edition*, there are no references for ICF code e525 Housing Services, Systems, and Policies.

In *Recreational Therapy Basics, Techniques, and Interventions, First Edition*, there are no references for ICF code e525 Housing Services, Systems, and Policies.

### e530 Utilities Services, Systems, and Policies

Services, systems, and policies for publicly provided utilities, such as water, fuel, electricity, sanitation, public transportation, and essential services.

Exclusion: civil protection services, systems, and policies (e545)

- *e5300 Utilities Services*
  Services and programs supplying the population as a whole with essential energy (e.g., fuel and electricity), sanitation, water, and other essential services (e.g., emergency repair services) for residential and commercial consumers, including those who provide these services.

- *e5301 Utilities Systems*
  Administrative control and monitoring mechanisms that govern the provision of utilities services, such as health and safety boards and consumer councils.

- *e5302 Utilities Policies*
  Legislation, regulations, and standards that govern the provision of utilities services, such as health and safety standards governing delivery and supply of water and fuel, sanitation practices in communities, and policies for other essential

services and supply during shortages or natural disasters.

- *e5308 Utilities Services, Systems, and Policies, Other Specified*
- *e5309 Utilities Services, Systems, and Policies, Unspecified*

Recreational therapists do not typically address services, systems, and policies related to utilities. However, there may be times when certain groups of recreational therapists are a part of utility advocacy, such as working with a mission program that advocates for better drinking water. If a service, system, or policy is identified as a barrier to engagement in a life activity, recreational therapists probably will work with other health professionals who can intervene and provide further guidance. Other health professionals will most often use these e-codes as descriptors.

### Cross References

In *Recreational Therapy for Specific Diagnoses and Conditions, First Edition*, there are no references for ICF code e530 Utilities Services, Systems, and Policies.

In *Recreational Therapy Basics, Techniques, and Interventions, First Edition*, there are no references for ICF code e530 Utilities Services, Systems, and Policies.

### e535 Communication Services, Systems, and Policies

Services, systems, and policies for the transmission and exchange of information.

- *e5350 Communication Services*
  Services and programs aimed at transmitting information by a variety of methods such as telephone, fax, surface and air mail, electronic mail, and other computer-based systems (e.g., telephone relay, teletype, teletext, and internet services), including those who provide these services.

Exclusion: media services (e5600)

- *e5351 Communication Systems*
  Administrative control and monitoring mechanisms, such as telecommunication regulation authorities and other such bodies, that govern the transmission of information by a variety of methods, including telephone, fax, surface and air

mail, electronic mail, and computer-based systems.

- *e5352 Communication Policies*
  Legislation, regulations, and standards that govern the transmission of information by a variety of methods including telephone, fax, post office, electronic mail, and computer-based systems, such as eligibility for access to communication services, requirements for a postal address, and standards for provision of telecommunications.

- *e5358 Communication Services, Systems, and Policies, Other Specified*
- *e5359 Communication Services, Systems, and Policies, Unspecified*

Recreational therapists do not typically address services, systems, and policies related to communication. If a service, system, or policy is identified as a barrier to engagement in a life activity, recreational therapists probably will work with other health professionals who can intervene and provide further guidance. Other health professionals will most often use these e-codes as descriptors. If the service barrier is on a local level and pertains directly to engagement in a specific activity, the recreational therapist will commonly intervene, such as a recreational therapist working with a client who is deaf. The therapist may place a call to the phone company to gather information on policies for setting up a TTY service for the client.

### Cross References

In *Recreational Therapy for Specific Diagnoses and Conditions, First Edition*, there are no references for ICF code e535 Communication Services, Systems, and Policies.

In *Recreational Therapy Basics, Techniques, and Interventions, First Edition*, there are no references for ICF code e535 Communication Services, Systems, and Policies.

### e540 Transportation Services, Systems, and Policies

Services, systems, and policies for enabling people or goods to move or be moved from one location to another.

- *e5400 Transportation Services*
  Services and programs aimed at moving persons or goods by road, paths, rail, air, or water, by

public or private transport, including those who provide these services.

Exclusion: Products and Technology for Personal Indoor and Outdoor Mobility and Transportation (e120)

- *e5401 Transportation Systems*
  Administrative control and monitoring mechanisms that govern the moving of persons or goods by road, paths, rail, air, or water, such as systems for determining eligibility for operating vehicles and implementation and monitoring of health and safety standards related to use of different types of transportation.

Exclusion: social security services, systems, and policies (e570)

- *e5402 Transportation Policies*
  Legislation, regulations, and standards that govern the moving of persons or goods by road, paths, rail, air, or water, such as transportation planning acts and policies, policies for the provision and access to public transportation.

- *e5408 Transportation Services, Systems, and Policies, Other Specified*
- *e5409 Transportation Services, Systems, and Policies, Unspecified*

Recreational therapists advocate for services, systems, and policies related to transportation. They also work to ensure that policies are carried out correctly. There may also be times when certain groups of recreational therapists are a part of transportation advocacy, such as in the independent living movement. If a service, system, or policy is identified as a barrier to engagement in a life activity, recreational therapists provide the client with relevant information that might be used to make a change, including information about the Americans with Disabilities Act. They also work with other health professionals who can intervene and provide further guidance. Both recreational therapists and other health professionals use these e-codes as descriptors. If the service barrier is on a local level and pertains directly to engagement in a specific activity, the recreational therapist will commonly intervene, such as a recreational therapist working in the independent living movement helping a client make a call to the local paratransit company to find out about its policies for scheduling rides.

*Cross References*

In *Recreational Therapy for Specific Diagnoses and Conditions, First Edition*, ICF code e540 Transportation Services, Systems, and Policies is listed in two chapters: Cerebral Palsy and Obesity.

In *Recreational Therapy Basics, Techniques, and Interventions, First Edition*, there are no references for ICF code e540 Transportation Services, Systems, and Policies.

## e545 Civil Protection Services, Systems, and Policies

Services, systems, and policies aimed at safeguarding people and property.

Exclusion: utilities services, systems, and policies (e530)

- *e5450 Civil Protection Services*
  Services and programs organized by the community and aimed at safeguarding people and property, such as fire, police, emergency, and ambulance services, including those who provide these services.

- *e5451 Civil Protection Systems*
  Administrative control and monitoring mechanisms that govern the safeguarding of people and property, such as systems by which provision of police, fire, emergency, and ambulance services are organized.

- *e5452 Civil Protection Policies*
  Legislation, regulations, and standards that govern the safeguarding of people and property, such as policies governing provision of police, fire, emergency, and ambulance services.

- *e5458 Civil Protection Services, Systems, and Policies, Other Specified*
- *e5459 Civil Protection Services, Systems, and Policies, Unspecified*
  Recreational therapists do not typically address services, systems, and policies related to civil protection. However, there may be times when certain groups of recreational therapists are a part of civil protection advocacy, such as in the independent living movement. If a service, system, or policy is identified as a barrier to engagement in a life activity, recreational therapists probably will work with other health professionals who can intervene and provide further guidance. Other health professionals will most

often use these e-codes as descriptors. If the service barrier is on a local level and pertains directly to engagement in a specific activity, the recreational therapist will commonly intervene. This might include a recreational therapist working in the independent living movement helping a client make a call to the local firehouse to alert the fire company that a person with a disability lives in the house so they can respond appropriately should there ever be a fire in the home.

*Cross References*

In *Recreational Therapy for Specific Diagnoses and Conditions, First Edition*, ICF code e545 Civil Protection Services, Systems, and Policies is listed in one chapter: Obesity.

In *Recreational Therapy Basics, Techniques, and Interventions, First Edition*, there are no references for ICF code e545 Civil Protection Services, Systems, and Policies.

## e550 Legal Services, Systems, and Policies

Services, systems, and policies concerning the legislation and other law of a country.

- *e5500 Legal Services*
  Services and programs aimed at providing the authority of the state as defined in law, such as courts, tribunals, and other agencies for hearing and settling civil litigation and criminal trials, attorney representation, services of notaries, mediation, arbitration, and correctional or penal facilities, including those who provide these services.

- *e5501 Legal Systems*
  Administrative control and monitoring mechanisms that govern the administration of justice, such as systems for implementing and monitoring formal rules (e.g., laws, regulations, customary law, religious law, international laws, and conventions).

- *e5502 Legal Policies*
  Legislation, regulations, and standards, such as laws, customary law, religious law, international laws and conventions, that govern the administration of justice.

- *e5508 Legal Services, Systems, and Policies, Other Specified*
- *e5509 Legal Services, Systems, and Policies, Unspecified*

Recreational therapists do not typically address services, systems, and policies related to legal services. If a service, system, or policy is identified as a barrier to engagement in a life activity, recreational therapists probably will work with other health professionals who can intervene and provide further guidance. Other health professionals will most often use these e-codes as descriptors. If the service barrier is on a local level and pertains directly to engagement in a specific activity, the recreational therapist will commonly intervene, such as a recreational therapist helping a client process a parking placard application.

### Cross References

In *Recreational Therapy for Specific Diagnoses and Conditions, First Edition*, there are no references for ICF code e550 Legal Services, Systems, and Policies.

In *Recreational Therapy Basics, Techniques, and Interventions, First Edition*, there are no references for ICF code e550 Legal Services, Systems, and Policies.

## e555 Associations and Organizational Services, Systems, and Policies

Services, systems, and policies relating to groups of people who have joined together in the pursuit of common, noncommercial interests, often with an associated membership structure.

- *e5550 Associations and Organizational Services*
  Services and programs provided by people who have joined together in the pursuit of common, noncommercial interests with people who have the same interests, where the provision of such services may be tied to membership, such as associations and organizations providing recreation and leisure, sporting, cultural, religious, and mutual aid services.

- *e5551 Associations and Organizational Systems*
  Administrative control and monitoring mechanisms that govern the relationships and activities of people coming together with common noncommercial interests and the establishment and conduct of associations and organizations such as mutual aid organizations, recreational and leisure

organizations, cultural and religious associations, and not-for-profit organizations.

- *e5552 Associations and Organizational Policies*
  Legislations, regulations, and standards that govern the relationships and activities of people coming together with common noncommercial interests, such as policies that govern the establishment and conduct of associations and organizations, including mutual aid organizations, recreational and leisure organizations, cultural and religious associations, and not-for-profit organizations.

- *e5558 Associations and Organizational Services, Systems, and Policies, Other Specified*
- *e5559 Associations and Organizational Services, Systems, and Policies, Unspecified*

Recreational therapists advocate for services, systems, and policies related to associations and organizational services including inclusion of people with disabilities into mainstream recreation associations. This may be done for a particular client or through support and involvement in professional organizations. If a service, system, or policy is identified as a barrier to engagement in a life activity, recreational therapists provide the client with relevant information that might be used to make a change, including information about the Americans with Disabilities Act. They also work with other health professionals who can intervene and provide further guidance. Both recreational therapists and other health professionals use these e-codes as descriptors. If the service barrier is on a local level and pertains directly to engagement in a specific activity, the recreational therapist will commonly intervene, such as educating the priest at the church about reasonable accommodations for a client to be able to participate at mass.

### Cross References

In *Recreational Therapy for Specific Diagnoses and Conditions, First Edition*, there are no references for ICF code e555 Associations and Organizational Services, Systems, and Policies.

In *Recreational Therapy Basics, Techniques, and Interventions, First Edition*, there are no references for ICF code e555 Associations and Organizational Services, Systems, and Policies.

### e560 Media Services, Systems, and Policies

Services, systems, and policies for the provision of mass communication through radio, television, newspapers, and internet.

- **e5600 Media Services**
  Services and programs aimed at providing mass communication, such as radio, television, closed captioning services, press reporting services, newspapers, Braille services, and computer-based mass communication (world wide web, internet), including those who provide these services.

  Exclusion: communication services (e5350)

- **e5601 Media Systems**
  Administrative control and monitoring mechanisms that govern the provision of news and information to the general public, such as standards that govern the content, distribution, dissemination, access to, and methods of communicating via radio, television, press reporting services, newspapers, and computer-based mass communication (world wide web, internet).

  Inclusions: requirements to provide closed captions on television, Braille versions of newspapers or other publications, and teletext radio transmissions

  Exclusion: communication systems (e5351)

- **e5602 Media Policies**
  Legislation, regulations, and standards that govern the provision of news and information to the general public, such as policies that govern the content, distribution, dissemination, access to, and methods of communicating via radio, television, press reporting services, newspapers, and computer-based mass communication (world wide web, internet).

  Exclusion: communication policies (e5352)

- **e5608 Media Services, Systems, and Policies, Other Specified**
- **e5609 Media Services, Systems, and Policies, Unspecified**
  Recreational therapists do not typically address services, systems, and policies related to media. If a service, system, or policy is identified as a barrier to engagement in a life activity, recreational therapists

probably will work with other health professionals who can intervene and provide further guidance. Other health professionals will most often use these e-codes as descriptors. If the service barrier is on a local level and pertains directly to engagement in a specific activity, the recreational therapist will commonly intervene, such as a recreational therapist working in the independent living movement helping a client make a call to the local newspaper to find out if a Braille copy is available.

### Cross References

In *Recreational Therapy for Specific Diagnoses and Conditions, First Edition*, there are no references for ICF code e560 Media Services, Systems, and Policies.

In *Recreational Therapy Basics, Techniques, and Interventions, First Edition*, there are no references for ICF code e560 Media Services, Systems, and Policies.

### e565 Economic Services, Systems, and Policies

Services, systems, and policies related to the overall system of production, distribution, consumption, and use of good and services.

Exclusion: social security services, systems, and policies (e570)

- **e5650 Economic Services**
  Services and programs aimed at the overall production, distribution, consumption, and use of goods and services, such as the private commercial sector (e.g., businesses, corporations, private for-profit ventures), the public sector (e.g., public, commercial services such as cooperatives and corporations), financial organizations (e.g., banks and insurance services), including those who provide these services.

  Exclusions: utilities services (e5300); labor and employment services (e5900)

- **e5651 Economic Systems**
  Administrative control and monitoring mechanisms that govern the production, distribution, consumption, and use of goods and services, such as systems for implementing and monitoring economic policies.

Exclusions: utilities systems (e5301); labor and employment systems (e5901)

- *e5652 Economic Policies*
  Legislation, regulations, and standards that govern the production, distribution, consumption, and use of goods and services, such as economic doctrines adopted and implemented by governments.

  Exclusions: utilities policies (e5302); labor and employment policies (e5902)

- *e5658 Economic Services, Systems, and Policies, Other Specified*
- *e5659 Economic Services, Systems, and Policies, Unspecified*

Recreational therapists do not typically address services, systems, and policies related to economic services. If a service, system, or policy is identified as a barrier to engagement in a life activity, recreational therapists probably will work with other health professionals who can intervene and provide further guidance. Other health professionals will most often use these e-codes as descriptors. If the service barrier is on a local level and pertains directly to engagement in a specific activity, the recreational therapist will commonly intervene. An example might be a client out with a recreational therapist for integration training who has his money access card eaten by the ATM machine. The recreational therapist can assist the client in going to the bank and finding out what happened to the card and what procedures need to be followed to have it returned.

### Cross References

In *Recreational Therapy for Specific Diagnoses and Conditions, First Edition*, ICF code e565 Economic Services, Systems, and Policies is listed in one chapter: Obesity.

In *Recreational Therapy Basics, Techniques, and Interventions, First Edition*, treatment for ICF code e565 Economic Services, Systems, and Policies is discussed in one chapter: Adaptive Sports.

## e570 Social Security Services, Systems, and Policies

Services, systems, and policies aimed at providing income support to people who, because of age, poverty, unemployment, health condition, or disability,

require public assistance that is funded either by general tax revenues or contributory schemes.

Exclusion: economic services, systems, and policies (e565)

- *e5700 Social Security Services*
  Services and programs aimed at providing income support to people who, because of age, poverty, unemployment, heath condition, or disability, require public assistance that is funded either by general tax revenues or contributory schemes, such as services for determining eligibility, delivering or distributing assistance payments for the following types of programs: social assistance programs (e.g., non-contributory welfare, poverty, or other needs-based compensation), social insurance programs (e.g., contributory accident or unemployment insurance), and disability and related pension schemes (e.g., income replacement), including those who provide these services.

  Exclusions: health services (e5800)

- *e5701 Social Security Systems*
  Administrative control and monitoring mechanisms that govern the programs and schemes that provide income support to people who, because of age, poverty, unemployment, health condition, or disability, require public assistance, such as systems for implementation of rules and regulations governing the eligibility for social assistance, welfare, unemployment insurance payments, pensions, and disability benefits.

- *e5702 Social Security Policies*
  Legislation, regulations, and standards that govern the programs and schemes that provide income support to people who, because of age, poverty, unemployment, health condition, or disability, require public assistance, such as legislation and regulations governing the eligibility for social assistance, welfare, unemployment insurance payments, disability, and related pensions and disability benefits.

- *e5708 Social Security Services, Systems, and Policies, Other Specified*
- *e5709 Social Security Services, Systems, and Policies, Unspecified*

Recreational therapists do not typically address services, systems, and policies related to social security. If a service, system, or policy is identified as a barrier to engagement in a life activity, recreational therapists probably will work with other health professionals who can intervene and provide further guidance. Other health professionals will most often use these e-codes as descriptors.

### Cross References

In *Recreational Therapy for Specific Diagnoses and Conditions, First Edition*, ICF code e570 Social Security Services, Systems, and Policies is listed in one chapter: Rheumatoid Arthritis.

In *Recreational Therapy Basics, Techniques, and Interventions, First Edition*, there are no references for ICF code e570 Social Security Services, Systems, and Policies.

### e575 General Social Support Services, Systems, and Policies

Services, systems, and policies aimed at providing support to those requiring assistance in areas such as shopping, housework, transport, self-care, and care for others, in order to function more fully in society.

Exclusions: personal care providers and personal care assistants (e340); social security services, systems, and policies (e570); health services, systems, and policies (e580)

- *e5750 General Social Support Services*
  Services and programs aimed at providing social support to people who, because of age, poverty, unemployment, health condition, or disability, require public assistance in the areas of shopping, housework, transport, self-care, and care of others, in order to function more fully in society.

- *e5751 General Social Support Systems*
  Administrative control and monitoring mechanisms that govern the programs and schemes that provide social support to people who, because of age, poverty, unemployment, health condition, or disability, require such support, including systems for the implementation of rules and regulations governing eligibility for social support services and the provision of these services.

- *e5752 General Social Support Policies*
  Legislation, regulations, and standards, that govern the program and schemes that provide social support to people who, because of age, poverty,

unemployment, health condition, or disability, require such support, including legislation and regulations governing eligibility for social support.

- *e5758 General Social Support Services, Systems, and Policies, Other Specified*
- *e5759 General Social Support Services, Systems, and Policies, Unspecified*

Recreational therapists advocate for services, systems, and policies related to general social support, such as support services for recreational activities, mostly through support and involvement in professional organizations. If a service, system, or policy is identified as a barrier to engagement in a life activity, recreational therapists provide the client with relevant information that might be used to make a change, including information about the Americans with Disabilities Act. They also work with other health professionals who can intervene and provide further guidance. Both recreational therapists and other health professionals use these e-codes as descriptors. If the service barrier is on a local level and pertains directly to engagement in a specific activity, the recreational therapist will commonly intervene, such as educating the supervisor at the supermarket about reasonable accommodations under the Americans with Disabilities Act to reduce or eliminate barriers at the supermarket for the client.

### Cross References

In *Recreational Therapy for Specific Diagnoses and Conditions, First Edition*, ICF code e575 General Social Support Services, Systems, and Policies is listed in two chapters: Epilepsy and Schizophrenia Spectrum and Other Psychotic Disorders.

In *Recreational Therapy Basics, Techniques, and Interventions, First Edition*, treatment for ICF code e575 General Social Support Services, Systems, and Policies is discussed in one chapter: Adaptive Sports.

### e580 Health Services, Systems, and Policies

Services, systems, and policies for preventing and treating health problems, providing medical rehabilitation, and promoting a healthy lifestyle.

Exclusion: general social support services, systems, and policies (e575)

- *e5800 Health Services*

  Services and programs at a local, community, regional, state, or national level, aimed at delivering interventions to individuals for their physical, psychological, and social well-being, such as health promotion and disease prevention services, primary care services, acute care, rehabilitation, and long-term care services; services that are publicly or privately funded, delivered on a short-term, long-term, periodic, or one-time basis, in a variety of service settings such as community, home-based, school, and work settings, general hospitals, specialty hospitals, clinics, and residential and non-residential care facilities, including those who provide these services.

- *e5801 Health Systems*

  Administrative control and monitoring mechanisms that govern the range of services provided to individuals for their physical, psychological, and social well-being, in a variety of settings including community, home-based, school, and work settings, general hospitals, specialty hospitals, clinics, and residential and non-residential care facilities, such as systems for implementing regulations and standards that determine eligibility for services, provision of devices, assistive technology, or other adapted equipment, and legislation such as health acts that govern features of a health system such as accessibility, universality, portability, public funding, and comprehensiveness.

- *e5802 Health Policies*

  Legislation, regulations, and standards that govern the range of services provided to individuals for their physical, psychological, and social well-being, in a variety of settings including community, home-based, school, and work settings, general hospitals, specialty hospitals, clinics, and residential and non-residential care facilities, such as policies and standards that determine eligibility for services, provision of devices, assistive technology, or other adapted equipment, and legislation such as health acts that govern features of a health systems such as accessibility, universality, portability, public funding, and comprehensiveness.

- *e5808 Health Services, Systems, and Policies, Other Specified*

- *e5809 Health Services, Systems, and Policies, Unspecified*

Recreational therapists advocate for services, systems, and policies related to health at their worksite and through professional organizations. If a service, system, or policy is identified as a barrier to engagement in a life activity, recreational therapists provide the client with relevant information, such as information on the Americans with Disabilities Act, and then work with other health professionals who can intervene and provide further guidance.

This code poses an interesting situation for therapists who identify residual needs for a client that are not addressed because of a health service, system, or policy, such as a client who would benefit from outpatient transportation training but the funding source does not cover the service. In our current health system, there is a danger of using the codes in this category too liberally because health care professionals usually want more for their clients than is available. Therapists must be careful to not use this code routinely as a way to advocate for their profession by judiciously choosing these codes as barriers only when well informed about the service, policy, or system and evaluating the total health care services being received by the client, not just recreational therapy.

If the therapist is well informed about the specific service, policy, or system that is a barrier and the client is not able to receive the service from any other health care professional, the therapist can use the codes in this category to reflect the specific barrier. For example, a client with a stroke desires to return to playing golf. He used to play golf five times a week as a primary source of exercise for health promotion. He currently has moderate difficulty overall with the game. At this level of difficulty, the client refuses to return to the game of golf. He has no other forms of physical activity in his current lifestyle. In the clinical judgment of the therapist, the client can progress to no difficulty with individual outpatient therapy on the golf course along with support from his fellow players. The client states that he would return to golf if he could achieve this level of playing. The therapist petitions for outpatient recreational therapy services and it is denied by the health insurance company. The therapist speaks with the occupational and physical therapists to review whether their outpatient therapy recommendations might include the recreational therapy objectives for golf. It is determined that it is unrealistic for the other therapies to absorb the golf objectives. In this case, the therapist could score e5801 Health Systems as a barrier to d9201 Sports and possibly d5701 Managing Diet and Fitness.

### Cross References

In *Recreational Therapy for Specific Diagnoses and Conditions, First Edition*, ICF code e580 Health Services, Systems, and Policies is listed in six chapters: Borderline Personality Disorder, Burns, Hearing Loss, Osteoarthritis, Rheumatoid Arthritis, and Visual Impairments and Blindness.

In *Recreational Therapy Basics, Techniques, and Interventions, First Edition*, there are no references for ICF code e580 Health Services, Systems, and Policies.

### e585 Education and Training Services, Systems, and Policies

Services, systems, and policies for the acquisition, maintenance, and improvement of knowledge, expertise, and vocational or artistic skills. See UNESCO's International Standard Classification of Education (ISCED-1997).

- *e5850 Education and Training Services*
  Services and programs concerned with education and the acquisition, maintenance, and improvement of knowledge, expertise, and vocational or artistic skills, such as those provided for different levels of education (e.g., preschool, primary school, secondary school, post-secondary institutions, professional programs, training and skills programs, apprenticeships, and continuing education), including those who provide these services.

- *e5851 Education and Training Systems*
  Administrative control and monitoring mechanisms that govern the delivery of education programs, such as systems for the implementation of policies and standards that determine eligibility for public or private education and special needs-based programs; local, regional, or national boards of education or other authoritative bodies that govern features of the education systems, including curricula, size of classes, numbers of

schools in a region, fees and subsidies, special meal programs, and after-school care services.

- *e5852 Education and Training Policies*
  Legislation, regulations, and standards that govern the delivery of education program, such as policies and standards that determine eligibility for public or private education and special needs-based programs, and dictate the structure of local, regional, or national boards of education or other authoritative bodies that govern features of the education system, including size of classes, numbers of schools in a region, fees and subsidies, special meal programs, and after school care services.

- *e5858 Education and Training Services, Systems, and Policies, Other Specified*
- *e5859 Education and Training Services, Systems, and Policies, Unspecified*

Recreational therapists do not typically address services, systems, and policies related to education. However, there may be times when certain groups of recreational therapists are a part of education advocacy, such as recreational therapists who work in the school system. If a service, system, or policy is identified as a barrier to engagement in a life activity, recreational therapists provide the client with relevant information, such as information on Individualized Education Plans. They also work with other health and education professionals who can intervene and provide further guidance. Both recreational therapists and other professionals use these e-codes as descriptors. If the service barrier is on a local level and pertains directly to engagement in a specific activity, the recreational therapist will commonly intervene, such as a recreational therapist working in the school system who advocates for a student to receive recreational therapy services.

### Cross References

In *Recreational Therapy for Specific Diagnoses and Conditions, First Edition*, ICF code e585 Education and Training Services, Systems, and Policies is listed in two chapters: Cerebral Palsy and Obesity.

In *Recreational Therapy Basics, Techniques, and Interventions, First Edition*, there are no references for ICF code e585 Education and Training Services, Systems, and Policies.

## e590 Labor and Employment Services, Systems, and Policies

Services, systems, and policies related to finding suitable work for persons who are unemployed or looking for different work, or to support individuals already employed who are seeking promotion.

Exclusion: economic services, systems, and policies (e565)

- *e5900 Labor and Employment Services*
  Services and programs provide by local, regional, or national governments, or private organizations to find suitable work for persons who are unemployed or looking for different work, or to support individuals already employed, such as services of employment search and preparation, reemployment, job placement, outplacement, vocational follow-up, occupational health and safety services, and work environment services (e.g., ergonomics, human resources and personnel management services, labor relations services, professional association services), including those who provide these services.

- *e5901 Labor and Employment Systems*
  Administrative control and monitoring mechanisms that govern the distribution of occupations and other forms of remunerative work in the economy, such as systems for implementing policies and standards for employment creation, employment security, designated and competitive employment, labor standards and law, and trade unions.

- *e5902 Labor and Employment Policies*
  Legislation, regulations, and standards that govern the distribution of occupations and other forms of remunerative work in the economy, such as standards and policies for employment creation, employment security, designated and competitive employment, labor standards and law, and trade unions.

- *e5908 Labor and Employment Services, Systems, and Policies, Other Specified*
- *e5909 Labor and Employment Services, Systems, and Policies, Unspecified*
  Recreational therapists do not typically address services, systems, and policies related to labor and employment. However, there may be times when certain groups of recreational therapists are a part of

education and employment advocacy, such as in the independent living movement. If a service, system, or policy is identified as a barrier to engagement in a life activity, recreational therapists provide the client with relevant information that might be used to make a change, including information about the Americans with Disabilities Act. They also work with other health professionals who can intervene and provide further guidance. Both recreational therapists and other health professionals use these e-codes as descriptors. If the service barrier is on a local level and pertains directly to engagement in a specific activity, the recreational therapist will commonly intervene, such as a recreational therapist working in the independent living movement who assists the client in talking with an employer about job responsibilities and abilities.

### Cross References

In *Recreational Therapy for Specific Diagnoses and Conditions, First Edition*, there are no references for ICF code e590 Labor and Employment Services, Systems, and Policies.

In *Recreational Therapy Basics, Techniques, and Interventions, First Edition*, there are no references for ICF code e590 Labor and Employment Services, Systems, and Policies.

## e595 Political Services, Systems, and Policies

Services, systems, and policies related to voting, elections, and governance of countries, regions, and communities, as well as international political organizations.

- *e5950 Political Services*
  Services and structures such as local, regional, and national governments, international organizations, and the people who are elected or nominated to positions within these structures, such as the United Nations, European Union, governments, regional authorities, local village authorities, traditional leaders.

- *e5951 Political Systems*
  Structures and related operations that organize political and economic power in a society, such as executive and legislative branches of government, and the constitutional or other legal sources from which they derive their authority, such as political organizational doctrine, constitu-

tions, agencies of executive and legislative branches of government, the military.

- *e5952 Political Policy*
  Laws and policies formulated and enforced through political systems that govern the operation of the political system, such as policies governing election campaigns, registration of political parties, voting, and members in international political organizations, including treaties, constitutional and other law governing legislation and regulation.

- *e5958 Political Services, Systems, and Policies, Other Specified*
- *e5959 Political Services, Systems, and Policies, Unspecified*

Recreational therapists do not typically address services, systems, and policies related to political policy. If a service, system, or policy is identified as a barrier to engagement in a life activity, recreational therapists probably will work with other health professionals who can intervene and provide further guidance. Other health professionals will most often use these e-codes as descriptors. One exception might be helping to enforce voting rights for a person in a long-term care facility when local regulations are in conflict with federal law.

### Cross References

In *Recreational Therapy for Specific Diagnoses and Conditions, First Edition*, ICF code e595 Political Services, Systems, and Policies is listed in one chapter: Cerebral Palsy.

In *Recreational Therapy Basics, Techniques, and Interventions, First Edition*, there are no references for ICF code e595 Political Services, Systems, and Policies.

## e598 Services, Systems, and Policies, Other Specified

## e599 Services, Systems, and Policies, Unspecified

### References

Hammel, J., Jones, R., Gossett, A., & Morgan, E. (2006). Examining barriers and supports to community living and participation after stroke from a participatory action research approach. *Topics in Stroke Rehabilitation, 13*(3), 43-58.

# Personal Factors

*Yoshitaka Iwasaki, Ph.D.*

Personal Factors (PF) are things that have to do with a person's life and living. They are not part of a health problem, but rather are attributes of a person and his/her way of life that could affect his/her health and functioning. Examples of PF identified by the ICF include gender, race, age, other health conditions, fitness, lifestyle, habits, upbringing, coping styles, social background, education, profession, past and current experience, overall behavior patterns and character style, individual psychological assets, and other characteristics.

Personal factors and environmental factors are the two major groups of contextual factors. Personal factors represent individual characteristics and backgrounds unique to each person. Given the very diverse nature of our societies and the communities in which people live, the scope of personal factors is extremely diverse. In addition to socio-demographic factors such as gender, race/ethnicity, age, and social class, it is important to give attention to lifestyle factors and experience-based and meaning-oriented factors. Each of these aspects is described in this chapter, as supported by the ICF framework from a holistic, humanistic, and strengths-based perspective with the aim of better meeting the unique needs and aspirations of individuals.

Personal factors, although recognized by the ICF as being influential on a person's health and functioning, are not currently coded in the ICF. There is talk, however, that personal factors codes will eventually be developed. Consequently, it is important for therapists to understand personal factors and the impact they have on functioning, health, and disability.

## Socio-Demographic Factors

Socio-demographic factors should be conceptualized as more than simply human categories. This means that one's gender, race/ethnicity, age, social class, etc. embrace deeper meanings because these socio-demographic factors reflect the challenges and advantages that a person faces in life. They also represent personal ways people use to cope with challenges or use as advantages. For example, it is necessary to pay attention to the availability of and access to socio-economic resources, such as income, social support, educational, and employment, that contextualize a person's life because lacking or limited socio-economic resources present a significant disadvantage. On the other hand, strengthening personal resources such as stress-coping resources and strategies for resilience; family, social, and community support that promotes a sense of belonging; and human development resources, including education, is essential to better address and overcome these life challenges.

Also, we need to recognize that an individual's gender, race/ethnicity, age, class, disabilities, and sexual orientation are the basis for different forms of discrimination, stigma, and oppression in our society. These are specifically called sexism, racism, ageism, classism, ableism, and heterosexisim or homophobia, respectively. Thus, it is crucial to consider power imbalance in our society that leads to disadvantages for those in a lower hierarchical position such as women as opposed to men, colored vs. white, older persons vs. younger persons, those in lower social class vs. those in higher social class, people with disabilities vs. those without disabilities, and lesbians and gay men vs. heterosexual women and men.

Typically, those non-dominant groups of people who belong to a lower hierarchical position in our society are marginalized. Our social system does not often cater directly to the needs of those disfranchised population groups, compared to more dominant groups of people having a higher hierarchical position. Furthermore, the intersection of these different "isms" should be considered because a person may simultaneously face multiple forms of discrimination and stigma. For example, a racial/ethnic minority person with disability faces the double jeopardy of racism and ableism. For another example, an older Hispanic lesbian woman with disability living under poverty may encounter all of sexism, racism, ageism, ableism, classism, and heterosexisim or homophobia.

### Cultural and Identity-Oriented Factors

Extending from the above notion of socio-demographic factors, we must give attention to cultural and identity-oriented factors not only because our society is culturally diverse, but also because everything we do in our life is cultural in nature. Respectfully acknowledging cultural uniqueness of an individual is a must since the implementation of people-friendly practices and services to cater to the unique needs of different cultural groups is considered a high priority for scholarly and professional activities. Culture is a way of life of individuals in a society or community and represents more than just race and ethnicity. It also encompasses the aspect of identity to say who we are as persons. Thus, we should recognize different forms of culture including race/ethnicity-based culture, gender-specific culture, disability culture (e.g., deaf culture, autistic culture), age-based culture, gay culture, etc. Many people identify themselves with a specific form of culture that can be a key source of collectivity, community, empowerment, and human development.

### Lifestyle Factors

People's lifestyles should be also recognized as key personal factors. One of the most significant lifestyle aspects relevant directly to the ICF framework represents the notion of active living or actively engaged living. Active living, however, should be conceptualized as more than just a way of life focused on integrating physical activity into daily routines, as it is often defined. It should be considered more broadly as a potentially enjoyable, joyful, meaningful, and enriching way of life, in which one is actively engaged in living all aspects of life both personally and in families and communities as part of a more holistic and humanistic perspective. Based on the extent to which one maintains active living, one's lifestyle can be defined along the continuum of actively engaged living versus an inactive or sedentary lifestyle. Lifestyle consideration should also be given to the degree to which one maintains healthy versus unhealthy lifestyle in, for example, diet, exercise, smoking, and at-risk behavior.

An often ignored and undervalued, yet potentially significant notion, is that leisure and recreation, which is more than just physical activity and exercise, represent key elements of active living and a major pathway toward health promotion. Research points to the importance of leisure and recreation for the pursuit of active living and the promotion of health and life quality for various population groups including individuals with disabilities (Fullagar, 2008; García-Villamisar & Dattilo, 2010; Iwasaki, Coyle, & Shank, 2010; Lante, Reece, & Walkley, 2010). Thus, it is important to consider integrating the pursuit of leisure and recreation into an active living and health promotion intervention program especially for those who are concerned with weight-related and lifestyle issues. Furthermore, acknowledging coping style as a key lifestyle factor is important, as noted earlier, because the ways people cope with life challenges significantly influence their well-being and life quality. Since a completely stress-free life is almost impossible, coping with stress represents a major lifestyle issue for many people for their survival and thriving in life.

### Experience-Based and Meaning-Oriented Factors

Personal factors include more than just behavioral aspects. It is necessary to give attention to experience-based and meaning-oriented aspects that are uniquely personal to each individual. When engaging in activity, people think, feel, and experience, along with showing personal behavior. Thinking, feeling, and experience can be positive, negative, or neutral. Thus, considering cognitive, emotional, and experiential make-ups of personal activity is a must. It is also necessary to realize that a person's past and present, as well as his/her aspirations toward the future, significantly influence the life story that is unique to each individual from a human development perspective.

Important consideration should also be given to personal meanings that people gain from activities. Specific meanings sought and gained from an activity may be psychological, emotional, social, spiritual, and cultural. For example, a nature walk with friends can provide an opportunity to gain social (e.g., companionship), emotional (e.g., positive moods), and spiritual (e.g., spiritual renewal) benefits in a natural environment. These are in addition to the physiological benefits of a nature walk. Another example is a culturally meaningful, spiritually refreshing, and/or creative leisure activity such as art, crafts, music, dance, gardening, and martial arts that can promote self-expression and identity within a unique cultural context.

These examples deal with psychological and emotional meanings including self-expression, identity, and positive moods; social meanings of companionship or friendship; spiritual meanings of renewal and rejuvenation; and cultural meanings from culturally expressive activities such as appreciating and/or performing ethnic dance and music. As illustrated in these examples, the pursuit of various leisure and recreation activities plays a key role in the personal meaning-making process by promoting a sense of connection and identity (Heintzman, 2008; Iwasaki, 2008; Porter, Iwasaki, & Shank, 2011). These pursuits also promote coping with stress and healing, active living, and health and life quality (García-Villamisar & Dattilo, 2010; Iwasaki et al., 2006; Kleiber & Hutchinson, 2010). It is a human's natural tendency to seek a meaningful and enriching life. Thus, it is very important to consider what meanings people try to gain and how the process of meaning-making operates and functions in various life activities.

### Application

Therapists should understand that personal factors act as either facilitators or barriers to meaningful leisure engagements. In particular, giving attention to the promotion of positive personal factors as facilitators is a must, while, at the same time, helping clients overcome negative (or lacking and limited) personal factors as barriers. As described in this chapter, personal resources include socio-demographic, cultural, and identity-oriented factors, as well as lifestyle and experience/meaning-based factors. A combination of all of these personal resources represents an individual's uniqueness and context of his/her life. Respectfully acknowledging these personal resources helps professionals better understand who the person is and what individual characteristics s/he possesses. Because no two individuals are identical, professionals must consider personalizing their therapeutic approach to effectively meet the unique needs, characteristics, and life context of each person.

In particular, identifying a client's personal strengths and resources is important. For example, these personal strengths may include identification and connection with a social or cultural group, such as disability culture, youth culture, race- or ethnicity-based culture, or gay culture. Promoting personal identification and connection with a social or cultural group can act as a key facilitator in the pursuit of actively engaged, enjoyable, and meaningful leisure.

One such approach is to systematically structure a series of recreation-based therapeutic sessions in order to promote identification and connection with a disability culture among a group of persons with disability. During sessions involving various enjoyable, expressive, and meaningful activities, participants may actively engage in both personal and group-based recreation and leisure to facilitate their journey toward self- and collective-discovery and learning about the important role of: (1) identity (e.g., disability pride as opposed to disability shame), (2) social, mutual support, (3) the celebration of human strengths and uniqueness, and (4) self- and collective-advocacy and empowerment for positive social change in potentially enhancing overall quality of life.

On the other hand, personal factors may act as barriers to meaningful leisure in other situations. Examples include various forms of discrimination against oppressed groups and inactive, sedentary, or unhealthy lifestyles, as described earlier. Consequently, professionals must consider implementing an intervention or some form of accommodation to address and overcome these potential barriers. For instance, accommodating the needs of persons with disabilities who are using assistive technology and adaptive recreation and sports is important. It addresses ableism by ensuring access. An active-living health promotion intervention can be implemented to address an inactive, sedentary, or unhealthy lifestyle. Similar to the case of environmental factors, giving attention to personal factors that can act as facilitators or barriers is needed. By focusing on the promotion of personal facilitators and the reduction or elimination of personal barriers, therapists can enhance clients' experiences in leisure and recreation.

### Conclusion

As supported by the ICF framework, we must envision and conceptualize personal factors from a holistic, humanistic, and strengths-based perspective by respectfully appreciating the abilities, resources, and potentials of each individual. Consistent with this vision, the ICF is considered as a universal model to reflect the diverse nature of our societies and communities. Therefore, paying attention to personal factors is essential to appropriately meet the unique needs and aspirations of each individual.

These personal factors should be conceptualized as an interrelated and interdependent component of the ICF framework. For example, race or ethnicity should be considered in relation to the contextual element of organizational or systemic racism described in environmental factors, while also recognizing its impact on participation in activities, body functions, and body systems. Lacking or limited opportunities in educational, occupational, and community life for marginalized and underserved population groups is a significant social and health issue. This issue should be addressed by substantially improving those people's access to these domains of life.

The effective use of facilitators, such as assistive technology, universal design, adaptive recreation and sports, disability culture, and stress-coping strategies, is as important as significantly reducing or eliminating barriers for enhancing access and meaningful experiences for each individual. Therapists must fully understand personal features such as race or ethnicity, gender, social class, age, abilities or disabilities, and sexual orientation. They must also acknowledge cultural and identity-oriented factors associated with these personal features. In addition, the scope of personal factors is very diverse, encompassing such notions as people's lifestyles; experiential and behavioral make-ups of personal activities; and psychological, emotional, social, spiritual, and cultural meanings that people seek to achieve through these activities.

Therapists need to take a perspective that considers each person's development and journey through life. Appropriately recognizing all of these personal factors and their interrelationships is critical for therapists to promote health, well being, and quality of life for their clients. Therapists need to help their clients reach their full potential through the pursuit of actively engaged, enjoyable, and meaningful leisure and recreation.

### *References*

Fullagar, S. (2008). Leisure practices as counter-depressants: Emotion-work and emotion-play within women's recovery from depression. *Leisure Sciences, 30*(1), 35-52.

García-Villamisar, D. A. & Dattilo, J. (2010). Effects of a leisure programme on quality of life and stress of individuals with ASD. *Journal of Intellectual Disability Research, 54*(7), 611-619.

Heintzman, P. (2008). Leisure-spiritual coping: A model for therapeutic recreation and leisure services. *Therapeutic Recreation Journal, 42*(1), 56-73.

Iwasaki, Y. (2008). Pathways to meaning-making through leisure in global contexts. *Journal of Leisure Research, 40*, 231-249.

Iwasaki, Y., Coyle, C., & Shank, J. (2010). Leisure as a context for active living, recovery, health, and life quality for persons with mental illness in a global context. *Health Promotion International. 25*(4), 483-494.

Iwasaki, Y., MacKay, K., Mactavish, J., Ristock, J., & Bartlett, J. (2006). Voices from the margins: Stress, active living, and leisure as a contributor to coping with stress. *Leisure Sciences, 28*, 163-180.

Kleiber, D. A. & Hutchinson, S. L. (2010). Making the best of bad situations: The value of leisure in coping with negative life events. In L. Payne, B. Ainsworth, & G. Godbey (Eds.), *Leisure, health, and wellness: Making the connections* (pp. 155-164). State College, PA: Venture Publishing, Inc.

Lante, K., Reece, J., & Walkley, J. (2010). Energy expended by adults with and without intellectual disabilities during activities of daily living. *Research in Developmental Disabilities, 31*(6), 1380-1389.

Porter, H. R., Iwasaki, Y., & Shank, J. (2011). Conceptualizing meaning-making through leisure experiences. *Society & Leisure/Loisir et Societe, 33*(2), 167-194.

# *Index*

# About the Author/Editor

Heather R. Porter, Ph.D., CTRS

Heather Porter, Ph.D., CTRS, is a faculty member in the Rehabilitation Sciences Department at Temple University in Philadelphia, PA. She has a dual BS in Recreational Therapy and Sport/Recreation Management, an MS in Counseling Psychology with a Certificate in Marriage and Family Counseling, and a Ph.D. in Health Studies (Recreational Therapy and Public Health). She has a strong clinical background in inpatient and outpatient physical rehabilitation and has been teaching recreational therapy in higher education for over 18 years. She is committed to strengthening recreational therapy research and disseminating research information to practitioners, consumers, payers, legislators, and the general public. Most notably, she coordinates an annual Recreational Therapy Evidence-Based Practice Conference and maintains an open-access database for recreational therapy research and resources that has been utilized by over 60 countries (www.rtwiseowls.com). Dr. Porter also provides consultations to recreational therapy academic programs on how to integrate evidence-based research into academic coursework, and is recognized as a leader in the community seeking to integrate the World Health Organization's *International Classification of Functioning, Disability, and Health* into healthcare practice.